Respiratory Critical Care

David W. Chang

Gary C. White

Jonathan B. Waugh

Ruben D. Restrepo

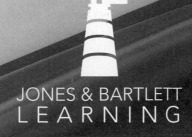

JONES & BARTLETT
LEARNING

World Headquarters
Jones & Bartlett Learning
5 Wall Street
Burlington, MA 01803
978-443-5000
info@jblearning.com
www.jblearning.com

Jones & Bartlett Learning books and products are available through most bookstores and online booksellers. To contact Jones & Bartlett Learning directly, call 800-832-0034, fax 978-443-8000, or visit our website, www.jblearning.com.

Substantial discounts on bulk quantities of Jones & Bartlett Learning publications are available to corporations, professional associations, and other qualified organizations. For details and specific discount information, contact the special sales department at Jones & Bartlett Learning via the above contact information or send an email to specialsales@jblearning.com.

20217-5

Production Credits

VP, Product Management: Amanda Martin
Director of Product Management: Cathy L. Esperti
Product Specialist: Rachael Souza
Project Manager: Kristen Rogers
Digital Products Manager: Jordan McKenzie
Digital Project Specialist: Angela Dooley
Director of Marketing: Andrea DeFronzo
Marketing Manager: Michael Sullivan
Production Services Manager: Colleen Lamy
VP, Manufacturing and Inventory Control: Therese Connell

Composition: S4Carlisle Publishing Services
Project Management: S4Carlisle Publishing Services
Cover Design: Scott Moden
Text Design: Scott Moden
Senior Media Development Editor: Troy Liston
Rights Specialist: Rebecca Damon
Cover Image (Title Page, Part Opener, Chapter Opener):
   © s_maria/Shutterstock
Printing and Binding: LSC Communications
Cover Printing: LSC Communications

Library of Congress Cataloging-in-Publication Data

Names: Chang, David W., author. | White, Gary C., 1954- author. | Waugh,
   Jonathan B., author. | Restrepo, Ruben D. (Ruben Dario), author.
Title: Respiratory critical care / David W. Chang, Gary C. White, Jonathan B.
   Waugh, Ruben D. Restrepo.
Description: Burlington, Massachusetts : Jones & Bartlett Learning, [2020]
   | Includes bibliographical references and index.
Identifiers: LCCN 2019032816 | ISBN 9781284177503 (paperback)
Subjects: MESH: Respiration, Artificial | Critical Care
Classification: LCC RC87.9 | NLM WF 145 | DDC 615.8/362--dc23
LC record available at https://lccn.loc.gov/2019032816

6048

Printed in the United States of America
23 22 21 20 19   10 9 8 7 6 5 4 3 2 1

To all respiratory therapists who go beyond the traditional roles of RT and willingly work with other critical care clinicians for better patient care and outcomes. ∽

—David W. Chang

To my wife, Carolyn, who has supported my writing avocation for over 33 years. ∽

—Gary C. White

To my wife, Linda, and my children, Alia, Ian, and Adria, who support me with their love. To my past and future students who motivate me to learn. And to my dear Lord Jesus, who makes everything possible. ∽

—Jonathan B. Waugh

To my amazing "best half," Diana, a respiratory therapist and great educator who has supported me on every project. To my three princesses, Andrea, Natalia, and Valentina. They know well that this book has been on my bucket list for years. ∽

—Ruben D. Restrepo

Brief Contents

Contents

Preface

Since the inception of mechanical ventilation, the roles of respiratory therapists (clinicians) in critical care settings have changed a great deal. The days of performing "vent checks" and "ABGs" as the primary tasks are gone forever. Instead, respiratory therapists are expected to perform as a member of the critical care team. They must be able to select useful clinical data, perform appropriate patient assessments, and communicate the findings to the physician and other critical care clinicians. For these reasons, all critical care clinicians should have a fundamental and solid knowledge of mechanical ventilation, critical care procedures, pharmacotherapy in critical care, medical and trauma critical care issues, and current clinical practice guidelines pertaining to critical care.

There are 15 chapters in this new text. Nine chapters focus on the key elements of mechanical ventilation, ranging from principles of mechanical ventilation to weaning from mechanical ventilation. One chapter covers the fundamentals of neonatal and pediatric mechanical ventilation. The other five chapters cover a broad range of critical care topics: critical care procedures, pharmacotherapy in critical care, medical critical care issues, traumatic critical care issues, life support, and clinical practice guidelines.

The primary audience of this text is respiratory therapy students. This text has incorporated the essential content in the Therapist Multiple-Choice (TMC) and Adult Critical Care Specialty (ACCS) exam matrices by the National Board for Respiratory Care (NBRC). This text is also a useful resource guide and quick reference for clinicians caring for critically ill patients. It is my intent that this new text will help broaden the traditional roles of respiratory therapy in the critical care settings. More important, a knowledgeable and cohesive critical care team will deliver evidence-based patient care and produce better patient outcomes.

David W. Chang, EdD, RRT

How to Use This Book

- Each chapter of the book begins with a list of **Objectives** to help you focus on the most important concepts in that chapter.
- **Tables** are used to highlight important information, such as **Table 8-15** "Characteristics and Recovery Time for First-, Second-, and Third-Degree Burns."

TABLE 8-15
Characteristics and Recovery Time for First-, Second-, and Third-Degree Burns

Degree of Burn	Characteristic	Recovery
First-degree burn	Reddening of the skin surface Patient feels pain	Within days
Second-degree superficial dermal burn	Blister; dermis below blister is red Patient feels pain	1–2 weeks
Second-degree deep dermal burn	Blister; dermis below blister is white and anemic Patient may not feel pain	3–4 weeks
Third-degree burn	Necrosis through the dermis; white or brown leatherlike appearance or completely charred skin Patient does not feel pain	Up to 3 months

- This text is highly **illustrated** with diagrams and photos demonstrating a variety of concepts, such as the illustration of sniffing position in **Figure 4-18**.

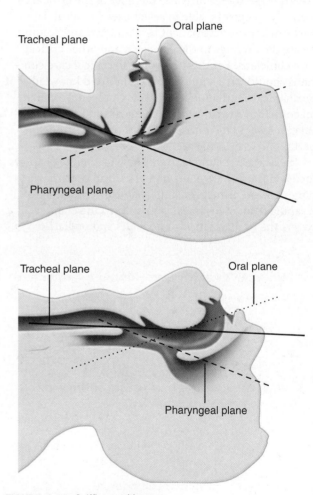

FIGURE 4-18 Sniffing position.

■ Throughout the text, **Boxes** highlight key points and important information, to ensure comprehension and to aid the study of critical materials.

BOX 6-9 Calculation of SVR

$$SVR = \frac{(MAP - CVP) \times 80}{CO}$$

CO, cardiac output; CVP, central venous pressure; MAP, mean arterial pressure; SVR, systemic vascular resistance.

■ Every chapter concludes with a **Case Study** to help readers review and put into practice what they have learned.

CASE STUDY

Mr. King, a patient with chronic obstructive pulmonary disease (COPD) in severe respiratory distress, is picked up by an ambulance. During transport and upon arrival at the hospital, he is receiving noninvasive ventilation via an oronasal mask. Patient assessment shows patient-ventilator dyssynchrony. Mr. King is complaining of "not getting enough air."

1. **What is the cycle mechanism of this noninvasive ventilator?**

2. **What can be done to provide more ventilation to the patient?**

   Mr. King is subsequently admitted to the intensive care unit (ICU) for acute exacerbation of COPD and severe hypoxemia. He is intubated and placed on volume-controlled ventilation.

3. **What is the cycling mechanism of this type of mechanical ventilation?**

4. **The physician orders positive end-expiratory pressure (PEEP) of 5 cm H_2O for Mr. King. What type of ventilator variable is PEEP?**

5. **What is the primary reason for applying this baseline variable?**

Instructor and Student Resources

Qualified instructors will receive a full suite of instructor resources, including:

For the Instructor

■ Comprehensive, chapter-by-chapter slides in PowerPoint format
■ A Test Bank containing questions on a chapter-by-chapter basis
■ Answers to the Case Studies

For the Student

■ Case Studies are embedded into the eBook as writeable PDFs
■ Concept Maps are available online and break down key concepts within every chapter

About the Authors

David W. Chang, EdD, RRT is a Professor for the Department of Cardiorespiratory Care at the University of South Alabama, Mobile. Over the years, he has served in different capacities in the American Association for Respiratory Care (AARC), Commission on Accreditation for Respiratory Care (CoARC), and National Board for Respiratory Care (NBRC). He has published many textbooks, including *Respiratory Care Calculations* and *Clinical Application of Mechanical Ventilation*.

Gary C. White, MEd, RRT, RPFT, FAARC is Program Director of Respiratory Therapy at Spokane Community College (Washington). He has served as a board member and in many other capacities in the Commission on Accreditation for Respiratory Care (CoARC). He has published many textbooks, including *Basic Clinical Lab Competencies for Respiratory Care: An Integrated Approach* and *Equipment Theory for Respiratory Care*.

Jonathan B. Waugh, PhD, RRT, RPFT, FAARC is a Professor for the Respiratory Therapy program at Liberty University in Lynchburg, Virginia. He received a BS in Respiratory Therapy from the Cardiopulmonary Sciences program at the University of Central Florida in 1985. He earned an MS in Health Science (1990) and a PhD in Cardiopulmonary Sciences (1994) from The Ohio State University. He conducts research in ventilatory monitoring, capnography, high-flow therapy, medical device testing, and tobacco prevention and treatment.

Ruben D. Restrepo, MD, RRT is a Tenured Professor and Coordinator of Research for the Division of Respiratory Care at the University of Texas Health Science Center in San Antonio. He earned his diploma as Physician and Surgeon from Colombia, South America. He graduated from the Respiratory Therapy program at Georgia State University in 1994. In 2007, he was recognized as a Fellow of the American Association for Respiratory Care and in 2017 as Fellow of the American College of Chest Physicians. He is a member of the editorial board for *Respiratory Care,* the *Open Journal of Allergy,* and the *World Journal of Critical Care Medicine.* He is a well-known international speaker with over 60 peer-reviewed publications.

Acknowledgments

I sincerely thank my coeditors and contributing authors for their dedication in making this new text a reality. Their expertise in the respective content areas make this text a very useful learning resource for students and clinicians. I am grateful to the editorial and production team members of Jones & Bartlett Learning for their talents and experience in making this a text that students and clinicians will enjoy reading.

David W. Chang

Contributors

Michael W. Canfield, MAEd, RRT, CCT
Director of Clinical Education
Cardiopulmonary Sciences
Samford University
Birmingham, Alabama

Lisa A. Conry, MA, RRT
Program Director
Respiratory Therapy
Greenville Technical College
Greenville, South Carolina

Crystal L. Dunlevy, EdD, RRT
Professor-Clinical
The Ohio State University
Columbus, Ohio

Shannon Harris, DNP, FNP, CCRN
Assistant Professor
College of Nursing
University of South Alabama
Mobile, Alabama

1

Principles of Mechanical Ventilation

David W. Chang, EdD, RRT

© S_maria/Shutterstock

OUTLINE

OBJECTIVES

1. Define and explain the clinical significance of airflow resistance.
2. Define and explain the clinical significance of static compliance and dynamic compliance.
3. Describe the clinical application of plateau pressure and peak inspiratory pressure.
4. Describe the clinical application of pressure-volume (compliance) slope.
5. Describe the clinical application of PIP-Pplat pressure gradient.
6. Describe the relationship between dead space ventilation and rapid shallow breathing pattern.
7. Define and describe the causes leading to ventilatory failures.
8. Define and describe the causes leading to oxygenation failures.
9. List the pulmonary and nonpulmonary conditions leading to mechanical ventilation.

KEY TERMS

airflow resistance
dead space ventilation
dynamic compliance
hypoxemia
hypoxia
intrapulmonary shunting
oxygenation failure
peak inspiratory pressure

plateau pressure
pressure-volume slope
static compliance
ventilation-perfusion
  mismatch
ventilatory failure

Introduction

Mechanical ventilation is an invasive procedure to provide partial or full support of a patient's ventilation and oxygenation needs. Indications for mechanical ventilation include numerous clinical conditions that fail to meet these gas exchange requirements. Examples include abnormal functioning of the respiratory drive (e.g., drug overdose, postanesthesia recovery, traumatic brain injury), ventilatory pump (e.g., flail chest, diaphragm), airway (e.g., epiglottitis, status asthmaticus), and lung parenchyma (e.g., acute respiratory distress syndrome [ARDS], chronic obstructive pulmonary disease [COPD]).

Durations of mechanical ventilation range from less than an hour (e.g., postanesthesia recovery) to years (e.g., high spinal cord injury). Locations for use of mechanical ventilation include acute care units, mass casualty situations, long-term care facilities, and at home. This chapter covers the essential principles of normal and abnormal respiratory physiology for spontaneous breathing and how they relate to the use of mechanical ventilation.

Airway Resistance

Airway resistance (Raw) is a mechanical factor affecting the airflow in the airways. **Airflow resistance** has a similar definition, except it can be used to describe the condition in the airways or in the lungs. Airway resistance is considered the nonelastic airflow resistance, because the airway diameter changes minimally during respiration. The elastic recoil of the lungs contributes to the elastic resistance to gas flow. The total airflow resistance is the sum of nonelastic and elastic resistance. The degree of airway resistance is primarily determined by the length, internal diameter, and patency of the airway. The patency of the airway may be reduced in conditions of retained secretions, bronchospasm (nonelastic airflow resistance), or compression of the lung parenchyma (i.e., elastic airflow resistance). For mechanically ventilated patients, the endotracheal (ET) tube and ventilator circuit impose additional airflow resistance to the airways.

Factors Affecting Airway Resistance

Airflow obstruction causes different degrees of resistance in the airways. It is increased when the patency or diameter of the airways is reduced. Airflow obstruction may be caused by changes inside the airway (e.g., retained secretions), in the wall of the airway (e.g., neoplasm of the bronchial muscle structure), or outside the airway (e.g., tumors surrounding and compressing the airway). These conditions reduce the internal diameter of the airway and increase the airway resistance. The simplified Poiseuille's law shows that when the radius of a circle is reduced by 50%, the driving pressure (ΔP) must increase by a factor of 16-fold to maintain the same airflow ($\dot{V}$).

Simplified form of Poiseuille's law: $\Delta P = \dot{V}/r^4$

There are many conditions that can increase the airway resistance. Two common diseases with increased airway resistance are asthma and COPD (e.g., emphysema, chronic bronchitis, and bronchiectasis). Mechanical factors that increase airway resistance include foreign body aspiration, main stem intubation, and artificial airways for mechanical ventilation. Infectious processes include laryngotracheobronchitis (croup), epiglottitis, and bronchiolitis.

The normal airway resistance (of the natural airways) in adults is between 0.5 and 2.5 cm H_2O/L/sec. The total resistance of all airways in the tracheobronchial tree is referred to as *airways* resistance. It is higher in intubated patients due to the small diameter of the ET tube. Airway resistance varies directly with the length and inversely with the diameter of the airway or ET tube. A shortened ET tube or tracheostomy tube facilitates airway management and removal of secretions. It also reduces mechanical dead space and airway resistance. However, the main determinant of increased airway resistance is the internal diameter of the ET tube. For this reason, the largest but appropriately sized ET tube should be used for mechanical ventilation. Once the patient is intubated, patency of the ET tube must be maintained as secretions inside the ET tube greatly increase the airway resistance.

Besides the ET tube, the ventilator circuit and condensation collected in it also contribute to the airflow resistance. Pressure support ventilation (PSV) is often used to compensate for airflow resistance and to augment spontaneous breathing efforts.

Airway Resistance and Work of Breathing

Airway resistance (Raw) is calculated by pressure gradient (ΔP)/flow:

$$Raw = \frac{\text{Pressure gradient } (\Delta P)}{\text{Flow}}$$

The pressure gradient (ΔP) in the equation reflects the work of breathing. Since Raw is directly related to ΔP, an increase in airway resistance will increase the work of breathing. If the work of breathing remains unchanged in the presence of increased airway resistance, the flow (or volume) will decrease. In essence, an increase in airway resistance will lead to an increase in work of breathing or a decrease in flow (or volume). In a clinical setting, relief of airflow obstruction is an effective way to improve ventilation and to reduce the work of breathing.

Effects on Ventilation and Oxygenation

An increase in airway resistance hinders ventilation and oxygenation. If an abnormally high airway resistance is sustained over a long time, respiratory muscle fatigue may occur. This leads to eventual ventilatory and oxygenation failure. **Ventilatory failure** occurs when the patient's minute alveolar ventilation cannot keep up with the metabolic rate or CO_2 production. Oxygenation failure usually follows when the cardiopulmonary system cannot provide adequate oxygen needed for metabolism.

Waveform Displays

The airflow resistance of a patient-ventilator system may be monitored using the pressure-volume (compliance) loop on the ventilator waveform display. An increased bowing of the pressure-volume loop (**Figure 1-1**) suggests an overall increase in airflow resistance. The increase in airflow resistance may be due to excessive inspiratory flow or increased expiratory flow resistance.

Another method to evaluate the airflow resistance of a patient-ventilator system is to use the peak inspiratory pressure-plateau pressure (PIP-Pplat) gradient on the pressure-time waveform obtained by a brief end-inspiratory pause. **Figure 1-2** shows the PIP and Pplat (duration of Pplat = pause time). PIP is the total pressure needed to overcome the airflow resistance (nonelastic resistance) in the airways *and* the elastic recoil forces (elastic resistance) of the lung parenchyma. Since Pplat is the pressure needed to overcome the recoil forces of the lungs, the PIP-Pplat gradient reflects the airflow resistance characteristic of each volume-controlled breath.

The PIP-Pplat gradient is a steady indicator of airflow resistance and is not influenced by changes of the lung compliance. As the lung compliance is decreased, the Pplat will increase causing the PIP to increase by the

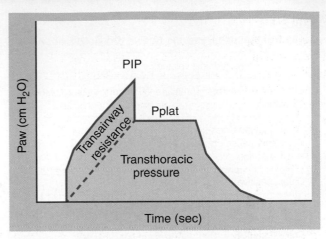

FIGURE 1-2 Pressure-time waveform. PIP-Pplat gradient reflects airflow resistance. PIP, peak inspiratory pressure; Pplat, plateau pressure.

same proportion. Likewise, when the lung compliance is increased, the Pplat will decrease causing the PIP to decrease by the same proportion.

Compliance

Lung compliance (C_L) describes the distensibility of the lung parenchyma. The opposite of compliance is elastance. Compliance is calculated by dividing the change in volume (ΔV) by change in pressure (ΔP), or $\Delta V/\Delta P$. In volume-controlled ventilation, ΔV is the mechanical tidal volume and ΔP is the pressure needed to deliver the tidal volume. In pressure-controlled ventilation, ΔP is the set peak inspiratory pressure and ΔV is the volume delivered by the pressure. It should be noted that the required pressure (during volume-controlled ventilation) and delivered volume (during pressure-controlled ventilation) are variable for each breath, and they are influenced by the changing airflow resistance and lung compliance.

The compliance equation is a very useful tool in mechanical ventilation. During volume-controlled ventilation, a rising plateau pressure indicates a decreasing compliance (and vice versa). (Note: A rising peak inspiratory pressure may be due to a decreasing compliance or an increasing airflow resistance.) During pressure-controlled ventilation, a decreasing volume indicates a decreasing compliance (and vice versa).

Measurement of Compliance

In mechanical ventilation, the compliance measurement can be separated into dynamic and static compliance. **Dynamic compliance** (Cdyn) is measured during a mechanical breath with gas movement (thus the term *dynamic*). The ΔP used to calculate dynamic compliance is the **peak inspiratory pressure** (PIP). **Static compliance** (Cst) is measured during an end-inspiratory pause where gas movement is *absent* (thus the term *static*). The ΔP in static compliance measurement is the

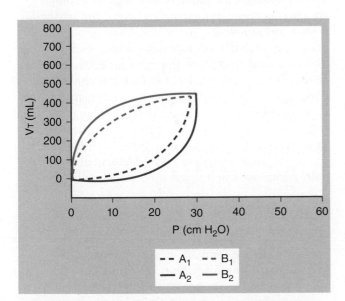

FIGURE 1-1 Pressure-volume (compliance) loop shows increased bowing (from dotted to solid lines) suggesting an increase in airflow resistance due to presence of excessive inspiratory flow or increased expiratory resistance. Bowing from A1 to A2 could be due to excessive flow during inspiration, and since expiration is passive the bowing from B1 to B2 is likely due to expiratory flow obstruction.

TABLE 1-1
Steps to Measure Dynamic and Static Compliance

1. Calculate corrected tidal volume.
2. Obtain peak inspiratory pressure (PIP) during volume-controlled ventilation.
3. Obtain plateau pressure (Pplat) by applying a brief end-inspiratory pause or manually occluding the exhalation port at end inspiration.
4. Obtain positive end-expiratory pressure (PEEP), if any.
5. Dynamic compliance (Cdyn) = Corrected tidal volume/ (PIP − PEEP) Static compliance (Cst) = Corrected tidal volume/ (Pplat − PEEP)

plateau pressure (Pplat), also known as static pressure. Most ventilators can measure and display the dynamic and static compliance values. A manual method to measure and calculate static and dynamic compliance is outlined in **Table 1-1**.

Dynamic and Static Compliance

Since Cdyn is measured during a mechanical breath, the rise and fall of PIP is determined by two main factors: airflow resistance (ventilator circuit, ET tube, airways) and total compliance (chest wall and lung parenchyma). In clinical practice, monitoring the PIP or Cdyn does not offer enough details for optimal patient care. This is because an increase in PIP (or a decrease in Cdyn) could be caused by an increase in airflow resistance or a decrease in lung compliance, or both. In most cases, careful patient assessment can isolate the cause for the PIP and Cdyn changes. For objective evaluation of a patient's status during mechanical ventilation, the Pplat and Cst should be measured along with the PIP and Cdyn.

Pplat is measured during a brief end-inspiratory pause. When flow is stopped momentarily, there is no airflow resistance. For this reason, the Pplat is the pressure needed to overcome the lung compliance (or elastic force of the lungs) during a mechanical breath. Since Pplat is used in the Cst equation (see Table 1-1), Cst reflects the lung compliance characteristics. In this chapter, discussion on compliance refers to the total compliance (chest wall and lungs) unless it is specified as dynamic compliance (airway and lungs) or static compliance (lungs).

Abnormal Lung Compliance

Abnormally low or high lung compliance affects the work of breathing and hinders the normal process of ventilation and oxygenation. Low compliance means high elastance (tendency to recoil to size at rest), and it is a problem affecting the respiratory mechanics during the inspiratory phase. This condition greatly increases the alveolar opening pressure and makes lung inflation and expansion difficult. The work of breathing is increased, and the patient typically adopts a rapid shallow breathing pattern. High compliance means diminished elastic recoil. This abnormal condition becomes evident during the expiratory phase, and it may lead to incomplete exhalation, incomplete CO_2 elimination, CO_2 retention, air trapping, and auto positive end-expiratory pressure (PEEP). Extreme low or high compliance abnormalities are two contributing factors to increased work of breathing and ventilatory failure.

Low Lung Compliance

In low lung compliance (high elastance) conditions, a higher than normal inspiratory pressure is required to inflate the lungs and deliver a set volume. The lungs are stiff or noncompliant. The work of breathing is increased proportionally to the decrease in compliance. Atelectasis and ARDS are two examples that produce low lung compliance. They are associated with refractory hypoxemia, the type of hypoxemia that responds poorly to oxygen therapy alone. Low lung compliance is usually related to conditions that reduce the patient's functional residual capacity. Patients with noncompliant lungs often have a restrictive lung defect, low lung volumes/capacities, and low minute ventilation.

High Lung Compliance

High lung compliance means low elastance (less elastic recoil during exhalation). The lungs are easily opened and inflated at a given inspiratory pressure. Unlike low lung compliance, the problem with high lung compliance occurs during the expiratory phase. The exhalation is often incomplete due to the low elastic recoil property of the lung parenchyma. Emphysema is an example of high lung compliance with impaired gas exchange. This condition typically leads to CO_2 retention, chronic air trapping, destruction of lung tissues, and enlargement of terminal and respiratory bronchioles. The lung functions will show increased residual volume, functional residual capacity, and total lung capacity. Patients with extremely compliant lungs often develop ventilatory failure and require noninvasive or invasive mechanical ventilation.

Plateau Pressure and Peak Inspiratory Pressure

Pplat and PIP are common measurements on the pressure-time waveform. During volume-controlled ventilation, these pressure readings increase or decrease in response to the breath-by-breath changes in airflow resistance or compliance. Conditions leading to changes in plateau pressure and static compliance invoke similar changes in peak inspiratory pressure and dynamic compliance. For example, atelectasis causes an increase in plateau pressure and a decrease in static compliance. These changes will lead to an increase in peak inspiratory pressure and a decrease in dynamic compliance (**Figure 1-3** [A to B]). With resolution of atelectasis, the plateau and peak inspiratory pressures return to normal (see Figure 1-3 [B to A]). When the plateau pressure and peak inspiratory pressure change by the same proportion (increase or decrease), the lungs are responsible for the changes. In some cases, the chest wall compliance may invoke similar changes as in lung compliance.

In conditions where the airway resistance is increased (e.g., bronchospasm), the peak inspiratory pressure is increased and the dynamic compliance is decreased. It is important to note that the plateau pressure and static compliance remain unchanged (**Figure 1-4** [A to B]). The plateau pressure and static compliance stay unchanged because the lung parenchyma is not involved in the increase of airway resistance. When bronchospasm is resolved, the peak inspiratory pressure and dynamic compliance measurements return to normal (see Figure 1-4 [B to A]). **Table 1-2** shows examples of clinical conditions leading to changes in plateau pressure and peak inspiratory pressure.

TABLE 1-2
Conditions Leading to Changes in Plateau Pressure (Pplat) and Peak Inspiratory Pressure (PIP)

Pplat	PIP	Conditions
↑	↑	↓ lung compliance (proportional changes in PIP and Pplat)
↑	↑↑	↓ lung compliance + ↑ airway resistance
↓	↓	↑ lung compliance (proportional changes in PIP and Pplat)
↓	↓↓	↑ lung compliance + ↓ airway resistance
No change	↑	↑ airway resistance
No change	↓	↓ airway resistance
↑	No change	↓ lung compliance and ↓ airway resistance
↓	No change	↑ lung compliance and ↑ airway resistance

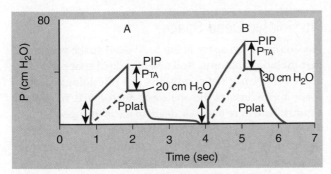

FIGURE 1-3 Changes in plateau pressure (Pplat) and peak inspiratory pressure (PIP). In atelectasis, both Pplat and PIP increase by the same proportion (from A to B). Upon resolution of atelectasis, both Pplat and PIP return to normal (from B to A).

Chang, DW. *Respiratory Care Calculations.* revised 4th ed. Jones and Bartlett Learning; 2021.

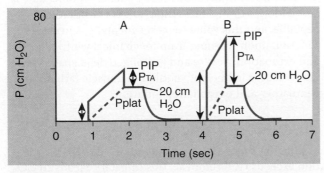

FIGURE 1-4 Changes in peak inspiratory pressure (PIP). Increase in airway resistance will increase the PIP, but not the plateau pressure (Pplat) (from A to B). When the airway resistance is corrected, the PIP returns to normal (from B to A).

Chang, DW. *Respiratory Care Calculations.* revised 4th ed. Jones and Bartlett Learning; 2021.

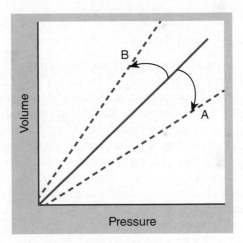

FIGURE 1-5 Pressure-volume (P-V) display. Shifting of the P-V slope toward the pressure axis (from solid line to dotted line A) indicates a decrease in compliance. Shifting of the P-V slope toward the volume axis (from solid line to dotted line B) indicates an increase in compliance.

Pressure-Volume Slope

On the ventilator graphic, the pressure-volume (P-V) display represents the compliance because $C = \Delta V/\Delta P$. The P-V slope shows the patient's compliance characteristics during mandatory breaths. **Figure 1-5** shows a P-V slope. A shift of the slope toward the pressure axis (from solid line to dotted line A) indicates a decrease in compliance. A shift of the slope toward the volume axis (from solid line to dotted line B) indicates an increase in compliance.

Interpretation of compliance should be made over time using a trend of serial measurements. In general, gradual changes in compliance are usually related to progressive conditions such as consolidation, atelectasis, and retained secretions. Sudden changes in compliance are often due to urgent conditions such as tension pneumothorax, main stem intubation, and mucus plugs.

Effects on Ventilation and Oxygenation

Abnormal compliance impairs gas exchange. When an abnormally low or high compliance is uncorrected and prolonged, muscle fatigue may occur and lead to the development of ventilatory and oxygenation failure. Ventilatory failure develops when the patient's minute ventilation cannot keep up with the CO_2 production. Oxygenation failure usually follows when the cardiopulmonary system cannot provide the oxygen demand for metabolism and increased work of breathing.

Dead Space Ventilation

Dead space ventilation is defined as the portion of tidal volume that does not take part in gas exchange. It is also called *wasted ventilation* or *ventilation in excess of perfusion*. Dead space ventilation has three distinct types: anatomic, alveolar, and physiologic.

Anatomic Dead Space

Normally, the conducting airways make up about 30% of dead space ventilation. A tidal volume (V_T) of 500 mL normally has about 150 mL of anatomic dead space volume (V_D). This anatomic V_D (i.e., volume in nasal cavity, trachea, and main stem bronchi) does not contribute to gas exchange because it is not in contact with the pulmonary capillaries where gas exchange takes place. The V_D/V_T can be measured or estimated (1 mL/lb predicted body weight). Decrease in tidal volume (shallow breathing) results in a relatively higher V_D/V_T %. For example, if the tidal volume was decreased from 500 mL to 300 mL, the V_D/V_T% would increase from 30% (150 mL/500 mL) to 50% (150 mL/300 mL). In conditions leading to a shallow breathing pattern, the spontaneous breathing frequency is often increased to maintain the minute ventilation. This rapid shallow breathing pattern is inefficient for gas exchange. It causes increased work of breathing, respiratory muscle fatigue, and eventual ventilatory failure. In mechanical ventilation, the rapid shallow breathing index is used as an indication for mechanical ventilation and for making weaning and extubation decisions.

Alveolar Dead Space

Alveolar dead space also contributes to wasted ventilation. This occurs when alveoli receive normal ventilation but it is *not* adequately perfused by pulmonary circulation. This high ventilation-perfusion ($\dot{V}/\dot{Q}$) mismatch may be due to (1) absence of regional pulmonary

TABLE 1-3
Clinical Conditions That Increase Physiologic Dead Space Ventilation

Cause of Increased Physiologic Dead Space	Example
↓ spontaneous tidal volume (V_T)	Neuromuscular diseases Respiratory suppressing drug overdose Respiratory muscle fatigue Postanesthesia recovery
↑ alveolar dead space (due to lack of matching pulmonary perfusion)	Decreased cardiac output (e.g., congestive heart failure, blood loss) Obstruction or constriction of pulmonary vessels (e.g., pulmonary embolism, hypoxic vasoconstriction)

perfusion in conditions such as pulmonary embolism, (2) decreased of global pulmonary perfusion in conditions such as congestive heart failure and hypovolemia, and (3) constriction of pulmonary blood vessels as in hypoxic vasoconstriction.

Physiologic Dead Space

Physiologic dead space is the total dead space volume that includes anatomic and alveolar dead space volumes. Under normal conditions, the physiologic dead space approximates the anatomic dead space. In clinical conditions where alveolar dead space is increased, physiologic dead space becomes higher than anatomic dead space. **Table 1-3** shows clinical conditions that increase physiologic dead space ventilation.

Physiologic dead space to tidal volume ratio (V_D/V_T) can be calculated as follows:

$$V_D/V_T = (Pa_{CO_2} - P_{\bar{E}CO_2})/Pa_{CO_2}$$

Pa_{CO_2} is arterial carbon dioxide tension and $P_{\bar{E}CO_2}$ is P_{CO_2} of a mixed expired gas sample. These two samples are collected simultaneously. In patients on mechanical ventilation, V_D/V_T of less than 60% is considered acceptable, and this value suggests adequate ventilatory function upon weaning from mechanical ventilation and extubation. Severe and prolonged dead space ventilation causes inefficient ventilation, muscle fatigue, and ventilatory and oxygenation failure.

Ventilatory Failure

Ventilatory failure is a condition in which CO_2 production exceeds CO_2 removal. This imbalance leads to CO_2 retention, increase in Pa_{CO_2}, and respiratory acidosis. In mild cases, the Pa_{CO_2} exceeds its upper normal limit (45 mm Hg). In severe ventilatory failure, the Pa_{CO_2} may exceed 80 mm Hg. It is important to note that evaluation of ventilatory failure or respiratory acidosis requires an arterial blood gas sample. The $Paco_2$ is the measurement used to evaluate how well a patient is ventilating (i.e., $\uparrow$ $Paco_2$ = hypoventilation and $\downarrow$ $Paco_2$ = hyperventilation). A patient's spontaneous frequency or tidal volume cannot be used to evaluate hypoventilation or hyperventilation.

Hypercapnia (increase in $Paco_2$) is the key feature of hypoventilation or ventilatory failure. Since ventilation is a key factor in gas exchange, hypoventilation almost always leads to hypoxemia. In general, hypoxemia due to hypoventilation responds well to ventilation and low concentration of supplemental oxygen. Without supplemental oxygen, the degree of hypoxemia correlates with the severity of ventilatory failure.

The primary conditions leading to ventilatory failure include (1) hypoventilation, (2) $\dot{V}/\dot{Q}$ mismatch, (3) intrapulmonary shunting, and (4) diffusion defects. If uncorrected, these conditions inevitably lead to increased work of breathing, hypercapnia, respiratory acidosis, ventilatory failure, and mechanical ventilation.

Hypoventilation

Hypoventilation is defined as a condition that results in an increased $Paco_2$. It may be caused by a variety of clinical conditions, including high spinal cord injury, neuromuscular disorders, overdose of analgesics or sedatives, severe airway obstruction, and central sleep apnea. In a clinical setting, hypoventilation is characterized by a reduction of minute alveolar ventilation ($\dot{V}A$) and an increase of $Paco_2$. The following equation shows inverse relationship between $\dot{V}A$ and $Paco_2$:

$$\dot{V}A = \dot{V}co_2 / Paco_2$$

Minute alveolar ventilation is the product of respiratory frequency and the difference between tidal volume and dead space volume $\dot{V}A = f \times (V_T - V_D)$. A decrease in frequency or tidal volume, or an increase in dead space volume will reduce the minute alveolar ventilation and raise the $Paco_2$. In essence, CO_2 production, respiratory frequency, tidal volume, and dead space volume are the main determinants of the adequacy of ventilation.

During mechanical ventilation, hypoventilation can be corrected by increasing the frequency or tidal volume (in volume-controlled ventilation) or the peak inspiratory pressure (in pressure-controlled ventilation). Unlike tidal volume, dead space volume is difficult to manage because anatomic dead space stays rather constant and physiologic dead space is due to high $\dot{V}/\dot{Q}$ mismatch (inadequate pulmonary perfusion).

Ventilation-Perfusion Mismatch

The $\dot{V}/\dot{Q}$ ratio is the percent proportion of ventilation in L/min to pulmonary perfusion in L/min. Since blood flow is gravity dependent, the $\dot{V}/\dot{Q}$ ratio ranges from about 0.4 in the lower lung zone (more perfusion) to 3.0 in the upper lung zone (less perfusion). When

ventilation is in excess of perfusion, this high $\dot{V}/\dot{Q}$ mismatch leads to dead space ventilation. Pulmonary embolism is an example of conditions leading to dead space ventilation. On the other extreme, low $\dot{V}/\dot{Q}$ mismatch causes intrapulmonary (right-to-left) shunting. Atelectasis is an example of conditions leading to intrapulmonary shunting. Severe $\dot{V}/\dot{Q}$ mismatch is responsible for the development of hypoxemia. With sufficient pulmonary reserve, a patient can usually compensate for the hypoxemic condition by increasing the heart rate or spontaneous respiratory frequency. These cardiopulmonary compensations require work expenditure. If the patient cannot sustain this additional workload over a long period of time, ventilatory failure may result. The key management strategy for $\dot{V}/\dot{Q}$ mismatch is to identify its cause and to implement appropriate treatment plan before decompensation occurs. In uncomplicated $\dot{V}/\dot{Q}$ mismatch, oxygen therapy can be very effective. If refractory hypoxemia develops on $F_{IO_2} > 0.5$, presence of intrapulmonary shunting should be investigated.

Intrapulmonary Shunting

Unlike dead space ventilation (high $\dot{V}/\dot{Q}$ mismatch), **intrapulmonary shunting** is a condition in which perfusion is present but ventilation is diminished or absent (low $\dot{V}/\dot{Q}$ mismatch). Intrapulmonary shunting is more difficult to manage because oxygen therapy alone cannot correct refractory hypoxemia. Delivery of oxygen to the lungs requires ventilation—a component lacking in intrapulmonary shunting. Shunted pulmonary blood flow is ineffective in gas exchange because the collapsed alveoli at the alveolocapillary interface are not ventilated or do not carry oxygen.

In healthy individuals, the physiologic shunt is about the same as the anatomic shunt (<5%). For noncritically ill patients, the normal (acceptable) physiologic shunt is less than 10%. In other disease states, the physiologic shunt may be greater than 30%. **Table 1-4** provides interpretation of shunt percent in critically ill patients.

The shunt percent can be calculated (classic shunt equation) or estimated (estimated shunt equation). The classic shunt equation is more accurate, but it requires arterial and mixed venous blood gas samples. The

TABLE 1-4
Interpretation of Physiologic Shunt Percent in Critically Ill Patients

Physiologic Shunt	Interpretation
<10%	Normal
10% to 19%	Mild shunt
20% to 29%	Moderate shunt
≥30%	Critical and severe shunt

estimated shunt equation is easier to use as it requires only an arterial blood gas sample. See Appendix B for these two shunt equations.

In significant or severe physiologic shunts, the cardiopulmonary system typically cannot sustain the workload to compensate for the refractory hypoxemia. Over time, respiratory muscle fatigue and ventilatory failure are the end results. This is usually followed by oxygenation failure if ventilatory interventions are unsuccessful. In intrapulmonary shunting, lack of adequate ventilation is due to collapsed or fluid-filled lung units. PEEP and continuous positive airway pressure (CPAP) are two methods to reopen and ventilate these lung units. Other chapters describe the use of PEEP or CPAP and other strategies to manage intrapulmonary shunting.

Diffusion Defects

Diffusion of oxygen and carbon dioxide across the alveolocapillary (A-c) membrane is mainly dependent on the gas pressure gradients. Oxygen diffuses from the alveoli (P_{AO_2} = 109 mm Hg) to the pulmonary capillaries ($P\bar{v}_{O_2}$ = 40 mm Hg) with a pressure gradient of 69 mm Hg. Carbon dioxide diffuses from the pulmonary capillaries ($P\bar{v}_{CO_2}$ = 46 mm Hg) to the alveoli (P_{ACO_2} = 40 mm Hg) with a net pressure gradient of only 6 mm Hg. This low-pressure gradient for CO_2 diffusion is possible because the CO_2 diffusion coefficient is about 20 times higher than the diffusion coefficient for oxygen.

Diffusion of oxygen is greatly impaired in environments with low barometric pressure (P_B) and low inspired oxygen tension (P_{IO_2}). Two examples show the importance of adequate P_B and P_{IO_2} for proper gas diffusion: At high altitude, the barometric pressure and inspired oxygen tension are lower than that at sea level. This leads to hypoxic hypoxia. Fire in an enclosure reduces the P_{IO_2} because combustion consumes oxygen in the air. Patients with smoke inhalation are at risk of developing hypoxic hypoxia (low P_{IO_2}) as well as anemic hypoxia (carbon monoxide inhalation).

In addition to the pressure gradient and diffusion coefficient, the gas diffusion rate is also affected by the thickness of the A-c membrane, surface area of the A-c membrane, and time available for diffusion. **Table 1-5** outlines the clinical conditions that reduce gas diffusion rate. Similar to other chronic cardiopulmonary diseases, persistent reduction of gas diffusion rate may lead to hypoxemia, hypoxia, hypoxic vasoconstriction, pulmonary hypertension, right ventricular hypertrophy, and cor pulmonale.

Oxygenation Failure

Oxygenation failure is defined as severe hypoxemia due to any condition (e.g., high altitude, smoke inhalation, cardiopulmonary diseases) that lead to persistent

TABLE 1-5
Clinical Conditions That Reduce Gas Diffusion Rate

Type of Diffusion Defect	Clinical Condition
↓ P(A – a)O_2 gradient (due to ↓P_{AO_2})	High altitude (↓P_B) Fire combustion (↓F_{IO_2})
↓ Surface area of alveolo-capillary membrane	Emphysema Pulmonary fibrosis
↑ Thickness of alveolar-capillary membrane	Pulmonary edema Retained secretions
Insufficient time for gas diffusion	Tachycardia

cellular and tissue hypoxia. Regardless of the cause, mechanical ventilation may be indicated to reduce the work of breathing, prevent depletion of oxygen reserve, and provide oxygenation to vital organs.

Hypoxemia and Hypoxia

Hypoxemia is defined as lower than normal levels of oxygen in blood, and this can be evaluated directly by performing arterial blood gases or transcutaneous blood gases (neonates) or indirectly by using pulse oximetry (an estimation). **Hypoxia** is lack of sufficient oxygen in the tissues or organs. Presence of hypoxia may not be apparent but it should be implied whenever hypoxemia is present. It should be noted that hypoxia can occur without hypoxemia. For example, anemic hypoxia can occur with a reduced hemoglobin level (e.g., anemia, sepsis) or an increased level of dysfunctional hemoglobins (e.g., ↑ carboxyhemoglobin due to carbon monoxide poisoning). Histotoxic hypoxia and circulatory hypoxia can occur with cyanide poisoning and decreased cardiac output, respectively. Hypoxia due to dysfunctional hemoglobins typically shows normal or near normal P_{aO_2} because this value is measured from the dissolved oxygen in the plasma. It is a grave oversight if the patient's oxygenation status is based on the P_{aO_2} (dissolved oxygen) alone because over 98% of available oxygen is bounded to functional hemoglobin. If the P_{aO_2} is normal and the patient shows signs of hypoxia (e.g., complaint of dyspnea, deterioration of vital signs, diminished mental status, cyanosis), arterial oxygen content (C_{aO_2}) measured by CO-oximetry should be evaluated because it includes the oxygen combined with hemoglobin and the oxygen dissolved in the plasma.

With some exceptions noted, hypoxemia and hypoxia are closely related. Since P_{aO_2} is often used to evaluate a patient's oxygenation status, **Table 1-6** provides a quick reference for interpretation of oxygenation status based on P_{aO_2} at sea level and 6000 ft above sea level (Denver, CO).

TABLE 1-6
Interpretation of Oxygenation Status Based on Pao_2 at Sea Level and 6000 ft Above Sea Level

Status	Pao_2 (P_B = 760 mm Hg)	Pao_2 (P_B = 609 mm Hg)
Normal	80 to 100 mm Hg	60 to 79 mm Hg
Mild hypoxemia	60 to 79 mm Hg	50 to 59 mm Hg
Moderate hypoxemia	40 to 59 mm Hg	40 to 49 mm Hg
Severe hypoxemia	<40 mm Hg	<40 mm Hg

TABLE 1-7
Early and Late Signs and Symptoms of Hypoxia

Category	Early Phase	Late Phase
Assessment findings	Pallor Nasal flaring Mouth breathing	Cyanosis Respiratory arrest Cardiac arrest
Vital signs	↑ Respiratory frequency ↑ Heart rate ↑ Blood pressure	↓ Respiratory frequency ↓ Heart rate ↓ Blood pressure
Blood gases and oximetry	↓ Pao_2 ↓ Spo_2 ↓ Cao_2	↓ Pao_2 ↓ Spo_2 ↓ Cao_2 Metabolic (lactic) acidosis Combined acidosis with hypoventilation
Neurologic signs	Anxiety Agitation Restlessness	Confusion Loss of consciousness

Table data from Considine J. Emergency assessment of oxygenation. Acutecaretesting.org. https://acutecaretesting.org/en/articles/emergency-assessment-of-oxygenation. Published January 2007; Rochester DF. Respiratory muscles and ventilatory failure. *Am J Med Sci.* 1993;205(6):394–402.

Clinical Signs of Hypoxia

Results of arterial blood gases and pulse oximetry are commonly used to evaluate how well a patient is ventilating and oxygenating. Under certain hypoxic conditions, Pao_2 and Spo_2 do not accurately reflect a patient's oxygenation status, especially at the tissue level. Normal cellular metabolism under aerobic condition produces up to 38 adenosine triphosphate (ATP) molecules (energy units). Under hypoxic condition, only 2 ATPs are produced. This drastic reduction of energy unit shows the importance of adequate oxygenation at the cellular level. Recognition of the presence of hypoxia is therefore an important assessment tool, especially in the early stage of hypoxia. Early intervention of hypoxia is crucial for patient outcomes because untreated hypoxia is one main reason for hospital and intensive care unit (ICU) admissions. **Table 1-7** outlines the early and late signs and symptoms of hypoxia.

Conditions Leading to Mechanical Ventilation

Mechanical ventilation is frequently used to support a patient's ventilation and oxygenation needs. Hypoventilation will lead to immediate respiratory acidosis and hypoxemia. Severe and prolonged hypoventilation often results in ventilatory failure, oxygenation failure, cellular and tissue hypoxia, anaerobic metabolism, lactic acidosis, hypoxic brain, and cardiopulmonary arrest. Severe hypoxia results in similar adverse outcomes. Mechanical ventilation is often necessary to manage oxygenation failure.

Inadequate ventilation or oxygenation may be caused by pulmonary or nonpulmonary conditions. ARDS is an example of a pulmonary condition commonly associated with mechanical ventilation. This condition produces severe and progressive hypercapnia and refractory hypoxemia. Nonpulmonary conditions leading to hypoventilation and hypoxemia include postanesthesia recovery, neuromuscular diseases, and brain injury. In general, pulmonary conditions leading to mechanical ventilation usually have more ventilator-associated problems. Unless complications occur, nonpulmonary conditions usually have an uneventful course of mechanical ventilation. The next sections describe the pathophysiology of ventilatory failure and the rationales for initiation of mechanical ventilation.

Gas Exchange Abnormalities

Severe or prolonged gas exchange abnormalities (dead space ventilation, diffusion defect, and shunting) often lead to ventilatory and oxygenation failure and the need for mechanical ventilation. Dead space ventilation is a perfusion problem. Lack of perfusion produces dead space ventilation or "wasted ventilation." A classic example of dead space ventilation is pulmonary embolism in which the amount of ventilation is not matched proportionally by the amount of pulmonary blood flow. Diffusion defects occur at the alveolocapillary level and they impede the normal gas diffusion functions—mainly oxygen diffusion from alveoli to pulmonary capillaries. Emphysema is an example of diffusion defect due to loss of surface area for gas exchange. Pulmonary fibrosis is another example of diffusion defect in which the reduction in gas diffusion is due to the increased thickening of A-c membrane. Absolute shunt (true shunt, capillary shunt) occurs when the capillary blood flow is not matched by alveolar ventilation (i.e., complete or near complete absence of ventilation as in atelectasis). Relative shunt (shuntlike effect) refers to a condition in which capillary perfusion is in excess of ventilation (i.e., ventilation is present but at lesser degrees). Therefore, shunting is a ventilation problem. Classic examples of absolute shunt include atelectasis and consolidation. Examples of relative shunt include hypoventilation, **ventilation-perfusion mismatch,** and diffusion defects. It should be noted that relative shunts respond very well to supplemental ventilation and oxygenation. On the other hand, absolute shunts do not respond well to traditional methods of ventilation and oxygenation.

Venous admixture is the end result of shunting where the shunted, nonoxygenated blood is mixed with reoxygenated blood distal to the alveoli with adequate ventilation. Conditions resulting in venous admixture usually respond well to traditional methods of oxygenation.

Depressed Respiratory Drive

Depressed or absent respiratory drive often leads to hypoventilation and hypoxemia. In spontaneously breathing patients, the tidal volume and frequency are decreased. Patients with reversible neurologic impairment typically have normal lung functions in the early stage. The lung functions may quickly worsen with complications from intubation and mechanical ventilation. For reversible causes, mechanical ventilation is needed to support the ventilation and oxygenation needs until the cause of insufficient respiratory drive has been identified and resolved. **Table 1-8** summarizes the clinical outcomes as a result of depressed respiratory drive.

Excessive Ventilatory Workload

Under normal conditions, the ventilatory workload is in balance with metabolic and oxygenation needs. However, the workload is increased in conditions with high airflow resistance (e.g., bronchospasm), low compliance (e.g., ARDS), and high metabolic rate or oxygen consumption (e.g., fever). Other conditions may include increased dead space ventilation (e.g., rapid shallow breathing pattern), congenital heart disease, cardiovascular decompensation, and shock. When the workload exceeds the patient's physical ability or endurance, ventilatory and oxygenation failures are the eventual outcomes. The patient will show cyanosis, tachycardia, and a rapid shallow breathing pattern. Arterial blood gases will show progression from respiratory alkalosis with hypoxemia, respiratory acidosis, impending ventilatory failure, ventilatory failure, and oxygenation failure. **Table 1-9** outlines common clinical conditions leading to excessive ventilatory workload.

Failure of Ventilatory Pump

The ventilatory pump includes the diaphragm, thoracic skeletal structure, respiratory muscles, and lung parenchyma. Failure of one or more mechanical components will lead to increased work of breathing due to $\dot{V}/\dot{Q}$ mismatch. If uncorrected, failure of the ventilatory pump can result in ventilatory and oxygenation failure. Clinical

---

TABLE 1-8
Outcomes and Examples of Depressed Respiratory Drive

Type	Outcome/Example
Anesthesia or drug overdose	Central hypoventilation (narcotics, sedatives) Acute respiratory insufficiency (cocaine, heroin, methadone, propoxyphene, phenothiazine, alcohol, barbiturates) Severe pulmonary complications (poisons and toxins such as paraquat, petroleum distillates, organophosphates, mushrooms of *Amanita* genus, hemlock, botulism)
High spinal cord injury	Apnea (tetraplegic with injury at C1–C3 level)
Traumatic head injury	Abnormal respiratory patterns (apnea, tachypnea, Cheyne-Stokes respiration, apneustic breathing, ataxic breathing) Neurogenic pulmonary edema (increase in intracranial pressure) Delayed pulmonary dysfunction (intrapulmonary shunt, increased pulmonary vascular resistance, $\dot{V}/\dot{Q}$ mismatch)
Neurologic dysfunction	Coma (anoxic brain) Reduced sensorium (hypoxic brain) Cerebrovascular accident (stroke)
Sleep disorders	Sleep apnea (central, obstructive, mixed)

Table data from Bach JR. Alternative methods of ventilatory support for the patient with ventilatory failure due to spinal cord injury. *J Am Paraplegia Soc.* 1991;14(4):159–174; Greene KE, Peters JI. Pathophysiology of acute respiratory failure. *Clin Chest Med.* 1994;15(1):1–12; Kelly BJ, Matthay MA. Prevalence and severity of neurologic dysfunction in critically ill patients—influence on need for continued mechanical ventilation. *Chest J.* 1993;104:1818–1824; Parsons PE. Respiratory failure as a result of drugs, overdoses, and poisonings. *Clin Chest Med.* 1994;15(1):93–102; Pierson DJ. Indications for mechanical ventilation in adults with acute respiratory failure. *Respir Care.* 2002;47(2):249.

TABLE 1-9
Clinical Conditions Leading to Excessive Ventilatory Workload

Type	Clinical Condition
Increased airflow resistance	Bronchospasm Asthma Chronic obstructive pulmonary disease (COPD) Acute epiglottitis Endotracheal tube intubation
Decreased lung and chest wall compliance	Acute respiratory distress syndrome (ARDS) Atelectasis Tension pneumothorax Chest trauma Obesity Postthoracic surgery
Increased dead space ventilation	Rapid shallow breathing pattern Pulmonary embolism Decreased cardiac output Congestive heart failure Emphysema
Increased oxygen demand	Fever Increased work of breathing Sepsis Patient-ventilator dyssynchrony
Congenital heart disease	Hypoplastic left heart syndrome Tetralogy of Fallot Persistent pulmonary hypertension Left-to-right intra-atrial or intraventricular shunt
Hypovolemic shock	Blood loss Sepsis Congestive heart failure
Drug	Acute pulmonary edema (e.g., narcotics, salicylates, nonsteroidal anti-inflammatory agent, naloxone, thiazide diuretic, insulin, contrast media) Bronchospasm (e.g., salicylates, nonsteroidal anti-inflammatory agent, hydrocortisone, β-blocker, neuromuscular blocking agents, contrast media)

Table data from Bach JR. Alternative methods of ventilatory support for the patient with ventilatory failure due to spinal cord injury. *J Am Paraplegia Soc.* 1991;14(4):159–174; Greene KE, Peters JI. Pathophysiology of acute respiratory failure. *Clin Chest Med.* 1994;15(1):1–12; DiCarlo JV, Steven JM. Respiratory failure in congenital heart disease. *Pediatr Clin North Am.* 1994;41:525–542; Hinson JR, Marini JJ. Principles of mechanical ventilator use in respiratory failure. *Ann Rev Med.* 1992;43:341–361. doi:10.1146/annurev.me.43.020192.002013; Kraus P, Lipman J, Lee CC, et al. Acute lung injury at Baragwanath ICU, an eight-month audit and call for consensus for other organ failure in the adult respiratory distress syndrome. *Chest.* 1993;103:1832–1836.

conditions that may lead to ventilatory pump failure include chest trauma (e.g., flail chest, pneumothorax), prematurity (respiratory distress syndrome), electrolyte imbalance (e.g., hyperkalemia), and geriatric patients (e.g., fatigue or dysfunction of respiratory muscles).

Summary

Mechanical ventilation is an invasive tool commonly used to support a patient's failing breathing efforts.

Ventilatory and oxygenation failures are two main reasons for mechanical ventilation. In turn, these failures can be caused by pulmonary and nonpulmonary conditions. Identification of the causes of ventilatory and oxygenation failure is important because the strategies for implementing mechanical ventilation are often patient specific. The chapter covers the fundamental concepts in mechanical ventilation, including airflow resistance, compliance, dead space ventilation, and shunting. Clinicians should apply these concepts during mechanical ventilation for better patient outcomes.

Case Study

You are evaluating patients in the intensive care unit (ICU). The first patient, 55-year-old Bill, is on volume-controlled ventilation. Over the past 6 hours, the peak inspiratory pressure (PIP) has increased from 40 cm H_2O to 44 cm H_2O.

1. What is the meaning of this increase in PIP?

The second patient, Pam, a 50-year-old with a recent onset of ARDS, has the following ventilator parameters during volume-controlled ventilation (VT 500 mL, f = 18/min): At 6:00 a.m., PIP 50 cm H_2O, plateau pressure (Pplat) 36 cm H_2O. At 8:00 a.m., PIP 46 cm H_2O, Pplat 32 cm H_2O.

2. What is the main reason for the changes in PIP and Pplat?

The third patient, Hero, a 33-year-old, was recently admitted to the ICU for overdose. The toxicology panel is pending. He is breathing spontaneously on a high-flow nasal cannula (HFNC). The flow is set at 30 L/min with an FIO_2 of 40%. Over the past 30 minutes, his spontaneous frequency has changed from 18/min to 30/min.

3. This change in breathing pattern (not considering the effects of FIO_2 and HFNC) will most likely result in which outcome? (A) increase in compliance, (B) decrease in compliance, (C) increase in dead space ventilation, (D) decrease in dead space ventilation.

4. If Hero's spontaneous breathing pattern persists, what is the likely outcome? (A) ventilatory failure due to respiratory muscle fatigue, (B) respiratory arrest due to decrease in compliance, (C) ventilatory failure due to overdose of an unknown drug, (D) oxygenation failure due to inadequate flow by nasal cannula.

Bibliography

Airway Resistance

Blanch L. Bernabe F, Lucangelo U. Measurement of air trapping, intrinsic positive end-expiratory pressure, and dynamic hyperinflation in mechanically ventilated patients. *Respir Care.* 2005;50(1):110–123.

Chang DW. *Clinical Application of Mechanical Ventilations.* 4th ed. Clifton Park, NY: Delmar-Cengage Learning; 2014.

Myers TR. Use of heliox in children. *Respir Care.* 2006;51(6):619–631.

Rochester DF. Respiratory muscles and ventilatory failure. Am J Med Sci. 1993;205(6):394–402.

Waugh JB, Deshpande VM, Brown MK, et al. *Rapid Interpretation of Ventilator Waveforms.* 2nd ed. Upper Saddle River, NJ: Pearson Education; 2007.

West JB. *Pulmonary Pathophysiology—The Essentials.* 6th ed. Baltimore, MD: Lippincott Williams & Wilkins; 2007.

Compliance

Chang DW. *Clinical Application of Mechanical Ventilations.* 4th ed. Clifton Park, NY: Delmar Cengage Learning; 2014.

Rochester DF. Respiratory muscles and ventilatory failure. *Am J Med Sci.* 1993;205(6):394–402.

Waugh JB, Deshpande VM, Brown MK, et al. Rapid Interpretation of Ventilator Waveforms. 2nd ed. Upper Saddle River, NJ: Pearson Education; 2007.

Dead Space Ventilation

Chang DW. *Clinical Application of Mechanical Ventilations.* 4th ed. Clifton Park, NY: Delmar-Cengage Learning; 2014.

Shapiro BA, Kacmarek RM, Cane RD, et al. *Clinical Application of Respiratory Care.* 4th ed. St. Louis, MO: Mosby; 1991.

Ventilatory Failure

Greene KE, Peters JI. Pathophysiology of acute respiratory failure. *Clin Chest Med.* 1994;15(1):1–12.

Rochester DF. Respiratory muscles and ventilatory failure. *Am J Med Sci.* 1993;205(6):394–402.

Shapiro BA, Kacmarek RM, Cane RD, et al. *Clinical Application of Respiratory Care.* 4th ed. St. Louis, MO: Mosby; 1991.

Shapiro BA, Peruzzi WT, Kozlowski-Templin R. *Clinical Application of Blood Gases.* 5th ed. St. Louis, MO: Mosby; 1994.

West JB. *Pulmonary Pathophysiology—The Essentials.* 6th ed. Baltimore, MD: Lippincott Williams & Wilkins; 2007.

Wilkins RL, Dexter JR. *Respiratory Disease—Principles of Patient Care.* 2nd ed. Philadephia, PA: FA Davis; 1998.

Oxygenation Failure

Considine J. Emergency assessment of oxygenation. Acutecaretesting.org. Available at https://acutecaretesting.org/en/articles/emergency-assessment-of-oxygenation Accessed May 14, 2019. Published January 2007.

Rochester DF. Respiratory muscles and ventilatory failure. *Am J Med Sci.* 1993;205(6):394–402.

Shapiro BA, Kacmarek RM, Cane RD, et al. *Clinical Application of Respiratory Care.* 4th ed. St. Louis, MO: Mosby; 1991.

Conditions Leading to Mechanical Ventilation

Bach JR. Alternative methods of ventilatory support for the patient with ventilatory failure due to spinal cord injury. *J Am Paraplegia Soc.* 1991;14(4):159–174.

Blanch L, Bernabe F, Lucangelo U. Measurement of air trapping, intrinsic positive end-expiratory pressure, and dynamic hyperinflation in mechanically ventilated patients. *Respir Care.* 2005;50:110–123.

DiCarlo JV, Steven JM. Respiratory failure in congenital heart disease. *Pediatr Clin North Am.* 1994;41(3):525–42.

Freeman SJ, Fale AD. Muscular paralysis and ventilatory failure caused by hyperkalemia. *Br J Anaesth.* 1993;70:226–227.

Greene KE, Peters JI. Pathophysiology of acute respiratory failure. *Clin Chest Med.* 1994;15(1):1–12.

Hinson JR, Marini JJ. Principles of mechanical ventilator use in respiratory failure. *Ann Rev Med.* 1992;43:341–361. doi:10.1146/annurev.me.43.020192.002013

Kelly BJ, Matthay MA. Prevalence and severity of neurologic dysfunction in critically ill patients—influence on need for continued mechanical ventilation. *Chest J.* 1993;104:1818–1824.

Kraus P, Lipman J, Lee CC, et al. Acute lung injury at Baragwanath ICU, an eight-month audit and call for consensus for other organ failure in the adult respiratory distress syndrome. *Chest.* 1993;103(6):1832–1836.

Krieger BP. Respiratory failure in the elderly. *Clin Geriatr Med.* 1994;10(1):103–119.

Parsons PE. Respiratory failure as a result of drugs, overdoses, and poisonings. *Clin Chest Med.* 1994;15(1):93–102.

Pierson DJ. Indications for mechanical ventilation in adults with acute respiratory failure. *Respir Care.* 2002;47(2):249.

2

Classification of Mechanical Ventilation

Gary C. White, MEd, RRT, RPFT, FAARC

© s_maria/Shutterstock

OUTLINE

OBJECTIVES

1. Describe the normal physiology of ventilation, including inhalation and exhalation.
2. Define pulmonary compliance.
3. Differentiate between the elastic and nonelastic forces of ventilation.
4. Describe ventilatory work and relate the equation of motion of the respiratory system to pulmonary physiology.
5. Describe the elements of Chatburn's classification of mechanical ventilators.

KEY TERMS

baseline variable
control circuit
control variable
cycle variable
drive mechanism
flow controller
limit variable
neurally adjusted ventilatory
  assist (NAVA®)

pressure controller
pulmonary compliance
time controller
trigger variable
volume controller
volume cycling

Introduction

Mechanical ventilation plays an important role in the management of critically ill patients. The proper application of mechanical ventilators to support these patients requires an understanding of mechanical ventilator classification and, conversely, how the classification can affect the management of these patients. A respiratory care education program does not have the resources to provide examples of every type of ventilator. Knowing the classification system equips the operator to become quickly familiar with and be able to operate a new ventilator encountered in the clinical setting. It is not uncommon for clinicians to be thrust into a situation in the critical care setting where they have never operated or been responsible for the care of a patient on a ventilator they have never used before. A solid understanding of the classification system will equip clinicians to succeed in this seemingly impossible situation.

Human physiology of ventilation must be understood thoroughly prior to being able to understand how ventilatory work is supported with mechanical ventilation. Understanding how pleural, alveolar, and transairway pressure changes result in lung expansion and contraction allows clinicians to substitute a mechanical ventilator for the work of ventilation.

Robert Chatburn has authored numerous articles on the classification of mechanical ventilation. His classification system remains as relevant today as when it was first described in 1991. Chatburn's classification system has the advantage of using the equation of motion of the respiratory system as the basis of its design. The fundamental knowledge of the physiology of ventilation will remain constant throughout the foreseeable future to be applied as technology evolves. The classification system will change as technology evolves; the basics of the system, which is rooted in physiology and physics, will remain relatively constant.

Physiology of Spontaneous Ventilation

Normal spontaneous ventilation occurs because inspiratory and expiratory muscles create a pressure difference between the atmospheric pressure and the alveolar pressure. Fluids, including gases, will always move from an area of high pressure to an area of low pressure whenever a pressure gradient exists.

Inhalation

Inspiration occurs when the diaphragm contracts, descending in the thoracic cavity. The inferior movement of the diaphragm results in an increase in the volume of the thorax. Diaphragmatic motion is responsible for 75% of the thoracic volume change (for erect versus supine position when tidal breathing). The increase in thoracic volume causes the pleural pressure to decrease owing to the thin elastic nature of the pulmonary parenchyma. The lungs expand outward in response to the falling pleural pressures, resulting in the alveolar pressures falling relative to the atmospheric pressure.

Pressure falls in the alveoli according to Boyle's law. As the volume in the lungs increases, pressure falls while temperature remains constant. Once alveolar pressure is less than atmospheric pressure, gas begins to flow into the lungs.

Gas flow continues to fill the lungs so long as the thoracic cage continues to expand, which creates a pressure gradient between the atmosphere and the alveoli. Once thoracic and atmospheric pressures become equal at the end of inspiration, gas flow stops because there is no longer a pressure gradient.

Exhalation

The diaphragm relaxes during exhalation. The elastic properties of the chest wall and the lung parenchyma cause the thoracic volume to decrease. Alveolar pressures increase as the thoracic volume decreases. The thoracic pressure increases as the volume of the thorax decreases, while temperature remains constant (Boyle's law). The alveolar pressure becomes greater than the atmospheric pressure, which results in gas flowing out of the lungs.

Gas flow out of the lungs continues until the diaphragm has completely relaxed and the inward recoil of the lung parenchyma matches the corresponding outward tension created by the chest wall. This point is termed the resting functional residual capacity (FRC). At resting FRC alveolar pressure once again is equal to atmospheric pressure, and gas flow out of the lungs stops.

Pulmonary Compliance

Pulmonary compliance is the measure of the lungs' ability to stretch or to distend. Compliance is defined by the following equation.

$$C_L = \frac{\Delta V}{\Delta P}$$

where
ΔV = change in volume
ΔP = change in pressure

This equation describes the fact that the lungs accept a given volume of gas in response to a given change in pressure. At rest, the average total compliance is 100 mL/cm H_2O. When pleural pressure decreases by −5 cm H_2O, the lungs expand by 500 mL.

Elastic and Nonelastic Forces of Ventilation

Gas must not only overcome pressure gradients to move into and out of the lungs, but elastic and nonelastic forces influence gas flow as well. The elastic forces that oppose ventilation include the properties of the chest wall and the lung parenchyma. The bones and cartilaginous structure and muscles of the chest wall create a force that tends to tether the chest wall outward, resulting in thoracic expansion.

The lung parenchyma has its own elastic properties. The natural tendency of the lung parenchyma is to recoil inward. The lung parenchyma has a natural tendency to collapse. What balances this inward force is the subambient pleural pressure. The tendency of the chest wall to expand and the resulting subambient pleural pressures overcome this force, keeping the lungs filled even after a complete exhalation.

Airway resistance is the primary nonelastic force that airflow must overcome when air is flowing into or out of the lungs. Airflow depends on the number of parallel pathways present. For this reason, the large and particularly the medium-sized airways provide greater resistance to flow than do the more numerous small airways.

Equation of Motion of the Respiratory System

The nonelastic (airway) and elastic (muscle) forces are combined into an equation describing the total work of breathing (Paw + Pmus), as follows.

$$Paw + Pmus = (Flow \times Resistance)$$
$$+ (Volume / Compliance)$$

Muscle energy must overcome both elastic forces (volume and compliance) and nonelastic forces (resistance and flow) for gas to flow into the lungs. The pathology associated with pulmonary fibrosis causes the compliance to decrease, which then increases the muscle work required to inflate the lungs. Bronchospasm results in airway narrowing, which increases resistance and thus muscle work to inflate the lungs. The equation of motion of the respiratory system can help clinicians to understand how pathophysiology affects their ability to apply the ventilator in the care of patients.

Mechanical ventilators substitute for the muscle work, either taking the place of all muscle work (full ventilatory support) or partially relieving that workload (partial ventilatory support).

Chatburn's Classification of Mechanical Ventilators

Chatburn proposed his system of classifying mechanical ventilators almost three decades ago. Prior to his work, ventilator classification largely fell to those companies manufacturing them. A ventilator manufacturer's interest, however, is in distinguishing how its ventilator is different from another manufacturer's ventilator, to facilitate marketing. Therefore the classification systems of the past were largely based on a manufacturer's trademarked names and other proprietary terms used in sales and marketing.

Chatburn's classification system is based on the equation of motion of the respiratory system and other concepts grounded in physics. As stated, physiology and physical principles will not change in the near future even though ventilator manufacturers and their proprietary names will. The original classification system has been updated many times and has withstood the test of time. Learning the classification system is important so that clinicians can describe a ventilator's operation or mode in a language that is universally understood, similar to learning medical terminology.

Input Power

Input power describes the power source used to power the mechanical ventilator. Modern ventilators may be powered by pneumatics, electricity, or a combination of both. Pneumatically powered ventilators have a distinct advantage in the transport setting. They can be truly portable, only needing a compressed gas cylinder for operation (**Figure 2-1**).

The example ventilator in Figure 2-1 is pneumatically powered and controlled and will function in any position. Percussionaire Corporation also manufactures a critical care ventilator, the VDR-4, which is pneumatically powered and controlled but utilizes an electrically powered monitoring unit (**Figure 2-2**).

Electricity may also be used as a power source for mechanical ventilators. Electrically powered ventilators are well suited for home care applications. In the home care setting, few domiciles are equipped with medical gases without renting or purchasing medical gas cylinders. Supplemental oxygen is frequently supplied using oxygen concentrators and bleeding

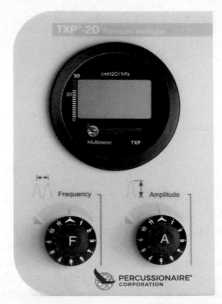

FIGURE 2-1 The Percussionaire TXP-2D neonatal transport ventilator.
Courtesy of Percussionaire Corporation.

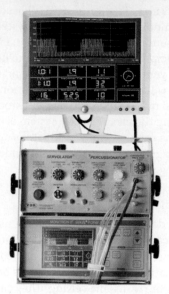

FIGURE 2-2 The Percussionaire Corporation VDR-4 critical care ventilator.
Courtesy of Percussionaire Corporation.

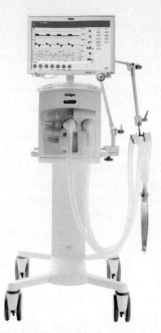

FIGURE 2-4 The Dräger Evita Infinity V500 ventilator.

Ventilators may also be powered by a combination of pneumatics and electricity. These ventilators typically use the pneumatics to power the gas delivery system while electricity powers the microprocessor control system. The Dräger V500 is an example of a combined power (pneumatic and electric) critical care ventilator (**Figure 2-4**). The majority of advanced critical care ventilators (e.g., Puritan Bennett 840, SERVO-i, Viasys AVEA) utilize a combined power source.

Drive Mechanism

The **drive mechanism** for a mechanical ventilator describes the method used by the ventilator to convert the input power into ventilatory work. Pneumatically powered ventilators use needle valves and reducing valves to reduce line pressure from 50 pounds per square inch to safe levels for ventilation.

Electrically powered ventilators typically use that energy to power electric motors. Those motors are then connected to turbine type blowers or to pistons, which use the rotary energy of the electric motor to produce positive pressure gas. The Respironics V60 ventilator (**Figure 2-5**) is an example of a noninvasive ventilator that is powered by a rotary blower or compressor.

Combined input-powered ventilators use the electrical power to run the microprocessor control systems. The microprocessor control systems regulate the operation of all aspects of the ventilator, with electricity providing the input power to do so. The pneumatic power (air and oxygen) is typically routed through reducing valves and then proportional solenoid valves, which regulate the inspiratory phase and the proportion of air and oxygen (FIO_2). The pneumatic system provides the drive mechanism.

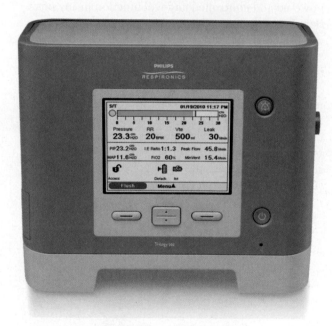

FIGURE 2-3 The Respironics Trilogy 202 ventilator.
Couresy of Philips Healthcare.

in oxygen at a flow that achieves acceptable oxygen saturations. An electrically powered ventilator can simply be connected to a 120-V/60-Hz power source (**Figure 2-3**). The electrical power is then used to power a compressor, or piston mechanism, to provide the positive pressure needed for ventilation. The electrical power for these ventilators may also be supplied via a direct current (DC) battery. Many ventilators incorporate a backup battery that is automatically charged when the ventilator is plugged into an alternating current (AC) outlet. Most backup batteries will power the ventilator for a minimum of 4 hours.

Pressure Delivery

The purpose of a mechanical ventilator is to fully support a patient's ventilation (full ventilatory support) or to partially support a patient's ventilation (partial ventilatory support). The ventilator can accomplish this support in one of two ways. The ventilator can apply pressure within the patient's chest through either a tight-fitting mask (noninvasive ventilation) or a cuffed artificial airway (invasive ventilation). **Figure 2-6** illustrates noninvasive and invasive positive pressure ventilation. In both examples, positive pressure is applied within the lungs to expand them, reducing muscle work.

Exhalation is passive. The elastic recoil of the lungs and the chest wall creates a pressure gradient such that the pressure in the lungs exceeds atmospheric pressure, and gas flows out of the lungs passively.

A mechanical ventilator may also apply subambient pressure outside of the chest, creating a pressure gradient that causes gas to flow into the lungs. The earliest form of this type of negative pressure ventilator was the iron lung that had widespread use in the 1940s and 1950s. Today,

negative pressure ventilators are rarely used in the home and acute setting by the application of a cuirass or shell that surrounds the anterior chest wall. **Figure 2-7** is an example of a biphasic (subambient inhalation and positive pressure exhalation) cuirass ventilator.

Control Circuit

The **control circuit** is the mechanism the ventilator uses to control its drive mechanism. The control circuit determines the characteristics of the ventilator's output. This includes the morphology or shape of the inspiratory waveforms (pressure, flow, and volume) as well as how quickly these variables change during inhalation. Control circuits may be divided into several subclassifications, including open and closed loop, mechanical, pneumatic, electric, and electronic.

In open loop control circuits the clinician sets the desired output. The mechanical ventilator then achieves that desired output without further intervention by the clinician or by monitoring changes in the patient's parameters (pressure, flow, or volume).

In closed loop control circuits the clinician sets the desired output and the ventilator monitors pressure, flow, or volume and adjusts its output based on the continuously monitored variable. These control systems may also be referred to as servo controlled.

Mechanical control circuits are the simplest type of control mechanisms. These are mechanical devices such as levers, cams, wheels, and pulleys that are used to alter the ventilator's drive mechanism. Today, these systems have been replaced by microprocessor controlled proportioning valves.

Pneumatic control systems use needle valves, spring-loaded diaphragms, pneumatic cartridges, and other devices to regulate the output of the ventilator's pneumatic system. Needle valves are the functional part of an oxygen flowmeter. Adjusting oxygen flow requires opening or closing a needle valve. Pressure can be regulated by balancing gas pressure against spring tension across a diaphragm. Adjusting the pressure on a medical gas cylinder is achieved by increasing or decreasing spring tension, which increases or decreases pressure. An advantage of pneumatic control systems is that they

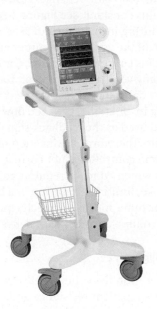

FIGURE 2-5 The Respironics V60 ventilator.
Courtesy of Philips Healthcare.

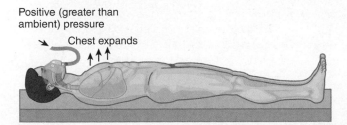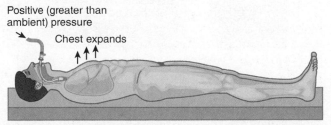

FIGURE 2-6 An illustration of noninvasive and invasive positive pressure ventilation.

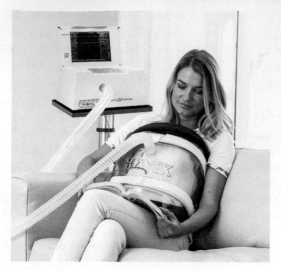

FIGURE 2-7 The Hayek Biphasic Cuirass Ventilator (BCV).
Courtsey of Hayek Medical.

are fully portable, so only a source of pressurized gas (cylinder, for example) is required for their operation.

Electric control may include limit switches to control the ventilator's drive system. Limit switches can be used to control the stroke of an electrically powered piston, which then determines the tidal volume. Some home care ventilators may use these systems because they are simple and generally reliable.

Electronic control systems today are primarily microprocessor control systems. Microprocessor technology has allowed the development of highly sophisticated control and monitoring systems in current generation ventilators. With backup battery power, these ventilators may also be portable as long as the battery has sufficient power for the duration of time it is not connected to AC power.

Control Variables

A mechanical ventilator can control one of four variables during breath delivery. These variables are pressure, volume, flow, and time. A **control variable** is a variable that is measured and used as feedback to control the

ventilator's output. In Chatburn's first article describing his classification system, he presented an algorithm used to determine which of the four variables is the control variable. That algorithm is replicated in **Figure 2-8**.

Pressure Controller

A ventilator functions as a pressure controller if pressure is measured during inspiration and is used as a feedback signal to control the ventilator's output. According to Figure 2-8, if the pressure remains constant during inspiration when subjected to changes in patient resistance and compliance, that ventilator is termed a **pressure controller**. A ventilator that is a pressure controller can be identified by observing the inspiratory pressure waveform. If inspiratory pressure remains constant even under changes in ventilator load (resistance or compliance), it is a pressure controller.

Volume Controller

When a ventilator is classified as a **volume controller**, pressure varies during inspiration when the patient's resistance and compliance change. However, volume delivery remains constant (see Figure 2-8). If volume is measured during inspiration and used as a feedback signal to control the ventilator's output and the volume delivery remains constant, the ventilator is a volume controller. Many ventilators are called *volume ventilators*, because tidal volume is set by the clinician and delivered during inspiration. However, flow is frequently measured and used as the feedback signal to determine volume output. Therefore classification of these ventilators as a volume controller is not correct. Volume must be measured, which typically requires adjustment of a piston's stroke, limiting expansion of a bellows drive mechanism or other means of directly measuring and determining volume during breath delivery.

Flow Controller

If during inspiration the volume delivery remains unchanged when patient resistance and compliance

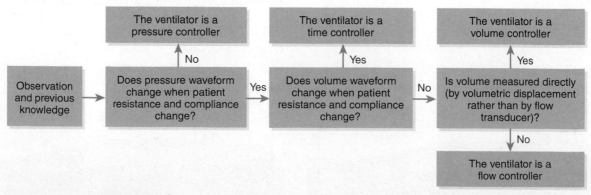

FIGURE 2-8 The criteria to determine the control variable during ventilator-assisted inspiration.
Reproduced from Hess D, Kacmarek R. *Essentials of Mechanical Ventilation.* 2nd ed. New York, NY: McGraw-Hill Professional; 2002.

change, and if volume is not measured and used to control the ventilator's output, it is classified as a **flow controller** (see Figure 2-8). Many microprocessor controlled ventilators measure inspiratory flow, using it as a feedback signal to control the ventilator's output. Some of these ventilators use dedicated internal flow sensors, while others measure the pressure drop across the proportional flow control valves, which is directly proportional to flow.

Time Controller

When the volume and pressure waveforms change during inspiration when subjected to changes in the patient's resistance and compliance, the ventilator is termed a **time controller**. Inspiration is controlled by measuring inspiratory and expiratory times, which then controls the breath rate, inspiratory time, and expiratory time.

Phase Variables

Ventilator-assisted breaths may be divided into four distinct phases: the change from inspiration to exhalation, inspiration, the change from exhalation to inspiration, and exhalation or baseline. Evaluating pressure, volume, flow, and time during these four phases will give more detail regarding the ventilator's characteristics.

Trigger Variable

The **trigger variable** describes how the ventilator changes from exhalation to inspiration. Ventilators can measure pressure, volume, flow, or time during the expiratory phase. When one of these variables reaches a preset value, inspiration begins.

Time is a common trigger variable. Breaths are delivered by the ventilator at preset intervals independent of the patient's spontaneous efforts. For example, setting the rate at 10 breaths per minute ensures that a breath will be delivered every 6 seconds.

Pressure may also be a trigger variable. If airway pressure is monitored, and airway pressure falls to a preset value (below baseline pressure), then a ventilator breath will be delivered. Some ventilators allow this variable to be adjusted by the clinician, while other ventilators use a preset trigger (typically 2 cm H_2O less than baseline pressure).

Flow may also be measured during exhalation. When flow reaches a preset value, the ventilator begins inspiration. Some contemporary ventilators use external flow sensors that are integrated into the circuit at the patient's airway. External sensors help to detect subtle changes in flow that might be missed if using a flow sensor that is internal to the ventilator.

Volume may also be measured during the expiratory phase. Once a preset volume change is detected, a ventilator breath is delivered. As described, many contemporary ventilators use an external flow sensor for this purpose. When flow is multiplied by the time over which that flow is measured, volume is derived.

Neurally Adjusted Ventilatory Assist

Maquet SERVO-i ventilator, when equipped with the **neurally adjusted ventilatory assist (NAVA®)** option, uses neurologic (electrical) signals from the patient's diaphragm contraction to trigger inspiration. A specialized esophageal catheter is placed at the level of the diaphragm. Diaphragmatic activity is detected as a change in an electrical signal, which then initiates inspiration. Neurologic triggering can help to eliminate some of the delay seen with other ventilators because of the distal placement of flow or pressure sensors relative to the patient.

Limit Variable

The **limit variable** describes the variable that remains constant during the inspiratory phase. A pressure controller, for example, delivers a constant pressure during the ventilator-assisted breath. Pressure rises to a preset level and doesn't change in the face of changing resistance or compliance on the part of the patient. Since the variable (pressure) does not change, it is said to be limited. **Figure 2-9** provides an algorithm that is useful in determining the limit variable.

Volume becomes the limit variable if volume reaches a preset value and remains constant during the inspiratory phase. Volume is normally not a limit variable, but it can become one if the clinician adds an inspiratory pause or selects the inspiratory hold feature. In both situations, the expiratory and inspiratory valves of the ventilator are closed, trapping the delivered volume in the patient's lungs for the duration of the inspiratory pause or the manual breath hold.

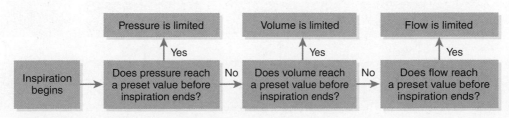

FIGURE 2-9 An algorithm to determine the limit variable.

Flow becomes the limit variable if flow rises to a preset value and then remains constant for the duration of the inspiratory phase. In any mode of ventilation for which the clinician sets the maximum inspiratory flow (volume control, for example), flow becomes the limit variable. Flow is limited at the set flow rate in liters per minute.

Cycle Variable

The **cycle variable** describes how the ventilator changes from inspiration to exhalation. Cycle variables may include pressure, volume, and time. To be considered a cycle variable, the variable must be measured by the ventilator and then used as a feedback signal to terminate or end the inspiratory phase. Cycle variables may include pressure, volume, flow, or time (**Figure 2-10**).

Pressure becomes the cycle variable if pressure is measured during inspiration and used as a feedback signal to end the inspiratory phase of ventilation (see Figure 2-10). A classic example of a mechanical ventilator using pressure cycling is the Bird Mark 7 IPPB ventilator. Once pressure reaches the value established by the pressure control, inspiration ends. Pressure may also become a cycle variable in volume control if the pressure limit is reached. When the pressure limit is reached, the breath ends (prior to complete volume delivery), and the breath becomes pressure cycled.

Volume cycling can occur only if volume is measured and used as a feedback signal to end the inspiratory phase (see Figure 2-10). The Medtronic/Covidien Newport HT70 ventilator is volume cycled during volume-controlled breaths. Volume is determined by the stroke of the piston pump and is directly measured. Once volume reaches the preset value, the ending inspiratory phase ends. Many ventilators may be incorrectly classified as being volume cycled, when internally the ventilator is measuring flow, and volume becomes the product of flow multiplied by inspiratory time.

Flow may also become the cycle variable if it is measured and inspiration is terminated once a preset flow is reached (see Figure 2-10). Flow cycling is common among noninvasive ventilators delivering bilevel positive airway pressure. The ventilator delivers a preset pressure during the inspiratory phase. Once the pressure level is established, inspiratory flow is monitored. When flow decays to a preset value, the inspiratory phase is ended. Flow is the variable that is measured and used as a feedback signal to end inspiration.

Time becomes the cycle variable when it is measured and used to determine the end of the breath (see Figure 2-10). During pressure control ventilation, the clinician sets an inspiratory pressure, inspiratory time, and rate. The length of inspiration is determined by the inspiratory time. Once the inspiratory time has been met, the ventilator terminates inspiration and begins the expiratory phase.

Baseline Variables

The **baseline variable** describes what occurs between the end of one ventilator breath and the start of the next ventilator breath, or the expiratory phase of ventilation. Mechanical ventilators use pressure as the baseline variable. During the expiratory phase for both ventilator-assisted breaths and spontaneous breaths, pressure may be increased above baseline (ambient pressure).

Elevated baseline pressure, termed *positive end-expiratory pressure* (PEEP) for mandatory or ventilator breaths and *continuous positive airway pressure* (CPAP) for spontaneous breaths, increases the patient's FRC. Increasing the FRC improves surface area for oxygenation and is one strategy used by clinicians to improve oxygenation.

Conditional Variables

Conditional variables describe the patterns that a ventilator uses and the control and phase variables during a particular ventilator cycle. During one phase of ventilation, a ventilator may control tidal volume, rate, and inspiratory flow. During another spontaneous phase of ventilation, the ventilator may control inspiratory pressure. The conditional variables describe how the ventilator logic uses some preset conditions to determine what control and phase variables to use. Microprocessor systems use if-then rules to determine if the preset conditions have been met.

Output Waveforms

Much can be learned by the evaluation of a ventilator's output waveforms. Waveforms are typically presented in the order of pressure, flow, and volume versus time. These are referred to as scalar waveforms. A typical graphic representation is presented in **Figure 2-11**.

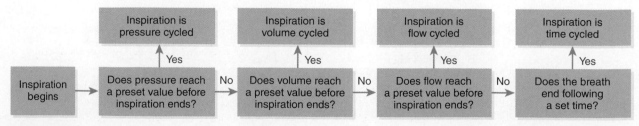

FIGURE 2-10 An algorithm to determine the cycle variable.

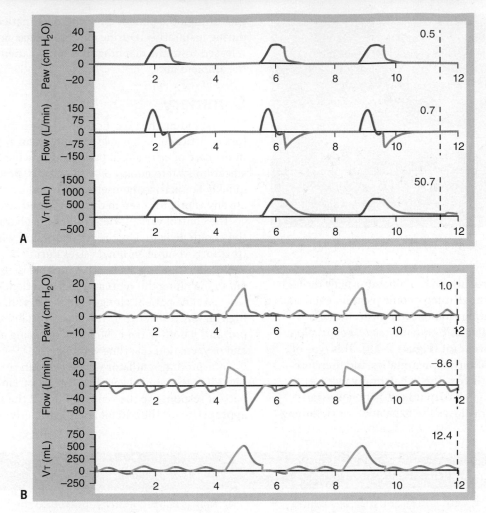

FIGURE 2-11 Ventilator output waveforms depicting (**A**) pressure-controlled inspiration and (**B**) volume-controlled inspiration.

By observing a specific variable (pressure, flow, or volume), the clinician may determine the limit variable for the breath (it increases, then plateaus during inspiration). Depending on the mode setting and the internal control circuitry of the ventilator, the control variable may also be assessed using waveform analysis. As with learning auscultation of breath sounds, waveform analysis requires practice and repetition. However, once mastered, it is an important aspect of patient-ventilator management.

Patient Circuit Design

Contemporary mechanical ventilators all use a single circuit design. The single patient circuit implies that the gas that powers or drives the ventilator is the same gas that enters the patient circuit and is delivered to the patient. The differences among the patient circuit designs today involve the placement of the exhalation valve.

When the ventilator incorporates a servo controlled exhalation valve, there is no exhalation valve in the

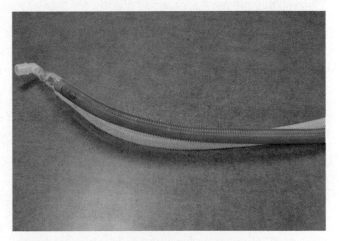

FIGURE 2-12 A ventilator circuit without an exhalation valve.

patient circuit (**Figure 2-12**). In this circuit, when the exhalation valve is closed and the inspiratory valve is opened, gas flows to the patient. When the inspiratory valve is closed and the exhalation valve is opened, the

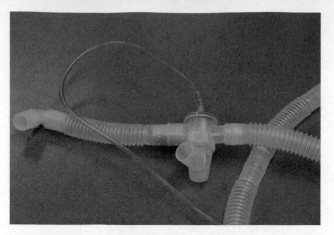

FIGURE 2-13 A ventilator circuit with an exhalation valve.

patient exhales through the circuit and usually through both a filter (to remove microscopic particles) and a gas conditioner (a heating element to remove water).

Transport ventilators frequently use an exhalation valve built into the circuit (**Figure 2-13**). This type of circuit minimizes internal pneumatics and therefore the size of the ventilator. The exhalation valve is a pneumatically actuated diaphragm. When pressurized, the diaphragm closes the exhalation port, forcing gas through the patient circuit into the patient's lungs during inspiration. During exhalation, gas pressure is released from the diaphragm, and the patient exhales to the ambient air.

Summary

Understanding the classification of mechanical ventilators is critical in being able to apply them at the bedside in the care of critically ill patients. Knowing the classification system equips respiratory care practitioners to quickly familiarize themselves with and be able to operate any ventilator used in the clinical setting.

The control variable determines the characteristic of the breath delivered by the ventilator and what variable (pressure, volume, or flow) varies during breath delivery. Understanding the control variable is also important in matching the ventilator to the patient's pathology (e.g., Are the patient's lungs compliant, stiff, or showing high airway resistance?). The phase variables are important in both patient comfort (triggering and cycle) and oxygenation (baseline variable).

Interpreting ventilator waveforms can reveal much regarding the control variables, phase variables, and patient response to the ventilator and if the settings are appropriate for the patient and the underlying disorder.

Case Study

Mr. King, a patient with chronic obstructive pulmonary disease (COPD) in severe respiratory distress, is picked up by an ambulance. During transport and upon arrival at the hospital, he is receiving noninvasive ventilation via an oronasal mask. Patient assessment shows patient-ventilator dyssynchrony. Mr. King is complaining of "not getting enough air."

1. **What is the cycle mechanism of this noninvasive ventilator?**

2. **What can be done to provide more ventilation to the patient?**

Mr. King is subsequently admitted to the intensive care unit (ICU) for acute exacerbation of COPD and severe hypoxemia. He is intubated and placed on volume-controlled ventilation.

3. **What is the cycling mechanism of this type of mechanical ventilation?**

4. **The physician orders positive end-expiratory pressure (PEEP) of 5 cm H_2O for Mr. King. What type of ventilator variable is PEEP?**

5. **What is the primary reason for applying this baseline variable?**

Bibliography

Chatburn RL. A new system for understanding mechanical ventilators. *Respir Care J.* 1991;36:1123–1155.

Chatburn RL. Classification of mechanical ventilators. *Respir Care J.* 1992;37:1009–1025.

Chatburn RL. Classification of ventilator modes: update and proposal for implementation. *Respir Care J.* 2007;52:301–323.

Chatburn RL. Determining the basis for a taxonomy of mechanical ventilation. *Respir Care J.* 2014;59:1747–1763.

Chatburn RL. A taxonomy for mechanical ventilation: 10 fundamental maxims. *Resp Care J* 59:1747–1763.

DesJardins TR. *Cardiopulmonary Anatomy & Physiology Essentials of Respiratory Care.* 6th ed. Clifton Park, NY: Delmar-Cengage Learning.4; 2013.

CHAPTER

3

Modes of Mechanical Ventilation

Gary C. White, MEd, RRT, RPFT, FAARC

OUTLINE

OBJECTIVES

1. Differentiate between the spontaneous modes of ventilation.
2. Differentiate between continuous positive airway pressure (CPAP) and positive end-expiratory pressure (PEEP).
3. Differentiate between pressure support, volume assured pressure support, and bilevel positive airway pressure (BiPAP).
4. Describe the characteristics of volume control ventilation.
5. Describe the characteristics of pressure control ventilation.
6. Describe the possible targeting schemes for both within a breath delivery and between breath delivery.
7. Classify the modes of ventilation using Chatburn's classification system.
8. Describe the high-frequency ventilation modes.

KEY TERMS

adaptive targeting
bilevel positive airway pressure
biovariable targeting
continuous positive airway pressure (CPAP)
control variable
flow triggering
intelligent targeting
limit variable
mandatory breath
optimal targeting
pressure control

pressure target
pressure triggering
servo targeting
set-point targets
spontaneous breath
synchronized intermittent mandatory ventilation
time triggering
Volume control—continuous mandatory ventilation
volume control
volume triggering

Introduction

A mode of mechanical ventilation is defined as a predetermined pattern of ventilation between a patient and a ventilator. That pattern is determined by a specific combination of control variable(s), breath sequence (mechanical or spontaneous), and specified targeting schemes. Today, modes of mechanical ventilation are selected by the user interface (touch screen, knobs, or other controls), and that specific mode or pattern is built into the ventilator software and gas delivery system.

Understanding modes of mechanical ventilation can be very complex and confusing. Ventilator manufacturers over many decades have worked diligently to trademark proprietary names for common modes such that their ventilator is unique from another manufacturer's ventilator. Clinicians also add to the confusion, in that many do not understand the basics of Chatburn's ventilator classification system (see Chapter 2), and therefore lack a standardized vocabulary to describe a ventilator's operational scheme (control variable, set point, trigger, etc.).

It is important that the respiratory care practitioner fully understand the various modes, how to simply and concisely describe their operation and function, and the advantages and disadvantages for the patient. A sound understanding of Chatburn's classification system and the content of this chapter is an important start. The ability to use an institution's particular ventilator with an active test lung will further improve the clinician's understanding of the various ventilator modes. By changing resistance and compliance of the active test lung (ventilator load), the clinician can observe the waveforms, pressures, and flows to fully understand how that particular ventilator behaves under those specific circumstances.

Spontaneous Ventilation Modes

Although it appears intuitive, there is much confusion about how to classify spontaneous ventilation: Is the patient's breath completely spontaneous, without any mechanical ventilator assistance? Does the patient's ventilatory effort cause the ventilator to initiate a breath (trigger)? Does the ventilator partially support the patient during a spontaneous breathing effort? Is the patient's baseline pressure elevated above ambient pressure during spontaneous ventilation? Does the patient both trigger and cycle the spontaneous breath? Answers to these questions are important in classifying spontaneous ventilation.

Continuous Spontaneous Ventilation

A **spontaneous breath** is defined as a breath in which the patient initiates the breath, determines the aspiratory flow and tidal volume, and determines when the breath ends. These criteria must be met without any ventilator or mechanical assistance. The patient determines the breath rate, depth, inspiratory flow, and duration of the breath without ventilator assistance. A clinical example a clinician may encounter in critical care is measurement of the rapid shallow breathing index (RSBI).

$$RSBI = \frac{\text{Respiratory rate}}{\text{Tidal volume (L)}}$$

In determining the RSBI, the patient is breathing unassisted or with minimal pressure support ventilation (up to 5 cm H_2O) while the clinician measures the patient's minute ventilation and ventilatory rate. This determination is made without the patient receiving any mechanical assistance from a ventilator or other device.

Continuous Positive Airway Pressure

Continuous positive airway pressure (CPAP) is the application of positive baseline pressure (pressure is elevated above ambient pressure), during continuous spontaneous ventilation (**Figure 3-1**). The positive baseline pressure increases the patient's functional residual capacity (FRC), recruiting previously unventilated or underventilated alveoli, which improves oxygenation. Before initiation of CPAP, it is important to determine that the patient is capable of sustaining eucapnic ventilation, as documented by an appropriate partial pressure of carbon dioxide ($Paco_2$) and pH from an arterial blood gas.

The patient interface for CPAP may include a mask, artificial airway (endotracheal or tracheostomy tube), and, in the neonate, nasal prongs. The key to the patient interface is that it must seal to allow the pressure to build above ambient pressure. Leaks can result in pressure loss and a fall in FRC, oxygen saturation (Spo_2), and partial pressure of oxygen (Pao_2).

Bilevel Positive Airway Pressure

Bilevel positive airway pressure (BiPAP) is the application of positive airway pressure during inspiration and exhalation (baseline pressure) during spontaneous ventilation (**Figure 3-2**). The inspiratory positive airway pressure (IPAP) and the expiratory positive airway pressure (EPAP) are set independently of one another. The IPAP must always be set higher than the EPAP.

The IPAP level improves ventilation ($Paco_2$) and oxygenation in conditions due to hypoventilation. The EPAP level functions much like CPAP, recruiting underventilated alveoli during exhalation, which increases FRC and oxygenation.

The difference between the two pressures (IPAP − EPAP) is sometimes termed the *drive pressure* or *pressure support*. Increasing the drive pressure improves ventilation ($Paco_2$) and measures how much assistance (pressure) the patient requires to maintain adequate ventilation ($Paco_2$ and pH).

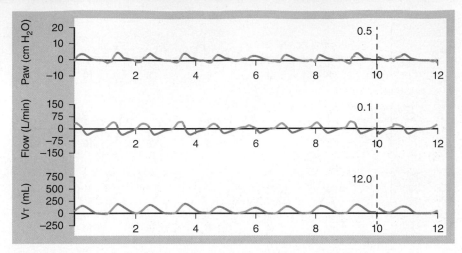

FIGURE 3-1 Application of continuous positive airway pressure (CPAP) during continuous spontaneous ventilation. Paw, airway pressure; V_T, tidal volume.

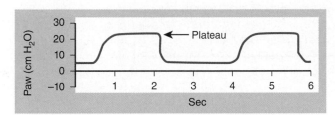

FIGURE 3-2 Application of bilevel positive airway pressure (BiPAP) during spontaneous ventilation. Note the two different pressure levels (inspiratory positive airway pressure [IPAP] and expiratory positive airway pressure [EPAP]). Paw, airway pressure.

BiPAP Modes

Within the spontaneous umbrella of BiPAP are two distinct modes, spontaneous and spontaneous timed. Spontaneous mode is the patient's continuous spontaneous ventilation supported by both IPAP and EPAP. The patient determines the ventilatory rate, while the ventilator controls the IPAP and EPAP by varying the flow rate. The breath is spontaneously triggered (flow) and flow cycled.

Spontaneous-timed mode of BiPAP allows the clinician to set a backup rate. In the event the patient's spontaneous rate falls below the rate threshold, the ventilator initiates a breath independent of the patient's effort. Should the patient resume spontaneous breathing at a rate above the rate threshold, no additional breaths are triggered by the ventilator. Spontaneous-timed mode provides a "safety" in the event the patient becomes apneic (if the clinician becomes aware that patient apnea exists, the patient should be converted to invasive ventilation).

Pressure Support

Pressure support is a form of assisted or augmented (ventilator) spontaneous breath when, during inspiration, pressure is applied. Pressure support is a mode in which all breaths are pressure or flow triggered, pressure targeted, and flow cycled. The patient triggers the breath by meeting a pressure threshold (**pressure triggering**) or flow threshold (**flow triggering**).

Pressure support is a spontaneous breath. The patient triggers the breath (pressure or flow), tidal volume delivery varies depending upon the patient's effort (inspiratory flow demand), the inspiratory time lasts only as long as the patient is actively inhaling, and the breath is terminated when the patient's inspiratory flow decays to a preset value (**Figure 3-3**).

Augmentation of the patient's spontaneous breath with pressure improves alveolar ventilation. It helps to reduce hypercapnia and improve oxygenation. The degree to which alveolar ventilation is improved is proportional to the amount of the pressure support setting.

Once inspiration begins, the ventilator targets a set pressure during inspiration. Flow increases to building pressure in the circuit. Throughout the inspiratory phase, flow will vary. Once the pressure target is approached, flow begins to decay. The breath is cycled when the inspiratory flow drops to a preset threshold (usually a percentage of peak flow).

Synchronized Intermittent Mandatory Ventilation

Synchronized intermittent mandatory ventilation (SIMV) is a mode of ventilation whereby, between ventilator breaths (**mandatory breaths**), the patient can breathe spontaneously for a short window of time. The term *synchronized* means that the next mandatory breath (ventilator breath) is synchronized or matched with the patient's spontaneous breath to avoid having the ventilator "stack" a mandatory breath on top of a spontaneous breath (**Figure 3-4**).

The mandatory breaths may be time or patient triggered in the event the patient has an inspiratory effort during the synchronization window for the next mandatory breath.

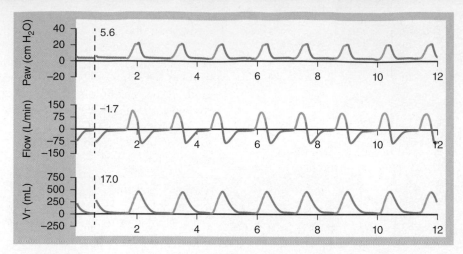

FIGURE 3-3 Pressure support ventilation (PSV). Note that the baseline is elevated 5 cm H₂O. Paw, airway pressure; Vᴛ, tidal volume.

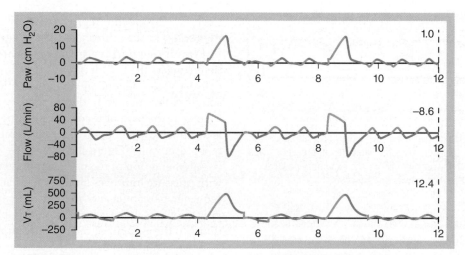

FIGURE 3-4 Synchronized intermittent mandatory ventilation (SIMV). Paw, airway pressure; Vᴛ, tidal volume.

The synchronization window is the time period just prior to when the ventilator would normally deliver a time triggered breath. During this short time frame, the ventilator is monitoring for a change in pressure or flow, indicating a spontaneous inspiratory effort. If that change is detected during that trigger window, a mandatory breath is delivered.

The tidal volume delivered during the spontaneous portion of SIMV is purely dependent upon the patient. Patient effort is what determines the volume delivered during the spontaneous portion of SIMV. The patient determines the rate, inspiratory flow, breath duration, and tidal volume.

The tidal volume during the spontaneous portion of SIMV may be augmented further by the addition of pressure support (described previously). The baseline pressure may be elevated during both the mandatory and spontaneous portions to increase FRC and improve oxygenation. If the baseline pressure is elevated, it is termed *positive end-expiratory pressure* (PEEP) during

the mandatory (ventilator) breaths and CPAP during the spontaneous breaths.

Volume Control Ventilation Modes

Volume control modes are ventilator modes in which the control variable is volume, and that variable is used as a feedback signal to control inspiration (pressure, volume, or flow). Remember, as described in Chapter 2, not all ventilators measure volume directly. Most ventilators measure flow (internal flow sensor or the pressure drop across the flow control valves), and derive volume indirectly as a product of flow multiplied by inspiratory time.

Volume control modes allow inspiratory pressure to vary. Flow and volume delivery are directly set by the clinician and controlled by the ventilator. Pressure will vary depending upon the patient's pulmonary compliance and resistance (ventilator load). If tidal volume delivery remains constant, and pressure varies from breath to breath, the ventilator is operating in a volume control mode.

Volume Control—Continuous Mandatory Ventilation

Volume control—continuous mandatory ventilation (VC-CMV) is a mode of ventilation in which the clinician sets the delivered tidal volume, inspiratory flow, and flow pattern. Pressure varies during inspiration depending upon the patient's pulmonary compliance and resistance. Volume is the control variable. All breaths are mandatory (ventilator delivered). Triggering may be time or patient triggered.

The trigger variable during VC-CMV may be time, pressure, flow, or volume depending upon the ventilator and its manufacturer. **Time triggering** occurs in the absence of any spontaneous patient efforts to breathe. Without any patient effort, the ventilator will deliver mandatory (ventilator) breaths at the set rate. Pressure triggering occurs when the ventilator detects a drop in circuit pressure below a preset threshold value. When pressure reaches the trigger threshold, a mandatory breath is delivered. Flow may also be set as a trigger variable. The ventilator monitors flow during the expiratory phase. If flow falls below the trigger threshold, a mandatory breath is delivered. In some ventilators, volume may also be used as a trigger variable. Ventilators incorporating **volume triggering** use an external flow sensor that attaches to the patient's artificial airway. When volume reaches the trigger threshold (Volume = Flow × Time), a mandatory breath is delivered. In all spontaneously triggered breaths, the breath delivered is a mandatory (ventilator) breath with a set tidal volume and inspiratory flow.

Flow may be a **limit variable** if the inspiratory flow pattern is set to a square wave. When the ventilator is operating in the square wave flow pattern, flow rises quickly to the peak flow setting established by the clinician. Once that flow is reached, it remains constant until the breath is cycled (volume cycled). When using the square wave pattern, it is important to set the peak flow high enough to meet the patient's inspiratory demands. If the peak flow is too low, the patient may exert extra work attempting to draw the flow that the ventilator is not providing.

The **cycle variable** during VC-CMV is volume. Once the set tidal volume has been delivered, inspiration ends. Volume may be directly measured, or more likely indirectly measured as a product of flow multiplied by inspiratory time.

The baseline pressure (PEEP) may be applied during VC-CMV. The purpose is to increase the FRC, improving alveolar ventilation and therefore oxygenation.

Volume Control—Synchronized Intermittent Mandatory Ventilation

Volume control—synchronized intermittent mandatory ventilation (VC-SIMV) combines volume-controlled mandatory breath delivery with spontaneous ventilation between mandatory breaths (**Figure 3-5**). Mandatory breaths are synchronized with the patient, such that a mandatory breath is not delivered on top of a spontaneous breath taken by the patient. A synchronization window (time interval) of approximately 0.5 second is active before mandatory breath delivery. During this synchronization window, the ventilator is monitoring for any spontaneous effort (pressure, flow, or volume change). If there isn't any patient effort during the threshold window, a mandatory breath is delivered at a set volume and flow.

The spontaneous portion of VC-SIMV allows patients to determine their own rate, tidal volume, and spontaneous minute ventilation. Tidal volume and minute ventilation are determined by the patient's effort and ventilatory drive.

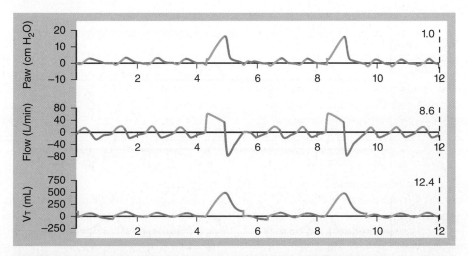

FIGURE 3-5 A graph showing volume control—synchronized intermittent mandatory ventilation (VC-SIMV). Paw, airway pressure; Vᴛ, tidal volume.

During both mandatory and spontaneous portions of VC-SIMV, baseline pressure may be elevated. PEEP is provided during the mandatory portion of VC-SIMV, while CPAP is provided during the spontaneous portion of VC-SIMV. In both cases, elevated baseline pressure (PEEP and CPAP) is to increase the FRC, improving alveolar ventilation and therefore oxygenation.

Pressure support may be added during the spontaneous portion of VC-SIMV to augment the patient's spontaneous breaths. Pressure support provides an additional pressure assist during the spontaneous portion, augmenting tidal volume and the spontaneous minute ventilation. Pressure support may be added during VC-SIMV to improve minute ventilation to help maintain a desired Pa_{CO_2} without increasing the mandatory portion of the minute ventilation.

Pressure Control Ventilation

Pressure control modes are ventilator modes where the control variable is pressure, and this variable is used as a feedback signal to control inspiration (pressure, volume, or flow). To be classified as a **control variable**, this variable must be measured and used as a feedback signal to control inspiration.

Pressure control modes are characterized by the pressure remaining constant during inspiration. The pressure does not vary in the face of changing patient compliance or resistance. Flow and volume delivery, however, will vary during the breath delivery in pressure-controlled ventilation.

Pressure Control—Continuous Mandatory Ventilation

Pressure control—continuous mandatory ventilation (PC-CMV) is a mode of ventilation in which the clinician sets the ventilatory rate, inspiratory pressure, inspiratory time, and baseline pressure. In this mode of ventilation, all breaths are mandatory (ventilator)

breaths and may be time or patient triggered. Pressure will remain constant during inspiration, even when pulmonary compliance and resistance vary (**Figure 3-6**). This mode of ventilation can be helpful in reducing ventilator induced lung injury (VILI) by limiting pressure to a preset value.

The trigger variables for PC-CMV include time, pressure, flow, and in some ventilators volume. Time triggering occurs when the patient makes no spontaneous efforts to breathe. Without patient effort, the ventilator will deliver mandatory (ventilator) breaths at the set rate. Patient triggered breaths in PC-CMV may include pressure, flow, or volume (if the ventilator has this capability).

Besides pressure being the control variable, in this mode of ventilation it is also the limit variable. The pressure set by the clinician is maintained and held at that value until the end of inspiration.

The cycle variable during PC-CMV is time. Inspiratory time determines the length of the inspiratory phase and when exhalation begins. Flow increases during early inspiration until the set pressure level is achieved. The ventilator controls the flow output, to maintain the established pressure until the end of the inspiratory time. Once the inspiratory time is complete, flow ceases and the ventilator cycles into exhalation.

Baseline pressure (PEEP) can be applied during PC-CMV. PEEP increases the FRC and alveolar ventilation, improving oxygenation.

Pressure Control—Synchronized Intermittent Mandatory Ventilation

Pressure control—synchronized intermittent mandatory ventilation (PC-SIMV) combines pressure-controlled mandatory breath delivery with spontaneous ventilation between mandatory breaths (**Figure 3-7**). Mandatory breaths are synchronized with the patient such that a mandatory breath is not delivered on top of

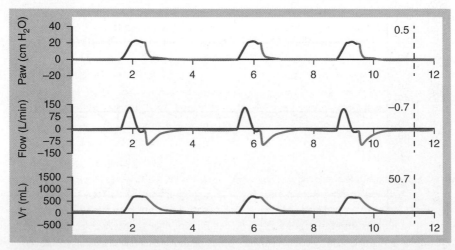

FIGURE 3-6 A graph showing pressure control—continuous mechanical ventilation (PC-CMV). Paw, airway pressure; VT, tidal volume.

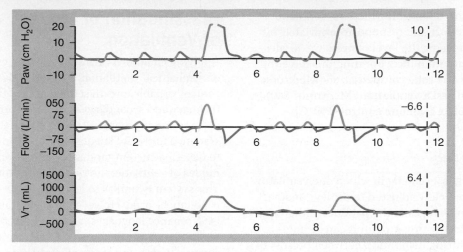

FIGURE 3-7 A graph showing pressure control—synchronized intermittent mandatory ventilation (PC-SIMV). Paw, airway pressure; VT, tidal volume.

a spontaneous breath taken by the patient. A synchronization window (time interval) of approximately 0.5 second is active before mandatory breath delivery. During this synchronization window, the ventilator is monitoring for any spontaneous effort (pressure, flow, or volume change). If the patient effort exceeds the threshold window, a mandatory breath is delivered at a set volume and flow, preventing breath delivery after the patient has taken a spontaneous breath.

The spontaneous portion of PC-SIMV allows patients to determine their own rate, tidal volume, and spontaneous minute ventilation. Tidal volume and minute ventilation are determined by the patient's effort and ventilatory drive.

Options during PC-SIMV include baseline pressure (PEEP/CPAP), patient triggering (pressure, flow, or volume), and pressure support during the spontaneous portion of the breath.

Ventilator Targeting Schemes

The ventilator targeting scheme describes the relationship between the ventilator operator's inputs and the ventilator's output that achieves the desired ventilatory pattern. The target can be considered a predetermined goal for the ventilator's output. A target may occur within a breath (the set volume, pressure, or flow) or between breath targets that modify the within-breath target or the overall ventilatory pattern.

Set-Point Targeting

Set-point targets are those that are established by the clinician. If setting PC-CMV, the clinician would set the inspiratory pressure (**pressure target**) and inspiratory time. If setting VC-CMV, the clinician would set the tidal volume and inspiratory flow rate, establishing the ventilatory pattern for those breaths. Conceptually, set-point targets are the easiest to understand, in that

these targets establish the framework for pressure or volume control modes.

Dual Targeting

Dual targeting allows the ventilator to switch from pressure control to volume control or from volume control to pressure control during a single inspiration or breath. The Dräger Evita Infinity V500, when operating in pressure-limited ventilation, can switch from volume control to pressure control to maintain the set target pressure. In volume assured pressure support, a ventilator can switch from pressure control to volume control within a breath to deliver the desired tidal volume (target).

Biovariable Targeting

Biovariable targeting allows the ventilator to adapt its output (tidal volume, for example) to mimic normal physiologic spontaneous ventilation. The Dräger Evita Infinity V500, when operating in variable pressure support, will vary the delivered pressure. The clinician establishes the inspiratory pressure set point and a percentage of variability from 0% to 100%. If the variability is 0%, the ventilator delivers the set inspiratory pressure. As the variability percentage increases, so does the delivered pressure. At the 100% setting, inspiratory pressure would randomly vary from the baseline pressure (PEEP/CPAP) to the pressure support setting.

Servo Targeting

Servo targeting allows the output of the ventilator (pressure, volume, or flow) to automatically follow a varying input. The input typically followed is the patient's inspiratory effort. The ventilator must be able to monitor the patient's respiratory effort signal. The level of pressure delivered is proportional to the patient's effort. If the patient's effort is high, the pressure delivery will be high, providing more ventilatory assistance. This is the only targeting scheme in which the ventilator will track patient effort and respond appropriately by increasing or decreasing the level of pressure. Modes of mechanical ventilation incorporating this targeting scheme are automatic tube compensation (Medtronic 840), proportional assist ventilation (Medtronic 840), and pressure-regulated volume control (PRVC) (Maquet SERVO-i).

Adaptive Targeting

Adaptive targeting is a scheme in which one ventilator set point is automatically adjusted to achieve another set point based on changes in the patient's pathophysiology. For example, the pressure limit can be automatically varied during inspiration between breaths to achieve a target tidal volume. Examples of this include pressure-regulated volume control (Maquet SERVO-i) and volume control plus (VC+) (Medtronic 840). Automatic adjustment of other set points includes inspiratory time or mandatory breath rate (mandatory minute ventilation).

Optimal Targeting

Optimal targeting allows a ventilator set point to be adjusted to optimize another ventilator set point. Adaptive support ventilation (ASV) (Hamilton Galileo) uses this targeting scheme. The clinician sets the patient's body weight, which the ventilator uses to estimate dead space. Next the clinician adjusts the percentage of minute volume (20% to 200% for adults). The ventilator delivers test breaths and measures compliance, airway resistance, and any intrinsic PEEP. Once these parameters have been measured by the ventilator, the pressure limit, breath rate, and inspiratory time are automatically adjusted to achieve the optimal minute ventilation and tidal volume.

Intelligent Targeting

Intelligent targeting automatically adjusts ventilator set points using rule-based systems. If-then statements are an example of rule-based logic: If the patient's spontaneous tidal volume does this, then adjust the pressure limit. Smart Care (Dräger Evita Infinity V500) automatically adjusts the pressure limit (tidal volume) and breath rate. The patient's end tidal CO_2 and pulmonary compliance and resistance are factored into the algorithm. The ventilator then adjusts the set points to maintain an appropriate minute ventilation and P_{ECO_2}.

Intelligent ASV is another mode incorporating intelligent targeting (Hamilton Medical). The clinician sets a target minute ventilation. Tidal volume and rate are determined by measurement of the patient's ventilatory mechanics by means of an external flow sensor. Tidal volume and rate are optimized for the patient's mechanics while the target minute ventilation is preserved.

Classification of Modes of Ventilation

Applying Chatburn's classification system for the modes of mechanical ventilation, a mode is classified by its control variable, breath sequence, and targeting scheme (primary and secondary) as outlined previously in this chapter and in Chapter 2. By applying this classification system, a universal language or method may be used to describe current modes of ventilation and future modes of ventilation not yet released for clinical use. This system is similar to learning Latin, a language that is no longer used. However, French, Italian, and Spanish (romance languages) all have their roots in Latin. If one understands the basis of Chatburn's classification system (Latin), any mode of ventilation (any romance language) may be described in a way that is universally understood by all clinicians familiar with the classification system.

Classification of Volume Control Modes

Many of the volume control modes have been previously described in this chapter and will be included in **Table 3-1** for classification purposes. Those modes not thoroughly described previously include mandatory minute ventilation, automatic tube compensation, and automode.

Mandatory Minute Ventilation

Mandatory minute ventilation (MMV) is a mode of ventilation in which the ventilator provides predetermined minute ventilation in the event that the patient's spontaneous minute ventilation fails to meet the specified threshold value. For example, if a patient were to experience a short period of apnea, the patient's minute ventilation would decrease. If the patient's minute ventilation fell below a preset threshold, the ventilator would automatically increase the rate to compensate and to increase the total minute ventilation until it exceeds the set threshold. As long as the patient's spontaneous minute ventilation exceeds the set threshold, no additional ventilator breaths are delivered. Classifying MMV volume is the control variable, IMV would be the breath sequence, the targeting scheme would be adaptive, and the secondary breath targeting scheme would be the set point (see Table 3-1).

Automatic Tube Compensation and Spontaneous Tube Compensation

Automatic tube compensation and spontaneous tube compensation are similar modes offered by two ventilators, Dräger Evita Infinity V500 and Medtronic PB 840. These may be applied in both volume and pressure control modes. Automatic tube compensation compensates for the increased resistance caused by the artificial airway. By compensating for this resistance, it is almost as

TABLE 3-1
Classification of Volume Modes

Mode	Control Variable	Breath Sequence	Primary Breath Targeting Scheme	Secondary Breath Targeting Scheme
Volume control—continuous mandatory ventilation (VC-CMV)	Volume	CMV	Set point	N/A
Volume control—synchronized intermittent mandatory ventilation (VC-SIMV)	Volume	SIMV	Set point	Set point
Volume control—synchronized intermittent mandatory ventilation with pressure support (VC-SIMV with PS)	Volume	SIMV	Set point	Servo
Volume control—mandatory minute ventilation (VC-MMV)	Volume	SIMV	Adaptive	Set point
Volume control—automatic tube compensation (VC-ATC)	Volume	SIMV	Set point	Servo
Automode (volume control to volume support)	Volume	SIMV	Dual	Dual/adaptive

TABLE 3-2
Classification of Pressure Control Modes

Mode	Control Variable	Breath Sequence	Primary Breath Targeting Scheme	Secondary Breath Targeting Scheme
Pressure control—continuous mandatory ventilation (PC-CMV)	Pressure	CMV	Set point	N/A
Pressure control—synchronized intermittent mandatory ventilation (PC-SIMV)	Pressure	SIMV	Set point	Set point
Bilevel and airway pressure release ventilation (APRV)	Pressure	SIMV	Set point	Set point
Proportional assist ventilation (PAV)	Pressure	CMV	Servo	N/A
Volume control plus (VC+)	Pressure	SIMV	Adaptive	Set point
Volume support	Pressure	SIMV	Adaptive	N/A
Pressure-regulated volume control (PRVC)	Pressure	CMV	Adaptive	Set point
Adaptive support ventilation (ASV)	Pressure	SIMV	Optimal/intelligent/servo	Set point/servo

if the patient were able to breathe spontaneously without the artificial airway's resistance. Pressure increases during inspiration, compensating for the resistance of the airway. Automatic tube compensation is classified in Table 3-1.

Automode (Volume Control to Volume Support)

Automode is a mode available on the Maquet SERVO-i ventilator. Automode provides a preset tidal volume and frequency with volume as the control variable (when set for the dual mode of volume control to volume support). If the patient's spontaneous effort is large enough, the ventilator will switch from volume control to pressure control (dual mode) with flow cycling. In the absence of any spontaneous efforts, the ventilator

defaults to PRVC breaths that are time triggered. When operating in volume control to volume support, dual mode volume is the control variable, SIMV is the breath sequence, with dual targeting scheme and dual/adaptive secondary breath targeting scheme (see Table 3-1).

Automode can also be set as a dual mode between pressure-regulated volume control and volume support and pressure control and pressure support (both pressure control modes, which will be described in the next section).

Classification of Pressure Control Modes

Many of the pressure control modes have been described in this chapter and are included in **Table 3-2** for classification purposes. Those modes not thoroughly described previously include bilevel, airway pressure release ventilation (APRV), proportional assist ventilation (PAV), volume control plus, volume support, pressure-controlled ventilation plus, pressure-regulated volume control, and adaptive support ventilation.

Bilevel and Airway Pressure Release Ventilation Modes

Both bilevel ventilation and APRV modes allow the clinician to set two distinct pressure levels, a high pressure limit (P_{high}) and a low pressure limit (P_{low}) independent of one another. P_{high} may be set to either the plateau pressure (volume control modes) or peak airway pressure (pressure controlled modes). It is recommended that the P_{high} be kept at no more than 30 to 35 cm H_2O. The P_{low} pressure is set to avoid alveolar collapse during exhalation or set at zero with a very short expiratory time (T_{low}) to achieve intentional (therapeutic) gas trapping or auto PEEP.

T_{high} is often set at a time interval that achieves the desired frequency for mandatory breaths.

T_{low} is more problematic to adjust. There is a tradeoff between allowing sufficient time for exhalation and risking lung derecruitment (long T_{low}) and being too short (excess gas trapping and auto PEEP). Peak expiratory flow and the patient's time constants may be used to attempt to fine-tune the T_{low} setting. There is no "magic bullet" or setting that empirically works every time, as pathology changes rapidly.

Both inspiratory and expiratory times may be manipulated as well. The patient is able to breathe spontaneously at both the high pressure and low pressure level (**Figure 3-8**).

The mandatory breaths (switch from P_{low} to P_{high}) may be time triggered (mandatory) or patient triggered (pressure or flow triggered).

Bilevel and APRV may be used with tube compensation to overcome airway resistance of the artificial airway and pressure support, to augment the patient's spontaneous breathing efforts. The classification of bilevel and APRV is in Table 3-2.

Proportional Assist Ventilation

PAV permits the sharing of ventilatory work between the ventilator and the patient. Ventilatory work may be entirely provided by the ventilator (CMV) or entirely provided by the patient (CSV), or provided by any range of shared work between those extremes. PAV is a pure spontaneous mode of ventilation in that the patient determines rate, inspiratory time, and tidal volume. The ventilator provides a proportional pressure support, depending upon the characteristics of the patient's lungs. The breaths may be flow or pressure triggered. The clinician sets the amount of tube compensation (resistance) and the amount of volume assistance (elastance to be supported). The ventilator uses the equation of motion of the lungs (see Chapter 2) to calculate the total pressure needed to overcome the resistive and elastic properties of the system. The clinician then sets the percentage of PAV to be provided by the ventilator. Any remaining percentage (up to 100%) must then be provided by the patient. The breath cycles into exhalation once the patient's volume or flow demands have been met. PAV is classified in Table 3-2.

Volume Control Plus

VC+ is a form of pressure-controlled ventilation whereby the ventilator adjusts its output to achieve a target tidal volume. In this mode, the clinician sets frequency, rise time, inspiratory time, PEEP and oxygen percentage, and the target tidal volume. The ventilator delivers a test breath using volume control with a decelerating flow pattern and an inspiratory plateau to determine the system compliance.

The ventilator then switches to pressure control, adjusting the inspiratory pressure to achieve the target tidal volume. The inspiratory pressure varies between

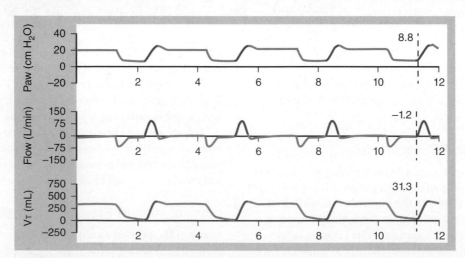

FIGURE 3-8 A graph of airway pressure release ventilation (APRV) mode. Paw, airway pressure; VT, tidal volume.

breaths, as does the inspiratory flow. This mode is classified in Table 3-2.

Volume Support

Volume support mode is a form of pressure-limited ventilation. The clinician sets a target tidal volume, rise time, trigger sensitivity (pressure or flow), and expiratory sensitivity (percent of peak inspiratory flow). The ventilator delivers a pressure support breath, varying inspiratory pressure breath to breath to achieve the target tidal volume. There are no mandatory breaths in volume support. All breaths are patient triggered and cycled. Volume support is classified in Table 3-2.

Pressure-Regulated Volume Control

PRVC is a mode of pressure control in which the clinician sets the breath rate, baseline variable (PEEP), rise and inspiratory time, and the target tidal volume. The ventilator varies inspiratory pressure between breaths to achieve the target tidal volume. Pressure is constantly adjusted by the ventilator responding to changes in the patient's compliance and resistance. In conditions of reduced compliance or increased resistance, the pressure is kept low by a lower flow rate and the same volume is maintained by a longer inspiratory time (Volume = Inspiratory flow × Inspiratory time). The goal of this mode of ventilation is to achieve the desired tidal volume at the lowest pressure delivery. PRVC is classified in Table 3-2.

Adaptive Support Ventilation

ASV is a pressure control mode. The clinician sets the patient's height, gender, the percentage target for minute ventilation (20% to 200%), oxygen percentage, PEEP, pressure rise time, flow trigger (spontaneous triggering), expiratory trigger sensitivity, and maximum pressure limit. ASV is classified in Table 3-2.

The ventilator measures the system compliance and airway resistance and any intrinsic PEEP. The ventilator now automatically adjusts frequency, inspiratory pressure, inspiratory time, and I:E ratio. The ventilator adjusts these parameters to meet the target minute ventilation in the absence of any spontaneous efforts by the patient.

If the patient has spontaneous effort and ventilation, the ventilator delivers pressure support breaths to meet the target minute ventilation. During spontaneous ventilation, as the patient assumes more ventilatory work, the mandatory breaths decrease and the pressure support level for the spontaneous portion is adjusted to maintain the target minute ventilation.

High-Frequency Mechanical Ventilation

High-frequency ventilation delivers breath rates of greater than 150 breaths per minute. The concept behind high-frequency ventilation is to provide the lowest tidal volume at the lowest mean airway pressure. By reducing tidal volumes and mean airway pressures, the incidence of ventilator-associated lung injury may also be reduced.

Conventional ventilation uses tidal volumes that exceed the physiologic (anatomic and alveolar) dead space. Once effective ventilation has been achieved, gas exchange occurs through bulk flow of gas into and out of the alveoli.

High-frequency ventilation uses tidal volumes that are much smaller than physiologic dead space. The increased frequency and low tidal volume result in an asymmetric velocity profile in the airway, such that the inspiratory gas forms a parabolic front down the center of the airway. Gas velocity slows at the perimeter of the airway due to increased friction at the boundary layer of the airway's wall (**Figure 3-9**). The differential velocities result in fresh gas delivery down the airway's center and exhaled air passively moving up around the perimeter of the airway. This is similar to pouring a constant stream of water into the center of a drinking glass with overflow around the rim of the glass. Flow into the glass (down the center) and flow out of the glass (along the sides) occur at the same time.

High-Frequency Jet Ventilation

High-frequency ventilators are classified as to their method of gas delivery. One technique of gas delivery is jet ventilation. A high-frequency jet ventilator (HFJV) delivers high-frequency pulses (jets) of gas through a modified endotracheal tube or through a special adapter

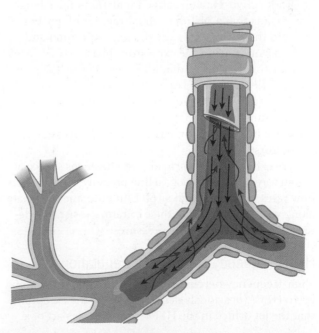

FIGURE 3-9 A line drawing illustrating asymmetric velocity profile in the airway. Note that fresh gas moves down the airway's center while exhaled CO_2 moves up the periphery.

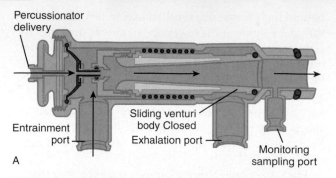

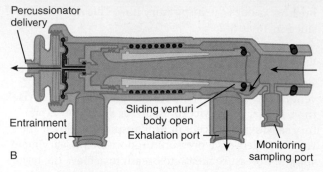

FIGURE 3-10 A line drawing illustrating the operation of the Phasitron: (**A**) inspiration, (**B**) exhalation.

that is attached to the endotracheal tube. Some of these ventilators are used in tandem with a conventional ventilator that provides a fresh gas flow (CPAP) past the patient's airway.

The HFJV creates the asymmetric velocity profile described previously in this section. Fresh gas moves through the more rapid parabolic flow in the center of the airway. Exhaled gas moves upward passively around the periphery of the airway. The jet pulses of gas are small, less than the anatomic dead space, and are delivered at lower mean airway pressures than are possible by conventional positive pressure ventilation. HFJV is provided in the Bunnell Life Pulse ventilator.

High-Frequency Oscillatory Ventilation

High-frequency oscillatory ventilation (HFOV) is different from HFJV in that inhalation and exhalation are both active. Having active inhalation and exhalation means that a piston or diaphragm both pushes gas into the patient's airway during inspiration and pulls gas out during the expiratory phase. HFOV uses both pistons and large diaphragms to create the pressure gradients. HFOVs operate at frequencies of 3 to 15 Hz (180 to 900 breaths/minute), delivering low tidal volumes at low mean airway pressures. HFOV is provided by CareFusion's 3100A and 3100B oscillator ventilators.

A bias flow (CPAP) provides the fresh gas source at the airway as well as the baseline pressure (CPAP). Bias flow rates may be as high as 60 L/minute. Bias flow rate along with adjustment of the expiratory resistance determines the mean airway pressures.

High-Frequency Percussive Ventilation

High-frequency percussive ventilation (HFPV) is similar to HFJV (previously described), with the exception that the jet orifice in the HFPV ventilator is part of a

sliding venturi, which is directly attached to the patient's airway. The sliding venturi mechanism is termed the Phasitron. During inspiration, the gas supplied by the high-frequency pulse generator displaces a diaphragm toward the patient's airway, closing the exhalation port while the high-velocity gas simultaneously entrains ambient air at a ratio of 5:1, augmenting flow (**Figure 3-10**). HFPV is provided by the Percussionaire Corporation's VDR-4 ventilator.

Summary

The modes of ventilation may be classified as spontaneous, volume control, pressure control, and high-frequency ventilation. Spontaneous modes of ventilation include CPAP, BiPAP, and pressure support. In spontaneous modes, the patient determines the start of the breath, the tidal volume, flow delivery, and when the breath ends.

Volume control modes use volume as the control variable. Under normal conditions, this mode guarantees a clinician-set tidal volume, while pressure varies. This mode is best when the clinician wants to provide a specific minute ventilation to ensure adequate CO_2 removal.

Pressure control modes use pressure as the control variable. These modes ensure a fixed constant inspiratory pressure, while both volume and flow vary. Pressure control modes are best when the clinician is concerned with excessive pressures and wants to minimize ventilator-induced lung injury.

High-frequency ventilation is defined as respiratory rates greater than 150 breaths per minute. High-frequency ventilation delivers gas via diffusion and asymmetric gas velocity profiles rather than bulk convective gas flow as in conventional ventilation. High-frequency ventilation may accomplish adequate gas exchange at lower pressures when compared with conventional ventilation.

Case Study

Mr. J. is a 55-year-old patient presenting in your emergency department (ED) in respiratory distress. The ED physician greets you on the way to see Mr. J. and states, "He's in respiratory distress and I think this is another round for his renal failure. Do what you can, but he has an advance directive and does not want to be intubated."

Assessing Mr. J., you note a respiratory rate of 35, with shallow labored breathing. He's on oxygen at 5 L/min via nasal cannula, with an SpO$_2$ of 85%. He's diaphoretic and appears very frightened. He can only speak in short bursts of words without gasping for breath. His heart rate is 135 and he has a normal sinus rhythm. Answer the three questions below.

1. **What are your options for Mr. J. considering the do-not-intubate advanced directive?**

2. **Assuming you select BiPAP to ventilate Mr. J., what are your goals?**

3. **What would you try for initial ventilator setting?**

Bibliography

Chatburn RL. Classification of ventilator modes: update and proposal for implementation. *Respir Care J.* 2007;52:301–323.

Chatburn RL. A taxonomy for mechanical ventilation: 10 fundamental maxims. *Respir Care J.* 2014;59:1747–1763.

Daoud E, Hany F, Chatburn R. Airway pressure release ventilation: what do we know? *Respir Care J.* 2012;57:282–292.

Kacmarek RL. Proportional assist ventilation and neurally adjusted ventilatory assist. *Respir Care J.* 2011;56:140–152.

Miller K. High frequency ventilation. What is the best choice? *RT for Decision Makers in Respir Care.* http://www.rtmagazine.com/2012/02/high-frequency-ventilation-what-is-the-best-choice. Published February 7, 2012.

Norman MA, Coselli JS. Ventilator management in the surgical intensive care unit. *Texas Heart Inst J.* 2010;37:681–682.

Standardized vocabulary for mechanical ventilation. *Resp Care J.* appendix 2. http://rc.rcjournal.com/content/respcare/suppl/2015/01/13/respcare.03057.DC1/Supplemental_-_Standardized_Vocabulary_v2-20-14.pdf.

4

Invasive and Noninvasive Airway Management

Michael W. Canfield, MAEd, RRT, CCT

©s_maria/Shutterstock

OUTLINE

OBJECTIVES

1. Compare and contrast the management of invasive and noninvasive airways.
2. Describe the advantages and disadvantages to invasive and noninvasive airway management.
3. List the criteria and indication for intubations.
4. List the essential equipment needed to complete an intubation.
5. Describe methods of assessment for confirmation of endotracheal tube placement.
6. Explain the reason for monitoring the cuff pressure on an endotracheal tube.
7. Describe the assessment for extubation readiness and explain the typical extubation procedure.
8. Provide indications for the use of a tracheostomy tube and the variations in tube size and design.

KEY TERMS

carina
Cook catheter
endotracheal intubation
endotracheal tube
extubation
laryngoscope
Macintosh blade
Mallampati classification
Miller blade

pilot balloon
radiopaque line
rapid sequence intubation
sniffing position
stylet
tracheostomy tube
vallecula
vocal cords

Introduction

Airway management implies establishing proper function of an airway. Managing the airway of a person who has become compromised in some manner is serious, and controlling the crisis means the difference between survival and death. Securing the airway is an immediate concern. The clinician needs to be aware of the underlying issue that may have caused the respiratory distress. The first step is to properly evaluate the situation, then institute the proper techniques to intervene and avert a crisis. In this chapter, the means by which to establish, maintain, and discontinue airways is elucidated.

Airway Management, What It Means

Management of the airway is key in the survival of the patient. The clinician must have knowledge of airway management and be competent with the procedure to establish control of the airway. It may seem somewhat simple to establish an airway, but patients still die because of inadequate initiation of support. Airway management is to be performed proficiently and in a timely manner. Practice and skill development are necessary to truly be competent. Intubation skills are considered psychomotor skills; they must be practiced to maintain expertise. Airway management requires dexterity for the mechanical manipulation needed for airway stabilization or intubation. The ability to recognize the symptoms of airway compromise plays an important role in physical assessment. The goal is reestablishment of ventilation, oxygenation, and respiration. Generally speaking, brain damage occurs when the body has been deprived of oxygen for about 6 minutes. Given this time limit, the airway must be established and confirmed quickly.

Causes of Respiratory Failure

While trying to maintain the airway, the clinician must also determine the cause of respiratory compromise. There are many factors that can affect breathing in general. Muscle fatigue, physiologic incompetence, and cardiovascular arrest are common causes. There are many disease processes that can contribute to respiratory demise that are not necessarily limited to the respiratory system alone. Airway management begins by assessing how well a patient is oxygenating and ventilating and then ascertaining the next step.

Establishing an airway is fundamental in proper care of the patient who is in respiratory failure; yet, deciding the route of support is not always clear. The goal for airway management is maintaining patency so the patient survives a period of instability. Destabilization of the airway may be the prelude to complete respiratory failure. The human body can progress to a state of exhaustion while trying to maintain homeostasis in the presence of a compromised airway. The type of airway management will need to be determined, starting with whether noninvasive or invasive support is needed.

Airway/ventilatory support without intubation could be invasive or noninvasive intervention. For example, the patient many need a nasopharyngeal airway, bag-valve-mask (BVM), or other type of support; this will be based on the patient's level of consciousness, orientation, and oxygenation status.

Main Goals of Airway Management

The clinician needs to establish the plan for supporting the patient whose airway is compromised. Is it an option to position the patient in such a way as to ensure proper air movement and possibly use noninvasive support? Or will the attending clinician take a step further and establish an invasive airway? Whether the clinician chooses to use noninvasive means or invasive means of ventilatory support, the main goal for either form is *to restore the patient to a homeostatic condition.*

The first priority is to establish if noninvasive ventilation or invasive ventilation will be needed to provide intervention to patient under distress. To help understand this, the difference between noninvasive and invasive airway support needs clarification. A noninvasive airway is limited to placement in the upper airway (does not enter into the trachea through the **vocal cords**). Conversely, invasive airway support involves any artificial airway that extends through the vocal cords and enter the trachea or main-stem bronchus (**Figure 4-1**).

Anatomical Review

This section is an anatomical review of the airways and oral cavity (consisting of the tongue, teeth, tonsils, and uvula). See **Figure 4-2**.

This review of the upper oropharynx to the lower conducting airways is intended as a brief refresher because the reader already has this foundational knowledge (**Figure 4-3**).

The respiratory system consists of the nose, nasal cavity, pharynx, larynx, trachea, bronchi, and lungs. It is divided into the upper and lower respiratory systems.

Upper Oral Airway Anatomy

The upper portion of the airway has the primary functions to filter, warm, and moisten inspired air. The nose is composed of bone and cartilage and may play a vital role in establishing an artificial airway. The nose has two external openings called *nares*. The overall nasal cavity is lined with epithelial tissue, and this mucosa is largely covered by a mucous blanket of varying thickness.

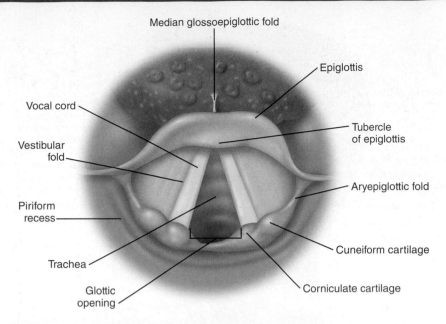

FIGURE 4-1 Vocal cords.

Margolis G, American Academy of Orthopedic Surgeons. *Paramedic: Airway Management.* Sudbury, MA: Jones & Bartlett; 2004.

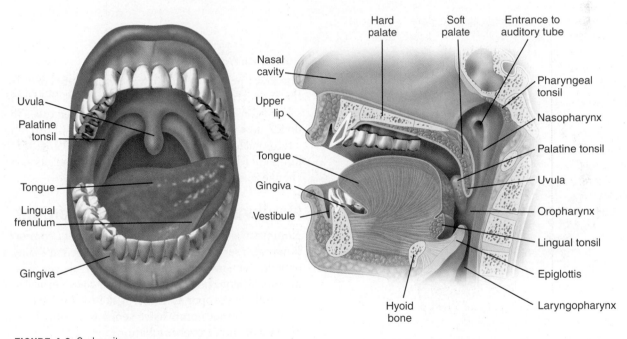

FIGURE 4-2 Oral cavity.

Margolis G, American Academy of Orthopedic Surgeons. *Paramedic: Airway Management.* Sudbury, MA: Jones & Bartlett; 2004.

Figure 4-4 shows the nasal sinuses. Goblet cells scattered throughout the epithelial lining serve to produce mucus. The narrow nasal passages and considerable surface area of the mucous lining serve as a filter for particulate matter. Hairlike projections termed *cilia* provide the movement of foreign material from the upper and posterior nasal cavity. If the mucosal area becomes dehydrated, then the mucus can dry and become thickened or crusted. Dried mucus can impede the airway passages, which is why it is critical to maintain

proper humidification. Properly maintaining the mucociliary blanket allows for cleansing of the mucosa to ensure patency.

A specific insertion procedure is used for nasal intubation. Extreme caution needs to be exercised during the procedure because the upper airway and the nose can play a major part in establishing stability but can be damaged in the process. Each side of the nose has a lateral and medial wall formed by the ethmoid and vomer bones. These bones are thin and sometimes damaged

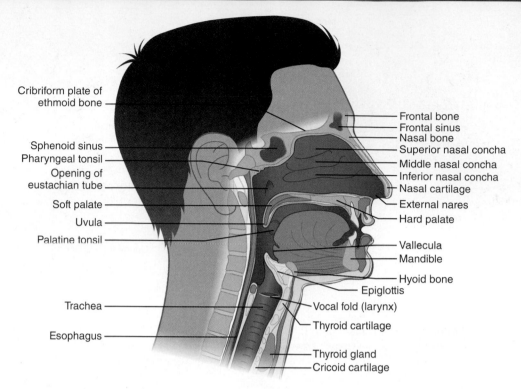

FIGURE 4-3 Anatomy of airway.

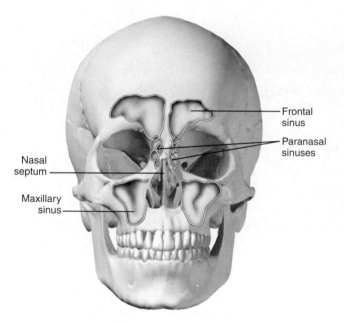

FIGURE 4-4 Nasal sinuses.

Margolis G, American Academy of Orthopedic Surgeons. *Paramedic: Airway Management.* Sudbury, MA: Jones & Bartlett; 2004.

either by trauma of an accident or the process of nasal intubation. The medial wall is also known as the nasal septum and is a structure that may be deviated in some patients. This will be very important to consider when placing airway devices into the nares. If when advancing a nasal airway resistance is met, the clinician must gingerly manipulate and try to reposition. Nasal intubation is avoided if possible because of the complication of associated sinus infection.

Lower Airway Anatomy

The lower portion of the airway (**Figure 4-5**) consists of the conducting airways. This portion of the respiratory system consists of a series of interconnected tubes that divide subsequently into the lung tissue until reaching a terminal location of the alveoli. The distal areas of the lungs are where the delivered air reaches the gas exchange zones.

Noninvasive Airway Management

Noninvasive ventilation can increase patient comfort. It may also serve as an effective means for stabilizing a patient. Remember, this application is truly noninvasive, meaning it does not pass beyond the vocal cords. However, utilizing proper assessment skills is the best way to evaluate whether noninvasive ventilation should be the method of choice over intubation.

Options and Limitations

Addressing noninvasive ventilation requires a wide perspective on what options are available to the clinician. Noninvasive oxygenation or ventilatory support could be continuous positive airway pressure (CPAP), high flow nasal cannula, or bag valve mask (BVM) system (**Figures 4-6** and **4-7**). (BVM is the generic term; the device category is sometimes referred to as an Ambu, which is a brand name used as a generic term as well.) The clinician may use a laryngeal mask airway (LMA) as an alternative. The decision must be made quickly to evaluate whether the patient has the ability to

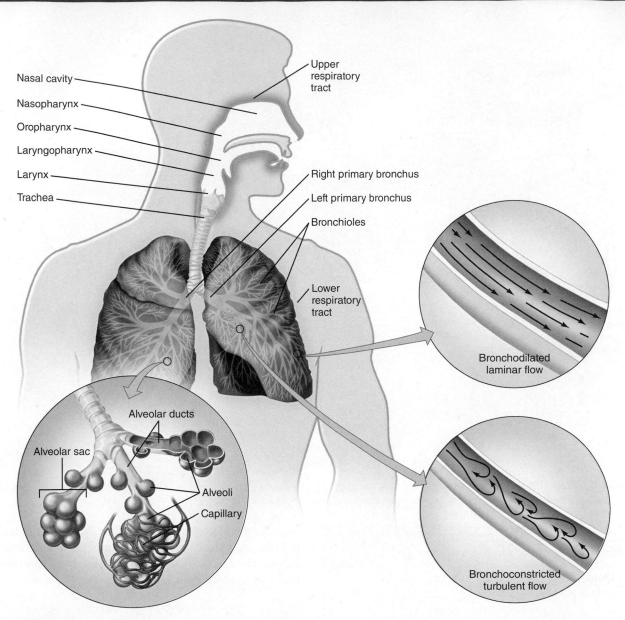

Nasal cavity

Nasopharynx

Oropharynx

Laryngopharynx

Larynx

Trachea

Upper
respiratory
tract

Right primary bronchus

Left primary bronchus

Bronchioles

Lower
respiratory
tract

Bronchodilated
laminar flow

Bronchoconstricted
turbulent flow

Alveolar ducts

Alveolar sac

Alveoli

Capillary

FIGURE 4-5 Lower airways.

Margolis G, American Academy of Orthopedic Surgeons. *Paramedic: Airway Management*. Sudbury, MA: Jones & Bartlett; 2004.

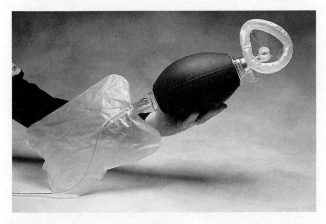

FIGURE 4-6 Bag-valve-mask system.

compensate. See **Table 4-1**. The LMA sits over the glottis as a drain tube to aid gastric suctioning; some versions may allow an endotracheal (ET) tube to be passed to aid in intubation.

When to Transition to Invasive

Some situations may require transition to an invasive airway. If noninvasive ventilation can adequately meet a patient's needs, then it should remain. Noninvasively supporting the patient may create less trauma and allow the period of time needed for ventilation to be shorter. The less time spent with artificial support to meet the patient's needs, the better. However, if a patient needs to be intubated, prolonged use of

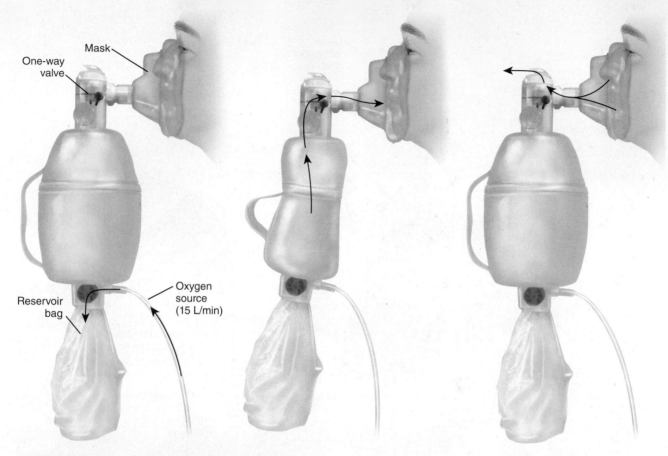

FIGURE 4-7 Proper bag-valve-mask placement and reservoir usage.
Margolis G, American Academy of Orthopedic Surgeons. *Paramedic: Airway Management*. Sudbury, MA: Jones & Bartlett; 2004.

TABLE 4-1
Indications for Mask Ventilation

Indications
- Apnea of any cause

Contraindications
- None in an emergency

Advantages
- Physical barrier between rescuer and patient's blood or body fluids
- One-way valve prevents blood or body fluids from splashing onto the paramedic
- May be easier to obtain face seal

Disadvantages
- Useful only if readily available

Complications
- Hyperinflation of patient's lungs
- Hyperventilation of rescuer
- Gastric distention

Margolis G, American Academy of Orthopedic Surgeons. *Paramedic: Airway Management*. Sudbury, MA: Jones & Bartlett; 2004.

noninvasive airway only delays the needed invasive airway. Transition to an invasive airway may be necessary if the patient do not have the muscular strength to keep their own head upright. This physical sign may indicate the patients have spent too much energy trying to compensate for their respiratory failure. As they enter into complete exhaustion, opting to go directly to invasive ventilation is prudent.

Clinical Note

Tell the patient what is going to happen and the sequence of events to obtain patient compliance during airway placement.

Make eye contact, speak clearly, use short explanations, and assure that proper care will be given.

These few steps can help alleviate the anxiety that is likely to accompany the respiratory distress.

Invasive Airway Management

Aspects of **endotracheal intubation** (placement of a tube into the trachea to maintain an patent airway) with regard to indications, contraindications,

TABLE 4-2
Endotracheal Intubation

Indications
- Decreased level of consciousness
- Risk of regurgitation
- Depressed or absent gag reflex
- Respiratory failure
- Respiratory arrest or cardiac arrest

Contraindications
- None in emergency situations

Advantages
- Ensures a patent airway
- Reduces the risk of regurgitation or aspiration
- Improves ventilation
- Provides route for the administration of oxygen

Disadvantages
- Bypasses the function of the upper airway

Complications
- Hypoxia during insertion
- Dysrhythmia
- Tracheal trauma
- Laryngospasm
- Barotrauma
- Bronchial intubation
- Esophageal intubation

Margolis G, American Academy of Orthopedic Surgeons. *Paramedic: Airway Management.* Sudbury, MA: Jones & Bartlett; 2004.

disadvantages, and complications is addressed in this section (**Table 4-2**).

Intubation Kit: The Equipment Needed

The persons performing an intubation should come prepared to conduct it from start to finish. There are routine preparations that should be maintained to ensure readiness for emergency airway placement. Intubation kits are often prepackaged, so the problem is who determines what will be placed in the intubation kit (**Figure 4-8**). Is it the supply department, the hospital staff in different areas of the hospital, or the respiratory therapy department? Each intubation tray, kit, or box (named differently depending on the institution) needs to have an inventory list of required equipment and supplies within the container. The specific equipment for intubation can vary by institution; however, the categories of equipment and supplies should be relatively standard across institutions.

Typical intubation items include the following:

Gloves
ET tubes, typically sizes 5 through 9 with a stylet
  (**Figure 4-9**)
10-mL syringe
Laryngoscope handle
BVM

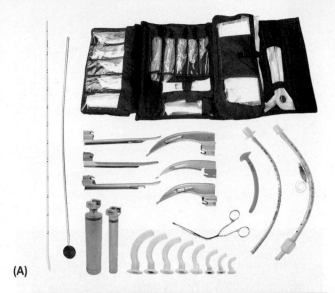

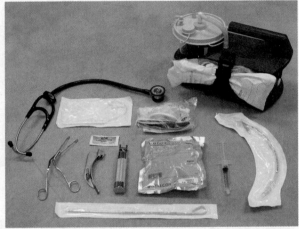

(A)

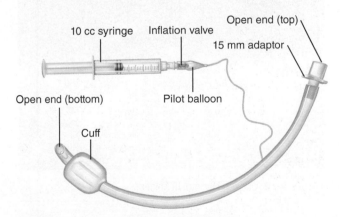

(B)

FIGURE 4-8 (**A**) Intubation kit. (**B**) Assembled equipment.
(**A**) Courtesy of SunMed; (**B**) © Jones and Bartlett Publishers. Courtesy of MIEMSS.

FIGURE 4-9 Endotracheal tube prepped for use.
Margolis G, American Academy of Orthopedic Surgeons. *Paramedic: Airway Management.* Sudbury, MA: Jones & Bartlett; 2004.

Series of different blades, both Miller (straight) and
  Macintosh (curved) (**Figures 4-10, 4-11, 4-12**)
Carbon dioxide detector (disposable)
Nasopharyngeal airway of different sizes

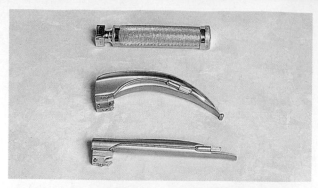

FIGURE 4-10 Laryngoscope blades Macintosh and Miller.

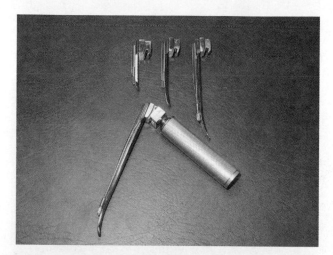

FIGURE 4-11 Straight (Miller) blades.

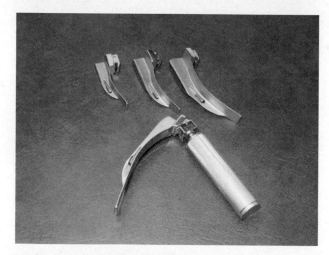

FIGURE 4-12 Curved (Macintosh) blades.

Oropharyngeal airway of different sizes
Water-based lubricant
Gauze tape
Extra batteries for the handles
ET tube holder (this could be cloth tape or other
    means of securing the ET tube)
Stethoscope (which every respiratory therapist
    should have on hand—a crucial item)

Blades and handles for the oral **laryngoscope** can also present a challenge. There must be a conscious effort to ensure that the handles have batteries, that they work, and that the blades interlock into the handle prior to placing them in the tray.

Choosing the ET Tube

The most primary piece of equipment is the **endotracheal tube**. The basic components of the ET tube incorporate a proximal end, the tube, the **pilot balloon**, and the end of the tube, which is tapered and has a bevel tip. The end proximal to the patient will have a standard 15/22-mm adapter, which is considered universal. This allows connection to a BVM system or mechanical ventilator circuit. The tube length is indicated by graduated markers with numbers printed to indicate the millimeter length. The ET tube is designed with a **radiopaque line** (a line that runs the length of the tube), so the clinician can verify placement within the airway on a chest radiograph. ET tubes vary in size from 2 to 10 mm (internal diameter). Typically, the ET tube size 5 or greater will have a cuff, whereas tubes smaller than 5 are typically cuffless. The cuff is inflated once the ET tube has been inserted in the patient's airway through the pilot balloon with a syringe (**Figure 4-13**). The pilot balloon usually has a one-way valve that is spring loaded to keep the cuff inflated with air until it is extracted intentionally.

Tube Types

There are many different types of ET tubes, and they are selected depending upon the specific needs of a patient's condition. The individual tube to choose may come in variety of types. One may be a high-volume low-pressure cuff. Another, although not as commonly used, could be a low-volume high-pressure cuff. The tubes will be labeled on the packaging. There may be a Hi-Lo Evac tube, which has a suction port as well as a pilot balloon integrated into the ET tube. The tube is

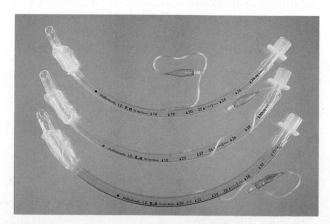

FIGURE 4-13 Endotracheal tubes with pilot balloon.

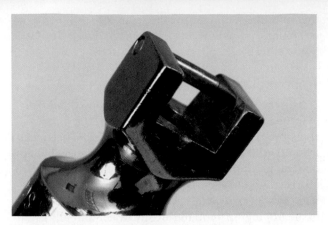

FIGURE 4-14 The laryngoscope handle.

made from medical grade silicone. Remember, selecting the correct size is crucial when intubating the patient. Smaller tubes may be easier to pass through the vocal cords but create additional airway resistance. When resistance increases because of the ET tube, this increases the work of breathing. The size range for females is 7 to 7.5 mm, and for males the size range is 7.5 to 8.5 mm. The size selection can vary depending on the sizing standard used and the degree to which an individual deviates from the average sizing.

Blades and Handles

A universal standard for laryngoscopes and blades would be expected, but that is not the case. It is essential for these items to be prechecked to ensure that the laryngeal blade in the intubation kit connects to the handle (**Figure 4-14**).

Some laryngoscopes are disposable and have fixed blades that cannot be removed. Others have a permanent handle but a disposable blade. Being aware of what is in the intubation kit will increase efficiency. Most often, a reusable handle with a reusable blade and disposable bulb will be the standard equipment because of cost savings. There are some electronic options that are very helpful, such as a GlideScope (Verathon, Bothell, WA). The advantage of this device is its electronic visual display. However, they are still quite costly and may not be readily available in an emergency situation.

Macintosh Versus Miller

Controversy over which blade to use has continued over many years among the clinicians. Each clinician will have a preference, but all clinicians should become familiar and proficient in using different types of intubation devices.

A basic intubation kit consists of a laryngoscope handle, laryngoscope blade, ET tube, water soluble lubricant, 10-mL syringe, and optional flexible **stylet**. **Figure 4-15** shows the laryngoscope handle (top), **MacIntosh blade** (middle), and **Miller blade** (bottom).

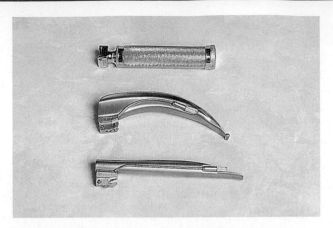

FIGURE 4-15 Choose Macintosh or Miller blades. Laryngoscope handle (top), Macintosh curved blade (middle), and Miller straight blade (bottom).

When performing the intubation with a Miller blade, the clinician captures the epiglottis with the tip of the blade and lifts it up and away to visualize the vocal cords. When performing the intubation with a Macintosh blade, the clinician will insert the tip of the blade into the **vallecula** and then lift up to visualize the vocal cords.

Intubation Procedure

Box 4-1 outlines the main signs of respiratory failure that often leads to intubation and mechanical ventilation. The decision to intubate is a timing challenge. Intubation done too early may subject the patient to unnecessary complications related to use of an invasive airway. Intubation done too late often leads to prolonged hypercapnia, hypoxemia, and duration of mechanical ventilation.

Controlled Versus Uncontrolled

There are two basic aspects of endotracheal intubation controlled and uncontrolled environments.

The controlled environment is a situation in which most if not all factors (i.e., patient position, availability of high oxygen supply, or assistance from other medical providers) can be precisely manipulated and modified. The example of a controlled environment would be a surgical suite. The situation that occurs most often, however, is the uncontrolled environment.

The uncontrolled environment is a situation in which most factors cannot be modified. Slight variations can complicate the overall procedure. An example of the uncontrolled environment is when a patient is far away from critical care personnel, equipment, and supplies. This situation proves to be a challenge because of limitations related to the help available and accessibility of equipment.

Quick Airway Assessment

When considering the anatomical structure of the airway, it is important to do a quick airway assessment to help determine what will be the best route of airway management. Part of the quick assessment is to consider if there has been any physical damage to the face, nasal sinus, mandible, and neck. During this initial assessment the clinician also will need to be mindful of any cervical damage due to trauma (**Figure 4-16**).

Trouble Signs and Mallampati Score

One of the most important clues to potential difficulty in intubating a patient is the patient's overall physical appearance and body habitus (body build, in particular). Patients who have a short, stocky build are usually more difficult to intubate. Patients who have large neck diameters can be a challenge to intubate. If a patient is obese, there may also be issues because of the additional fat tissue impinging upon the airway. When initially evaluating the oral cavity for intubation, the clinician must consider the **Mallampati classification** (**Table 4-3**).

This designation is a way to grade the potential difficulty when intubating a patient. It was named after the anesthesiologist who established the class designations. To view the anatomic features using the Mallampati classification, the patient sits upright with head in neutral position. The patient is asked to open the mouth as wide as possible and extend the tongue. Mallampati grade I is ideal and it shows the hard palate, soft palate, entire uvula with space between uvula and tongue

---

BOX 4-1 Signs of Respiratory Failure: Quick Reference

No one sign indicates respiratory failure. Look at the entire clinical picture and consider combinations of the following signs/symptoms to suggest respiratory failure.

- Look of anxiety
- Signs of sympathetic overactivity (dilated pupils, sweating)
- Acute dyspnea—especially when it results in the inability to talk
- Use of accessory muscles
- Self-PEEP (breathing against pursed lips, expiratory grunting, groaning)
- Cyanosis
- Restlessness and fidgeting, progressing to apathy or coma
- $SpO_2 < 90\%$ despite ventilatory support with 100% oxygen
- $PaO_2 < 60$ mm Hg despite ventilatory support with 100% oxygen
- $PaCO_2 > 60$ mm Hg despite ventilatory support with 100% oxygen
- Uncompensated respiratory acidosis

PEEP, positive end-expiratory pressure.
Margolis G, American Academy of Orthopedic Surgeons. *Paramedic: Airway Management.* Sudbury, MA: Jones & Bartlett; 2004.

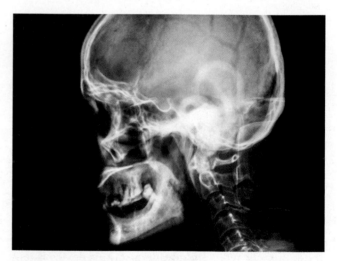

FIGURE 4-16 Cervical neck injury.
© Puwadol Jaturawutthichai/Shutterstock.

TABLE 4-3
Mallampati Class Designation

Mallampati Class	Laryngoscopic View			
	Grade 1: Entire glottis fully exposed	Grade 2: Glottis partially exposed	Grade 3: Glottis cannot be exposed, corniculate cartilages can be visualized	Grade 4: Neither the glottis nor corniculate cartilages can be visualized
Class I (74%)	80%	20%		
Class II (19%)	30%	35%	25%	10%
Class III (7%)		7%	60%	33%

Margolis G, American Academy of Orthopedic Surgeons. *Paramedic: Airway Management.* Sudbury, MA: Jones & Bartlett; 2004.

and pillars. (Note: Palatine uvula is the soft round tissue structure that hangs at the back of throat). Grade II shows most of uvula with tongue blocking part of it. Grades I and II offer easy access to the vocal cords and intubation attempts typically do not require anesthesia assistance. Grade III only shows the base of uvula. In Grade IV, the entire uvula is not visible. Grades III and IV require anesthesia assistance for intubation. The size of tongue and mouth opening dictate the Mallampati grading. As the size of the tongue broadens it takes up more space in the oral cavity and can obscure the view into the airway. In this instance when the glottis is partially exposed it would be assigned a grade 2. When looking into the airway, if the glottis and uvula cannot be visualized and obstruct the view of the opening of the oral cavity, this would be considered a grade 3. Finally, if the glottis or the corniculate cartilages cannot be viewed and the tongue is excessively wide and obtrusive, then this is considered a grade 4. Performing this evaluation can help the clinician anticipate how difficult the intubation is likely to be. This will allow preparation for other interventions and provide for guidance as to how to proceed in establishing the airway. Although a numerical rating is assigned, it is still a subjective evaluation.

Sniffing Position

To attain a proper **sniffing position**, the neck must be flexed toward the chest, typically by elevating the head with a cushion under the occiput and extending the head on the atlanto-occipital joint (**Figure 4-17**). **Figure 4-18** shows the proper airway alignment for intubation when the sniffing position is properly performed.

Adjunctive Devices Prior to Intubation

Initially there may be a need for adjunctive devices to facilitate intubation. Examples of these assisting items

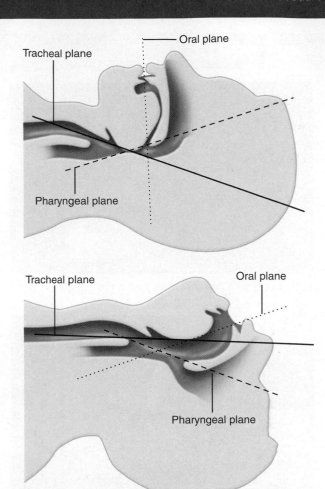

FIGURE 4-18 Sniffing position.

Margolis G, American Academy of Orthopedic Surgeons. *Paramedic: Airway Management.* Sudbury, MA: Jones & Bartlett; 2004.

are discussed in the following section. Although these are not absolutely necessary, it is strongly suggested to consider these devices as important parts of the intubation equipment: the nasopharyngeal airway, oropharyngeal airway, a tube exchanger, and a naso-oral suction catheter (also called a Yankauer device).

Oropharyngeal Airway

The appropriate size of an oropharyngeal airway is determined by the measurement from the corner of the patient's mouth to the angle of the jaw (**Skill Drill 4-1**, Step 2). The sizes range from 0 to 5, with 0 being the smallest and 5 the largest. This device holds the airway and tongue into position from the posterior pharynx, but it does not isolate the trachea. The oral airway is inserted with the curve toward the side of the mouth and rotated so that the curve of the airway matches the curve of the tongue (see **Figure 4-19**). **Table 4-4** outlines the key indications, contraindications, advantages, disadvantages, and complications of an oral airway.

Nasopharyngeal Airway

If a nasopharyngeal airway is to be used, measure the size needed in a similar fashion as the oral airway.

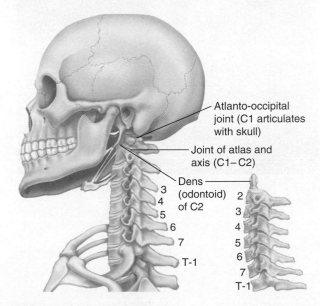

FIGURE 4-17 Atlanto-occipital joint.

SKILL DRILL 4-1 Oral Airway Insertion Technique 1 for Adults Only

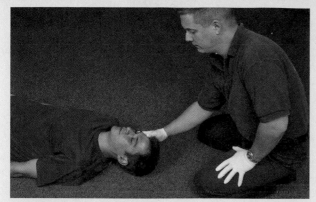

STEP 1 Approach the patient from the top of the head.

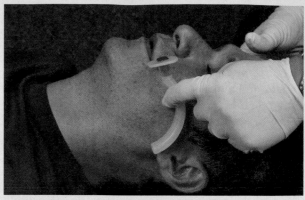

STEP 2 Select the correct sized airway for the patient.

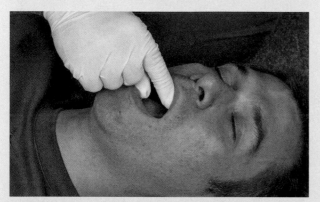

STEP 3 Using the nondominant hand, tilt the patient's head back and open mouth. The latter can be accomplished by placing the side of your thumb just below the lower lip and pushing gently toward the feet, or by using the crossfinger maneuver, in which you cross your thumb and index finger and place the tip of your thumb on the lower incisors and the tip of your index finger on the upper incisors.

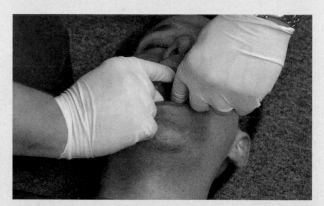

STEP 4 Remove any visible obstructions.

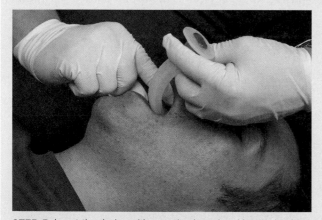

STEP 5 Insert the device with your dominant hand by placing its distal tip toward the palate (concavity cephalad) and inserting the device until you feel a slight resistance.

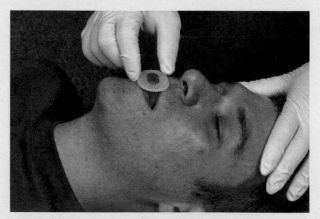

STEP 6 Turn the device 180° until the flange comes to rest at the patient's incisors.

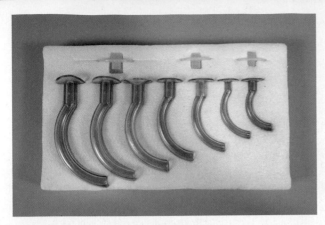

FIGURE 4-19 Oral airway measurement

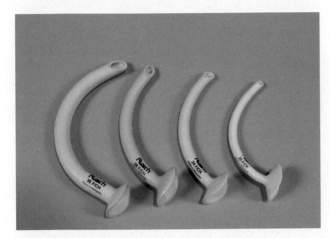

FIGURE 4-20 Nasal airways.

The measurement will begin from the nare to the bottom of the ear canal. This point will be slightly above the earlobe. Remember this is an estimation, and the clinician may have to adjust it based on the anatomy of the patient. Even though patients are the same anatomically, they are still very different when it comes to anatomical representation because these structures may be different sizes or in a slightly different position than expected. The clinician will need to anticipate this variation.

Prior to insertion, the nasopharyngeal airway (**Figure 4-20**) should be lubricated with a water-soluble lubricant. Using this adjunctive device in the airway will provide an enhanced means of BVM support. It is short enough to not trigger the gag reflex when the patient may still be semiconscious.

The bevel tip should be directed toward the nasal septum, and the natural curvature of the nasopassage should be used to gently slide the nasopharyngeal tube into place (**Figure 4-21**). This should come to rest in the posterior pharynx. If resistance is met when trying to place the tube into the nasal passage, gently pull back a

TABLE 4-4
Oral Airways

Indications
- Deeply unconscious patients
- Absent gag reflex

Contraindication
- Presence of a gag reflex

Advantages
- Noninvasive
- Easily placed
- Prevents blockage of glottis by tongue

Disadvantages
- Does not prevent aspiration
- Unexpected gag may produce vomiting and/or laryngospasm
- Still may require a head tilt

Complications
- Gagging and retching, which may cause vomiting, laryngospasm, and increased intracranial pressure
- Pharyngeal or dental trauma with poor technique

Margolis G, American Academy of Orthopedic Surgeons. *Paramedic: Airway Management.* Sudbury, MA: Jones & Bartlett; 2004.

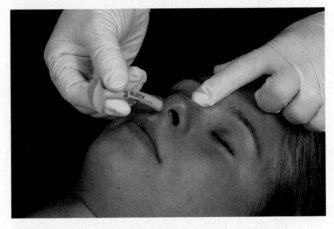

FIGURE 4-21 Inserting nasal airway.
© Jones and Bartlett Publishers. Courtesy of MIEMSS.

few centimeters, twist slightly, and re-advance. If resistance is met once again, then consider use of the opposite nasal passage.

Medications Needed

Medications used during a **rapid sequence intubation** (RSI) can vary widely, but there are typically certain standards that are used almost universally (**Figure 4-22**). **Box 4-2** lists some medications that are used during intubation.

Vecuronium bromide (Norcuron): Duration of action 15 to 30 minutes; onset of action less than 1 minute; can be given intravenous (IV) push 0.04 to 0.06 mg/kg

SKILL DRILL 4-2 Inserting a Nasal Airway

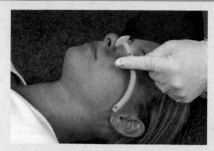

STEP 1 Selecting the correct sized airway for the patient.

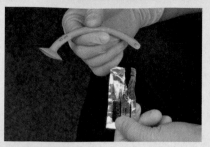

STEP 2 Lubricate the airway with a water-soluble lubricant.

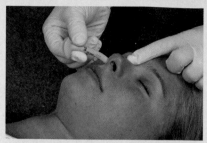

STEP 3 With the bevel toward the septum, gently insert the device straight back (toward the ear, not the eye) until the flange rests at the nostril.

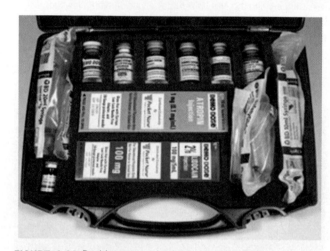

FIGURE 4-22 Rapid sequence intubation medication kit.

BOX 4-2 Medication Agents for Rapid Sequence Intubation

Butyrophenones: Sedative

Haloperidol (Haldol)

Droperidol (Inapsine)

Benzodiazepine: Sedative-Hypnotic

Diazepam (Valium)

Midazolam (Versed)

Barbiturate: Sedative-Hypnotic

Thiopental (Pentothal)

Methohexital (Brevital)

Opioids: Sedative-Analgesic

Fentanyl (Sublimaze)

Alfentanil (Alfenta)

Propofol (Diprivan): Sedative-Hypnotic

Etomidate (Amidate): Sedative-Hypnotic

Ketamine (Ketalar): Sedative-Analgesic-Hypnotic

Margolis G, American Academy of Orthopedic Surgeons. *Paramedic: Airway Management.* Sudbury, MA: Jones & Bartlett; 2004.

Etomidate: Duration of action 3 to 12 minutes; onset of action less than 45 seconds (most hemodynamically neutral); can be given IV push 0.3 to 0.6 mg/kg over 30 to 60 seconds

Etomidate does not affect cardiac metabolism; no depression of cardiac output or of peripheral or pulmonary circulation is indicated but it may cause some drop in blood pressure.

Ketamine analgesia and anesthetic sedative: Duration of action 10 to 20 minutes; onset of action 45 to 60 seconds; IV dose 1 to 2 mg/kg (if patient is not alert or awake at all); an option of one-half dose (0.25 to 0.5 mg/kg IV push) may be effective and still potent.

*Ketamine is a great way to accommodate a sympathetic surge (excessive sympathetic nervous system response). This is also a medication that will have a first pass response with push. (All drug dose absorbed from the gastrointestinal tract is **first** delivered to the **liver** by the portal vein. A fraction of the drug can then be metabolized in the **liver** before it even reaches the systemic circulation.)*

Propofol (given with ketamine during RSI): Duration of action is effective for approximately 10 minutes; onset of action is immediate; IV push 1.5 to 3 mg/kg *unless in shock* and hemodynamically unstable; in this instance the practitioner would use no more than 15 mg.

Succinylcholine—neuromuscular blocker: Higher doses are recommended when a patient is in shock (2 mg/kg); duration of action 3 to 5 minutes; onset of action less than 30 seconds.

Remember that the time for the onset of chemical action may be longer owing to a significant decrease in cardiac output, and a patient in shock/vascular failure will not respond as quickly.

Some medications may not be as easy to work with and have other effects that may preclude their use. Two such medications are midazolam and fentanyl, and although midazolam is still widely used for procedural sedation it is not a good choice to assist intubation. If this is a standard at the facility it should be carefully considered, and best practices should be researched prior to making it part of the formulary for intubations.

Patients who are hypotensive or in septic shock are of concern when determining what medication to use to sedate. All sedative medications will physiologically cause some decrease in blood pressure. Using a sedative with a patient who is already hypotensive is inviting trouble. Patients in this situation should be readily transfused with fluids to increase the blood pressure. It is better to be slightly hypertensive prior to intubation because many of the medications given will typically drop blood pressure. The last thing that is needed is to intubate the patient and then code the same patient because his or her pressures bottom out.

Performing the Intubation

To prepare patients for intubation, preoxygenate and manually ventilate them once they are medicated and ready to intubate. It is important to use 100% oxygen. **Box 4-3** provides protocol for RSI for hemodynamically stable and unstable patients.

Using the BVM, make a proper seal to the patient's face and ventilate while assembly of equipment is being completed. An adjunctive airway may be useful during this step (**Figures 4-23** and **4-24**).

The equipment must be checked and assembled prior to placing the patient in the preferred sniffing position.

Hold the laryngoscope in the left hand and gradually insert the blade into the right side of the patient's mouth so that the tongue can be shifted to the left (**Figure 4-25**).

Next, lift up and away (this means toward the ceiling and away from the intubating individual). Once the vocal cords are observed, insert the ET tube (with stylet in place) into the mouth and visualize it passing through the vocal cords. Performing this step as indicated, up and away from the patient, is critical. If the clinician instead rocks the laryngoscope backward or pulls it toward oneself, dental trauma may occur (**Figure 4-26**).

Lastly, remove the blade from the patient's mouth and inflate the cuff on the ET tube with a 10-mL syringe attached to the pilot balloon connector (cuff pressure can be adjusted after the tube has been secured) and secure the tube. Record the centimeter mark at which the

---

BOX 4-3 Protocol for Rapid Sequence Intubation (RSI)

For Hemodynamically Stable Patients

1. Prepare patient and equipment
2. Preoxygenate (Fio_2 1.0 for 3 to 5 minutes)
3. Consider defasciculating dose of nondepolarizing neuromuscular blocker, lidocaine, and/or atropine
4. Sedate
5. Administer succinylcholine
6. Apply cricoid pressure
7. Intubate, verify tube placement, release cricoid pressure
8. Administer nondepolarizing neuromuscular blocker and maintain adequate sedation

For Hemodynamically Unstable Patients

1. Prepare patient and equipment
2. Preoxygenate or ventilate as necessary
3. Consider sedation
4. Administer succinylcholine
5. Apply cricoid pressure
6. Intubate, verify tube placement, release cricoid pressure
7. Administer nondepolarizing neuromuscular blocker

Margolis G, American Academy of Orthopedic Surgeons. *Paramedic: Airway Management.* Sudbury, MA: Jones & Bartlett; 2004.

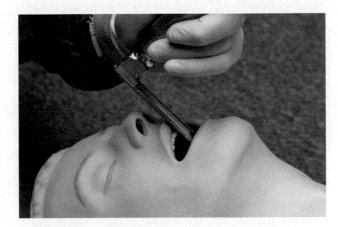

FIGURE 4-23 Improper technique.

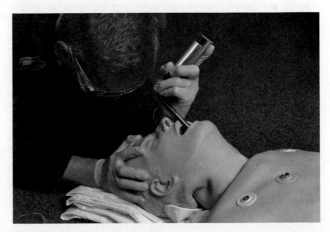

FIGURE 4-24 Proper technique.

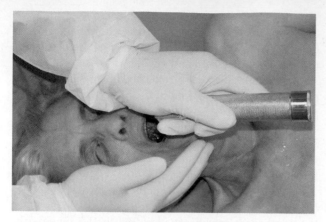

FIGURE 4-25 Proper laryngeal scope orientation.

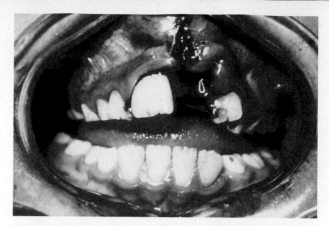

FIGURE 4-26 Dental trauma from improper technique.

ET tube exits the patient's lips. This can vary depending on the size of the patient. Taller patients in general will have longer airway anatomy. The tube is taped at the 21- to 23-cm mark on the average adult.

Auscultation is the more important aspect to determine if bilateral breath sounds exist. To be truly

effective, the clinician will need to listen to the chest in several places: right and left apical, right and left middle, and over the right and left bases (posterior chest wall).

SKILL DRILL 4-3 Intubation of the Trachea Using Direct Laryngoscopy

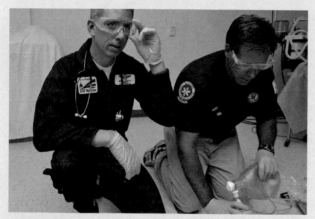

STEP 1 Use body substance isolation precautions (gloves and face shield).

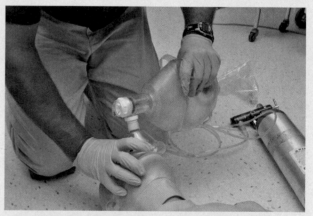

STEP 2 Preoxygenate the patient whenever possible with a bag-valve-mask device and 100% oxygen.

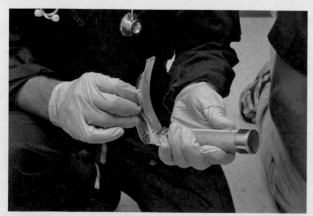

STEP 3 Check, prepare, and assemble your equipment.

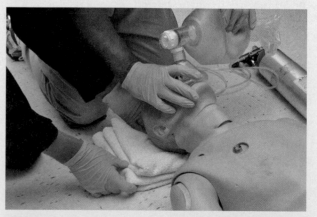

STEP 4 Place the patient's head in the sniffing position.

SKILL DRILL 4-3 Intubation of the Trachea Using Direct Laryngoscopy
(Continued)

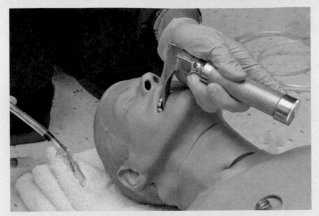

STEP 5 Insert the blade into the right side of the patient's mouth and displace the tongue to the left.

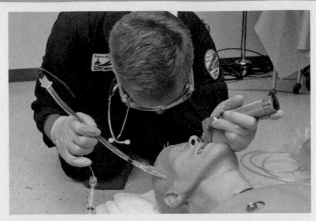

STEP 6 Gently lift the long axis of the laryngoscope handle until you can visualize the glottic opening and the vocal cords.

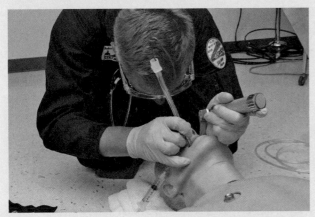

STEP 7 Insert the endotracheal tube through the right corner of the mouth and place it between the vocal cords.

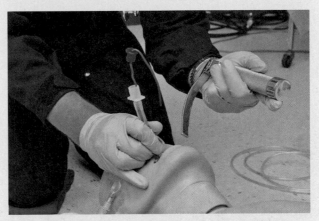

STEP 8 Remove the laryngoscope from the patient's mouth.

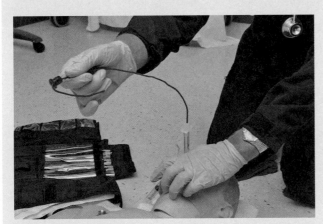

STEP 9 Remove the stylet from the endotracheal tube.

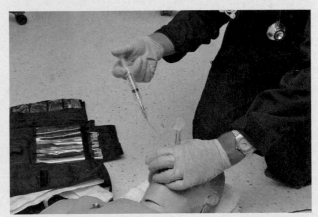

STEP 10 Inflate the distal cuff of the endotracheal tube with 5 to 10 mL of air and detach the syringe.

(continues)

SKILL DRILL 4-3 Intubation of the Trachea Using Direct Laryngoscopy (*Continued*)

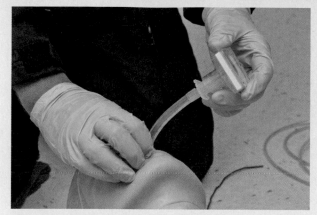

STEP 11 Attach the end-tidal carbon dioxide detector to the endotracheal tube.

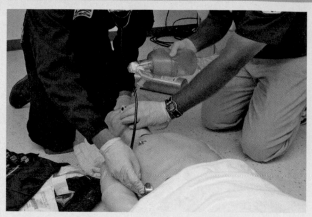

STEP 12 Attach the bag-valve device, ventilate, and auscultate over the apices and bases of both lungs and over the epigastrium.

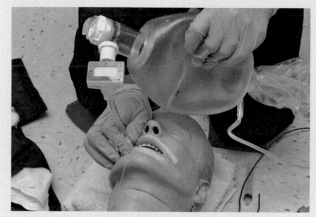

STEP 13 Secure the endotracheal tube.

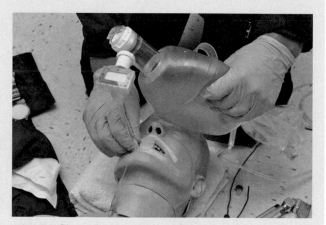

STEP 14 Place a bite block in the patient's mouth.

Stabilizing the Tube

Move the ET tube to the corner of the patient's mouth and stabilize it with tape or securing device. Proper care will require that the ET tube be moved routinely from one side of the mouth to the other to prevent tissue breakdown. This will depend on how many days the patient has been intubated. Reattach the manual resuscitator bag to the ET tube and give a couple deep breaths to determine that a proper tube placement was obtained. Using auscultation, determine bilateral breath sounds.

Airway Clearance

Once the patient is intubated and the therapist has secured the ET tube, follow-up airway care can commence. It is important to ensure that the patient is able to receive the proper amount of both oxygen and ventilation. Secretion production is normal in the upper airway and oral cavity, which is stimulated by the presence of the ET tube. It is important to maintain proper suctioning to clear the airway only as indicated.

Suction Procedure

Either fixed or portable suction devices can be used when performing suctioning procedures. Fixed suction devices typically are on a permanent fitting within a hospital room or a department. Portable devices may be indicated for those individuals who are being intubated either in the field or in a hospital area without a piped vacuum source (i.e., common areas or a psychiatric unit)

SKILL DRILL 4-4 Securing the Endotracheal Tube with Tape

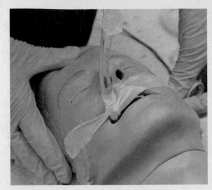

STEP 1 Note the cm marking on the tube at the level of the patient's teeth.

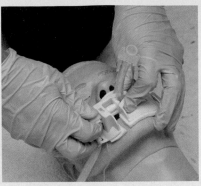

STEP 2 Remove the bag-valve device from the endotracheal (ET) tube.

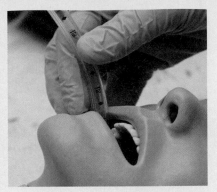

STEP 3 Move the ET tube to the corner of the patient's mouth.

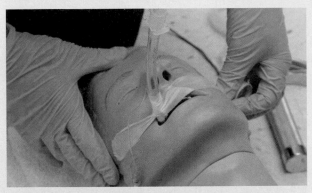

STEP 4 Encircle the ET tube with tape and secure the tape to the patient's maxilla (using tincture of benzoin to facilitate tape adhesion).

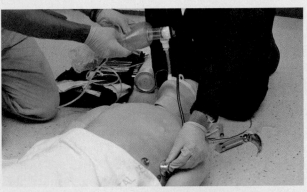

STEP 5 Reattach bag-valve device and auscultate again over the apices and bases of the lungs and over the epigastrium.

Securing an Endotracheal Tube with a Commercial Device

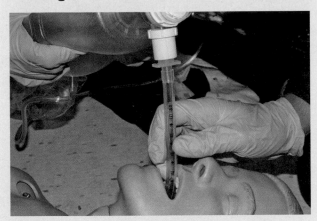

STEP 1 Note the cm marking on the tube at the level of the patient's teeth.

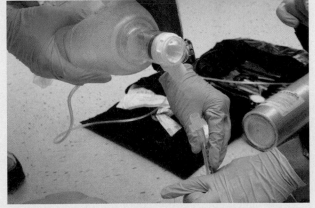

STEP 2 Remove the bag-valve device from the endotracheal tube.

(continues)

SKILL DRILL 4-4 Securing the Endotracheal Tube with Tape (*Continued*)

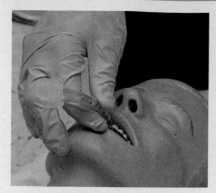

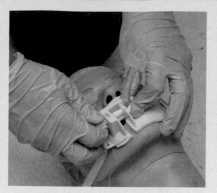

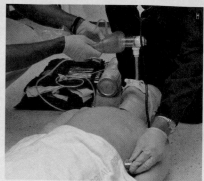

STEP 3 Position the endotracheal tube in the center of the patient's mouth.

STEP 4 Place the commercial device over the endotracheal tube and secure.

STEP 5 Reattach the bag-valve device and auscultate again over the apices and bases of the lungs over the epigastrium.

(**Figure 4-27**). Prior to any suction procedure, remember to preoxygenate the patient preferably for 3 to 5 minutes. By preoxygenating the patient, the clinician minimizes the risk of iatrogenic hypoxic events occurring.

When suctioning the patient, remember that normal saline instillation should be avoided unless you are unable to remove detected secretions. If using saline, instill about 3 to 5 mL and deliver a few breaths to loosen secretions in the airway before suctioning. Instilled fluid is quickly absorbed by the airway mucosa, so additional saline may be needed. Because saline installation is associated with transient deoxygenation, use with caution.

The suction catheter is advanced gently to the proper depth within the airway. The catheter will have incremental markings to provide a guide for depth. Many times, caregivers will attempt to forcefully push the catheter all the way into the tube until only the very end of the catheter connector is left protruding. If the catheter is completely inserted within the ET tube, it is very likely advanced too far into the trachea or it coils at the bifurcation. This aggressive maneuvering may cause airway trauma and bleeding. There is no reason to force excessive length of the suction catheter into the airway. The goal of suctioning is to remove secretions from the trachea, not the mainstem bronchi. The catheter should be introduced to the point of the **carina**, then slightly pulled back, then suction applied. Suction should only be instituted as the clinician is pulling the catheter back, not during advancement. A good rule of thumb for clinicians is to hold their breath when suctioning to help them remember that if they need a breath so does the patient.

Difficult Airways

Body Habitus

Difficult airways will inevitably be encountered. The clinician will have to anticipate and be prepared to deal

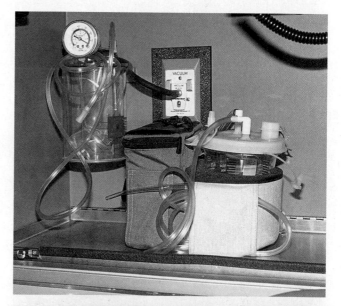

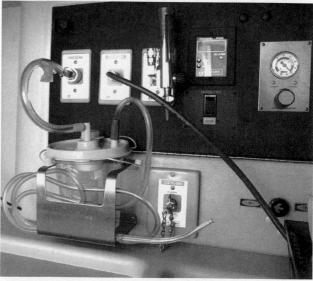

FIGURE 4-27 Vacuum suction devices.

SKILL DRILL 4-5 Performing Tracheobronchial Suctioning

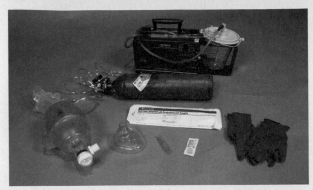

STEP 1 Check, prepare, and assemble your equipment.

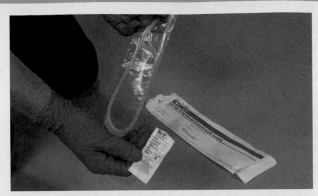

STEP 2 Lubricate the suction catheter (perform this step only for nasotracheal suctioning).

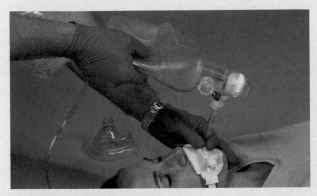

STEP 3 Preoxygenate the patient.

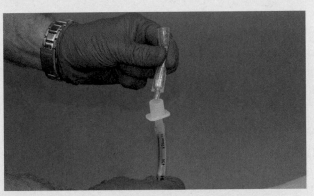

STEP 4 Detach the ventilation device and inject 3 to 5 mL of sterile water down the endotracheal tube (only as indicated).

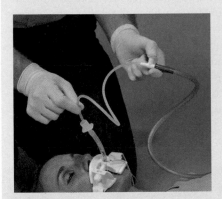

STEP 5 Gently insert the catheter into the endotracheal tube until resistance is felt.

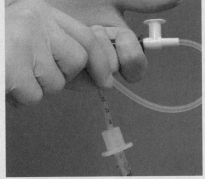

STEP 6 Suction in a rotating motion while withdrawing the catheter. Monitor the patient's cardiac rhythm and oxygen saturation during the procedure.

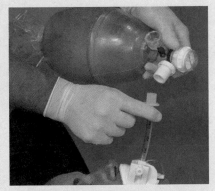

STEP 7 Reattach the ventilation device and resume ventilation and oxygenation.

with emesis, nonstandard patient positions, and head or neck injuries. The upper airway anatomy can be challenging, depending on the body habitus. The clinician should be looking for any signs of trouble and asking these important questions.

1. Does the patient have a large neck?
2. Is the patient obese?

3. Are there obvious anatomical variations that would make establishing an airway difficult?

Head or Neck Injuries

The other important challenge will be those patients who have a head or neck injury. Moving a patient with a neck injury is a difficult task; intubating a patient who has a neck injury may produce more complications. The clinician should ask these questions.

1. Has the patient suffered a traumatic event, motor vehicle accident, or bodily injury involving the neck?
2. Has the patient fallen, struck the head, lost normal color, become diaphoretic, or become unresponsive?

If a patient has been impacted by any of these life-threatening situations, then proper patient positioning is crucial to facilitate quality care and safe transport. Helpful Emergency Medical Services (EMS) guidelines can be referenced at https://www.ems1.com/cms-products/patient-handling/articles/1112498-Patient-positioning-is-a-critical-skill-for-EMS-providers.

Blind Insertions

Airways designed for blind insertions are sometimes an option. Two popular forms of blind insertion airways are discussed next.

Combitube and King

The esophageal tracheal Combitube (Sheridan Catheter Corp., Argyle, NY) is a multilumen airway that works whether it is inserted into the esophagus or into the trachea (**Figure 4-28**). It either blocks the esophagus above and below the glottis or by directly ventilating the trachea. This device is contraindicated in patients under 5 ft tall, under 14 years old, have ingested caustic substances, in patients with esophageal trauma or disease, and in patients with a gag reflex.

Unlike the Combitube, the King Airway (King Systems, Noblesville, IN) will work only if inserted into the esophagus. It is available in three sizes and is limited to patients at least 4 ft tall.

Nasal Intubation

Nasotracheal intubation in general is the procedure of using the ET tube in one of the nares (**Figure 4-29**). The process is completed through the nasopharynx and then through the glottis opening into the trachea through the vocal cords. In general, this works efficiently even though it has been passed a little differently, and not directly through the oral cavity. Typically, this is considered a semiblind type of intubation because it is difficult to see the passage of the end of the ET tube through the vocal cords (unless a laryngoscope or fiberoptic catheter is used). When performing this procedure, use the patient's spontaneous breathing to guide the tube into the trachea. One of the things the clinician is looking for is flashes of humidity within the ET tube as it is passed into the airway. Condensate can be seen inside the tube as moisture accumulates during exhalation.

One of the advantages of the nasal tracheal intubation is that it can be done on a patient who is awake and breathing. This can be done successfully because most of the gag reflex comes from the upper oral cavity in the throat, and by doing the nasal tracheal intubation the clinician bypasses this area.

Contraindications for nasotracheal suctioning include blood clotting abnormalities and patients who are on anticoagulants. This is because the tissue in the naso-pharyngeal area is soft and subject to bleeding. The patient may also have a deviated septum, which would prevent the ability to pass the tube through either nare. It could potentially perforate the naopharyngeal mucosa as well if excessive force is used to maneuver the tube into place. Nasotracheal intubations are usually short term because extended use carries the risk of sinus infections.

Stabilize the tube once it is in place. Note the centimeter marking on the tube at the patient's nare and record the information. Remember, the mark will be different than what would be recorded for an oral intubation. The nasotracheal ET tube marking ranges from 26 to 28 cm (5 to 6 cm longer than the oral ET tube marking.

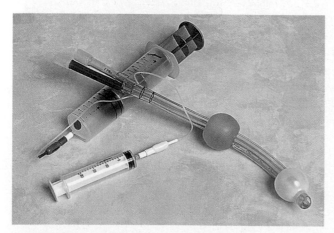

FIGURE 4-28 Combitube.

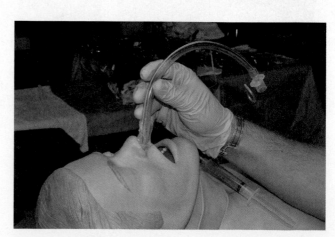

FIGURE 4-29 Nasal intubation.

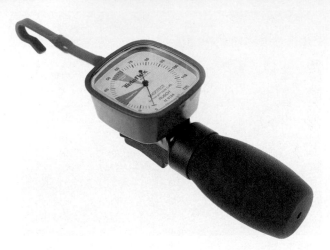

FIGURE 4-30 Cufflator.

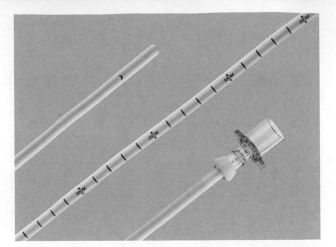

FIGURE 4-31 Cook catheter.

Complications with ET Tube and Cuff

A necessary function of the ET tube cuff is to seal the airway. By providing a seal, the patient's airway is protected by averting leaks and potential aspiration. Catastrophic consequences of ET tube cuff overinflation and inadequate inflation have been reported by Khan et al. (2016). Excessive cuff pressure decreases tracheal capillary perfusion, and insufficient cuff pressure can allow pulmonary aspiration of oropharyngeal content.

The ET tube cuff pressure must be in a range that ensures delivery of the set mechanical tidal volume. The clinician can use a device called the Cufflator (**Figure 4-30**).

By maintaining a proper pressure, the risk for aspiration of secretions that typically accumulate above the cuff is reduced. According to Seegobin and van Hasselt (1984), a cuff pressure of 20 to 30 cm H_2O is recommended for the prevention of aspiration and ventilator-associated pneumonia. The lower cuff pressures lessen the tendency to occlude capillary blood flow in the tracheal tissue and help prevent tissue necrosis. The cuff pressure should be the least amount necessary to ensure a proper seal (even less than 20 cm H_2O if possible).

If the pressure is excessive at the trachea (above 30 cm H_2O), it will result in obstructed mucosal blood flow. This leads to destruction of the columnar epithelium and exposure of the basement membrane, as reported by Khan et al., who also noted that when the standard ET tube cuff was injected with volumes between 2 and 4 mL, this usually produced cuff pressures between 20 and 30 cm H_2O, independent of tube size.

Cook Catheter Exchanger

It is extremely helpful to have a **Cook catheter** available at the bedside (**Figure 4-31**). The catheter is a hollow, semirigid type of tube with blunt tips, which can be used to exchange an ET tube with a leaking cuff. Unlike traditional stylets used to facilitate tube exchange, the Cook catheter airway exchangers are hollow to allow oxygen delivery if necessary. This is possible because of the 15-mm adapter that can be attached to oxygen tubing. They are also available in different size options and materials to accommodate varying clinical needs. Even with proper artificial airway care, there are occasional failures of the material components.

Cook catheters can provide additional safety for follow-up on procedures completed in emergency situations such as cricothyrotomy and transtracheal insertion. The Cook catheter can be used to more quickly and safely restore a patient's airway.

Ventilating Success

Signs of Endotracheal Intubation

An exhaled carbon dioxide detector can aid in determining proper intubation. A nonelectronic version, known as a colorimeter, is a small device attached in line between the ET tube and a manual resuscitator bag. If the chemically treated indicator disc turns yellow, there is a positive confirmation of the presence of carbon dioxide coming from the ET tube. If the color indicator remains purple, there is no confirmation of carbon dioxide production.

The most common limitation to this device is a false negative because of poor cardiovascular perfusion. This occurs frequently in patients in cardiac arrest, hence the reason not to rely on only one method to verify ET tube placement. When the intubation is completed it is important to have a chest x-ray to determine proper insertion depth of the ET tube. Electronic exhaled CO_2 monitors are also available

SKILL DRILL 4-6 Performing End-Tidal CO$_2$ Detection

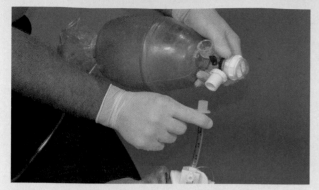

STEP 1 Detach the ventilation device from the endotracheal tube.

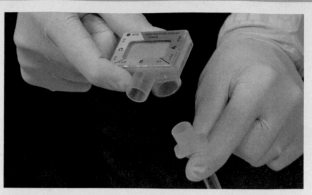

STEP 2 Attach in-line capnograph or capnometer to proximal adaptor of the endotracheal tube.

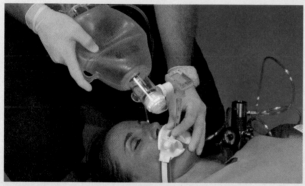

STEP 3 Reattach the ventilation device to the endotracheal tube and resume ventilations.

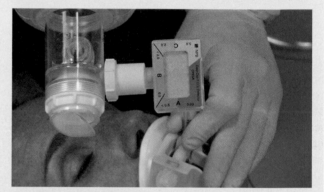

STEP 4 Monitor the capnograph for appropriate reading (appropriate color change or digital reading).

for use during intubation attempts. One handheld example is the EMMA device (Masimo Corporation, Irvine, CA).

Right Main Stem

One common issue occurs when the ET tube is put into place but advanced too far and is placed in the right main stem bronchus (**Figure 4-32**). This would need to be corrected by deflating the cuff slightly and gently pulling the tube back (until tip of ET tube is at least 1 in above the carina) and reflating the cuff, then re-securing the tube.

Signs of Esophageal Intubation

One sign that the ET tube is in the esophagus rather than the trachea is seen when the patient develops progressive hypoxemia and hypoxia that continues in spite of providing 100% oxygen and BVM ventilation. Additional signs are abnormal sounds that may be heard in the abdominal region (epigastric sounds during inspiration), no bilateral chest expansion, abdominal distention, and excessive difficulty ventilating the patient.

If esophageal intubation is not detected early, it may create distracting cardiovascular irregularities that will make it increasingly difficult to judge if the tube is properly placed. When performing intubation, always keep a suspicion of esophageal intubation, especially if the intubation was problematic.

Verification for Ventilation Success

Determining tube placement is important. Utilizing proper assessment skills, the clinician can evaluate the effective application of artificial ventilation (**Table 4-5**).

The standard procedure is to verify satisfactory positioning of the ET tube within the trachea with a chest x-ray. The ET tube tip should be about 1 in (2 to 3 cm) above the carina.

Extubation

Extubation is the process of removing the tube from an intubated patient. One of the main indications that patients are ready to be extubated is their level of consciousness and their ability to participate in some respiratory mechanics maneuvers.

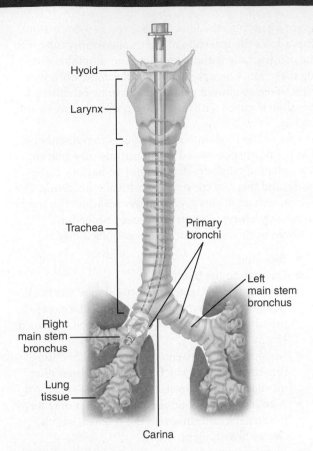

FIGURE 4-32 Right main stem intubation.

Margolis G, American Academy of Orthopedic Surgeons. *Paramedic: Airway Management.* Sudbury, MA: Jones & Bartlett; 2004.

TABLE 4-5
Evaluation of Effective Artificial Ventilation

Signs of Effective Ventilation
- Increasing SpO_2
- Improving skin color
- Increasing level of consciousness
- Adequate chest rise
- Quiet ventilation
- Improving blood gases
- Normalization of heart rate
- Good bilateral breath sounds

Signs of Ineffective Ventilation
- Falling or low SpO_2
- Poor skin color
- Decreasing level of consciousness
- Inadequate chest rise
- Noisy ventilation
- Low PaO_2 and/or high $PaCO_2$
- Abnormal heart rate
- Absent, diminished breath sounds

Margolis G, American Academy of Orthopedic Surgeons. *Paramedic: Airway Management.* Sudbury, MA: Jones & Bartlett; 2004.

Extubation Criteria

According to Sturgess et al. (2017), the patient ready for extubation should have an acceptable respiratory pattern and should be without a great deal of pain. The patient should also have cardiovascular stabilization and proper circulation, which should be satisfactory, and the patient should be stable. The patient should be awake, have adequate neurologic function, and be cooperative. The patient should also be superficially warm and well perfused. The patient should be awake and able to comprehend and communicate by some means. The arterial blood gas values should be acceptable on FIO_2 <0.5. Vital signs should indicate stability, and the arterial oxygen saturation should be greater than 94% (unless the patient has chronic obstructive pulmonary disease [COPD] or another pulmonary disease, then around 90% would be acceptable). The duration of time on mechanical ventilation may alter the criteria for acceptable values related to extubation.

Steps for Extubation

Patients are usually placed upright in a semi-Fowler position, where the head of the bed is raised to a 45-degree angle and the patient's knees are elevated slightly. It is advisable to have a towel available or emesis basin in case the patient vomits (forewarn the patient of the potential for momentary discomfort). Once it has been confirmed that the patient is responsive enough to protect his or her own airway, the clinician can now suction and remove any secretions from the tube. Begin by deflating the cuff, then on the next exhalation remove the tube in one steady, smooth motion.

Signs of Extubation Failure

Major airway and respiratory complications of extubation are common according to Epstein and Ciubotaru. The study conducted an anonymous postal survey of consultant anesthetists to investigate extubation techniques. Their retrospective survey revealed that 37% of anesthetists had experienced postextubation complications in the 3 months leading up to the survey. Laryngeal spasm accounted for 25% of all reported extubation complications. Desaturation was the next most frequently reported complication, which was defined as an SpO_2 of less than 94% and accounted for 22% of all reported complications.

According to Epstein, extubation failure, usually defined as the need for reintubation 24 to 72 hours after planned extubation, ranges from 2% to 25%. Also, decreased peak expiratory flow rates (<60 L/min) and increased sputum volume (>2.5 mL/hour in the 2 to 3 hours prior to extubation) were associated with relative risks for reintubation.

Tracheostomy Tubes

Variations

Tracheostomy tubes are available in a variety of metal and nonmetal materials. Metal tubes are made of silver or stainless steel. Metal is robust, impedes bacteria

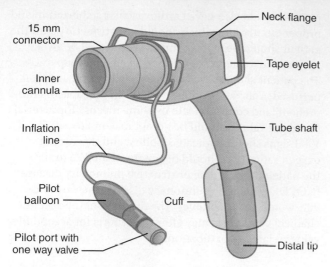

FIGURE 4-33 Components of a tracheostomy tube.

growth, deters biofilm development, is easy to clean, and can be sterilized with heat or steam, which is an advantage over any plastic tracheostomy tube, which would melt under steam. Hess reported that metal tubes are usually not a common prescription product because they are expensive, unbending in the construction, and deficient of a cuff and the usual medical standard 15-mm connector. Without a connector the clinician cannot attach a BVM or a ventilator (a rubber connector can be used if available, but it is less effective). **Figure 4-33** shows the components of a disposable tracheostomy tube.

The most commonly used tracheostomy tubes are made from polyvinyl chloride (PVC), silicone, or polyurethane. The two primary types of PVC and silicone tubes are Shiley (Medtronic, Minneapolis, MS) and Portex (Smiths Medical, Dublin, OH). PVC softens at body temperature, conforming to patient anatomy and centering the tube in the trachea. Silicone is naturally soft and unaffected by temperature, resists colonization and biofilm buildup, and can be sterilized.

Dimensions

The dimensions of tracheostomy tubes are given by their inner diameter, outer diameter, length, and curvature (**Table 4-6**). The sizes of some tubes are given by Jackson size, which was developed for metal tubes and refers to the length and taper of the outer diameter. These tubes have a gradual taper from the proximal to the distal tip.

Tracheostomy

Complications of Tracheostomy

Tracheostomies are generally safe, but they do have risks. Some complications are particularly likely during or shortly after surgery. A rounded-tip obturator is used to pass into the lumen of the tracheostomy tube. This allows the insertion of the tracheostomy tube into the ostomy hole without catching the skin folds during insertion. Once the tube is in place, the obturator is removed to allow a patent airway to be established. It is then secured with a standard tracheostomy tie or anchor.

One of the most important aspects to remember is that if a newly completed tracheostomy tube placement is accidentally dislodged, it will not go back in place easily, and this can constitute a critical emergency. The risk of such problems greatly increases when the tracheotomy is performed as an emergency procedure.

Some of the immediate complications include:

- Bleeding
- Damage to the trachea
- Air trapped in tissue under the skin of the neck (subcutaneous emphysema), which can cause breathing problems and damage to the trachea or esophagus
- Buildup of air between the chest wall and lungs (pneumothorax), which causes pain, breathing problems, or lung collapse
- A collection of blood (hematoma) that may form in the neck and compress the trachea, which causes breathing problems
- Misplacement or displacement of the tracheostomy tube

When a Tracheostomy Should Be Performed

There is some debate over when to perform a tracheostomy partly because it is a surgical procedure and there are risks involved. However, once a patient has been orally or nasally intubated for 7 days, the patient should have the tracheostomy performed according to Durbin. Thus there are differing recommendations on when the conversion to tracheostomy should be performed (3-week time limit according to the American College of Chest Physicians). The implementation requires input from the entire medical team, which includes nursing, respiratory, surgery group, and intensivists, among others. There is no absolute consensus at this time for when to initiate the tracheostomy. The decision will be based on the patient's clinical condition and prognosis.

Performing a tracheostomy is frequently an elective procedure, and there are 4 reasons for performing it. One reason is to relieve upper airway obstruction due to possible infection, obtrusive tissue (such as a tumor), or surgical necessity. A second reason is prolonged intubation, and to prevent laryngeal and upper airway damage due to the excessive duration of endotracheal intubation. A third reason is to allow easy, recurrent access to the lower airway for suctioning and excretion elimination. A final reason is to provide a stable airway in a patient who requires prolonged mechanical ventilation or oxygenation support.

TABLE 4-6
Tracheostomy Tube Measurements

Size	ID (mm)	ID with Inner Cannula (mm)	OD (mm)	Total Length	Proximal Length	Radial Length	Distal Length
Portex Blueline Ultra™ cuffed/uncuffed, fenestrated/non-fenestrated, with/without Suctionaid™							
6.0	6.0	5.0	9.2	64.5	-	-	-
7.0	7.0	6.0	10.5	70.0	-	-	-
8.0	8.0	7.0	11.9	75.5	-	-	-
9.0	9.0	8.0	13.3	81.0	-	-	-
Portex Uniperc™							
7.0	9.3	7.0	11.6	115.0	-	-	-
8.0	10.3	8.0	12.6	125.0	-	-	-
9.0	11.3	9.0	13.6	135.0	-	-	-
Tracoe Twist Plus™ fenestrated/non-fenestrated, with and without subglottic suction							
07	-	7.0	9.8	91.0	-	-	-
08	-	8.0	10.8	95.0	-	-	-
09	-	9.0	11.8	99.0	-	-	-
Shiley™ cuffless non-fenestrated (CFS), cuffless fenestrated (CFN), cuffed non-fenestrated (LPC) and cuffed fenestrated (FEN)							
4	-	5.0	9.4	65.0	-	-	-
6	-	6.4	10.8	76.0	-	-	-
8	-	7.6	12.2	81.0	-	-	-
Shiley XLT™ Distal							
50XLT	-	5.0	9.6	90.0	5.0	37	48.0
60XLT	-	6.0	11.0	95.0	8.0	38	49.0
70XLT	-	7.0	12.3	100.0	12.0	39	49.0
80XLT	-	8.0	13.3	105.0	15.0	40	50.0
Shiley XLT™ Proximal							
50XLT	-	5.0	9.6	90.0	20.0	37.0	33.0
60XLT	-	6.0	11	95.0	23.0	38.0	34.0
70XLT	-	7.0	12.3	100.0	27.0	39.0	34.0
80XLT	-	8.0	13.3	105.0	30.0	40.0	35.0
Shiley™ laryngectomy tube (LGT)							
6	-	6.4	11.1	50.0	-	-	-
8	-	7.6	12.6	50.0	-	-	-

Critical Care Airway Management. Tracheostomy. Retrieved from https://www.ccam.net.au/handbook/tracheostomy

Summary

Multiple areas of competency will be required to successfully care for the patient who is in respiratory failure. The clinician who is most prepared and skilled will be able to provide safe and proper support. The appropriate application and understanding of airway management will mean the difference between survival and death. It is the intention of this chapter to provide the essential foundation for airway management.

In summary, management of the airway is key in the survival of the patient. The clinician must have knowledge of airway management and be competent with the procedure to establish control of the airway. The first step for securing an airway is to properly evaluate the situation, then institute the proper techniques to intervene and avert a crisis. The clinician must have knowledge of airway management and be competent with the procedure to establish control of the airway. A noninvasive airway is limited to placement in the upper airway (does not go below the vocal cords). Conversely, invasive airway support involves any artificial airway that is placed below the vocal cords. The most primary piece of equipment when establishing an invasive airway is the ET tube. A necessary function of the ET tube cuff is to seal the airway. By providing a seal, the cuff protects the patient's airway by averting leaks and potential aspiration. Once the patient is stabilized and the emergent respiratory failure is corrected, then extubation can be performed. One of the main indications that the patient is ready to be extubated is the level of consciousness and the ability to participate in some respiratory mechanics maneuvers. If a patient is going to be intubated for longer than 1 week, there should be some conversation about potentially using a tracheostomy. The implementation requires input from the entire medical team, which includes nursing, respiratory, surgery group, and intensivists, among others. There is no absolute consensus at this time for when to initiate the tracheostomy. The decision will be based on the patient clinical condition and prognosis.

Case Study

Respiratory therapist Sarah is assigned to the emergency department (ED) in a 800-bed hospital. An unconscious patient in room 1 is in respiratory arrest, and endotracheal (ET) intubation is unsuccessful following four different attempts by two individuals. While waiting for anesthesia consult and assistance, the ED physician asks Sarah to place a temporary airway.

1. **What should be a suitable airway alternative for patients needing ET intubation?**

After taking care of the patient in room 1, Sarah is paged to room 4 for an urgent ET intubation on a conscious patient who has been exposed to smoke and chemical inhalation. During preintubation assessment, Sarah asks the patient to open the mouth as wide as possible. She sees a partially exposed glottis and uvula (but no gap between the uvula and tongue).

2. **Based on Sarah's observation, what is the Mallampati classification?**

The nurse asks Sarah what type of medications the patient should receive prior to intubation.

3. **For rapid sequence intubation, name the drugs for (a) neuromuscular blockade and (b) sedation.**

4. **Does the patient require an analgesic?**

Sarah begins assembling the intubation equipment. She notices that the intubation setup includes an assortment of ET tubes and accessories, but with only Miller laryngoscope blades.

5. **Where should Sarah place the tip of the blade during intubation?**

Sarah is paged to the intensive care unit (ICU) to reintubate a mechanically ventilated patient with a leaking ET tube cuff.

6. **What type of special catheter (ET tube exchanger) should Sarah bring with her?**

After exchanging the leaking ET tube with a new one, Sarah performs patient assessment to ensure that the new ET tube has not entered the esophagus.

7. **What are some signs of esophageal intubation?**

Bibliography

Adnet F, Baillard C, Borron SW, et al. Randomized study comparing the "sniffing position" with simple head extension for laryngoscopic view in elective surgery patients. *Anesthesiology.* 2001;95:836–841.

Amathieu R, Combes X, Abdi W, et al. An algorithm for difficult airway management, modified for modern optical devices (Airtraq laryngoscope; LMA CTrach): a 2-year prospective validation in patients for elective abdominal, gynecologic, and thyroid surgery. *Anesthesiology.* 2011;114:25–33.

American College of Chest Physicians. Available at https://www.chestnet.org/Guidelines-and-Resources.

Baillard C, Fosse JP, Sebbane M, et al. Noninvasive ventilation improves preoxygenation before intubation of hypoxic patients. *Am J Respir Crit Care Med.* 2006;174:171–177.

Barker SJ, Tremper KK, Hyatt J. Effects of methemoglobinemia on pulse oximetry and mixed venous oximetry. *Anesthesiology.* 1989;70:112–117.

Bishop MJ, Harrington RM, Tencer AF. Force applied during tracheal intubation. *Anesth Analg.* 1992;74:411–414.

Combes X, Jabre P, Margenet A, et al. Unanticipated difficult airway management in the prehospital emergency setting: prospective validation of an algorithm. *Anesthesiology.* 2011;114:105–110.

Durbin CG Jr. Early complications of tracheostomy. *Respir Care.* 2005a;50:511–515.

Durbin CG Jr. Techniques for performing tracheostomy. *Respir Care.* 2005b;50:488–496.

Durbin CG Jr. Tracheostomy: why, when, and how? *Respir Care.* 2010;55(8):1056–68.

El-Orbany M, Woehlck HJ. Difficult mask ventilation. *Anesth Analg.* 2009;109:1870–1880.

Epstein, SK. Extubation failure: an outcome to be avoided. *Crit Care.* 2004;8:310. doi:10.1186/cc2927

Epstein SK, Ciubotaru RL. Independent effects of etiology of failure and time to reintubation on outcome for patients failing extubation. *Am J Respir Crit Care Med.* 1998;158:489–493.

Epstein SK, Ciubotaru RL, Wong JB. Effect of failed extubation on the outcome of mechanical ventilation. *Chest.* 1997;112:186–192.

Graham DR, Hay JG, Clague J, et al. Comparison of three different methods used to achieve local anesthesia for fiberoptic bronchoscopy. *Chest.* 1992;102(3):704–707.

Henderson JJ, Popat MT, Latto IP, et al. Difficult Airway Society guidelines for management of the unanticipated difficult intubation. *Anaesthesia.* 2004;59:675–694.

Hess DR, Altobelli NP. Respiratory Care. 2014;59(6):956–973. doi:10.4187/respcare.02920

Imberti R, Bellinzona G, Riccardi F, et al. Cerebral perfusion pressure and cerebral tissue oxygen tension in a patient during cardiopulmonary resuscitation. *Intensive Care Med.* 2003;29:1016–1019. doi:10.1007/s00134-003-1719-x]

Isono S, Tanaka A, Ishikawa T, et al. Sniffing position improves pharyngeal airway patency in anesthetized patients with obstructive sleep apnea. *Anesthesiology.* 2005;103:489–494.

Dauphinee K. Nasotracheal intubation. *Emerg Med Clin North Am.* 1988;6:715–723.

Khan MU, Khokar R, Qureshi S, et al. Measurement of endotracheal tube cuff pressure: instrumental versus conventional method. *J Anaesth.* 2016;10:428–431.

Kheterpal S, Han R, Tremper KK, et al. Incidence and predictors of difficult and impossible mask ventilation. *Anesthesiology.* 2006;105:885–891.

Kheterpal S, Martin L, Shanks AM, et al. Prediction and outcomes of impossible mask ventilation: a review of 50,000 anesthetics. *Anesthesiology.* 2009;110:891–897.

Langeron O, Masso E, Huraux C, et al. Prediction of difficult mask ventilation. *Anesthesiology.* 2000;92:1229–1236.

Moore TJ, Walsh CS, Cohen MR. Reported adverse event cases of methemoglobinemia associated with benzocaine products. *Arch Intern Med.* 2004;164:1192–1196.

Mort TC, Waberski BH, Clive J. Extending the preoxygenation period from 4 to 8 mins in critically ill patients undergoing emergency intubation. *Crit Care Med.* 2009;37:68–71.

Novaro GM, Aronow HD, Militello MA, et al. Benzocaine-induced methemoglobinemia: experience from a high-volume transesophageal echocardiography laboratory. *J Am Soc Echocardiogr.* 2003;16:170–175.

Peterson GN, Domino KB, Caplan RA, et al. Management of the difficult airway: a closed claims analysis. *Anesthesiology.* 2005;103:33–39.

Racine SX, Solis A, Hamou NA, et al. Face mask ventilation in edentulous patients: a comparison of mandibular groove and lower lip placement. *Anesthesiology.* 2010;112:1190–1193.

Rouby JJ, Laurent P, Gosnach M, et al. Risk factors and clinical relevance of nosocomial maxillary sinusitis in the critically ill. *Am J Respir Crit Care Med.* 1994;150:776–783.

Rubes D, Klein AA, Lips M, et al. The effect of adjusting tracheal tube cuff pressure during deep hypothermic circulatory arrest: a randomised trial. *Eur J Anaesthesiol.* 2014;31:452–456.

Seegobin RD, van Hasselt GL. Endotracheal cuff pressure and tracheal mucosal blood flow: endoscopic study of effects of four large volume cuffs. *Br Med J (Clin Res Ed).* 1984;288:965–968.

Sturgess DJ, Greenland KB, Senthuran S, et al. Tracheal extubation of the adult intensive care patient with a predicted difficult airway—a narrative review. *Anaesthesia.* 2017;72:248–261. doi:10.1111/anae.13668

Yildiz TS, Solak M, Toker K. The incidence and risk factors of difficult mask ventilation. *J Anesth.* 2005;19:7–11.

CHAPTER

5

Initiating Mechanical Ventilation

Jonathan B. Waugh, PhD, RRT, RPFT, FAARC

© s_maria/Shutterstock

OUTLINE

OBJECTIVES

1. Differentiate between acute ventilatory failure (AVF) and respiratory insufficiency.
2. Differentiate between hypoxemic respiratory failure and hypercapnic respiratory failure.
3. Discuss the causes of acute respiratory failure.
4. Identify the goals of mechanical ventilation.
5. Explain how the need for mechanical ventilation is typically assessed.
6. Describe the benefits associated with using a protocol to initiate mechanical ventilation.
7. Select initial settings for volume and pressure-targeted mechanical ventilation.
8. Differentiate abnormal values from those that indicate the need for ventilatory support for relevant physiologic measurements.
9. Discuss modifications for initial settings for selected special conditions.

KEY TERMS

acute ventilatory failure
alveoloarterial oxygen
  pressure gradient
Biot's respirations
Cheyne-Stokes respirations
I:E ratio
impending ventilatory
  failure

maximal expiratory
  pressure (MEP)
maximal inspiratory
  pressure (MIP)
medical futility
P/F ratio
prophylactic support
therapeutic hyperventilation

Introduction

Purpose of Mechanical Ventilation

Mechanical ventilation is a technology that mimics the natural function of moving gas into and out of the lungs to facilitate the delivery of oxygen and removal of carbon dioxide from the body. The primary function of a mechanical ventilator is to provide ventilation with each breath so that gas exchange can occur at the cellular level. It can also perform secondary functions, but the main indication for mechanical ventilation is insufficient spontaneous breathing. This can result from an excessive breathing effort required, weakened respiratory muscles, disrupted control of respiratory muscles, or inefficiency in gas exchange. Mechanical ventilation is a lifesaving procedure, but it comes with risks that in some cases can be life threatening. This chapter addresses the process for deciding if someone should receive mechanical ventilatory support and the choices of implementation that are available. A systematic approach to selecting initial ventilation settings for oxygenation, ventilation, and acid-base balance is used to minimize hazards and complications. Ventilatory support is adjusted based on assessments of a patient's response (discussed in Chapter 8).

Support Versus Treatment

Mechanical ventilation comes in a variety of forms with the choice of many modes. It is an intervention that supports breathing and not a treatment. It sustains patients so that treatments can be administered to remedy what caused the need for artificial ventilation. When mechanical ventilation is initiated, it is almost always as positive pressure ventilation that pushes a breath into a patient's lungs rather than pulling it into the lungs, as with negative pressure spontaneous breathing. Even when mechanical ventilation is finely tuned to patient needs, it tends to produce stresses and complications that increase with its duration. Various lung protective ventilatory strategies have been proposed, and one of the most accepted is the use of small tidal volume (VT) and appropriate levels of positive end-expiratory pressure (PEEP). This approach has been most thoroughly investigated in patients with acute respiratory distress syndrome (ARDS). All patients requiring ventilatory support should be treated with a gentle, lung protective approach, but that does not mean every patient should be treated the same way.

The greater the difference in transpulmonary pressure during positive pressure ventilation, the more likely patient harm and structural damage will occur. The lower the transpulmonary pressure, the less likely the development of ventilator-induced lung injury. Measuring transpulmonary pressure at the bedside is involved, but the easily obtained plateau pressure (Pplat) measurement can serve as a reasonable indicator of it. Kacmarek (2005) contends that a plateau pressure ≤ 28 cm H_2O is considered acceptable, but some abnormal conditions (decreased thoracic compliance) may tolerate a slightly higher pressure without increased risk. Although ≤ 28 cm H_2O is the preferred upper limit, the lowest possible Pplat generally produces the best outcome. The peak inspiratory pressure (also known as peak airway pressure) should also have boundaries, but it represents the pressure within the upper airway, which is much more resilient than tissue at the alveolar level. There is a link between driving pressure (difference between the peak inspiratory pressure and baseline [PEEP]) and mortality rate. In the study by Esteban and colleagues, a driving pressure difference of >15 cm H_2O increased mortality. Another aspect of lung protective ventilation involves the "open lung" concept that seeks to minimize the injury caused by repetitive opening and closing of unstable lung units. This approach often pairs lung recruiting maneuvers with an appropriate level of PEEP to keep unstable alveoli open, reducing the likelihood of additional lung injury (although some clinicians choose to avoid recruiting maneuvers because of perceived risk of overdistension).

Another aspect of the supportive nature of mechanical ventilation is its use to allow sedation or paralysis for certain procedures (including stabilizing the chest wall with massive flail, chest), and to decrease muscle O_2 consumption to maximize O_2 delivery to the tissues. It can also be used for a limited time period to decrease intracranial pressure resulting from cerebral edema (by inducing hyperventilation to promote cerebral vasoconstriction). The most common causes of respiratory failure leading to mechanical ventilation include hypercapnia and associated respiratory acidosis, severe hypoxemia, and ventilatory muscle dysfunction. The next section explores current concepts on these conditions.

Causes of Ventilatory Failure

Hypercapnic Ventilatory Failure

The primary indication for mechanical ventilation is **acute ventilatory failure**. Attempts to define this precisely in terms of blood gas values are debated, but it is a sudden increase in the $Paco_2$ (>50 to 55 mm Hg or perhaps >55 to 60 mm Hg for chronic obstructive pulmonary disease [COPD]) accompanied by respiratory acidosis with a pH ≤ 7.25. In the COPD patient, mechanical ventilatory support is better indicated by an acute increase in the $Paco_2$ above the patient's normal baseline $Paco_2$ accompanied by a consequent respiratory acidosis. Some COPD patients typically live with a $Paco_2$ value that is well above 50 mm Hg, so the more important indicator is a coincident respiratory acidosis. As important as these values are, the decision to initiate mechanical ventilation cannot be based solely on $Paco_2$ and pH.

Other signs that may be associated with acute ventilatory failure include apnea, bradypnea, and other abnormal patterns. An oxygenation problem such as mild to moderate hypoxemia (Pao_2 <50 to 60 mm Hg or Sao_2 <85% to 90%) does not equate to a ventilatory deficit and therefore does not by itself indicate the need for ventilatory support. If a hypoxemic patient is able to maintain adequate ventilation as determined by the $Paco_2$, then supplemental oxygen (conventional or high flow), continuous positive airway pressure (CPAP), or bilevel positive airway pressure (BiPAP) would be the preferred initial options (selecting the simplest therapy that satisfactorily treats the condition).

Apnea (Trauma, Neuromuscular, Pharmaceutical)

Depression of the central nervous system (CNS) by medications or injury can decrease respiratory drive, leading to reductions in alveolar ventilation. Although gas exchange structures at the alveolar level may be normal, the reduction in ventilation to the alveoli produces accumulation of CO_2 and decreased availability of O_2 within the blood. Initial increases in $Paco_2$ have a stimulatory effect on the respiratory center, but when it reaches 70 mm Hg, it begins to depress the CNS, which further reduces respiratory drive and ventilation. Hypoxemia also occurs during this process and normally acts as a respiratory stimulant when Pao_2 drops to values in the 50s, but the response to hypoxemia is diminished at high $Paco_2$ levels. Abnormal breathing patterns can result from CNS disorders associated with tumors, stroke, or head trauma. Cerebral bleeding from trauma can lead to increased intracranial pressure (ICP), which in turn can compress the respiratory center in the brainstem and alter its function. **Cheyne-Stokes respirations**, **Biot's respirations**, apneustic, and ataxic respirations are some abnormal breathing patterns associated with CNS disorders. CNS disorders can also affect reflex responses of the upper airway, thus an artificial airway may be needed for protection from aspiration.

Patients with head trauma are sometimes provided with intentional hyperventilation at the initiation of mechanical ventilation. This action has a protective effect against cerebral edema that often develops with closed head injury. This "therapeutic" hyperventilation lowers the $Paco_2$ and increases the pH, resulting in reduced cerebral perfusion and therefore reduced ICP (**Figure 5-1**). The body eventually adapts to the reduced $Paco_2$ through renal compensation, so the effect only lasts about 24 hours. Although the rationale behind **therapeutic hyperventilation** seems reasonable, it is not a reason to start it prophylactically or on a head injury patient on mechanical ventilation who otherwise has adequate spontaneous breathing, nor should it be used within the first 24 hours of severe traumatic brain injury (sTBI), when the risk of ischemia is greatest. The Cochrane collaboration concluded that there is insufficient evidence to determine whether hyperventilation therapy in the management of sTBI is beneficial or detrimental. The Brain Trauma Foundation guidelines recommend a brief period of hyperventilation (15 to 30 minutes to target $Paco_2$ 30 to 35 mm Hg) and

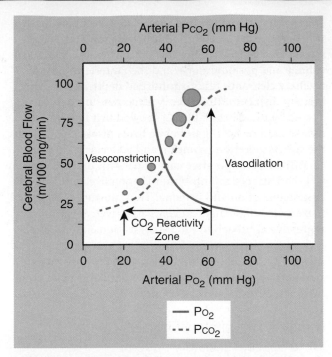

FIGURE 5-1 Effect of arterial CO_2 on cerebral perfusion (blue circles indicate vessel diameter).
Godoy DA, Seifi A, Garza D, et al. Hyperventilation therapy for control of posttraumatic intracranial hypertension. *Front Neurol.* 2017;8. doi:10.3389/fneur.2017.00250

cerebral perfusion pressure (CPP) target of 60 to 70 mm Hg coupled with close oxygenation neuromonitoring as an effective method of controlling intracranial hypertension during the acute phase of sTBI. Therapeutic hyperventilation may have temporary positive effects, but it does not appear to benefit patient outcomes.

Decreased Alveolar Ventilation (Atelectasis, Alveolar Surface Area, Gas Trapping, Muscle Weakness)

Decreased alveolar ventilation can also result from a loss of functional alveoli, which reduces the alveolar surface area available for gas exchange. Surface area loss due to alveolar collapse (atelectasis) is a common complication following procedures involving general anesthesia (particularly thoracic and upper abdominal surgery). Anesthesia gases have a mild inflammatory effect on lung tissue, and the risk of postanesthesia pulmonary edema increases with the duration of anesthesia. Thoracic surgery and cardiopulmonary bypass procedures can result in 50% or more of the lungs being collapsed several hours postsurgery. The effect can be even worse after abdominal surgery, with atelectasis persisting in some cases for several days. Lung recruitment maneuvers and PEEP applied at the conclusion of the procedure are not very effective at improving postoperative oxygenation, so reversal requires continued effort.

Postoperative atelectasis has many possible causes, starting with a weakened diaphragm leading to a reduced functional residual capacity, largely because it does not act as an effective barrier to prevent compression of the lungs by the abdominal organs. Postoperative medications for pain relief tend to suppress tidal volume and periodic sighs, and they interfere with mucociliary clearance. This diminished depth of breathing hinders surfactant function. Multivariate analysis conducted by Bonde et al. (2002) showed that being a current smoker or having ischemic heart disease increased the risk of secretion retention and atelectasis after surgery. Thus, postoperative care of patients on mechanical ventilation warrants a more aggressive approach to lung stabilization and hygiene. Thus, postoperative care of patients on mechanical ventilation warrants a more aggressive approach to lung stabilization and hygiene (airway clearance methods, including endotracheal suctioning should be utilized according to consensus guidelines available at https://www.aarc.org/wp-content/uploads/2014/08/06.10.0758.pdf).

Decreased Respiratory Efficiency (Dead Space, Ventilatory Pattern)

Dead space is the volume of each inspired breath that does participate in gas exchange, due either to the airway volume to conduct gas to the alveoli or mismatching of ventilation and perfusion in the alveolar regions. The dead space to tidal volume ratio (V_D/V_T) is a reasonably good indicator of ventilatory efficiency. Normally V_D/V_T ranges from 0.3 to 0.4 with typical tidal volumes during spontaneous breathing. The V_D/V_T value is expected to increase for patients who are intubated and receiving mechanical ventilation because of the changes in ventilation and lung perfusion that occur with positive pressure breaths. V_D/V_T values of more than 0.6 with mechanically ventilated patients indicate a critical increase in dead space. To compensate, the patient must increase the frequency and/or depth of breathing to maintain adequate gas exchange. Common causes of increased dead space ventilation include pulmonary emboli, pulmonary vascular injury, and diminished pulmonary perfusion. In the past, measurement of the V_D/V_T required the collection of expired gases and a simultaneous $PaCO_2$ value. This procedure was cumbersome and not well tolerated by critically ill patients. Measurement of V_D/V_T can now be performed with far easier noninvasive methods, such as volumetric capnometry. The arterial to end-tidal CO_2 pressure difference ($PaCO_2 - P_{ET}CO_2$) gradient is a simpler but less accurate indicator of V_D/V_T obtained with time-based capnography.

Hypoxemic Respiratory Failure

An oxygenation problem does not usually merit mechanical ventilation unless it is severe and not responsive to supplemental oxygen and CPAP therapy. The $P(A-a)$ O_2 value can be used to determine if respiratory failure is due to lung failure (abnormal alveolocapillary gas exchange) or respiratory pump failure (inadequate alveolar ventilation). The PaO_2/PAO_2 ratio uses the same measurements but shows them as the proportion of the alveolar oxygen that makes it to the capillary blood. The treatment for hypoxemia is based on its cause. Simple $\dot{V}/\dot{Q}$ mismatch typically responds to supplemental oxygen. Intrapulmonary shunting is an indication for mask CPAP therapy, and significantly decreased oxygen carrying capacity (anemia) may require a blood transfusion to improve oxygen content and transport. When hypoxemia is accompanied by an increase in work of breathing (WOB) or a significant respiratory acidosis, mechanical ventilation is required.

Impending Ventilatory Failure

Impending ventilatory failure is a term that means a patient may still be within normal ranges for blood gas values (usually marginal) but is progressing to ventilatory failure because of significant effort required to overcome increased WOB with blood gas values trending toward $PaCO_2 >50$ and pH ≤ 7.25. Usually the vital signs are abnormal due to the excess effort to breathe. Hypoxemia is the first sign of impending ventilatory failure. As the condition worsens, the respiratory system attempts to compensate by increasing minute ventilation. The $PaCO_2$ value may be normal or even low in the beginning when the respiratory muscle strength and endurance are adequate. If the cause of gas exchange deficiency is not corrected in time, respiratory muscles will fatigue and the $PaCO_2$ will rise and the pH will fall. This slow-motion version of ventilatory failure can usually be identified with the early clinical signs, which indicate that a patient has impending ventilatory failure (**Table 5-1**). These include changes in vital signs and physical signs of respiratory distress (anxiety, mouth breathing, nasal flaring, and use of accessory muscles of respiration). To minimize further increases in WOB, patients may utilize a tripod position (lean forward with the elbows resting on a bedside table or hands on the knees). Patients in cardiopulmonary distress may exhibit diaphoresis and may appear flushed, pale, or cyanotic. Signs of cardiac stress due to hypoxemia can include dysrhythmias and initial hypertension changing to hypotension. Advanced stages of ventilatory failure include abnormal breath sounds and paradoxical or abnormal movement of the thorax and abdomen.

Increased Work of Breathing

Normally WOB accounts for less than 5% of the body's total oxygen consumption at rest. Healthy individuals can tolerate temporary increases in WOB but if sustained it can lead to respiratory muscle fatigue. Some abnormal conditions can cause WOB to increase to as much as 40% of total oxygen consumption, usually resulting from increases in airway resistance, decreases in respiratory system compliance, or both. Traumatic injuries can impair the efficiency of breathing (flail chest, pneumothorax), yielding less gas movement for muscle effort. Tiring respiratory muscles lead to smaller, more

TABLE 5-1
Conditions Seen with Hypoxemia and Hypercapnia

Hypoxemia

	Mild to Moderate	Severe
Respiratory	Tachypnea, dyspnea, paleness	Tachypnea, dyspnea, cyanosis
Cardiovascular	Tachycardia, mild hypertension Peripheral vasoconstriction (cool extremities, numbness)	Tachycardia (eventually bradycardia, dysrhythmias) Hypertension (eventually hypotension)
Neurologic	Restlessness, disorientation Headaches, lethargy	Somnolence, confusion, delirium Blurred/narrowed vision Loss of coordination, slowed reactions Impaired judgment, altered personality Loss of consciousness, possible coma

Hypercapnia

	Mild to Moderate	Severe
Respiratory	Tachypnea, dyspnea	Tachypnea (eventually bradypnea)
Cardiovascular	Tachycardia, hypertension, vasodilation	Tachycardia Hypertension (eventually hypotension)
Neurologic	Headaches, drowsiness, dizziness, confusion	Hallucinations, euphoria/irritability Convulsions, unconsciousness, coma
Other	Sweating, skin redness	

frequent breaths (rapid shallow breathing pattern), producing further inefficiency from increased V_D/V_T and ultimately hypoxemia, hypercapnia, and acidosis.

When the diaphragm is exhausted, paradoxical breathing results, meaning the abdomen moves out during exhalation and moves in during inhalation while the chest wall moves out during inhalation and moves in during exhalation. This occurs when tidal breathing is mainly due to accessory muscles of respiration, and the fatigued diaphragm moves passively with changes in intrathoracic pressure. This is the reverse of normal breathing, where the chest wall and abdomen move outward together on inspiration and inward on exhalation.

Prophylactic Support (Shock, Head Injury, Burn Injury, Anesthesia)

Prophylactic support is indicated for patients with clinical conditions that have a high risk of ventilatory failure. This early intervention helps avoid complications due to extensive depletion of oxygen reserve. On rare occasion, a clinician may seek to provide prophylactic ventilatory support to avoid further injury to traumatized organ systems (ensuring sufficient oxygen to tissues and allowing rest and cellular repair). Patients with significant burn injuries have an increased metabolic rate and immune system activity that can benefit from ventilatory support (they also have a risk of developing airway and lung edema that may be difficult to anticipate). Indications for prophylactic ventilatory support are outlined in **Table 5-2**.

TABLE 5-2
Indications for Prophylactic Ventilatory Support

Indication	Examples
Reduce risk of pulmonary complications	Prolonged shock Head injury Smoke inhalation
Reduce hypoxia of major body organs	Hypoxic brain injury Myocardial hypoxia
Reduce cardiopulmonary stress	Prolonged shock Coronary artery bypass surgery Other thoracic or abdominal surgeries

Goals of Mechanical Ventilation

Mechanical ventilation provides ventilatory life support to allow time for determining the cause(s) of respiratory failure and treating the underlying pathology leading to the need for ventilator support. Besides reversing the pathologic condition that necessitated ventilator support, mechanical ventilation can help stabilize body functions (homeostasis), rehabilitate fatigued muscles, and enhance the effect of therapies. A coincident goal of mechanical ventilation is to avoid contributing additional injury and complications. The goals of mechanical ventilation are summarized in **Table 5-3**.

TABLE 5-3
Goals of Mechanical Ventilation

Goal	Target
1. Improve oxygenation and ventilation	Reverse hypoxemia (i.e., Paw), relieve acute respiratory acidosis (i.e., VMIN)
2. Reduce work of breathing, relieve respiratory distress	Reduce oxygen consumption by respiratory muscles, reduce CO_2 production, minimize dead space, reverse respiratory muscle fatigue
3. Improve pulmonary mechanics	Reduce airways resistance (manage secretions and bronchial tone/inflammation), improve compliance($\downarrow$atelectasis with PFFP/diuresis)
4. Permit lung and airway healing	Maintain lung and airway functions (i.e., surfactant production, minimize scar tissue)
5. Minimize damage to the lung and airways	Protect lung and airway (esp. minimize repetitive alveolar collapse/expansion), maintain respiratory muscle strength

Modified from Lodeserto F, Simplifying mechanical ventilation – Part 2: goals of mechanical ventilation & factors controlling oxygenation and ventilation, REBEL EM. 2019. Available at https://rebelem.com/simplifying-mechanical-ventilation-part-2-goals-of-mechanical-ventilation-factors-controlling-oxygenation-and-ventilation/; Tobin MJ. Mechanical ventilation. *N Engl J Med.* 1994;330(15):1056–1061.

Improve Gas Exchange

It may be appropriate to start mechanical ventilation on F_{IO_2} of 1.0 in emergent and extreme hypoxic situations. There is no danger from short-term use of a high level of inspired oxygen. Because blood gases will be analyzed soon after commencing mechanical ventilation, the patient's response to 100% oxygen concentration can provide useful diagnostic information to guide therapy. Poor Pao_2 increase to 100% oxygen indicates intrapulmonary shunting and the need for PEEP while the cause of the shunt can be investigated (i.e., pneumonia, heart failure, atelectasis, and pulmonary embolism). In some patients, PEEP causes no improvement or even a decrease in Pao_2. This effect is the result of increased dead space ventilation, diversion of blood flow from well-ventilated to unventilated regions, and decreased cardiac output (especially with hypovolemia). The effect of PEEP should be assessed in terms of oxygen delivery (or mixed venous Po_2 may serve as a substitute) because of its potential to reduce perfusion. While PEEP often improves oxygenation in many disease conditions, it can be very risky to implement with status asthmaticus patients due to air trapping concerns (some may benefit, but it varies by patient). Other interventions may be considered to improve hypoxemic respiratory failure, such as antibiotics for infections, diuretics for pulmonary edema, and inotropic medications to treat heart failure. The most difficult patients to ventilate (e.g., ARDS) may be treated with highly specialized therapies, such as nitric oxide supplementation, and prone positioning to enhance oxygenation. These strategies can increase oxygenation in patients with ARDS on a temporary basis, but none has improved patient outcome.

The goal of mechanical ventilation in patients with hypercapnic respiratory failure is to improve alveolar ventilation. This goal is more difficult to achieve in patients with a prolonged expiratory time requirement (COPD and asthma). Insufficient time for alveolar emptying leads to dynamic hyperinflation from gas trapping. Using small tidal volumes to shorten the time requirement for alveolar emptying may not achieve adequate alveolar ventilation because physiologic dead space is increased (less efficiency in ventilation). Some clinicians attempt to deliver adequate alveolar volumes and sufficient time to empty them by increasing ventilator inspiratory flow. The increase in flow decreases the time needed for inspiration; if respiratory frequency remains constant, this allows more time for exhalation.

Neuromuscular disorders, such as spinal cord injury, can cause hypercapnic respiratory failure, but these patients typically have normal lung mechanics so they are easier to ventilate than most other disease conditions. Perhaps the greater risk is excessive artificial ventilation that can cause complications, such as respiratory alkalosis, decreased cerebral perfusion, and cardiovascular instability. The negative consequences are amplified if a state of hypercapnia existed immediately prior to a swing toward alkalosis. When severe, alkalosis is occasionally associated with coronary artery spasm, confusion, myoclonus (muscle twitching), asterixis (hand tremor), and seizures.

Relieve Respiratory Distress

Connecting a patient to a ventilator and providing ventilator assistance should unburden the respiratory muscles and hopefully reduce muscle stress. A way to determine the desirable level of unburdening (and for how long) has not been identified for individual patients. Too much ventilatory support causes respiratory muscle atrophy and neurologic alterations, and insufficient support can lead to stress and fatigue. Although most patients in acute respiratory failure have increased work of breathing, there are often other coexisting problems contributing to physiologic and psychological aspects of respiratory distress. Most patients also have abnormal gas exchange, impaired muscle perfusion, and sepsis-induced muscle dysfunction. Unburdening patients of increased work of breathing by means of mechanical ventilation is intended to reduce O_2 consumption and CO_2 production, improving hypoxemia and hypercapnia, and hopefully feelings of discomfort. Using mechanical ventilation to rest the respiratory muscles and allow for sedation can help calm output of the sympathetic nervous system and improve tissue perfusion (especially helpful for patients suffering from shock).

Improve Pulmonary Mechanics

The application of PEEP with mechanical ventilation can do more than improve oxygenation. Lungs at risk for atelectasis can be stabilized with PEEP, but low-level

PEEP is not much help for reversing atelectasis that has already occurred. However, various interventions can help reclaim functional lung tissue and then PEEP can be used to help prevent it from collapsing again. Using PEEP to keep more alveoli open allows each breath to be distributed to more areas of the lungs. This is, in essence, like having larger lungs, which increases the compliance of the respiratory system. The improved compliance lowers the pressure required for the ventilator to deliver a breath and translates to a lower work of breathing for any spontaneous breaths taken by a patient.

Permit Lung and Airway Healing

Properly applied ventilatory support can minimize stress and rest respiratory muscles to allow for healing. Too much support can cause muscle atrophy and trauma from applied pressure and/or volume. Too little support can lead to lung stress and strain, especially when lung injury is severe. Injured lungs are also susceptible to another source of damage termed *pendelluft*. This occurs when strong spontaneous effort causes breath volume to shift from stable alveoli to unstable alveoli (usually in the dependent lung regions) at early inspiration. At the end of inspiration, the unstable alveoli collapse; if this cycle of opening and closing continues, it may lead to further lung injury. In this scenario, higher PEEP may stabilize the alveolar regions that are prone to collapse with tidal breathing and permit safer conditions for spontaneous breathing.

Avoid Complications

The potential hazards and complications associated with mechanical ventilation have been reported by many sources in the medical literature. They are categorized as shown in **Table 5-4**. Positive pressure ventilation distributes breath volume differently than spontaneous breathing, which can cause inflation injuries and alter cardiovascular function. Patient conditions, such as organ dysfunction/failure, can be aggravated by the stress of being on mechanical ventilation, and the risk of infection increases with duration of mechanical ventilation. Mishandling or maintenance of the ventilator, patient circuit, humidification, and artificial airway can result in many serious consequences. Injuries can arise from accidents or inappropriate care by clinicians (iatrogenic injuries), with cross-contamination among patients being one of the most serious and costly in terms of patient suffering and financial expense.

Barotrauma

Volutrauma is a term used to describe lung tissue injury or rupture that results from alveolar overdistention. *Barotrauma* is a term used to describe tissue injury that results from significant pressure differences within the body. It is assumed that volutrauma occurs with lung barotrauma, but volutrauma can occur even when ventilating pressures are within acceptable ranges if

TABLE 5-4
Hazards and Complications of Mechanical Ventilation

Condition	Examples
Positive pressure ventilation	Barotrauma (pneumothorax and other gas leaks) Hypotension, diminished cardiac output, dysrhythmia Oxygen toxicity (with extended duration FIO_2 >0.5) Bronchopleural fistula Bronchopulmonary dysplasia (in infants) Upper gastrointestinal hemorrhage
Related to patient condition	Infection (due to reduced immunity) Physical and psychological trauma Multiple organ failure (may be preexisting)
Related to equipment (ventilator and artificial airway)	Malfunction of ventilator or alarms Accidental patient disconnection or extubation Main stem bronchus intubation Endotracheal tube blockage Tissue damage (related to artificial airway/interface) Atelectasis (due to inadequate tidal volume)
Related to medical professionals	Hospital-acquired pneumonia (cross-contamination) Inappropriate ventilator settings Errors from poor understanding and communication

abnormal lung conditions exist. PIPs greater than 50 cm H_2O appear to increase the risk of barotrauma, but this is likely contingent upon the associated plateau pressure (Pplat). Bezzant and Slutsky reported that Pplat >35 cm H_2O, mean airway pressures >30 cm H_2O, and PEEP >10 cm H_2O may increase the risk of barotrauma. The risk of barotrauma also increases with the duration of positive pressure ventilation. Barotrauma may still occur below the stated pressure thresholds, they simply represent thresholds at which risk significantly increases. Patients with weakened parenchymal areas (such as lung blebs and bullae that may occur with COPD) or reduced lung tissue due to lobectomy or pneumonectomy are at greater risk for barotrauma. Other forms of barotrauma that may result from positive pressure ventilation include pulmonary interstitial emphysema, pneumomediastinum, pneumoperitoneum, pneumothorax, tension pneumothorax, and subcutaneous emphysema. In addition to barotrauma, air leaks within the lung parenchyma (interstitial emphysema) may occur.

Decrease in Cardiac Output and Blood Pressure

The most common hemodynamic instability associated with mechanical ventilation is cardiac embarrassment (hypotension due to decreased cardiac output). Application of positive pressure to chest by way of the lungs decreases venous return. There is a very small pressure gradient between the venous system and the right atrium to promote blood return to the heart. As the lungs are pressurized by positive pressure ventilation they press upon the surrounding tissues in the chest, including the heart. This squeezing of the heart raises the pressure within its chambers, including the central venous pressure (CVP; pressure within the vena cava and right atrium). The increase in CVP reduces the pressure gradient between the vena cava and right atrium, causing a decrease in cardiac output. Increases of the mean airway pressure have a greater detrimental effect on venous return and cardiac output than increases of the peak inspiratory pressure alone.

A patient with normal cardiovascular function and blood volume can compensate for small decreases in venous return and maintain cardiac output and blood pressure. Two compensatory mechanisms include an increased heart rate and systemic arterial vasoconstriction initiated by the cardiac baroreceptors. The magnitude of the increase in the CVP and the resultant decrease in venous return depends on how much of the positive pressure from mechanical ventilation is transmitted from the lungs to the intrathoracic space. The effect of the magnitude of airway pressure (best represented by mean airway pressure) is either increased or decreased depending on the patient's lung and chest wall compliances. Although lung and chest wall compliances both contribute to respiratory system compliance, they have opposite effects on intrathoracic pressure and venous return. Reduced lung compliance (stiff lungs) does not transmit ventilating (airway) pressure to the rest of the thorax. Therefore, although it is possible for low lung compliance conditions (such as ARDS) to experience significant decreases in venous return due to positive pressure ventilation, the reduction will likely not be as much as with normal lung compliance. The opposite is true with the example of more compliant lungs (COPD) that tend to transmit more of the airway pressure to the pleural space.

A reduced chest wall compliance puts the heart in the proverbial position of being between a "rock and a hard place." Reduced chest wall compliance means that the borders of the rib cage do not expand as easily as they should. In this situation, positive pressure ventilation causes the lungs to squeeze the heart against the rib cage, which does not give way as it normally would. This magnifies the adverse effect of positive pressure ventilation on venous return. Conditions in which the chest wall would be less compliant than normal include use of tight chest wall bandages, extensive chest wall burn injury, and increased intra-abdominal pressure from peritonitis.

Unintentional gas trapping is a possible consequence of positive pressure ventilation that results in auto-PEEP, another potential contributor to hypotension. All ventilator patients must be monitored for signs of cardiovascular instability; however, those with increased lung compliance, decreased chest wall compliance, or suspected or known preexisting cardiovascular disease are at greater risk for cardiac consequences and may require more frequent and thorough assessment.

Malfunction and Misuse of Alarms

Founded as Emergency Care Research Institute, the ECRI Institute is an international organization dedicated to patient safety that listed fatalities from missed alarms and injuries from failure to appropriately operate intensive care ventilators as two of the top 10 technology hazards for 2016. Federal safety reports indicated that from 2005 to 2011, at least 119 people died in the United States because of ventilator alarm-related problems, and the U.S. Food and Drug Administration reported about 800 alarm-related adverse events involving ventilator patients in the year 2010 alone. Causes of alarm-related adverse events can include incorrectly setting (or turning off) alarms, no alarm was available for certain disconnections, alarm testing was not performed, or response to an alarm was delayed or absent. Regular preventive maintenance and testing of alarm systems on ventilators and monitors should be ensured by routine auditing of departmental practices. The alarms must also be sufficiently audible with respect to the room design, distance, and noise level of the immediate patient care area. Overdependence on alarms should be avoided, and emphasis should be placed on frequent direct observation and assessment of the patient–ventilator system. Alarm fatigue is a growing concern, and steps should be taken to avoid it based on the unique context of each type of care environment.

Assessment of Need for Mechanical Ventilation

Predisposing Conditions

There are a multitude of disease states and conditions that may require mechanical ventilation. Some of the most common are categorized in **Table 5-5** (some conditions may fit under more than one category, regardless if shown). Many of the conditions with the potential to require mechanical ventilation depend on the severity of presentation. Even a condition such as a permanent cervical spine injury depends on the specific cervical vertebrae at which the injury occurred to determine the degree of support necessary. ARDS is often a serious lung condition with a high mortality rate, but not all cases (as defined by the Berlin definition) require mechanical ventilation. Despite the uncertainty, it is valuable to know what conditions have a high potential for requiring mechanical ventilation so proper monitoring and preparation can be planned. It should also be noted that short periods of intubation for secretion removal and airway stabilization may not require initiation of mechanical ventilation. However, prolonged use of an endotracheal tube will most likely require invasive ventilatory assistance.

Failure of Other Interventions to Avoid Invasive Ventilation

Other forms of support that can safely take the place of mechanical ventilation should be considered because

TABLE 5-5
Conditions That May Lead to Invasive Mechanical Ventilation

1. Apnea or impending respiratory arrest
   - Pneumothorax, trauma, shock, severe burns, near-drowning, sepsis
   - Severe asthma (unresponsive to treatment)
   - Phrenic nerve injury, diaphragmatic dysfunction
   - Drug overdose, general anesthesia, atelectasis

2. Exacerbation of chronic obstructive pulmonary disease (COPD) with dyspnea, tachypnea, and acute respiratory acidosis plus at least one of the following:
   - Acute cardiovascular instability
   - Altered mental status or persistent uncooperativeness
   - Inability to protect the lower airway
   - Copious or unusually viscous secretions
   - Abnormalities of the face or upper airway that would prevent effective noninvasive ventilation (NIV)

3. Acute ventilatory insufficiency in cases of neuromuscular disease accompanied by any of the following:
   - Acute respiratory acidosis (hypercapnia and decreased arterial pH)
   - Progressive decline in vital capacity to below 15 mL/kg predicted body weight (PBW)
   - Progressive weakening of maximal inspiratory pressure (MIP) (more positive than -20 cm H_2O)

4. Acute hypoxemic respiratory failure with tachypnea, respiratory distress, and persistent hypoxemia despite administration of a high fraction of inspired oxygen (FIO_2) with high flow oxygen devices or in the presence of any of the following:
   - Altered mental status
   - Acute respiratory distress syndrome (ARDS), severe pneumonia, pulmonary edema
   - Pulmonary embolism
   - Inability to protect the lower airway

5. Need for endotracheal intubation to maintain or protect the airway or to manage secretions, given the following factors:
   - Dyspnea, acute respiratory distress, upper airway obstruction
   - Exacerbation of COPD
   - Acute hypoxemic respiratory failure in immunocompromised patients
   - Traumatic brain injury
   - Flail chest

Modified from Karcz M, Vitkus A, Papadakos PJ, et al. State-of-the-art mechanical ventilation. *J Cardiothorac Vasc Anesth.* 2012;26(3):486-506; Pierson DJ. Indications for mechanical ventilation in adults with acute respiratory failure. *Respir Care.* 2002;47:249-262; Shapiro BA. *Clinical Application of Respiratory Care.* 4th ed. St. Louis: Mosby Year Book; 1991.

they may reduce the hazards and complications experienced by patients. Consider the simplest modality that satisfactorily treats the patient's condition. Mechanical ventilation can certainly treat severe hypoxemia, but if a patient has spontaneous breathing sufficient to maintain an acceptable $Paco_2$ then CPAP therapy may be worth trying first. CPAP is the first treatment to attempt with sleep apnea patients, reserving bilevel ventilation only if CO_2 retention is present. In addition, CPAP can be used to assist patients with COPD who have difficulty breathing. Spontaneously breathing COPD patients often have air trapping that results from early small airway collapse during exhalation. In many cases external CPAP can counterbalance the lung pressure, compressing small

airways and allowing them to remain open longer for greater alveolar emptying. This improves CO_2 removal and, though it is not a form of ventilation, it is enhances ventilation. Reducing gas trapping also decreases auto-PEEP, which lowers effort a patient has to generate for each breath, reducing diaphragmatic work and dyspnea.

Noninvasive ventilation (NIV) is often described as an intermediate step between oxygen/CPAP therapy and invasive ventilation. A newer intermediate step to be considered before NIV is the high flow nasal cannula (HFNC) (**Figure 5-2**). This device is able to deliver as much or higher inspired oxygen as oxygen masks to treat hypoxia but with greater comfort. At the higher end of the HFNC flow range (>30 L/min) a small amount of incidental CPAP is typically generated (<5 cm H_2O) but even more significant is its ability to flush exhaled gas from the anatomic dead space of the upper airway. This effectively reduces dead space ventilation and increases the efficiency of ventilation, making a patient's spontaneous breathing more effective.

Although NIV is not able to achieve the peak inspiratory pressures of invasive ventilation, it can be therapeutic for some patients and has fewer risks and complications than invasive positive pressure (and it avoids endotracheal intubation). NIV is the treatment of choice for acute-on-chronic ventilatory failure unless cardiovascular instability is present. The use of NIV for acute-on-chronic ventilatory failure has been shown to reduce the need for intubation, reduce complications of ventilation, shorten the hospital stay, and reduce hospital mortality rates. NIV is not for apneic patients, those requiring high ventilating pressures or when protection of the airway is needed.

Contraindications and Patient Advance Directive

The absolute contraindication for positive pressure ventilation is untreated tension pneumothorax. Other potential contraindications for mechanical ventilation are considered "relative" because they are contingent upon each patient's condition and circumstances. Campbell and Carlson. cited three considerations in which mechanical ventilation should not be started or in some cases may be withdrawn. They are based on (1) patient's informed request, (2) medical futility, and (3) reduction or termination of patient pain and suffering.

The meaning or legal definition of patient's informed request (consent) varies from state to state. In general, it means that a patient must be made aware of the potential benefits, risks, and alternatives involved with a medical procedure before and give written approval for it to be done. It is often explained and obtained by the individual who will order or perform the procedure but not always. Sometimes a family member, friend, or other individual legally empowered to give consent will act in a patient's place. Procedures that are routine and low risk typically do not require patient consent. Sometimes

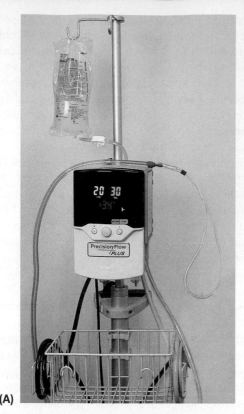

(A)

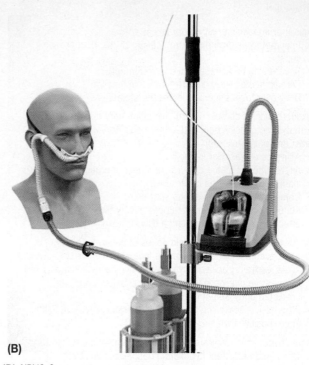

(B)

FIGURE 5-2 High flow nasal cannula devices. **(A)** Precision Flow Plus; **(B)** AIRVO 2

(A) Courtesy of Vapotherm Inc. (B) Courtesy of Fisher & Paykel Healthcare.

emergency conditions do not allow time to obtain consent. When in doubt, it is best to inquire from a knowledgeable colleague or risk management staff member. To protect both patients and caregivers, a protocol should be used to guide the process for deciding if ventilatory support should be started or discontinued.

Schneiderman et al. (1990) suggested that medical intervention may be futile if the clinicians have concluded that intervention was useless in the last 100 similar cases. Although this is one of the most commonly cited definitions of **medical futility**, it is not a law, nor has it been shown to be superior to other definitions. There is always uncertainty when it comes to making decisions about life support measures, including mechanical ventilation. The weight of the decision when deciding for another person is very great, even when the decision may seem straightforward. It is easier (legally and otherwise) to not begin mechanical ventilation than to withdraw it after it has been started (i.e., discovering an unconscious patient did not want it in an emergency situation). Patients with end-stage pulmonary fibrosis will at some point have a discussion with their clinician about whether they want to utilize mechanical ventilation near the end of their life or decline it. This often takes more than one conversation to come to a decision. It is a great help to family to know what a patient wants with regard to life support care.

A much less clear contraindication for mechanical ventilation is to reduce or terminate patient pain and suffering. This type of decision is best made with the input of knowledgeable professionals (medical, counseling, spiritual) who help inform but not decide. Discomfort alone is generally not viewed as sufficient cause on which to base such a decision, as powerful and sophisticated pain relief measures thankfully are available. Typically, a terminal condition is expected (i.e., multiorgan failure) for consideration (brain death may be another but it is not always certain). When discussing with family who is responsible for the decision, it sometimes helps to ask if the situation is extending the possibility of life or delaying death. Providing understandable explanations of the patient's condition and what is involved with ventilator support are very helpful to people making a decision. It must also be made clear that mechanical ventilation is a supportive measure, not a curative procedure.

Spontaneous Breathing Parameters

The spontaneous breathing parameters have poor predictive power for determining impending ventilatory failure and readiness to wean from mechanical ventilation but are still commonly used today. Even the best single predictors such as rapid shallow breathing index (RSBI or f/V_T) should be used in conjunction with other indicators. Progression to impending ventilatory failure is dependent on the ventilatory load (work of breathing) borne by a patient and the metabolic and physical capacity to handle that load. When work of breathing exceeds patient capacity, impending ventilatory failure is likely. Assessment of impending ventilatory failure relies on measurements related to the lung functions (i.e., tidal volume, frequency, minute volume, vital capacity, maximal inspiratory pressure). Although the spontaneous breathing parameters are used to estimate if a patient is capable of spontaneous breathing, the criteria for impending ventilatory failure can differ slightly from weaning criteria. That is because one is considering moving to ventilatory support and the other is considering leaving it, and that alters perspective of patient risk.

The order of measurement for the weaning parameters is important. The minute volume and frequency are recorded during resting ventilation, so they should be done first. The average tidal volume is calculated by dividing the minute volume by the frequency. Vital capacity requires momentary maximal effort, and if a passing value is achieved on the first effort there is no need to unnecessarily tire the patient by repeating it. Maximal inspiratory pressure is a sustained maximal effort and should be done last so it does not affect the other values. To be an accurate measure, the patient airway should be occluded continuously for a full 20 seconds unless it is agreed that the attempt can be ended early if any passing value is achieved.

Tidal Volume (Vτ)

A spontaneous tidal volume less than 3 to 5 mL/kg predicted body weight (PBW) is indicative of impending ventilatory failure. The range indicates uncertainty about what the threshold should be. A policy for monitoring patients suspected of impending ventilatory failure should specify the institutional criterion for this measure so there is consistency in patient care and decision making.

Frequency (f)

A spontaneous frequency greater than 30 breaths/min may indicate impending ventilatory failure, particularly when signs of increased work of breathing are present. Some clinicians prefer a threshold of 35 breaths/min, but the combination of frequency and tidal volume is a more powerful predictor (see f/Vτ ratio in the pulmonary mechanics section that follows).

Minute Volume (V̇E)

If the patient requires a spontaneous minute volume of greater than 10 L/min to achieve or maintain normal blood gases, impending ventilatory failure is likely. An increasing minute volume requirement is a sign of air hunger and increased work of breathing. The additional effort required will eventually fatigue the respiratory muscles, which can lead to eventual ventilatory failure. An increased minute volume achieved by a rapid shallow breathing pattern is less efficient because decreased tidal volumes mean a larger percentage of each breath is dead space (wasted) ventilation. This condition consumes more oxygen and produces more carbon dioxide, and this increases the burden on the patient's cardiopulmonary system.

Vital Capacity (VC)

If the patient's vital capacity is less than 15 mL/kg PBW, then impending ventilatory failure is likely. Measurement of vital capacity requires patient cooperation, which may be difficult to achieve during impending ventilatory failure. The maximal inspiratory pressure measurement can be used as an alternative if the patient is unable to perform the vital capacity maneuver. A measurement protocol does not have to require that all spontaneous breathing parameters have passing values.

Maximal Inspiratory Pressure

The **maximal inspiratory pressure (MIP)** is a measure of inspiratory muscle strength reflecting the patient's pulmonary reserves. It is obtained by measuring the maximum negative pressure that the patient can generate with a forced inspiratory maneuver against a negative manometer (pressure measuring device). Although the MIP maneuver can be performed using a facemask, a mouthpiece or mouth seal is often used (nose clips may be needed). If an artificial airway is in place, MIP can be measured by using a T-piece with one port attached to the endotracheal or tracheostomy tube, one port attached to the negative pressure manometer, and one port attached to a one-way valve that allows exhalation only. Although patients are often encouraged to exhale to residual volume, most patients do not require it and it may promote the development of atelectasis. Encourage inhalation to be as forceful as possible, but realize that even comatose patients can achieve passing results if the airway remains occluded for a full 20 seconds. Patients with a MIP of at least −25 cm H_2O obtained within 20 seconds can be assumed to have a vital capacity of 15 mL/kg PBW. MIP levels between 0 and −20 cm H_2O are consistent with impending ventilatory failure.

Blood Gases

Paco₂ Trend

A gradual but persistent increase of the Pa_{CO_2} to more than 50 mm Hg is indicative of impending ventilatory failure. The Pa_{CO_2} measurement should be done over a period of time and on an as-needed basis. The Pa_{CO_2} should be interpreted along with the patient's breathing pattern, as progressive tachypnea is common during impending ventilatory failure. End-tidal CO_2 (Et_{CO_2}) is a helpful noninvasive measurement of exhaled CO_2 that serves as an indicator of arterial CO_2 but not a direct substitute. It has the advantage of continuous monitoring and is arguably the quickest detector of apnea and hypoventilation.

Severe Hypoxemia

Hypoxemia is a common finding in lung diseases. When hypoxemia is severe, mechanical ventilation may be necessary to support the oxygenation deficit. ARDS, pulmonary edema, and carbon monoxide poisoning are examples that often require ventilatory support for the primary purpose of oxygenation. Hypoxemia can be assessed by measuring the PaO_2, or the **alveoloarterial oxygen pressure gradient** $(P(A - a)O_2)$. Severe hypoxemia is present when the PaO_2 is less than 60 mm Hg on 50% or more of inspired oxygen or less than 40 mm Hg at any FIO_2. $P(A-a)O_2$ is the difference of the PAO_2 and the PaO_2. The normal $P(A-a)O_2$ when breathing 21% oxygen should be less than 4 mm Hg for every 10 years of age. On 100% oxygen, every 50 mm Hg difference in the $P(A - a)O_2$ approximates 2% shunt.

Patients with ARDS have three common clinical manifestations: acute onset, bilateral infiltrates on frontal chest radiograph, and normal pulmonary artery occlusion pressure (PAOP) of ≤18 mm Hg. The distinguishing feature separating the severity of ARDS is the degree of hypoxemia or PaO_2/FIO_2 (P/F) ratio. The threshold for mild ARDS (formerly ALI) is a P/F value ≤300 mm Hg. For moderate and severe ARDS, the P/F thresholds are ≤200 mm Hg and ≤100 mm Hg, respectively (Berlin definition). Because severe hypoxemia is the hallmark of ARDS, the **P/F ratio** can be used to assess the degree of hypoxemia in critically ill patients. A summary of ventilation and oxygenation critical values is given in **Table 5-6**.

Hemodynamic Measurements

Hypercapnia and hypoxemia can each cause increases in sympathetic nervous system activity (greater effect if together), leading to hyperpnea and increases in heart rate and systemic blood pressure. Hypercapnia usually produces a greater effect on blood pressure than hypoxemia. The heart rate response to hypercapnia is less in elderly patients. Apnea amplifies the sympathetic activity produced by hypercapnia, and more so with hypoxemia.

Hypercapnia not only has a sympathetic vasoconstrictor effect to shunt blood to the body core but also has a direct vasodilator effect on some systemic arterioles (such as superficial facial vessels), which produces the skin "flush" often seen in these patients (lesser of the two effects). Hypercapnia causes vasodilation in the brain (proportional to the degree of hypercapnia). Like systemic perfusion, cerebrovascular reactivity to CO_2 depends on age.

Pulmonary Mechanics

The RSBI (f/V_T) is one of the most powerful single indicators of the sustainability of spontaneous breathing. The seminal study by Yang and Tobin reported a threshold value of 105 (breaths/minute/L), above which spontaneous breathing was unlikely to succeed unless conditions changed. Since then, the critical value is often rounded to 100, and it seems to make little difference in outcomes.

Maximal expiratory pressure (MEP) is the expiratory version of the MIP but does not have such stringent measurement requirements. The value is more indicative of cough strength and so is not often included in the monitoring of impending ventilatory failure.

Protocols
Evidence-Based Approach and Clinician-Driven Protocol

Evidence-based protocols are preferred when sufficient evidence is available. Even protocols based on expert consensus opinion can be of some benefit for helping to ensure more consistency in care and standards for monitoring and assessment. An example of clinician-driven protocol is shown in **Table 5-7**. It is not uncommon for specialized care units within the same institution to have different protocols for mechanical ventilation based on patient attributes and diseases.

Initial Settings

When it becomes necessary to provide mechanical ventilatory support for a patient, the following basic ventilator settings must be determined: mode, frequency, tidal volume, FIO_2, inspiratory: expiratory ratio, inspiratory flow pattern, and various alarm limits. These initial

TABLE 5-6
Ventilation and Oxygenation Critical Values

Criteria	Normal Values	Critical Values
Ventilation		
pH	7.35–7.45	≤7.25
$PaCO_2$ mm Hg	35–45	>50 (higher for COPD)
V_D/V_T	0.3–0.4	>0.6
f/V_T	<40	<105
Oxygenation		
PaO_2 mm Hg	80–100	<70 (on FIO_2 >0.6)
$P(A-a)O_2$ mm Hg	5–20	>450 (on O_2)
PaO_2/PAO_2	0.75	<0.15
PaO_2/FIO_2	475	<200

TABLE 5-7
Example of Clinician-Driven Protocol for Initial Ventilator Settings and Targets

A. Volume-controlled ventilation may be used for the majority of patients, but pressure ventilation (PV or PRVC) should be considered if peak pressures rise over 40 cm H_2O or plateau pressures rise >30 cm H_2O.

B. Tidal volume: 6–8 mL/kg predicted body weight (PBW), while maintaining plateau pressure < 30 cm H_2O and ΔP < 20 cm H_2O.

C. Minute ventilation ($\dot{V}E$): 4.0 x BSA (body surface area) = $\dot{V}E$ (L/min) for males and 3.5 x BSA = $\dot{V}E$ (L/min) for females adjusted for altitude and body temperature (DuBois BSA nomogram) while maintaining plateau pressure < 30 cm H_2O and ΔP < 20 cm H_2O.

D. Frequency: 10–20 breaths/minute adjusted to achieve optimum total cycle time and maintain desired minute ventilation, while maintaining plateau pressure < 30 cm H_2O and ΔP < 20 cm H_2O.

E. FIO_2: Initial setting of 1.0 until results from arterial blood gases (ABG) can be obtained and the setting adjusted.
   1. Initial ABG should be obtained 15–45 minutes from start of ventilation
   2. Pulse oximetry should be correlated with initial ABG and the patient subsequently monitored with continuous pulse oximetry to maintain SpO_2 at or above patient's normal or >90% SpO_2 (oxygen saturation by pulse oximetry)
   3. Positive end-expiratory pressure (PEEP) 5–15 cm H_2O. Set initial PEEP at 5 cm H_2O, unless otherwise indicated. Higher PEEPs may be required with acute respiratory distress syndrome (ARDS), according to ARDS Protocol

F. Pressure support (PS): 8–20 cm H_2O. Maintain Pplat < 30 cm H_2O and ΔP < 20 cm H_2O. PS should be adjusted to reduce work of breathing and patient fatigue and support effective ventilation.

G. I:E ratio greater than 1:1 (example 1:3). The I:E ratio should be optimized along with total cycle time (TCT) to provide optimum mean airway pressure, lung filling, lung emptying (minimizing air trapping/auto-PEEP), patient–ventilator synchrony.

From American Association for Respiratory Care, AARC-Adult Mechanical Ventilator Protocols from AARC Protocol Committee; Subcommittee Adult Critical Care Version 1.0a, Subcommittee Chair, Susan P. Pilbeam. Copyright © Sept. 2003 by American Association for Respiratory Care. Reprinted by permission of American Association for Respiratory Care.

TABLE 5-8
Initial Ventilator Setup

Initial ventilator setup includes the following key decisions:
   Noninvasive versus invasive ventilation
   Type and method of establishment of an airway
   Partial versus full ventilatory support
   Choice of ventilator
   Mode of ventilation
   Assist/control ventilation (volume controlled versus pressure controlled) versus synchronized intermittent mandatory ventilation (SIMV, with or without pressure support)
   Pressure support
   Other newer modes and adjuncts to ventilation
Next, the clinician must consider key ventilatory values:
   Trigger method (pressure or flow trigger) and sensitivity
   VT (volume-controlled ventilation) or pressure level (pressure support and control)
   Rate
   Inspiratory flow, inspiratory time, expiratory time, or I:E ratio
   Inspiratory flow pattern
   FIO_2
   Positive end-expiratory pressure (PEEP)
Last, the clinician must choose appropriate alarm and backup values:
   Low-pressure, low PEEP alarms
   High-pressure limit and alarm
   Volume alarms (low VT/high VT, high and low minute ventilation)
   High-frequency and low-frequency alarms
   Apnea alarm and apnea ventilation values
   High/low O_2 alarm
   High/low temperature alarm
   I:E ratio limit and alarm

ventilator settings are mainly based on a patient's body size, diagnosis, pathophysiology, and laboratory results. The settings only serve as a starting point, which should be adjusted according to changes in the patient's condition and requirements (**Table 5-8**).

Type of Ventilation

Volume-controlled ventilation (VCV) has the advantage of stable volume delivery; however, it has the disadvantage of increasing peak inspiratory pressure as lung compliance decreases or airway resistance increases. Overinflation of the more compliant lung areas is a risk. Pressure-controlled breaths have the advantages of providing flow that better matches the patient's demand and limiting pressures to better avoid overinflation of alveoli. With pressure-controlled breaths, VT varies as lung characteristics change. While each targeting approach has its own advantages and disadvantages, it has yet to be demonstrated that a clear advantage exists for one method over the other.

There are two ways to set the pressure in pressure-controlled breaths to provide the desired VT. One way is to deliver a volume-controlled breath to the patient at the desired VT and measure plateau and baseline pressures. Using the same baseline pressure, the breath can be switched to pressure-controlled breath using a set pressure equal to the plateau pressure. The resulting VT will be approximately equal to the VT during the volume breath, so long as inspiratory time is set appropriately. The pressure can then be adjusted as necessary to obtain the desired tidal volume delivery. A second method to initiate pressure ventilation is to start at a low pressure (10–15 cm H_2O), observe the resulting VT, and then incrementally adjust the pressure until the desired tidal volume is attained.

Mode

Most patients begin mechanical ventilation on full ventilator support (FVS) regardless of the mode chosen (for the most part). Full ventilatory support is achieved by any mode that assumes essentially all of the work of breathing. Controlled (time-triggered) ventilation is the closest to FVS and is appropriate only when a patient cannot make an effort to breathe. A patient should never be mechanically blocked from triggering breaths as this can cause great stress. For example, sedation and paralysis are used if seizure activity cannot be prevented or with a chemically induced coma to allow rest and healing in specific situations. Adequate alarms and monitors must be used to safeguard patients.

Assist/control ventilation allows time-triggered or patient-triggered mandatory breaths in which the operator sets a minimum breathing frequency, sensitivity level, and type of breath (volume or pressure controlled). Any patient-triggered breaths will be the same volume as machine-triggered breaths. The patient's ability to trigger additional breaths allows for a larger minute volume if metabolic needs increase, but it can also be undesirable if the patient has an abnormally fast breathing pattern (as might occur with a CNS abnormality), resulting in a respiratory alkalosis. Assist/control mode is a more commonly used mode for FVS because it has been shown that patients often exert some effort during what is meant to be FVS instead of relaxing as intended. The synchronized intermittent mandatory ventilation (SIMV) mode can function as either FVS (if set to provide all the ventilatory requirements of the patient, with no spontaneous breaths) or partial ventilatory support (PVS). By combining SIMV and pressure support ventilation (PSV), it is possible to come close to FVS but still allow some patient effort in a comfortable, assisted manner.

PVS is achieved by any mode that provides less than the total amount of the work of breathing. Patients usually transition from FVS to PVS in preparation to wean from mechanical ventilation. Allowing some degree of spontaneous breathing through a partial support mode can be useful for COPD patients because their disease tends to make them particularly susceptible to diaphragm atrophy from disuse. PSV is one PVS choice that is considered an assisted form of spontaneous breathing because the patient retains control over many aspects of each breath. Proportional assist ventilation (PAV) is another PVS choice that seeks to augment patient spontaneous efforts according to the effort made by the patient. The reality with most awake patients is that even if a mode is selected with the intention of delivering FVS, the patient will usually contribute some spontaneous effort so the ability to synchronize with patient efforts is important.

Control Mode

The equation of motion for ventilation specifies that only one variable can be controlled at a time during mechanical ventilation (e.g., either control of volume [VCV] or control of pressure [pressure-controlled ventilation, PCV]). Dual control mode ventilation attempts to control both volume and pressure during a breath. Although this may appear to happen, in reality there is a hierarchy of control so that ultimately there is one most important control variable. This seemingly dual control mode monitors patient feedback from the breaths delivered and switches between pressure-controlled and volume-controlled breaths. By combining VCV and PCV, the patient receives mandatory breaths that are volume controlled, pressure limited, and time cycled. Likewise, there are volume-controlled, pressure support breath modes that can be combined with the dual control mandatory breaths to allow greater synchrony and patient comfort. These modes do not guarantee a precise volume but can usually ensure a "minimum" volume. There are small differences in the operating characteristics among the various dual control mode offerings, but they all use some form of pressure breath to try to ensure a minimum volume. Dual control modes can be used with most patients to offer most of the benefits of both forms of ventilation.

Tidal Volume

Although there is no conclusive evidence for an ideal tidal volume, tidal volume on "initial" setting in the range of 6 to 8 mL/kg PBW is typical for patients with normal lungs. Tidal volumes as small as 4 mL/kg PBW may be used for patients with very low respiratory system compliance to maintain a safe Pplat value, but this extreme is not common at the initiation of mechanical ventilation. The most current literature indicates no need or benefit for a tidal volume >10 mL/kg PBW in general, and it is never indicated in critically ill patients.

If a patient's height cannot be measured for an estimated tidal volume calculation, arm span is an acceptable substitute. The primary reason for using lower tidal volumes (as with permissive hypercapnia) is to minimize the airway pressures and the risk of barotrauma. However, use of low tidal volume ventilation may lead to complications, such as acute hypercapnia, increased dead space ventilation and work of breathing, dyspnea, severe acidosis, and atelectasis. The following example shows how to calculate a patient's PBW.

PBW can be calculated as follows:

Male PBW in pounds = 106 + (6 × [Height in inches − 60])

Female PBW in pounds = 105 + (5 × [Height in inches − 60])

Convert PBW to kilograms by dividing PBW in pounds by 2.2.

COPD patients may also benefit from a reduced tidal volume setting. These patients have reduced expiratory flow rates due to decreased alveolar elastic recoil. For this reason, a longer expiratory time is needed for complete exhalation. If there is not enough time for complete exhalation, air trapping, ventilation-perfusion ($\dot{V}/\dot{Q}$) mismatch, hypoxemia, and hypercapnia may result. Decreasing the tidal volume by 100 to 200 mL in COPD patients reduces the expiratory time requirements and helps to prevent air trapping. A higher flow rate may also be used to shorten the inspiratory time and lengthen the expiratory time. For patients with a reduction of lung volumes due to lung resection, lower tidal volumes may also become necessary. Clinical conditions where lower tidal volume settings may be beneficial or necessary are discussed later in the chapter.

Most ventilators used in critical care automatically measure and adjust for volume lost to stretch of the patient–ventilator circuit (compressible volume). For the few that do not (i.e., certain transport and some strategic national stockpile ventilators), a method for calculating compressible volume of a ventilator circuit is as follows:

1. Using a ventilator that has passed its safety check, set the frequency at 10 per minute and the tidal volume between 100 and 200 mL with a low peak flow rate and the high pressure limit set to its maximum value. Ideally the ventilator circuit should be warmed to what will be used with the patient, as temperature affects tubing compliance.

2. Completely occlude the patient wye connection of the ventilator circuit.

3. Record the expired volume and peak inspiratory pressure while the circuit wye remains occluded.

4. To obtain the circuit compliance factor, divide the expired breath volume (mL) by the peak inspiratory pressure (cm H_2O) obtained while the circuit wye was occluded.

5. To calculate the compressible volume of the ventilator circuit (volume not delivered to the patient due to circuit expansion), multiply the circuit compliance factor (mL/cm H_2O) by the peak inspiratory pressure obtained from a patient breath (subtract any PEEP from peak inspiratory pressure).

Example:

Expired volume = 130 mL
Peak inspiratory pressure (during occlusion) = 45 cm H_2O
Peak inspiratory pressure (patient on mechanical ventilation) = 55 cm H_2O
PEEP 10 cm H_2O
Circuit compliance factor = 130 mL/45 cm H_2O = 2.9 mL/cm H_2O
Circuit compressible volume = (55 − 10) × 2.9 = 130.5 mL

Frequency and Minute Volume

The initial ventilator frequency is the number of breaths per minute that is intended to provide a $Paco_2$ within the normal range (35 to 45 mm Hg) or the patient's typical range (if chronic disease is present). The initial frequency is usually set between 10 and 12 per minute. This frequency, coupled with a tidal volume of 6 to 8 mL/kg, usually produces a minute volume that is sufficient to normalize the patient's $Paco_2$ at rest with a

normal metabolism (increased work of breathing usually requires an increased minute volume). Frequencies of 20 per minute or higher (with normal tidal volumes) are associated with auto-PEEP and should be avoided. In addition to high ventilator frequency, inadequate inspiratory flow and air-trapping disorders contribute to the development of auto-PEEP.

An alternative method of selecting the initial frequency is to estimate the patient's minute volume requirement and divide the estimated minute volume by the tidal volume.

$$\text{Frequency} = \text{Estimated minute volume} / \text{Tidal volume}$$

The estimated minute volume (L/min) for males is equal to 4.0 multiplied by the body surface area (BSA); for females, it is equal to 3.5 multiplied by the BSA. The BSA (in meters squared) can be obtained from a nomogram such as the Dubois BSA chart.

$$\text{Minute volume (male)} = 4 \times \text{BSA}$$

$$\text{Minute volume (female)} = 3.5 \times \text{BSA}$$

Adjusting the Frequency

The initial frequency setting of 10 to 12 breaths/min and the calculation just provided are based on the assumption that both CO_2 production and physiologic dead space are normal. If the CO_2 production is elevated (e.g., due to an increase in metabolic rate) or the physiologic dead space is increased (e.g., due to a decrease of pulmonary perfusion), the minute volume required to normalize the $Paco_2$ will need to be increased. Because increasing the tidal volume results in higher airway pressures on a volume-limited ventilator, it is usually more appropriate to increase the minute volume by increasing the ventilator frequency.

Blood gases should be obtained 15–45 minutes after initiation of mechanical ventilation (or after the patient has stabilized), to assess both ventilation and oxygenation. The proper response for a higher than normal $Paco_2$ (e.g., >45 mm Hg, or >50 mm Hg for patients with chronic CO_2 retention) would be to increase the minute volume by increasing the ventilator frequency (the tidal volume should already be set according to the patient's PBW). A lower than normal $Paco_2$ (e.g., <35 mm Hg, or <40 mm Hg for patients with CO_2 retention) indicates that the minute volume should be decreased, usually by decreasing the frequency.

Fraction of Inspired Oxygen

It is acceptable practice to place patients on an initial Fio_2 of 1.0. As mentioned, the patient response to 100% oxygen can assist with diagnosis of the cardiopulmonary condition. The Fio_2 can be adjusted according to the values of the arterial blood gas obtained after initiating mechanical ventilation. Further incremental titration of the F_{IO_2} can occur using pulse oximetry. It should be adjusted accordingly to maintain a Pa_{O_2} between 80 and 100 mm Hg (lower for patients with chronic CO_2 retention). Patients who are difficult to oxygenate may be allowed a Pa_{O_2} target as low as 60 mm Hg because that still provides about 90% oxygen saturation of hemoglobin, which provides acceptable if not normal oxygen delivery to the body tissues. If possible, the F_{IO_2} should be kept below 0.50 to minimize the risk of oxygen-induced lung injuries.

PEEP

PEEP increases the functional residual capacity (this improves lung compliance and reduces WOB in patients with low FRC) and is useful to treat refractory hypoxemia (low Pa_{O_2} not responding to high F_{IO_2}). The initial PEEP level may be set at 5 cm H_2O. Subsequent changes of PEEP should be based on the patient's blood gas results, F_{IO_2} requirement, tolerance of PEEP, and cardiovascular responses. Ventilator waveforms can also guide setting PEEP to counter auto-PEEP or titrate PEEP to achieve a minimal transpulmonary pressure at the end of expiration. For other methods to titrate optimal PEEP, see Chapter 8.

I:E Ratio

The **I:E ratio** is the ratio of inspiratory time to expiratory time. If tidal volumes, frequencies, and inspiratory times are within their respective normal ranges, the I:E ratio will usually be between 1:2 and 1:4. A larger I:E ratio may be used when additional time is needed for exhalation because of air trapping and auto-PEEP. The presence of air trapping during mechanical ventilation may be checked by noting if the flow scalar returns to baseline before the start of the next inspiration. If not, the amount of auto-PEEP can be measured by occluding the expiratory port of the ventilator circuit at the end of exhalation (an end expiratory breath hold). Any

additional positive pressure above the baseline pressure (i.e., 0 cm H_2O, or the PEEP level when PEEP is in use) at the end of expiration would be auto-PEEP. Many critical care ventilators will measure auto-PEEP when selected, but it can also be done manually using a simple device called a Braschi valve (or its equivalent).

Using inverse I:E ratios to correct refractory hypoxemia in ARDS patients has fallen out of favor and should never be attempted as an "initial" setting. Set (or external) PEEP is a safer and more uniform way to create expiratory distending pressure to improve oxygenation.

Depending on the features available on the ventilator, the I:E ratio may be altered by manipulating any one or a combination of the following controls: (1) flow rate, (2) inspiratory time, (3) inspiratory time%, (4) frequency, and (5) minute volume (tidal volume and frequency).

Effects of Flow Rate on I:E Ratio

Adjusting the flow rate is the most common method to change an I:E ratio because the flow rate control is a feature available on almost all ventilators. **Table 5-9** shows the effects of flow rate change on the I time, E time, and I:E ratio when the V_T and frequency are kept unchanged. Note that the I time and I:E ratio are inversely related. A longer I time leads to a lower I:E ratio.

Other Ventilator Controls That Affect the I:E Ratio

Besides the flow rate control, other settings available on some ventilators may also alter the I:E ratio. Table 5-9 shows the effects of tidal volume and frequency changes on the I time, E time, and I:E ratio.

Changing the I:E Ratio

Because the I:E ratio may be changed by altering different settings available on selected ventilators, different

TABLE 5-9
Effects of Flow Rate, Tidal Volume, and Frequency (f) Changes on I Time, E Time, and I:E Ratio

Parameter Change	Inspiratory (I) Time	Expiratory (E) Time	I:E Ratio
Increase flow rate	Decrease	Increase	Increase
Decrease flow rate	Increase	Decrease	Decrease
Increase tidal volume	Increase	Decrease	Decrease
Decrease tidal volume	Decrease	Increase	Increase
Increase f	Minimal change*	Decrease	Decrease
Decrease f	Minimal change*	Increase	Increase

*During volume-controlled ventilation, I time is determined by the tidal volume and flow rate.

methods to obtain a desired I:E ratio are provided as follows:

Example 1 Using Flow to Change the I:E Ratio
Given: Minute volume = 12 L/min
Desired I:E ratio = 1:3
Calculate: The flow rate for an I:E ratio of 1:3
Solution: Flow = Minute volume × Sum of I:E ratio
= 12 L/min × (1 + 3)
= 12 L/min × 4
= 48 L/min

Example 2 Using I Time to Change the I:E Ratio
Given: f = 16/min
Desired I:E ratio = 1:4
Calculate: The I time needed for an I:E ratio of 1:4
Solution: Since f = 16/min, time for each breath
= 60 sec/16 or 3.75 sec
I time = Time for each breath × (I ratio/Sum of I:E ratio)
= 3.75 sec × (1/[1 + 4])
= 3.75 sec × (1/5)
= 3.75 sec/5
= 0.75 sec

I Time% and I:E Ratio

Some ventilators (e.g., Hamilton Medical) permit the I:E ratio to be preset, usually by setting an I time% (percent inspiratory time). In these ventilators, the flow rate is automatically adjusted by the ventilator to maintain a constant I:E ratio regardless of changes in tidal volume or frequency. I:E ratios may be calculated by following Example 3.

Example 3 Using I Time% to Set the I:E Ratio
Given: Desired I:E ratio = 1:3.5
Calculate: The I time% needed for an I:E ratio of 1:3.5
Solution: I Time% = I Ratio/Sum of I:E ratio
= 1 / (1 + 3.5) = 1/4.5 = 22%

Flow Pattern

Most modern ventilators offer different inspiratory flow patterns. Although there are subtle variations, the principal flow patterns are (1) square (constant) flow pattern, (2) ascending flow pattern, (3) descending flow pattern, and (4) sine wave flow pattern. The waveforms for each of these flow patterns are shown in **Figure 5-3**. The terms *accelerating* and *decelerating* (negative acceleration) are no longer used because each term can represent two possible flow patterns (e.g., uniform and nonuniform acceleration), which is imprecise and produces confusion.

The square flow pattern may be used initially upon setting up the ventilator. This flow pattern provides an even, constant peak flow during the entire inspiratory phase. The initial peak flow at the very beginning of the inspiratory phase should help to overcome the airway resistance and parenchymal elastance, and the remaining peak flow throughout the inspiratory phase should enhance gas distribution in the lungs. Adjustment of

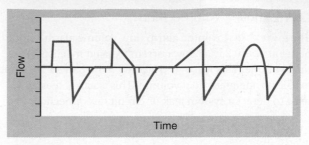

FIGURE 5-3 Flow pattern waveform examples. From left to right: Constant flow (aka square wave), descending ramp, ascending ramp, sinusoidal (aka sine).

the flow pattern may be made after stabilization of the patient. Note that the constant flow pattern is the only flow pattern in which the peak flow rate equals the mean flow rate. All other flow patterns will produce a mean flow rate that is less than the peak flow.

The ascending waveform is rarely found on the currently manufactured ventilators because it is typically not well tolerated by most patients. The descending flow pattern typically produces a high initial inspiratory pressure, and the decrease in flow may help improve distribution of volume and gas exchange. For patients with COPD, the decelerating flow may reduce the peak inspiratory pressure, mean airway pressures, physiologic dead space, and $Paco_2$. The sine wave flow pattern is considered more physiologic because it is similar to the flow pattern during spontaneous breathing (however, sine wave flow patterns produced by positive and negative pressure breaths are not equivalent). The sine wave may also improve the distribution of ventilation and therefore improve gas exchange. For ventilators that do not permit a preset inspiratory time, the inspiratory time may increase if the patient's peak inspiratory pressure (PIP) increases. This is because as the PIP increases, the pressure gradient between the ventilator and the patient's airway opening increases, resulting in an increased inspiratory time. However, on ventilators in which the inspiratory time is preset, the inspiratory time is held constant for any flow pattern selected.

In performing calculations that involve the inspiratory flow as a variable (e.g., resistance = pressure/flow), the mean inspiratory flow should be used. Because the only flow pattern in which the peak flow equals the mean inspiratory flow is the square wave pattern, the ventilator should be switched to a constant flow pattern prior to measurement.

Ventilator Alarm Settings

Although different ventilators have a variety of alarm systems, the following alarms should be basic to any ventilator: low exhaled volume alarm, low inspiratory pressure alarm, high inspiratory pressure alarm, apnea alarm, high-frequency alarm, and high and low Fio_2 alarm. These alarms should have a battery backup to prevent malfunction in the event of electrical failure.

Low Exhaled Volume Alarm

The low exhaled volume alarm (low volume alarm) should be set at about 25% below current exhaled mechanical tidal volume. This alarm is triggered if the patient does not exhale an adequate tidal volume. This alarm is typically used to detect a system leak or circuit disconnection.

Low Inspiratory Pressure Alarm

The low inspiratory pressure alarm (low pressure alarm) should be set at 10 cm H_2O below the observed peak inspiratory pressure. This alarm is triggered if the peak inspiratory pressure is less than the alarm setting. The low inspiratory pressure alarm complements the low exhaled volume alarm and is also used to detect system leaks or circuit disconnection.

High Inspiratory Pressure Alarm

The high inspiratory pressure alarm (high pressure limit alarm) should be set at 10 cm H_2O above the observed peak inspiratory pressure. This alarm is triggered when the peak inspiratory pressure is equal to or higher than the high pressure limit. Once the alarm is triggered by excess pressure (airflow obstruction or low compliance), inspiration is immediately terminated and the ventilator cycles to expiratory phase.

The patient must be evaluated to determine the cause of the excess airway pressure. Common causes that trigger the high inspiratory pressure alarm include water in the ventilator circuit, kinking or biting of the endotracheal rube, secretions in the airway, bronchospasm, mucous plugs, tension pneumothorax, decreases in lung compliance, increases in airway resistance, and coughing.

Apnea Alarm

The apnea low volume and low pressure alarms are triggered in apnea and circuit disconnection (i.e., inadvertent disconnection or during endotracheal suctioning). Inadvertent circuit disconnection is a common event in patients with a tracheostomy tube due to lack of allowance for airway flexibility as with an endotracheal tube. The apnea alarm should be set with a time delay of 15 to 20 seconds, with less time delay at higher ventilator frequency. On some ventilators, the apnea alarm also triggers an apnea backup ventilation mode in which the ventilator provides ventilatory support until the alarm condition no longer exists.

High-Frequency Alarm

The high-frequency alarm should be set at 10% to 20% greater than the current frequency. Triggering of the high-frequency alarm may indicate that the patient is experiencing respiratory distress. See Chapter 8 for a discussion on the causes and management of the high-frequency alarm.

High and Low FIO_2 Alarms

The high FIO_2 alarm should be set no more than 5% over the analyzed FIO_2, and the low FIO_2 alarm should be set at no more than 5% below the analyzed FIO_2.

Initial Settings for Special Patient Conditions

The initial settings for different unique patient conditions are discussed in the following sections. For subsequent setting changes due to changing patient conditions, refer to Chapter 8.

Advanced Chronic Obstructive Lung Disease

Basic guidelines for mechanically ventilating patients with COPD include the following:

> If possible, use NIV.
> Volume-control continuous mandatory ventilation (VC-CMV) or pressure-control continuous mandatory ventilation (PC-CMV) may unload the work of the respiratory muscles more than SIMV.
> Use the descending flow pattern when using VC-CMV with flow >60 L/min.
> Start with an initial VT of 6 to 8 mL/kg with a frequency of 8 to 16 breaths/minute, and TI 0.6 to 1.2 seconds.
> PEEP 5 cm H_2O or lower, or about 50% of auto-PEEP, should be used initially.
> Provide the longest expiratory time (TE) possible (decreasing TI, reducing f or VT).
> Maintain Pao_2 at 55 to 75 mm Hg or near the patient's normal Pao_2, with FIO_2 less than 0.5.

Severe Asthma

Patients presenting an exacerbation of acute severe asthma that requires mechanical ventilation are among the most difficult to manage. Increased airway resistance (Raw) from bronchospasm, increased secretions, and mucosal edema increase the incidence of air trapping. Trapped air can cause uneven overexpansion of various lung units, which can rupture or compress other areas of the lungs, leading to pneumothorax, pneumomediastinum, subcutaneous emphysema, and other forms of barotrauma.

The primary goal during mechanical ventilation of these patients is to focus on reversing the high Raw while avoiding or reducing air trapping. Sedation and possibly paralysis may be required if severe patient–ventilator dyssynchrony persists (paralytic agents come with serious hazards and should be considered with great caution).

The following guidelines provide suggestions for mechanically ventilating patients with asthma.

> VC-CMV and PC-CMV are acceptable modes (it is easier to control airway pressure with PC-CMV).
> PIP will be high, concentrate on maintaining acceptable plateau pressures (<30 cm H_2O).
> Ensure adequate oxygenation status, Pao_2 >60 mm Hg (may require FIO_2 ≥0.5).
> Monitor hemodynamic status to ensure cardiac output is stable.

Consider permissive hypercapnia ($PaCO_2$ 45 to 80 mm Hg) if pH is acceptable (i.e., $\geq$7.25).

If sedation or paralytic medications are used, discontinue as soon as possible.

The use of PEEP is perilous, use with extreme caution. Reduce the incidence of air trapping by providing long expiratory times:

Lowest possible frequency; V_T = 6 to 8 mL/kg; T_I = $\leq$1 sec; flow rate = 80 to 100 L/min; descending or constant flow pattern (depending on which is tolerated better)

Acute Respiratory Distress Syndrome

Guidelines for patients with ARDS continue to evolve, but the following represent reasonable "initial" options. Most often patients develop ARDS after they have been on mechanical ventilation for a while, not at the beginning of mechanical ventilation. Chapter 8 addresses protocols for mechanical ventilation for patient with ARDS in greater detail.

V_T of 6 to 8 mL/kg with a respiratory frequency of 15 to 25 breaths/minute (follow ARDSNet protocol).

Tidal volumes of 4 to 6 mL/kg may be necessary to maintain the Pplat <30 cm H_2O.

Choose a full support mode such as PC-CMV or VC-CMV.

Maintain SaO_2 at 88% to 90% or greater. Start at 100% oxygen.

Use ARDSNet PEEP/FIO_2 tables to support oxygenation.

Prone positioning may be indicated.

Cardiac output and hemoglobin levels should be optimized.

Permissive hypercapnia may be necessary, unless there is a risk of increased ICP.

If VC-CMV is selected, the descending flow waveform is preferred with flow rates >60 L/min.

Cardiogenic Shock and Pulmonary Edema

Patients with congestive heart failure (CHF) can rapidly develop acute pulmonary edema, and this can quickly lead to death if not treated quickly. Common causes of acute pulmonary edema include acute myocardial infarction, hypertension, rapid heart rates with inadequate filling time, valvular heart disease, and fluid overload. The following guidelines are recommended for mechanically ventilating patients with acute cardiogenic pulmonary edema and CHF.

Evaluate the effectiveness of CPAP/NIV before attempting invasive mechanical ventilation if possible.

NIV may buy time for pharmacologic treatment to become effective and avoid intubation.

Hemodynamic monitoring is important and may require a CVP line or other monitoring device.

VC-CMV or PC-CMV full support is recommended.

V_T range is moderate 6 to 8 mL/kg; set f $\geq$10/minute and flow rate > 60 L/min (descending).

PEEP of 5 to 10 cm H_2O and FIO_2 at 1.0 and titrate quickly by SpO_2 to maintain SpO_2 >90% to 92%.

Head Injury

Maintaining sufficient cerebral blood flow requires an adequate CPP. CPP is calculated by the equation: CPP = Mean arterial pressure (MAP) – ICP. Normal values for MAP are 90 to 95 mm Hg and ICP 8 to 12 mm Hg. There is no Class I evidence for the optimal CPP, but the low critical threshold is 70 to 80 mm Hg. Mortality increased about 20% for each 10 mm Hg drop in CPP. Low CPP is an indicator of poor cerebral perfusion. It is important to keep ICP low and MAP in the normal range to maintain CPP in brain-injured patients. The following guidelines are recommended for mechanically ventilating patients with closed head injuries.

Protect the airway (intubation) because there is a high risk for vomiting and aspiration.

PEEP can increase ICP so monitor carefully.

Monitor for increased ICP and hypoxemia to respond with extra breaths if needed.

Acute uncontrolled increased ICP may respond to $PaCO_2$ in 25 to 30 mm Hg range or titrate to ICP.

Ventilator settings include the following:

Provide full ventilatory support to start, either PC-CMV or VC-CMV can be used.

Maintain V_T 6 to 8 mL/kg ideal body weight (IBW) while maintaining Pplat at <30 cm H_2O.

Frequency of 15 to 20 breaths/minute to provide normal acid–base status, as long as auto-PEEP is avoided.

Initial FIO_2 of 1.0 titrate to keep PaO_2 $\geq$70 mm Hg to avoid hypoxemia.

♦ High inspiratory flow >60 L/min (descending), keep T_I short, about 1 sec (avoid auto-PEEP).

♦ PEEP = 0 to 5 cm H_2O, as long as ICP is being measured and is 10 mm Hg or less.

♦ Suctioning and chest physiotherapy can dramatically increase ICP, use extreme care.

Summary

Initiation of mechanical ventilation is best guided by evidence-based protocols and guidelines. There are many options to consider, which benefit from appropriate monitoring of patient status. Initial ventilator settings are often quickly changed, sometimes the mode of ventilation. Be ready to respond quickly to the needs of your patient and seek consultation when decisions are not clear. Systematic reviews of the literature (e.g., Cochrane Library Systematic Reviews) are excellent sources of information to guide clinical decisions. To summarize, **Table 5-10** outlines the indications for mechanical ventilation and **Table 5-11** provides on overview of the initial ventilator settings for an adult patient.

TABLE 5-10
Indications for Mechanical Ventilation

Indication	Parameters
Acute ventilatory failure	Pa_{CO_2} >50 mm Hg (higher for COPD) pH ≤7.25 Apnea
Impending ventilatory failure	Tidal volume <3–5 mL/kg PBW Frequency >35/minute Minute ventilation >10 L/min Vital capacity <15 mL/kg PBW MIP >–20 cm H_2O Rising Pa_{CO_2} >50 mm Hg
Severe hypoxemia	Pa_{O_2} <60 mm Hg at F_{IO_2} >0.5 or Pa_{O_2} <40 mm Hg at any F_{IO_2} Pa_{O_2}/F_{IO_2} (P/F ratio) ≤300 mm Hg

Prophylactic ventilatory support	Reduce risk of pulmonary complications:
	    Prolonged shock
	    Head injury
	    Smoke inhalation
	Reduce hypoxia of major body organs:
	    Hypoxic brain
	    Hypoxia of heart muscles
	Reduce cardiopulmonary stress:
	    Prolonged shock
	    Coronary artery bypass surgery
	    Other thoracic or abdominal surgeries

COPD, chronic obstructive pulmonary disease; MIP, maximal inspiratory pressure; PBW, predicted body weight.

TABLE 5-11
Initial Ventilator Settings for Normal Lungs

Parameter	Setting	Notes
Mode	Assist/control or SIMV	Provide ventilatory support
f	10–12/minute	Primary control to regulate ventilation that is guided by Pa_{CO_2}
V_T	6–8 mL/kg PBW (4–10 mL/kg in special circumstances)	Use lower V_T to reduce risk of pressure-related injuries. Very low compliance or previous lung resection may require 4 mL/kg PBW. Do not exceed 10 mL/kg PBW.
F_{IO_2}	1.0 for severe hypoxemia or compromised cardiopulmonary status	0.40 for mild hypoxemia or normal cardiopulmonary status
PEEP	≥5 cm H_2O for refractory hypoxemia	Monitor patient and note cardiovascular adverse effects
I:E	1:2–1:4	1:4 for patients needing longer E time due to gas trapping
Flow pattern	Constant or descending	Other flow patterns for a lower peak inspiratory pressure and better gas distribution (i.e., breath sounds)

E, expiratory; I, inspiratory; PBW, predicted body weight; SIMV, synchronized intermittent mandatory ventilation.

Case Studies

Case Study 5-1 Guillain-Barré Syndrome

A 7-year old boy was transferred from a small, rural hospital with a history of body aches and pains for the past week. He exhibited weakness and hypotonia (decreased muscle tone) the previous 4 days, inability to walk, drooling from the mouth, and inability to talk. On the previous day, his breathing difficulty increased to the point that mechanical ventilation was started. A diagnosis of Guillain-Barré syndrome (GBS) was made on the basis of progressive weakness of both upper and lower limbs, absence of fever at onset, areflexia, relative symmetry of signs, autonomic dysfunction, and the cerebrospinal fluid showing albuminocytologic dissociation (protein 5 g/L with no cells). A nerve conduction study showed grossly prolonged latencies with markedly reduced compound motor action potential amplitudes in all motor nerves of the upper and lower limbs. No sensory action potentials were elicited. The child received intravenous immunoglobulin and volume control ventilation with other supportive measures. After 29 days the child was successfully removed from ventilatory support and extubated.

1. **Was it appropriate to assign the diagnosis of GBS to this patient based on the information presented?**

2. **Was it appropriate to initiate mechanical ventilation based on the information presented?**

Case Studies

Case Study 5-2 Acute Respiratory Compromise with Multiple Difficulties

The patient is a 61-year-old white woman presenting to the emergency department with acute onset of shortness of breath. Approximately 2 days before, she started having symptoms that have progressively worsened with no associated, aggravating, or relieving factors noted. She had similar symptoms approximately 1 year ago with an acute chronic obstructive pulmonary disease (COPD) exacerbation requiring hospitalization. She uses noninvasive ventilatory support (bilevel positive airway pressure [BiPAP]) at night when sleeping and has requested to use this in the emergency department due to shortness of breath. The initial physical exam reveals temperature 97.3°F, heart rate 74 bpm, respiratory frequency 24, blood pressure (BP) 104/54, body mass index (BMI) 40.2, and SpO_2 90% on room air.

The patient reports difficulty breathing at rest, forgetfulness, mild fatigue, feeling cold (requests a blanket), increased urinary frequency, incontinence, and new swelling in her legs that is worsening. She has not ambulated from bed for several days except to use the restroom due to feeling weak, fatigued, and short of breath. She is confused with difficulty arousing on conversation and examination. The patient's husband revealed that she is poorly compliant with taking her medications. He reports that she "doesn't see the need to take so many pills."

Her family history includes significant heart disease, and her father had prostate cancer. Social history is positive for smoking tobacco use at 30 pack-years. She quit smoking 2 years ago due to increasing shortness of breath. She denies all alcohol and illegal drug use; she has no known food, drug, or environmental allergies.

Past medical history is significant for coronary artery disease, myocardial infarction, COPD, hypertension, hyperlipidemia, hypothyroidism, diabetes mellitus, peripheral vascular disease, tobacco usage, and obesity. Past surgical history is significant for an appendectomy, cardiac catheterization with stent placement, hysterectomy, and nephrectomy.

Based on physical examination, laboratory, and imaging studies, the following diagnoses were made:

Myxedema coma (severe hypothyroidism)
Pericardial effusion secondary to myxedema coma
COPD exacerbation
Acute-on-chronic hypoxic respiratory failure
Acute respiratory alkalosis
Bilateral community-acquired pneumonia
Small bilateral pleural effusions
Acute mild rhabdomyolysis
Acute chronic (stage IV) renal failure
Elevated troponin I levels, likely secondary to renal failure
Diabetes mellitus type 2, noninsulin dependent
Morbid obesity
Hepatic dysfunction

Initial arterial blood gases (ABGs) were: pH 7.491, $PaCO_2$ 27.6, PaO_2 53.6, HCO_3^- 20.6, and SaO_2 90% on room air. After starting BiPAP with 2 L/min oxygen, the repeat ABG values were: pH 7.397, $PaCO_2$ 35.3, PaO_2 69.4, HCO_3^- 21.2, and SaO_2 91%.

1. **Should this patient have been placed on her BiPAP machine, intubated, and started on invasive mechanical ventilation, or treated with some therapy other than mechanical ventilation?**

2. **Of the several ailments present that could affect ventilatory sufficiency, which one was likely causing the greatest impact on this patient's condition?**

Bibliography

Introduction

Brower RG, Matthay MA, et al. Ventilation with lower tidal volumes as compared with traditional tidal volumes for acute lung injury and the acute respiratory distress syndrome. *N Engl J Med.* 2000;342:1301–1308.

Chiumello D, Carlesso E, Cadringher P, et al. Lung stress and strain during mechanical ventilation for acute respiratory distress syndrome. *Am J Respir Crit Care Med.* 2008;178:346–355.

Esteban A, Ferguson ND, Meade MO, et al. Evolution of mechanical ventilation in response to clinical research. *Am J Respir Crit Care Med.* 2008;177:170–177.

Kacmarek RM. Lung protection: the cost in some is increased work of breathing. Is it too high? *Respir Care.* 2005;50:1614–1616.

Karcz M, Vitkus A, Papadakos PJ, et al. State-of-the-art mechanical ventilation. *J Cardiothorac Vasc Anesth.* 2012;26:486–506.

Lachmann B. Open up the lung and keep the lung open. *Intensive Care Med.* 1992;18:319–321.

Pierson DJ. Indications for mechanical ventilation in adults with acute respiratory failure. *Respir Care.* 2002;47:249–262.

Shapiro BA, Peruzzi WT, Kozelowski-Templin R. *Clinical Application of Blood Gases.* 5th ed. St. Louis, MO: Mosby; 1994.

Causes of Ventilatory Failure

Bonde P, McManus K, McAnespie M, et al. Lung surgery: identifying the subgroup at risk for sputum retention. *Eur J Cardiothorac Surg.* 2002;22:18–22.

Byrd RP, Roy TM. Mechanical ventilation. *Medscape.* 2018. Available at https://emedicine.medscape.com/article/304068-overview#showall

Karcz M, Vitkus A, Papadakos PJ, et al. State-of-the-art mechanical ventilation. *J Cardiothorac Vasc Anesth.* 2012;26:486–506.

Keenan SP, Heyland DK, Jacka MJ, et al. Ventilator-associated pneumonia. Prevention, diagnosis, and therapy. *Crit Care Clin.* 2002;18:107–125.

Lachmann B. Open up the lung and keep the lung open. *Intensive Care Med.* 1992;18:319–321.

Muizelaar JP, Marmarou A, Ward JD, et al. Adverse effects of prolonged hyperventilation in patients with severe head injury: a randomized clinical trial. *J Neurosurg.* 1991;75:731–739.

Otto CW. Ventilatory management in the critically ill. *Emerg Med Clin North Am.* 1986;4:635–654.

Tenling A, Hachenberg T, Tyden H, et al. Atelectasis and gas exchange after cardiac surgery. *Anesthesiology.* 1998;89:371–378.

Goals of Mechanical Ventilation

Bezzant TB, Mortensen JD. Risks and hazards of mechanical ventilation: a collective review of published literature. *Dis Mon.* 1994;40:581–638.

Pettenuzzo T, Fan E. 2016 year in review: mechanical ventilation. *Respir Care.* 2017;62:629–635.

Pipeling MR, Fan E. Therapies for refractory hypoxemia in acute respiratory distress syndrome. *JAMA.* 2010;304:2521–2527.

Rotheram EB Jr, Safar P, Robin E. CNS disorder during mechanical ventilation in chronic pulmonary disease. *JAMA.* 1964;189:993–996.

Slutsky AS. Consensus conference on mechanical ventilation—January 28–30, 1993 at Northbrook, Illinois, USA. Part I. European Society of Intensive Care Medicine, the ACCP and the SCCM. *Intensive Care Med.* 1994;20:64–79.

Tobin MJ. Mechanical ventilation. *N Engl J Med.* 1994;330:1056–1061.

Assessment of Need for Mechanical Ventilation

ARDS Definition Task Force, Ranieri VM, Rubenfeld GD, et al. Acute respiratory distress syndrome: the Berlin Definition. *JAMA.* 2012;307:2526–2533.

Byrd RP, Roy TM. Mechanical ventilation. *Medscape.* 2018. Available at https://emedicine.medscape.com/article/304068-overview#showall

Campbell ML, Carlson RW. Terminal weaning from mechanical ventilation: ethical and practical considerations for patient management. *Am J Crit Care.* 1992;1:52–56.

Caruso P, Friedrich C, Denari SD, et al. The unidirectional valve is the best method to determine maximal inspiratory pressure during weaning. *Chest.* 1999;115:1096–1101.

El-Khatib MF, Bou-Khalil P. Clinical review: liberation from mechanical ventilation. *Crit Care.* 2008;12:221.

Karcz M, Vitkus A, Papadakos PJ, et al. State-of-the-art mechanical ventilation. *J Cardiothorac Vasc Anesth.* 2012;26:486–506.

Pierson DJ. Indications for mechanical ventilation in adults with acute respiratory failure. *Respir Care.* 2002;47:249–262.

Schneiderman LJ, Jecker NS, Jonsen AR. Medical futility: its meaning and ethical implications. *Ann Intern Med.* 1990;112:949–954.

Shapiro BA, Peruzzi WT, Kozelowski-Templin R. *Clinical Application of Blood Gases.* 5th ed. St. Louis, MO: Mosby; 1994.

Shapiro BA. *Clinical Application of Respiratory Care.* 4th ed. St. Louis, MO: Mosby Year Book; 1991.

Yang KL, Tobin MJ. A prospective study of indexes predicting the outcome of trials of weaning from mechanical ventilation. *N Engl J Med.* 1991;324(21):1445–1450.

Protocols

(no references)

Initial Settings

Chang DW. *Respiratory Care Calculations.* 4th ed. Burlington, MA: Jones & Bartlett Learning; 2018.

Kallet RH, Corral W, Silverman HJ, et al. Implementation of a low tidal volume ventilation protocol for patients with acute lung injury or acute respiratory distress syndrome. *Respir Care.* 2001;46:1024–1037.

Kallet RH, Siobal MS, Alonso JA, et al. Lung collapse during low tidal volume ventilation in acute respiratory distress syndrome. *Respir Care.* 2001;46:49–52.

Shapiro BA, Peruzzi WT, Kozelowski-Templin R. *Clinical Application of Blood Gases.* 5th ed. St. Louis, MO: Mosby; 1994.

Tobin MJ. *Principles and Practice of Mechanical Ventilation.* 3rd ed. New York, NY: McGraw-Hill Education; 2013.

Waugh JB. *Rapid Interpretation of Ventilator Waveforms.* 2nd ed. Upper Saddle River, NJ: Pearson Prentice Hall; 2007.

Yang SC, Yang SP. Effects of inspiratory flow waveforms on lung mechanics, gas exchange, and respiratory metabolism in COPD patients during mechanical ventilation. *Chest.* 2002;122:2096–2104.

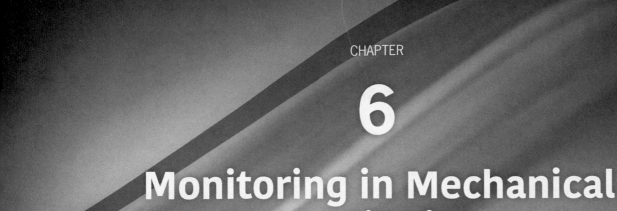

6

Monitoring in Mechanical Ventilation

Lisa A. Conry, MA, RRT

© s_maria/Shutterstock

OUTLINE

OBJECTIVES

1. Describe monitoring the ventilation of a patient receiving mechanical ventilation.
2. Explain how oxygenation and ventilation are monitored physiologically on a patient receiving mechanical ventilation.
3. Differentiate the effects of mechanical ventilation on other organ systems and how these effects are monitored.
4. Interpret capnography waveforms or gradients and explain their significance.
5. Describe the hemodynamic effects of mechanical ventilation and how they are monitored on a patient receiving mechanical ventilation.

KEY TERMS

anion gap
apnea test
auto-PEEP
bradypnea
bubble study
caloric test
capnogram
CO-oximetry
cuff leak test

doll's eyes test
pulse pressure
rise time
transesophageal
  echocardiography
vestibulo-ocular reflex

Monitoring the Ventilator Parameters

Once ventilator support has been initiated, monitoring of the ventilator and the patient helps ensure that it is being used safely and effectively. Monitoring of ventilator parameters is done to reduce dyssynchrony and to assess the patient's response to the settings. Physiologic monitoring yields further information about the patient and response to the ventilator. Adjustments may be made to decrease the detrimental effects of mechanical ventilation on the organ systems. Initial settings may over/underestimate the minute ventilation required by the patient's physiologic state. Monitoring the settings can help the therapist fine-tune the ventilator to meet the patient's needs.

Peak Inspiratory Pressure

Peak inspiratory pressure (PIP) is the highest pressure created during a positive pressure breath. It is the pressure required to overcome the elastic and resistive properties of the lung to deliver the breath. In volume-controlled ventilation, the PIP is reached at the end of inspiration.

Components of Peak Inspiratory Pressure

PIP must overcome the resistance of the airways to flow and the elastance of the lung, to fill the alveoli with air during inspiration. Because both resistive and elastic properties of the lung influence peak pressure, it will vary with changes in lung compliance and airway resistance.

Effects of Compliance on Peak Inspiratory Pressure

When the lung compliance is low, more pressure is required to overcome the opening pressure of the alveoli and fill them. Therefore, a decrease in lung compliance will result in an increase in PIP. As compliance improves, PIP will decrease. In volume-controlled ventilation, where pressure is variable, monitoring of the PIP may signal changes in compliance. PIP is used to calculate the dynamic lung compliance.

Effects of Resistance on Peak Inspiratory Pressure

The friction to airflow within the airways creates airway resistance. For a ventilator to fill the lungs with volume, this resistance must be overcome. The PIP is therefore influenced by the amount of airway resistance that is present. When a flow rate is set on a ventilator, an increase in airway resistance requires a greater applied pressure to maintain that flow. This means that PIP will increase with high airway resistance, and the reverse is also true. Lowering of airway resistance, such as with the application of a bronchodilator (i.e., β-adrenergic medication), will reduce the pressure required to maintain the flow because of a decrease in airway resistance. In volume-controlled ventilation, where PIP is variable based on the lung characteristics, changes in PIP may signal changing airway resistance.

In pressure-controlled ventilation, the PIP is typically achieved at the beginning of inspiration and is maintained at that pressure throughout inspiration. The peak pressure is set and cannot exceed the setting. Compliance and resistance changes do not affect the preset peak pressure limit when pressure-controlled ventilation is used.

Plateau Pressure

Plateau pressure is the pressure obtained when an inspiratory hold or pause is applied. This represents the pressure in the lungs (down to the alveoli) when airflow has stopped. To ensure a good measurement, the inspiratory pause must be long enough to achieve a pressure plateau.

Components of Plateau Pressure

Plateau pressure reflects the pressure required to overcome the elastic properties of the lungs. To determine the plateau pressure, an inspiratory pause is set or the inspiratory hold key is pressed until the value is obtained. Once the measurement has been taken, either the inspiratory hold is removed or the manual hold button is no longer pressed. It is generally a lower value than the PIP, but if airflow resistance is very low, the peak and plateau values may be very close. However, it is physiologically impossible for the plateau pressure to exceed the PIP. In this circumstance, the patient is most likely trying to actively exhale during the plateau measurement.

Effect of Compliance Changes on Plateau Pressure

Plateau pressure is used to calculate the static compliance. A decrease in lung compliance will result in an increase in the plateau pressure as it will take more pressure to overcome the elastic properties of the alveoli and fill them with volume. An improvement in lung compliance will decrease the plateau pressure. Monitoring the plateau pressure therefore allows the practitioner to track changes in lung compliance. Current recommendations are to keep the plateau pressure at or below 28 to 30 cm H_2O to reduce lung injury with mechanical ventilation. **Figure 6-1** shows a graphical representation of the peak and plateau pressures.

Effects of Resistance on Plateau Pressure

Because there is no airflow when the plateau pressure measurement is taken, airway resistance has no effect on the plateau pressure value (Figure 6-1).

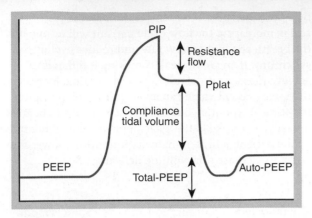

FIGURE 6-1 Peak inspiratory pressure (PIP) and plateau pressure (Pplat). PEEP, positive end-expiratory pressure.

BOX 6-1 Compliance Calculations

Dynamic Compliance = Tidal Volume / (PIP − PEEP)
Static Compliance = Tidal Volume / (Pplat − PEEP)

PIP = peak inspiratory pressure
Pplat = plateau pressure
PEEP = positive end-expiratory pressure

Dynamic Compliance

Dynamic compliance reflects the compliance of the lung when air is moving through the airways. It is calculated by dividing the tidal volume by the PIP minus the baseline pressure (see **Box 6-1**).

Components of Dynamic Compliance

Dynamic compliance includes components of both lung elasticity and airway resistance. It reflects how much pressure is required to overcome the resistance of the airways as well as how much pressure is required to overcome the elastic properties of the alveoli and fill them with air.

Normal Values for Dynamic Compliance

In a nonintubated patient, the dynamic compliance is normally 30 to 40 mL/cm H_2O. This means for every 1 cm H_2O of pressure change, 30 to 40 mL of volume will enter the lungs. Because the PIP is generally higher than the plateau pressure, dynamic compliance is usually a lower value than static compliance.

Effects of Lung Disease on Dynamic Compliance

Lung diseases that decrease lung compliance or increase airway resistance will result in a decrease in the dynamic compliance, as both of these conditions increase the PIP. As the patient improves, the dynamic compliance should increase. During volume-controlled ventilation, the dynamic compliance can be indirectly monitored by noting changes in the PIP (assuming set tidal volume remains the same).

Static Compliance

Static compliance reflects the pressure needed to overcome the elastic properties of the lung. It is calculated by dividing the exhaled tidal volume by the plateau pressure minus the baseline pressure (see Box 6-1).

Components of Static Compliance

Static compliance is calculated when there is no air movement in the lung. Only the elastic forces that must be overcome to fill the lung with volume are accounted for with static compliance.

Normal Value for Static Compliance

The normal for static compliance is 60 to 100 mL/cm H_2O. This value is higher than dynamic compliance because there is no airway resistance component to the static compliance.

Effects of Lung Disease on Static Compliance

Lung diseases that decrease lung compliance (increase lung elasticity) will result in a decrease in the static compliance. As a patient's lung improves, the static compliance will increase. The static compliance can be indirectly monitored by noting changes in the plateau pressure. The lower the plateau pressure, the higher the static lung compliance.

Use of Static Compliance in Determining Optimal PEEP

The static compliance can also be used to determine the optimal positive end-expiratory pressure (PEEP) setting for a patient. There are several methods that can be used to do so. One method is to increase the PEEP in small increments and calculate the static compliance at each level. The PEEP level that gives the highest static compliance is the optimal PEEP level. Another method is to recruit the lung fully and then decrease the PEEP in small increments until the static compliance decreases. The PEEP level just before the drop in compliance is the optimal PEEP. Optimal PEEP can also be set using dead space as a guide. In one study by El-Baraday and El-Shamaa (2014), using V_D/V_T to determine optimal PEEP resulted in a lower overall PEEP setting and a significantly higher Pao_2/Fio_2 ratio. Setting PEEP to achieve a transpulmonary pressure of 0 to 5 cm H_2O at end expiration and titrating to optimal hemodynamic values and oxygen delivery are other methods. Typically, more than one type of measurement is considered when setting PEEP. Regardless of method, the goal is to maintain alveolar recruitment without overdistention so that mechanical ventilation does not add injury to the patient's condition.

Flow Delivery

The ventilator will initiate the delivery of flow to a patient under two conditions. If a patient is not assisting (triggering breaths), the start of inspiratory flow will be determined by the total cycle time based on the frequency set. For example, if the mandatory rate is set to 12/min, inspiratory flow will be initiated every 5 seconds. If a patient is actively assisting breaths, flow is delivered when a breath is triggered by the patient.

Flow Patterns

Most ventilators offer different inspiratory flow patterns. The square (constant) flow pattern delivers the breath at a constant flow rate. The decelerating flow pattern delivers the fastest flow at the start of the breath and the flow decreases throughout inspiration. The sine flow pattern delivers the fastest flow in the middle of the breath. There has been no research to definitively support the use of any flow pattern over another. However, the descending ramp flow pattern is associated with a lower PIP than the square flow pattern and may meet initial flow demand better. In addition, descending ramp flow has been theorized to improve gas distribution and therefore oxygenation.

Rise Time

The **rise time** or slope control on a ventilator allows the practitioner to fine-tune how quickly the flow valve opens during inspiration, and peak flow and PIP are achieved when pressure ventilation modes are used. When the rise time is set on zero, or the slope on 100%, the flow valve opens as quickly as it can as inspiration begins, so the peak flow and PIP are rapidly achieved. Increasing the rise time setting, or decreasing the slope, will open the valve more slowly, and the rise to peak flow and PIP will be more gradual. If the valve is opening too quickly, there will be an overshoot in the pressure scalar followed by small spikes from airway turbulence. There may also be an overshoot in the flow scalar. If the opening of the valve is slowed too much, the pressure plateau is reduced and the tidal volume delivery may suffer. The rise time or slope should be set at a level that eliminates the pressure overshoot and turbulence without sacrificing pressure plateau and tidal volume delivery.

Cycle Percent

The cycle percent setting can be used to fine-tune when the flow valve closes to end inspiration. It is functional during spontaneous breaths that flow cycle (pressure support breaths). Most ventilators have a default percentage at which flow cycling occurs. Increasing the flow cycle percent would allow the breath to cycle to expiration sooner, while decreasing it would prolong inspiration. If a patient exhibits active exhalation, seen by a pressure spike at end inspiration on the pressure scalar, increasing the flow cycle percent will terminate the breath at a higher flow rate and reduce cycling dyssynchrony. If an airway leak is making it difficult to achieve the typical/default flow cycle setting, increasing the cycle percent value can avoid an extended inspiratory time. If spontaneous tidal volume needs to be maximized, a decrease in the cycle percent value, if tolerated by the patient, will terminate inspiration at a lower flow rate and increase tidal volume delivery.

I:E Ratio

The ratio between inspiration and expiration is monitored to avoid air trapping. It is normally at least 1:2, meaning that the expiration time is twice the length of inspiration. The adjustment of the I:E ratio is usually based on patient tolerance or lung condition. The I:E ratio normal range of 1:2 to 1:4 is based on a normal respiratory frequency (about 12 to 18/min).

How to Calculate I:E Ratio

The I:E ratio is calculated by determining the expiratory time and then dividing both the inspiratory time and the expiratory time by the smaller value. Usually, inspiratory time is shorter than expiratory time (1:2), so both inspiratory and expiratory time are divided by the inspiratory time (see **Box 6-2**).

Significance of the I:E Ratio

In patients prone to air trapping, it is advisable to have a shorter inspiratory time and a longer expiratory time to allow the patient to fully exhale. The time constant (TC), which is obtained by multiplying the airway resistance by the lung compliance, can be used as a guide when setting the I:E ratio. Allowing for at least 3 TCs for exhalation permits the majority of the tidal volume (95%) to exhale from the lung (4 TCs allow for 98% exhalation), thus avoiding air trapping. As the resistance or compliance increases, a longer expiratory time will be required.

For patients with severe air trapping, using a longer expiratory time as a remedy may not be the most effective strategy. This is because the *final* portion of

---

BOX 6-2 I:E Ratio Determination

60/rate = total cycle time

Expiratory time = Total cycle time − Inspiratory time

$$I:E = \frac{\text{Inspiratory time}}{\text{Inspiratory time}} : \frac{\text{Expiratory time}}{\text{Inspiratory time}}$$

If expiratory time is shorter than inspiratory time, divide by the expiratory time.

expiratory flow produces a very small volume due to expiratory flow decay (i.e., most volume is expired at the beginning of exhalation). In this case, reducing the rate or tidal volume may be more effective in reducing air trapping and auto-PEEP.

Reversing the I:E Ratio

Mean airway pressure is directly related to blood oxygenation. The inspiratory time can be manipulated to improve oxygenation of a patient by increasing it. A reverse ratio (or inverse ratio), in which inspiration is longer than expiration, may improve oxygenation in patients by increasing the diffusion time and the mean airway pressure. To reverse the ratio, the inspiratory time is slowly increased, over several hours, until a positive response in oxygenation occurs. Inverse ratio ventilation is not commonly used and carries many associated hemodynamic risks. Because it is uncomfortable, it requires sedation and sometimes paralyzation to be tolerated, depending on the increase in inspiratory time.

Airway Resistance

Airway resistance (the pressure required to maintain a flow) occurs whenever fluid flows through a tube. Gas (a compressible fluid) exhibits this same phenomenon when flowing through a tube, such as an airway.

Components of Airway Resistance

Because the walls of the airways are not smooth, gas flowing through an airway will encounter friction as it rubs the sides of the airways and encounters irregularities along the walls of the airway. These irregularities could be secretions on the walls of the airway or simply inflammation or narrowing of the walls of the airway. In addition, flow is altered at every bifurcation of the airway, which occurs with regularity in the lungs. All of these factors combine to cause airway resistance to flow.

Normal Value for Airway Resistance

Resistance through the natural airways is normally about 0.5 to 2.5 cm H_2O/L/sec in adult patients. The normal value for infants and children is much higher as their airways are much smaller. The expected value in an intubated patient is higher (at least double if not more) because of the resistance of the endotracheal (ET) tube.

Calculation of Airway Resistance

A patient's airway resistance can be calculated by dividing the difference between the peak and plateau pressure by a constant flow in L/sec (**Box 6-3**). As resistance increases, the difference between the peak and plateau pressures will increase. This occurs because PIP is influenced by airway resistance and lung compliance, while plateau pressure is only influenced by lung compliance.

BOX 6-3 Calculation of Airway Resistance

$$Raw \left(in \frac{L}{sec} \right) = \frac{(PIP - P_{plat})}{Flow}$$

To convert the flow to L/sec, divide the flow in L/min by 60.

PIP, peak inspiratory pressure; Pplat, plateau pressure; Raw, airway resistance.

How to Recognize Airway Resistance Without Calculating It

Trends in resistance can be tracked by noting the difference between the peak and plateau pressures. If resistance is increasing, the difference between the two will increase as PIP rises. When resistance decreases, the difference between the PIP and plateau pressure will decrease. If lung compliance alone is changing, both the peak and plateau pressures will increase with decreasing compliance (difference between peak and plateau pressures will remain relatively unchanged).

Auto-PEEP

At resting exhalation, the tendency of the rib cage to spring outward is normally offset by the tendency of the alveoli to recoil or collapse, and functional residual capacity (FRC) is attained. The lungs never completely empty of the air, even with maximal expiratory effort. When PEEP is set on a ventilator, the alveoli do not exhale to the usual FRC—some additional volume is retained in the lungs as a result of the PEEP pressure. Auto-PEEP occurs when unintended volume remains in the lungs at end-expiration.

Definition of Auto-PEEP

Auto-PEEP is the presence of unintended baseline pressure. It can exist with or without set (external) PEEP applied to the alveoli at end-expiration. When air that would normally be exhaled remains in the lungs at end exhalation, it exerts pressure within the thorax and results in auto-PEEP. It may also be called intrinsic, unintentional, latent, or occult PEEP, and it is caused by trapped air in the lungs. External PEEP delivered by a ventilator is applied evenly throughout the lungs, but auto-PEEP occurs unevenly in the lungs. It is important to monitor for auto-PEEP for several reasons. The extra pressure exerted in the thorax impedes venous return to the heart, according to Berlin (2014), potentially decreasing the cardiac output. In addition, extra pressure increases the risk of overdistention and barotrauma, especially due to the uneven distribution of auto-PEEP. Finally, the extra pressure increases the effort required for the patient to trigger the ventilator, increasing the work

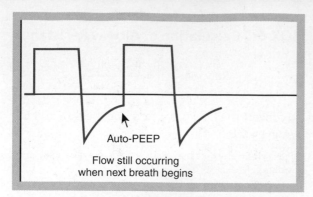

FIGURE 6-2 Air trapping (auto-PEEP) on the expiratory flow-time waveform. PEEP, positive end-expiratory pressure.

of breathing and patient–ventilator dyssynchrony. The presence of auto-PEEP is routinely monitored by assessing the end expiratory flow scalar. If the end expiratory flow is not zero, auto-PEEP may be present. **Figure 6-2** shows how auto-PEEP is recognized using ventilator graphical analysis. Once the presence of auto-PEEP has been detected, it can be measured by performing an end-expiratory pause. This allows pressure equilibration between the patient and the expiratory pressure manometer within the ventilator so the actual expiratory (baseline) pressure may be measured. (Figure 6-2).

Causes of Auto-PEEP

There are many causes of auto-PEEP. It will occur any time the expiratory time is insufficient to allow complete exhalation. It is also more common when airway resistance is high, as flow through the airways would be impeded. High minute ventilation is also associated with auto-PEEP (the result of dynamic hyperinflation). Gas trapping can also occur as a result of premature small airway collapse associated with chronic obstructive pulmonary disease (COPD).

How to Eliminate Auto-PEEP

Changes that reduce airway resistance can help reduce auto-PEEP. This includes suctioning the patient, administering a bronchodilator or anti-inflammatory agent, or replacing an artificial airway that is kinked or has dried accumulation of secretions. Shortening the inspiratory time and lengthening the expiratory time may also reduce auto-PEEP. Reducing an above-normal minute ventilation will often reduce the risk of auto-PEEP. This can be accomplished by a reduction in the respiratory rate or tidal volume, or by sedating the patient (assuming ventilation needs are met). Auto-PEEP associated with premature airway collapse is more likely to resolve with applied (external, therapeutic) PEEP than other causes of auto-PEEP.

Use of Auto-PEEP with Airway Pressure Release Ventilation

Airway pressure release ventilation (APRV) improves oxygenation in patients by intentionally creating auto-PEEP. The very short release times used do not allow for complete exhalation, causing air trapping and auto-PEEP. The shorter the release time, the greater the auto-PEEP that develops.

Patient Monitoring

Chest Inspection

After initiation of ventilation, a quick assessment of the chest helps evaluate the adequacy of the settings. This quick assessment does not eliminate the need for a more complete assessment. It is done to rapidly ensure patient safety once mechanical ventilation has been instituted. Even for this abbreviated assessment, one should never rely on a single method to confirm adequate settings.

Chest Movement

Bilateral chest rise should be observed with each breath following the application of mechanical ventilation. If it cannot be seen, the tidal volume setting may be too low or a leak may be present. If chest movement is uneven, ET tube position should be confirmed. If placement of the ET tube is correct, possibilities include pneumothorax, atelectasis, or mucous plugging.

Chest Percussion

Diagnostic chest percussion can be used to assess the adequacy of ventilation and the presence of abnormalities. Normal resonant percussion in all lobes implies adequate ventilation with no lung abnormalities. Dull percussion occurs over lung tissue with consolidation (increased density of lung tissue) caused by less air present in the lung (the result of atelectasis or edema). Hyperresonant percussion results from increased air in the lung, hyperexpansion, or air in the pleural space (pneumothorax). Monitoring for alterations in ventilation allows the practitioner to adjust ventilation parameters to better ventilate the patient.

Chest Radiograph

Monitoring the chest radiograph (x-ray film or image that is often referred to as simply "x-ray") is advisable to evaluate ET tube position and progression of the patient's lung disease. The ET tube should be visualized in the trachea with the tip approximately 3 to 5 cm above the carina. If the carina cannot be visualized, the tip of the tube should extend below the clavicles. As the patient's lung disease progresses, a chest radiograph can be used to evaluate interventions. Worsening of the disease state may be recognized by increasing opacities on

TABLE 6-1

Comparison of Findings in Normal and Abnormal Chest X-Rays

Normal Findings	Abnormal Findings
Trachea in the midline of the thorax.	Trachea shifted to either side, pushed away from a pneumothorax and pulled toward atelectasis/collapsed lung
Radiolucent lung fields (because x-rays freely pass through air)	Radio-opacities/infiltrates (because x-rays cannot easily pass through fluid/consolidated lung tissue)
Sharp costophrenic angle where the visceral pleura of the lung meets the parietal pleura of the chest wall near the diaphragm	Blunted costophrenic angle (pleural effusion) where the junction of the lung and chest wall is obscured because of fluid accumulated at the costophrenic angle
Heart size <60% of the horizontal distance from one side of the inner chest wall to the other	Heart size >60% (cardiomegaly) of the horizontal distance between the right and left sides of the inner chest wall border
Endotracheal tube 3 to 5 cm above carina or between T2 and T4 (or extending below the clavicles) if the carina cannot be visualized	Endotracheal tube too high above the carina or inserted too low (main stem intubation)

Modified from Oakes D, Jones S. *Oakes' ABG Instructional Guide*. 2nd ed. Orono, ME: Health Education Publications; 2017.

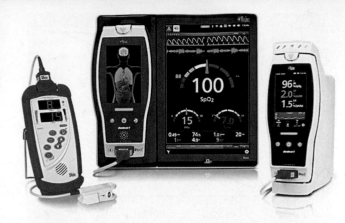

FIGURE 6-3 Masimo CO-oximeter devices integrating Masimo rainbow SET® technology.
Courtesy of Masimo Corporation.

the x-ray image, which may require higher PEEP levels to maintain recruitment and oxygenation. As the radiograph shows improvement, settings may be weaned to avoid overdistention of the lung. Monitoring of the chest x-ray, in conjunction with other information, helps the clinician make adjustments in ventilation to minimize the harmful effects of mechanical ventilation. **Table 6-1** outlines some normal and abnormal findings of chest radiography.

Saturation

Arterial oxygen saturation via pulse oximetry (SpO_2) is one method to monitor the oxygenation status of a ventilated patient. It is a noninvasive tool that allows reliable, rapid assessment.

How the Equipment Works

Pulse oximetry works by shining at least two wavelengths of light through a digit or ear, depending on the probe used (more wavelengths increase accuracy and allow for detection of abnormal hemoglobin variants). As described by Pope (2016), one of the wavelengths is in the red light zone, and this wavelength is absorbed by deoxygenated hemoglobin. The other wavelength of

light used is in the infrared zone, and this wavelength of light is better absorbed by oxygenated hemoglobin. By comparing the amount of red and infrared light absorbed, the oxygen saturation can be determined.

Normal Values

Oxygen saturation is normally 95% or greater, but in difficult-to-oxygenate patients an acceptable saturation is 90% or greater. It is important to understand that pulse oximetry using only two wavelengths of light is not accurate if dysfunctional hemoglobins are present. The pulse oximeter can only recognize hemoglobin in combination with oxygen (oxyhemoglobin) or hemoglobin in combination with hydrogen (deoxyhemoglobin). It will read falsely high in the presence of carboxyhemoglobin (COHb), sulfhemoglobin (SHb), methemoglobin (MetHb), or other abnormal forms of hemoglobin. In these cases, **CO-oximetry** with arterial blood sample is more accurate since it uses more wavelengths of light to measure other variants of hemoglobin. It is important to note that there are many manufacturers of pulse oximeters, and they each have their own unique characteristics. For example, devices integrating the Masimo rainbow SET® technology (**Figure 6-3**) uses additional wavelengths of light to monitor COHb as well as MetHb.

Significance of Changes

While adequate saturation is important to monitor, it does not completely evaluate a patient's oxygenation. As seen on the oxyhemoglobin curve in **Figure 6-4**, the PaO_2 must change by a large amount to increase or decrease the saturation by a small amount when the saturation exceeds 90%. If saturation is the only monitor of oxygenation, a patient could have a very large change in the PaO_2 before the saturation will change. This may not seem significant, consider this example: A patient with a PaO_2 of 500 mm Hg would have a saturation of 100%. If the PaO_2 drops by 400 mm Hg to 100 mm Hg, the saturation would change very little or not at all. It is

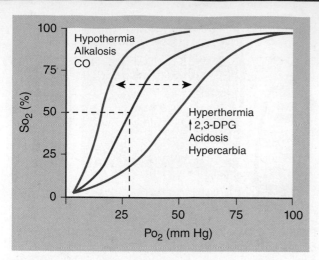

FIGURE 6-4 The oxyhemoglobin dissociation curve. 2,3-DPG, 2,3-diphosphoglycerate.

Reproduced from Crapo JD, Glassroth J, Karlinsky JB, King TE, eds. *Baum's Textbook of Pulmonary Diseases.* 7th ed. Philadelphia, PA: Lippincott Williams & Wilkins; 2003.

also important to note that a PaO_2 below 60 mm Hg causes a rapid drop in oxygen saturation (due to the steep portion of the oxyhemoglobin dissociation curve). Clinically, a PaO_2 of 60 mm Hg approximates an arterial oxygen saturation of 90%.

Respiratory Rate

Respiratory rate is monitored to evaluate the adequacy of ventilation. Ventilators are always set up to allow patient triggering so that the patient is never locked out and unable to trigger a breath (with the exception of control and intermittent mandatory ventilation modes). The type of breath the patient receives depends on the mode selected. If the mode is assist-control, or continuous mandatory ventilation, then all breaths delivered will be ventilator controlled, whether triggered by time or patient effort. When synchronized intermittent mandatory ventilation (SIMV) is the mode, then assisted breaths may be either ventilator or patient controlled. With spontaneous ventilation, all breaths are patient controlled; the patient determines the respiratory rate, the tidal volume, and the inspiratory time.

Normal Respiratory Rate

Normally, the initial set respiratory rate is between 12 and 18/min (ranges vary depending on the source). Lower rates may be set when weaning patients using the SIMV mode. Higher rates may be set when lung protective ventilation, which limits the tidal volume, is used.

Tachypnea

Patients may become tachypneic while on the ventilator and meet their minute ventilation needs in an attempt to maintain acid–base homeostasis, or a normal pH. This increases the patient's work of breathing, unless a full support mode is used. When a partial support mode, such as SIMV, or a fully spontaneous mode

is used, tachypnea may greatly increase the work of breathing through an ET tube. This can be mimicked by trying to breathe rapidly through a small straw—it is very difficult to get enough flow to meet breathing requirements when the rate is high. Increasing the level of support, by either changing to a full support mode or increasing the pressure support of spontaneous breaths, can help reduce the patient work of breathing. Tachypneic rates greater than 20/min should elicit a search for the cause. Pain, anxiety, fever, and increased metabolism could all lead to tachypnea. It also occurs as a physiologic response to severe hypoxemia. Sustained increases in respiratory rate signal the need for a detailed assessment of the patient and ventilator settings.

Bradypnea

When the ventilator rate is set below 12/min, such as when weaning in the SIMV mode, **bradypnea** may occur (a total respiratory rate less than 10/min). Patients who have had a head injury may exhibit uneven respiratory drive and become bradypneic or apneic. Additionally, if sedation is too high, bradypnea or apnea may occur. The set rate may need to be increased to meet the patient's physiologic needs.

Heart Rate

Mechanical ventilation can have profound effects on cardiovascular function, making heart rate monitoring a priority. Positive pressure applied to the thorax can interfere with venous return to the heart, as indicated by a rise in the central venous pressure due to mechanical ventilation. As central venous pressure increases, the gradient for blood flow back to the heart decreases, which can decrease preload of the heart. As preload drops, stroke volume (the amount ejected per beat) drops. The only way to maintain the cardiac output when the stroke volume decreases is for the heart rate to increase. While many other factors alter heart rate (e.g., hypoxemia, fever, pain, and stress), an alteration in cardiac output should be suspected if the heart rate increases in conjunction with initiation of mechanical ventilation or a change in ventilator settings.

Normal Heart Rate

Normally, the sinoatrial (SA) node controls the heart rate and maintains it between 60 and 100/min. The SA node can generate an electrical impulse in the heart without a nerve impulse from the central nervous system (CNS). While the CNS can influence the heart rate, it is a modifier and not the primary pacemaker.

Tachycardia

Tachycardia occurs when the heart rate exceeds 100/min. There are many causes of tachycardia, and it should signal an assessment to determine the cause when it is noted. Fever is a common cause of tachycardia. Anxiety, pain, hypoxia, and stress can also lead to tachycardia. It is also a side effect of some medications. Tachydysrhythmias of the atria may also cause tachycardia. Extreme tachycardia may lower the cardiac output because it shortens the filling time of the heart. In this instance, the tachycardia must be addressed with either medications to slow the heart rate or cardioversion to revert the rhythm back to a sinus rhythm.

Bradycardia

Bradycardia (a heart rate <60/min) is not usually a result of mechanical ventilation, but a failing heart may not be able to increase the heart rate in the face of decreased preload. Therefore, bradycardia may be a symptom of a diseased heart rather than a side effect of mechanical ventilation. It can, however, occur as a side effect of endotracheal suctioning, as a vagal response to the presence of the catheter in the airway. When this occurs, suctioning should be ceased and 100% oxygen administered to the patient. A dilated cardiomyopathy (enlarged heart) is one of the few conditions that may cause cardiac function to improve with positive pressure ventilation. The compression of the heart by positive pressure squeezes it to a more normal size that allows for better cardiac muscle fiber contraction (this reaction is variable).

Blood Pressure

Along with heart rate monitoring, blood pressure monitoring evaluates the hemodynamic stability of the patient. For tissues to be perfused and receive oxygen, adequate blood pressure must be maintained. Mechanical ventilation may potentially alter the blood pressure and therefore negatively affect tissue oxygenation. The brain and kidneys are especially sensitive to even brief drops in mean arterial blood pressure.

Normal Blood Pressure

The systolic blood pressure is normally less than 120 mm Hg. This is the peak pressure within the arteries when the ventricle contracts. The diastolic blood pressure is normally less than 80 mm Hg. This is the pressure exerted by the blood within the arteries when the heart is at rest. It is also the pressure that the ventricle must build up within it before the aortic valve will open and blood will flow into the aorta.

Hypertension

Hypertension is present when either the systolic or the diastolic blood pressure exceeds the normal value. It is usually idiopathic (no known cause) but may occur secondary to diseases (e.g., kidney or thyroid disease, obstructive sleep apnea) or use of medications (e.g., birth control pills, decongestants, illegal drugs). Many of the causes of tachycardia also increase the blood pressure.

Most clinicians treat blood pressure based on the diastolic value rather than the systolic value, because the diastolic value reflects how much work the heart has

TABLE 6-2
Blood Pressure Categories

Category	Systolic		Diastolic
Within normal limits	<120 mm Hg	plus	<80 mm Hg
Increased	120–129 mm Hg	plus	<80 mm Hg
Stage I hypertension	120–139 mm Hg	or	80–89 mm Hg
Stage 2 hypertension	140 mm Hg or higher	or	90 mm Hg or higher
Hypertensive crisis	>180 mm Hg	and/or	>120 mm Hg

Reprinted with permission Panchal AR, Berg KM, Kudenchuk PJ, et al. 2018 American Heart Association focused update on advanced cardiovascular life support use of antiarrhythmic drugs during and immediately after cardiac arrest: an update to the American Heart Association guidelines for cardiopulmonary resuscitation and emergency cardiovascular care. *Circulation.* 2018;138(23):e740–e749. ©2018 American Heart Association, Inc.

to do to open the aortic valve (**Table 6-2**). However, a high systolic blood pressure can be concerning as well. It is associated with cerebral vascular accidents (strokes) and vessel aneurysm.

Hypotension

If mechanical ventilation reduces preload and cardiac output, the response of the blood vessels is vasoconstriction, in an effort to maintain the blood pressure and organ perfusion. Hypotension may occur as a side effect of mechanical ventilation if the blood vessels are unable to constrict enough to maintain the blood pressure. If the hypotension occurs in conjunction with initiation of ventilation or with a change in the settings, mechanical ventilation should be suspected as the culprit.

Pulse Pressure

Pulse pressure is the difference between the systolic and diastolic blood pressure—the diastolic is subtracted from the systolic to obtain the pulse pressure. This determines the "felt" pulse strength, and it is an indirect monitor of the stroke volume. A patient may have high blood pressure values, but if the pulse pressure is narrow (small difference between systolic and diastolic pressures), it will feel like a weak pulse.

Normal Pulse Pressure

Normally, the pulse pressure is about 30 to 40 mm Hg, with a range of 30 to 50 mm Hg. This should be evaluated in light of the blood pressure, however. For example, a patient with a blood pressure of 120/80 mm Hg will have a pulse pressure of 40 mm Hg. A patient with a blood pressure of 200/160 mm Hg will also have a pulse pressure of 40, but clearly this patient has increased risk associated with the elevated blood pressure.

Significance of Changes

High pulse pressures are associated with increased stroke volume. Elevated pulse pressure is also common as the arteries become less elastic with aging (atherosclerosis). High pulse pressure is also found when heart valves are leaky. The presence of a high pulse pressure must be evaluated in concert with the patient's overall cardiac health. Low pulse pressure may occur when the heart is diseased and not contracting optimally. Monitoring the pulse pressure when mechanical ventilation is applied, or when changes are made, may indicate interference of the ventilator with heart function.

Breath Sounds

Evaluating the breath sounds is a way to monitor the effectiveness of ventilation. It is a rapid assessment of the adequacy of the ventilator settings as well as placement of the ET tube. Breath sounds should be assessed when ventilator monitoring is performed or when changes are noted in the patient's condition.

Normal Breath Sounds

There are three location-specific normal breath sounds. Bronchial breath sounds (high pitch and loud) are normal when they are heard over the anterior chest over the tracheal area. Bronchovesicular breath sounds (medium pitch) are normally heard anteriorly over the first and second intercostal spaces adjacent to the sternum and posteriorly between the scapulae. Vesicular breath sounds (low pitch and soft) are normal sounds heard over the lung periphery.

Adventitious Breath Sounds

Uneven breath sounds could signal a unilateral problem within the airways or the lung parenchyma or displacement of the ET tube. Diminished breath sounds may occur when airway resistance is high or when the lung is atelectatic. The diminished gas flow results in diminished breath sounds.

Wheezes are associated with airflow through a constricted airway. Very high resistance can reduce the flow so much that little to no air movement is heard. In this instance, the presence of wheezing would indicate a decrease in the airway resistance. Wheezes are heard when airflow continues through a restricted airway. Localized wheezing is usually associated with the aspiration of a foreign body. Generalized high-pitched wheezing is associated with a generalized increase in airway resistance. It should be noted that decreased air-flow in the lower lobes of the lungs should be assessed by auscultating the lateral (lower lobe anterior segments) and posterior aspects (all other lower lobe segments) of the thorax.

Crackles are affiliated with fluid or atelectasis. Fine crackles occur when alveoli pop open as they are recruited during inspiration. Atelectasis is best treated with PEEP to maintain alveolar patency. Coarse crackles occur with fluid in the alveoli and small airways. Alveolar fluid may be treated by eliminating the cause or by the use of diuretics to shift fluid volume from tissue spaces to the vascular space.

Stridor is a harsh inspiratory sound that may be heard following extubation or with infections causing severe upper airway inflammation (e.g., epiglottitis, croup). It signals the presence of glottic edema. Stridor may be treated with vasoconstricting medications, such as racemic epinephrine, or with steroids to reduce the inflammation. Cool mist aerosol may also relieve the edema and reduce the stridor. If the stridor is severely reducing airflow, reintubation is indicated. If there is severe glottic swelling, a smaller ET tube may be needed. In the case of extreme glottic swelling, a tracheostomy may be the airway of choice.

Arterial Blood Gases

The adequacy of ventilation can be assessed by monitoring the arterial blood gases (ABGs). This is an invasive test that withdraws blood from an artery to measure the values of hydrogen ion concentration (pH), partial pressure of oxygen (PaO_2), and partial pressure of carbon dioxide ($PaCO_2$). It is commonly performed to assess the ventilatory and oxygenation status of a patient receiving mechanical ventilation. The other values reported with pH, $PaCO_2$, and PaO_2 are calculated.

Assessing Ventilation

The $PaCO_2$ and the pH of the blood indicate if ventilation is meeting the patient's needs. If the minute ventilation provided by mechanical ventilation meets the patient's metabolic demand, the pH will be in the clinical range of 7.35 to 7.45. If the carbon dioxide production increases (such as with seizure or fever), the minute ventilation must increase to maintain a homeostatic pH. The focus is not on the $PaCO_2$, but on the pH. The goal of mechanical ventilation is to normalize the pH if possible. Many clinicians rely only on ABGs to assess ventilation rather than relying on their assessment findings. Inadequate ventilation is also associated with a rapid, shallow breathing pattern, confusion, and organ dysfunction.

ABGs should always be evaluated for accuracy before relying on them to make ventilator setting changes. The pH can be quickly verified by entering the $PaCO_2$ and HCO_3^- values into a predicted pH calculator—there are many available online.

Respiratory acidosis ensues if the pH falls below 7.35 while the $PaCO_2$ rises. It can occur if the CO_2 production increases without a compensatory increase in minute ventilation. It also occurs with an unchanged CO_2 production if the minute ventilation decreases. To reverse a respiratory acidosis, the minute ventilation must be increased. This can be done by either an increase in the respiratory rate or the tidal volume setting. While a change in tidal volume yields a larger change in Pa_{CO_2} and pH, it is only recommended if the tidal volume does not exceed 10 mL/kg predicted body weight (note: recommended 6 to 8 mL/kg) and the plateau pressure does not exceed 28 to 30 cm H_2O after the change. It should also be noted that if the patient is assisting at a rate higher than the set rate in an assist-control mode, an increase in rate will only be effective if it is set higher than the total rate. Respiratory acidosis can be compensated by retention of bicarbonate by the kidneys. This takes about 24–48 hours to begin to occur, so compensation implies a condition that is more chronic than acute.

Respiratory alkalosis occurs when ventilation is in excess of metabolic needs. This will cause an increase in the pH with a decrease in the Pa_{CO_2}. In this case, the minute ventilation can be reduced by either a reduction in rate or tidal volume. If the patient is assisting at a rate higher than the set rate in an assist-control mode, a decrease in the rate will have no effect. In this case, a change of mode to SIMV or spontaneous may be warranted. Respiratory alkalosis would be compensated by a decrease in bicarbonate by the kidneys. As with the compensation for respiratory acidosis, it will take the body 24–48 hours to see evidence of compensation (assuming normal kidney function). Most patients will either fatigue or have a reversal of the cause before compensation begins. Fatigue will lead to a respiratory acidosis. The only patients that may hyperventilate long enough to compensate a respiratory alkalosis would be those whose alkalosis is ventilator induced. Some patients with head injuries also may have an erratic breathing pattern that will lead to a respiratory alkalosis. Generally, once the cause of the respiratory alkalosis has been identified and treated, the alkalosis will resolve on its own, without intervention from the practitioner.

Acute Respiratory Alkalosis

During mechanical ventilation, acute respiratory alkalosis (alveolar hyperventilation) may occur due to different reasons (e.g., hypoxia, pain, anxiety). For hypoxia, the patient will typically increase the spontaneous rate or tidal volume as a compensatory mechanism for a higher Po_2. This type of respiratory alkalosis should be managed by identifying and resolving the cause of hypoxia. Acute respiratory alkalosis must *not* be managed by reducing the ventilator rate or tidal volume. By reducing ventilatory support, the patient will likely further increase the spontaneous work of breathing to make up the deficit from the ventilator. This can lead to undesirable events such as patient–ventilator dyssynchrony, tachycardia, arrhythmia, and respiratory muscle fatigue. Acute respiratory alkalosis is an

uncommon event when the ventilator settings are set appropriately. When the patient increases the spontaneous breathing effort, the causes of respiratory alkalosis must be investigated and resolved before making changes to the ventilator settings, especially the rate or tidal volume.

Metabolic alkalosis, in which the pH is alkalotic due to a rise in the bicarbonate level, has many causes. The pH becomes alkalotic from either a loss of acid or an increase in base. It is accompanied by a decrease in potassium and chloride, as the kidneys attempt to maintain electrical neutrality in the bloodstream. Compensated metabolic alkalosis is not seen clinically, unless the alkalosis is very mild, because the compensatory mechanism would be hypoventilation.

Metabolic acidosis occurs when the pH is acidotic due to a fall in the bicarbonate level. An increase in acids or a decrease in base would lead to a metabolic acidosis. Acids in the blood increase when the kidneys malfunction and cannot regulate acid–base balance. Ketoacids increase in the blood when fat is metabolized during diabetic ketoacidosis. Lactic acid builds up in the bloodstream when metabolism becomes anaerobic. The cause of a metabolic acidosis can be determined from the **anion gap**, a calculation that correlates cations and anions in the blood. Normally they are fairly well balanced with a gap of 10 to 14 mEq/L. An increased anion gap acidosis occurs with lactic acidosis, ketoacidosis, renal failure, and some drug toxicity. Metabolic acidosis with a normal anion gap is due to loss of bicarbonate and is associated with hyperchloremia (high chloride levels in the blood resulting from intracellular chloride shifting to the plasma to replace lost bicarbonate and maintain ionic balance). The compensation for metabolic acidosis is to hyperventilate and blow the CO_2 off. Because CO_2 is an acid, reducing it in the bloodstream will reduce the level of acidosis until the cause of the metabolic acidosis is found and reversed. **Table 6-3** summarizes ABG normal values, acidosis values, and alkalosis values.

Assessing Oxygenation

To assess the adequacy of oxygenation, several factors must be examined. Oxygen is carried through the bloodstream mainly bound to hemoglobin. Only a small

TABLE 6-3
Arterial Blood Gases

	Normal	Acidosis	Alkalosis
pH	7.35–7.45	<7.35	>7.45
P_{CO_2}	35–45	>45	<35
HCO_3^-	22–26	<22	>26

amount of oxygen (1% to 2% of total) is carried by the plasma. The Pa_{O_2} shows the amount of oxygen dissolved in the plasma, and it is normally 80 to 100 mm Hg. Mild hypoxemia occurs when the Pa_{O_2} falls below 80 mm Hg. While the Pa_{O_2} is insignificant in terms of oxygen carried, it is important because oxygen cannot combine with hemoglobin until it dissolves in the plasma, so a person must have an adequate Pa_{O_2} to have saturation of the hemoglobin.

About 98% of oxygen-carrying capacity is performed by hemoglobin. Hemoglobin is a blood protein that contains an iron group (heme) that can form a reversible reaction with oxygen. For optimal oxygenation, there must be adequate hemoglobin and sufficient oxygen saturation of hemoglobin.

Another component of adequate oxygenation is adequate cardiac output. Without blood flow, oxygen cannot be carried from the lungs to the tissues that require oxygen for metabolism. Cardiac output is normally 4 to 8 L/min and it varies with body size.

The Pa_{O_2} can be no higher than the PA_{O_2}—oxygen in the artery cannot be higher than oxygen within the alveolus. One rule of thumb to assess oxygenation is the 50/50 rule: If the FI_{O_2} is 0.5 or higher and the Pa_{O_2} is 50 mm Hg or lower, then a significant shunt is present (perfusion without ventilation).

Tissue oxygenation, which is the ultimate goal of mechanical ventilation, is assessed by looking for clinical signs or symptoms of hypoxia. Cyanosis is a sign of either tissue hypoxia or reduced tissue perfusion. When the cyanosis is seen in the mucous membranes, poor oxygenation is often the cause. Organ dysfunction can also point to hypoxia. Reduced level of consciousness, liver dysfunction, and reduced urine output could indicate the presence of tissue hypoxia in the absence of other causes of organ dysfunction. Several calculated values can also be used to assess oxygenation (**Table 6-4**).

CO-Oximetry

The major limitation of pulse oximeter and ABGs is that they cannot directly measure the oxygen saturation and different hemoglobin components of a blood sample. CO-oximetry uses the arterial blood sample and it can measure the levels of hemoglobin as well as other dysfunctional hemoglobins [e.g., COHb, SHb, and MetHb]. Dysfunctional hemoglobins have a limited capability to carry oxygen. For instance, patients with carbon monoxide poisoning ($\uparrow$ COHb) or methemoglobinemia ($\uparrow$ MetHb) would develop hypoxia refractory to oxygen therapy alone.

Interpretation of Superimposing Blood Gas Results

Correct interpretation of blood gas results relies on the knowledge of a patient's past and current diagnoses or clinical conditions. For example, initiation of mechanical ventilation on a patient with COPD would have combined blood gas data (compensated respiratory acidosis for COPD and acute respiratory alkalosis for mechanical ventilation). The combined superimposing blood gas results would have an "interpretation" of compensated metabolic alkalosis. The reason behind this incorrect interpretation is summarized in **Table 6-5**. The correct interpretation should be acute respiratory alkalosis superimposed on chronic respiratory acidosis. In general, patients with COPD usually have "baseline" preexisting blood gas results showing compensated respiratory acidosis. A similar method (by directional arrows to show increase or decrease) may be used to interpret other combined superimposing blood gas results.

Respiratory Acidosis and Compensated Metabolic Alkalosis

Respiratory acidosis is caused by hypoventilation. The most notable features of acute hypoventilation

---

TABLE 6-4
Assessment of Oxygenation

Parameter	Calculation	Normal	Abnormal	Significance of Abnormal Findings
P/F ratio	Pa_{O_2}/FI_{O_2}	>300	<300	Low arterial Pa_{O_2} for the FI_{O_2}, signals poor gas exchange across the alveolocapillary membrane. Low ratios (<300) are used to classify the severity of ARDS
Pa_{O_2}/PA_{O_2}	Pa_{O_2}/PA_{O_2}	0.8–1	<0.8	Values <0.8 indicate poor gas exchange across the alveolocapillary membrane
$P(A-a)_{O_2}$	$[(P_B - 47) \times FI_{O_2} - (Pa_{CO_2} \times 0.8)] - Pa_{O_2}$	5–10 on room air 30–60 on 100%	>60	Increased values signal poor gas exchange across the alveolocapillary membrane
Ca_{O_2}	$(Hb \times 1.34)Sa_{O_2} + Pa_{O_2} \times 0.003$	16–20 vol%	<16 vol%	Low values indicate low oxygen-carrying capacity of the arterial blood

ARDS, acute respiratory distress syndrome.
Adapted from Cairo JM. *Pilbeam's Mechanical Ventilation: Physiological and Clinical Applications.* 6th ed. St. Louis, MO: Elsevier; 2016; Chang D. *Clinical Application of Mechanical Ventilation.* 4th ed. Clifton Park, NY: Delmar-Cengage Learning; 2014.

TABLE 6-5
Interpretation of Combined Superimposing Blood Gas Results

	pH	P_{CO_2}	HCO_3^-
COPD (chronic respiratory acidosis)	Normal (7.35–7.45)	↑↑	↑↑
Mechanical ventilation (acute respiratory alkalosis)	↑	↓	Unchanged
Combined*	↑	↑	↑↑

*The combined blood gas results show partially compensated metabolic alkalosis, which does not describe the underlying clinical conditions. COPD, chronic obstructive pulmonary disease.

are increasing P_{CO_2} and decreasing pH. In partially or fully compensated metabolic alkalosis, the P_{CO_2} also shows an increase (thus an assumption of primary hypoventilation). In mechanical ventilation, an increase of P_{CO_2} in response to metabolic alkalosis should not be managed by increasing ventilatory support. Increasing ventilatory support (↑ f or ↑ V_T) is only appropriate when the increased P_{CO_2} is due to primary hypoventilation, not as a compensating mechanism for metabolic alkalosis.

Respiratory Alkalosis and Compensated Metabolic Acidosis

Respiratory alkalosis is caused by hyperventilation. This condition results in decreasing P_{CO_2} and increasing pH. In fully or partially compensated metabolic acidosis, the P_{CO_2} is decreased. This may give an impression that the patient has primary hyperventilation. A decreased P_{CO_2} in response to metabolic acidosis should not be managed by decreasing ventilatory support. Decreasing ventilatory support (↓ f or ↓ V_T) is only appropriate when the decreased P_{CO_2} is due to primary hyperventilation, not as a compensating mechanism for metabolic acidosis. The ventilator rate or tidal volume should not be used to manage out-of-range P_{CO_2} due to metabolic causes.

Transcutaneous Blood Gas Monitoring

Transcutaneous blood gas monitoring is a noninvasive method to estimate Pa_{O_2} and Pa_{CO_2} by measuring the oxygen and carbon dioxide that diffuses from the vessels through the skin (Ptc_{O_2} and Ptc_{CO_2}). These gases can diffuse through the skin to an electrode that measures their values. Transcutaneous monitors tend to work better on neonates than adults because adults have thicker skin layers. In adults, their usefulness is the ability to trend changes in oxygen and carbon dioxide rather than monitor actual levels in the blood. Transcutaneous oxygen monitoring may also be used to determine peripheral oxygenation, such as when determining blood flow to a limb (also useful for monitoring perfusion to grafted tissue and reattached body parts).

How the Equipment Works

The transcutaneous O_2 electrode is a modified Clark electrode, and the transcutaneous CO_2 electrode is a modified Severinghaus electrode. They both work by warming the skin at the application site to "arterialize" the area and liquefy the lipid layer in the cell membrane. Oxygen and carbon dioxide then diffuse through the skin to the electrodes, which measure their levels.

Significance of Changes

Transcutaneous monitors may be used to reflect changes in ventilation and oxygenation rather than yield actual values. For example, if the transcutaneous oxygen monitor is decreasing, then arterial oxygen must be decreasing. The actual value is not as important as recognizing the trend. The trend can be used in conjunction with assessment information to determine the oxygenation status of the patient and therefore avoid the invasive arterial stick. Because oxygen does not diffuse well, due to its low solubility coefficient, the transcutaneous oxygen monitor, which relies on diffusion of oxygen through the skin, is not very accurate. Carbon dioxide, with its higher solubility coefficient, diffuses much more readily than oxygen, making transcutaneous measurement more accurate for carbon dioxide than for oxygen. The monitor may more closely reflect the actual arterial carbon dioxide levels, but the monitor may also be used for trending of transcutaneous carbon dioxide. Increases in the transcutaneous value imply increases in the arterial value and point to a change in ventilation. Current American Association of Respiratory Care Clinical Practice Guidelines indicate that while transcutaneous carbon dioxide monitoring may be valuable, it should be correlated with an arterial blood gas upon institution.

Transcutaneous monitors also give an indication of perfusion to the site, which can assist in assessing cardiac output and tissue oxygenation. The power output on the transcutaneous monitor is used for this purpose. When blood flow is sluggish, the power output decreases, indicating that not as much power is required to maintain a heated site. The reverse is true when blood flow increases. In this instance, the power output must also increase to maintain a constant temperature.

V_D/V_T

The dead space to tidal volume ratio assesses the amount of the tidal volume that does not participate in gas exchange. Some portion of each breath remains in the airways and therefore is not involved in gas exchange. Unlike the lung parenchyma, conducting airways cannot take part in gas exchange because they do not have the alveolocapillary properties.

Normal Values for VD/VT

Normally VD/VT is about one-third with a normal range of 20% to 40%. Most of this normal dead space is anatomic dead space related to the airways. In patients receiving mechanical ventilation, dead space may be as high as 40–60% because the positive pressure within the thorax and lung parenchyma reduces the overall pulmonary capillary perfusion.

Significance of Changes

When ventilation exceeds perfusion, dead space increases. Mechanical ventilation can increase dead space if it causes alveolar overdistention that compresses the pulmonary capillaries. Pulmonary emboli, hypotension, or other causes of low pulmonary perfusion also increase the dead space volume. Increased dead space means less of each breath is participating in gas exchange and therefore VD/VT can serve as an indicator of ventilatory efficiency.

Exhaled CO₂/Capnography

Capnography is a noninvasive method to monitor ventilation by measuring the exhaled carbon dioxide pressure. Normally, the exhaled CO_2 level is slightly lower (1 to 5 mm Hg) than the arterial CO_2 level because of the effect of changing P_{CO_2} composition in the airways and alveoli during the exhalation maneuver.

Normal Capnogram

The shape of the exhaled CO_2 curve, the capnogram, yields information about ventilation and the condition of the airways. **Figure 6-5** shows a normal capnogram. At the start of exhalation, the CO_2 level should be zero, because at the beginning of exhalation the gas is coming from the airways that did not participate in gas exchange. As exhalation continues, gas from the

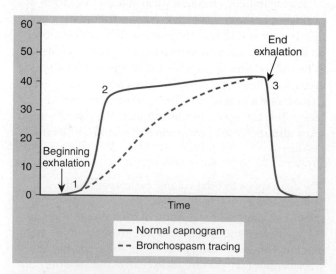

FIGURE 6-5 Normal capnogram.

conducting airways mixes with gas from proximal alveoli, and the CO_2 level begins to rise rapidly. Eventually, the airway gas portion is completely exhaled, and the remaining expiratory gas is all from the alveoli. At this point, the CO_2 level essentially plateaus. The end-tidal CO_2, the level at the very end of exhalation, is typically the highest value. When inspiration begins, the CO_2 level abruptly drops to zero, as the CO_2 level in room air is very low (about 0.3%). Normal end-tidal CO_2 is 35–40 mm Hg or 1 to 5 mm Hg lower than the Pa_{CO_2}.

Arterial End-Tidal Gradient

Normally there is a gradient between the arterial and the end-tidal CO_2, with the arterial being the higher of the two. This gradient occurs because ventilation and perfusion ($\dot{V}/\dot{Q}$) do not perfectly match in the lungs. Lung units that do not gas exchange, or have less perfusion, will dilute the end-tidal CO_2, resulting in a lower value.

Normal Gradient

The normal gradient between the arterial and end-tidal CO_2 is 1 to 5 mm Hg. Because $\dot{V}/\dot{Q}$ does not perfectly match in the lungs, units with little or no perfusion will have a CO_2 level near 0 mm Hg. Lung units with normal gas exchange function will have a CO_2 level closer to 40 mm Hg. These different lung units will mix and create an average end-tidal P_{CO_2} and establish a gradient between arterial and end-tidal values. In addition, there is a dilutional effect from the anatomic dead space that plays a major role in the normal gradient when lung function is normal. Finally, the end-tidal CO_2 level is a value at end-exhalation, whereas the arterial value is an average, which also contributes to the normal gradient.

Increased Gradient

The gradient between the arterial and end-tidal CO_2 increases with dead space diseases, such as pulmonary emboli or reduced cardiac output. Dead space also increases with overdistention of the alveoli, when tidal volume or application of PEEP is excessive. As dead space increases, more lung units do not gas exchange, influencing the end-tidal value. One application for monitoring the gradient is after cardiac surgery during which perfusion was routed through a heart-lung machine during the procedure. A rise in the end-tidal CO_2 indicates a reduction in dead space as the lung reperfuses following surgery. It signals when recovery is complete.

Decreased Gradient

The gradient between arterial and end-tidal CO_2 will decrease as $\dot{V}/\dot{Q}$ matching improves. Another

TABLE 6-6
Factors That Alter the P(a – ET)co_2 Gradient

Normal gradient	1 to 5 mm Hg
Increased gradient	Low cardiac output Decreased perfusion Cardiac arrest Pulmonary emboli Alveolar overdistention
Decreased gradient	Found in children

BOX 6-4 Physiologic Dead Space Calculation

$$\frac{Paco_2 - Peco_2}{Paco_2} = \frac{V_D}{V_T}$$

(Petco$_2$ is the end-tidal CO_2.)

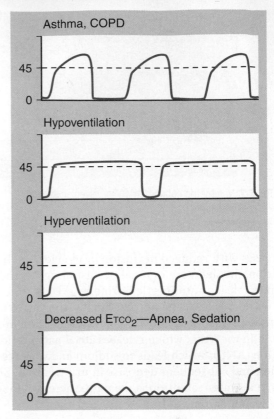

FIGURE 6-6 Abnormal capnograms. COPD, chronic obstructive pulmonary disease.

application of capnography is to monitor the effectiveness of CPR and the return of spontaneous circulation following a cardiac event. During compressions, if perfusion is effective, the end-tidal CO_2 will be close to the arterial level and the gradient should be close to the normal value. If compressions are ineffective, the end-tidal value will be low compared to the arterial. When spontaneous circulation returns, the end-tidal value should increase closer to the arterial level, decreasing the gradient. A decreased gradient occurs in children, as $\dot{V}/\dot{Q}$ matching is better than in adults. **Table 6-6** discusses factors that alter the P(a – ET)co_2 gradient.

Calculating Physiologic Dead Space

Physiologic dead space can be calculated from the arterial and end-tidal CO_2 values (**Box 6-4**). The difference between the arterial and end-tidal CO_2 is divided by the arterial to obtain the value. Physiologic dead space is the sum of anatomic dead space and alveolar dead space. An increase in physiologic dead space would indicate a reduction in pulmonary perfusion because the anatomic dead space is a fixed volume.

Abnormal Waveforms

Abnormal **capnogram** waveforms signal ventilation abnormalities or equipment problems. Referring to **Figure 6-6**, asthma and COPD reduce the plateau seen during exhalation such that the waveform resembles a shark fin in appearance. The peak exhaled CO_2 increases with hypoventilation or increased metabolism,

which both increase the arterial CO_2. In contrast, hyperventilation decreases the peak exhaled CO_2. The exhaled CO_2 drops to zero when there is a circuit disconnect. This may also be seen following an intubation attempt if the ET tube is placed in the esophagus. One exception may occur when esophageal intubation is done to a person who has recently consumed carbonated ($CO_2 + H_2O$) beverage. For this reason, occurrence of esophageal intubation should not rely on capnography alone. Other clinical signs of esophageal intubation must be evaluated (e.g., lack of bilateral breath sounds with assisted ventilation, desaturation, gastric distention, vomiting).

Volumetric Capnometry

Volumetric capnometry differs from end-tidal capnometry in that the horizontal axis is volume rather than time. Alveolar dead space can be determined from volumetric capnometry by subtracting out the anatomic dead space. Adding the anatomic and the alveolar dead space gives the physiologic dead space. **Figure 6-7** shows volumetric capnometry.

Urine Output

Mechanical ventilation may alter the urine output by several mechanisms. If cardiac output drops as a result of positive pressure ventilation, urine output

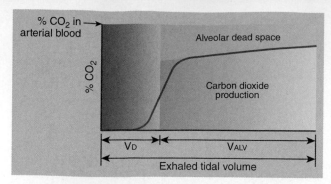

FIGURE 6-7 Volumetric capnometry. V$_{ALV}$, alveolar volume; V$_D$, deadspace volume.
Courtesy of Hamilton Medical Group.

decreases with reduced perfusion of the kidneys. In addition, the decrease in renal perfusion signals the brain to release antidiuretic hormone (ADH), which further decreases urine output. Finally, the decrease in venous return to the heart causes a reduction in stretch in the atria, which releases atrial natriuretic peptide (ANP), which leads to sodium and water retention and subsequent decrease in urine output. Sodium and water retention is meant to increase blood volume and cardiac output.

Assessment of Urine Output

Normal values for urine output range from 1 to 2 L/day, depending on the fluid intake and patient weight. Urine output may be monitored with an indwelling urine catheter in severely ill patients to closely monitor their fluid status. An hourly urine output of <0.5 mL/kg is concerning and may signal fluid retention. Assessment findings, such as hearing crackles during auscultation and observing edema in the extremities, in conjunction with a low urine output may indicate the development of pulmonary edema related to fluid retention. This patient may require a higher F$_{IO_2}$ or PEEP level to oxygenate adequately. If pulmonary edema is confirmed, a diuretic may be administered to improve fluid elimination.

Significance of Changes

In response to a reduction in cardiac output during mechanical ventilation, one of the body's responses is to retain fluid. In turn, fluid retention may lead to higher pulmonary pressures, which could result in an increase in interstitial fluid volume and potentially result in alveolar flooding. Both of these conditions would decrease oxygenation of the blood as the fluid interferes with diffusion. This may in turn result in an increase in mechanical ventilation settings, which could further impede the venous return and drop the cardiac output even more. A vicious cycle ensues. Recognizing mechanical ventilation as the source of the change in urine output may prevent this vicious cycle.

Kidney Function

As cardiac output drops during mechanical ventilation, kidney perfusion and function may be reduced. As discussed earlier, one of the most notable signs of decreased kidney function is a reduction in urine output. Other laboratory tests that correlate with decreased kidney function include elevated blood urea nitrogen (BUN; normal 7 to 20 mg/dL), serum creatinine (normal 0.6 to 1.2 mg/dL), and potassium (normal 3 to 5 mEq/L).

Drug Clearance

One of the kidney functions is to eliminate drugs and their metabolites. When the kidney function is reduced, clearance of drugs that rely on a normal kidney function is also reduced. This is an important consideration because accumulation of drugs may lead to a higher drug concentration over time. The drug intake dosage may need to be adjusted downward to factor in the inadequate kidney function. This caution also applies to patients with poor liver function when drugs are metabolized by the liver.

Liver Function

As cardiac output drops, and organ perfusion decreases, organ dysfunction may ensue as noted by Sun et al. (2013). Liver function reductions would interfere with drug metabolism, potentially requiring a reduction in dosing. Medications that are expected to be metabolized by the liver in a certain number of hours (the half-life) may have an extended/increased effect on a patient if the liver function is reduced.

Tests That Determine Liver Function

There are several blood tests that determine liver function (**Table 6-7**). Tests that monitor liver function include alanine transaminase (ALT), aspartate aminotransferase (AST), alkaline phosphatase (ALK), and bilirubin. Lactate levels, albumin levels, prothrombin time (PT), partial thromboplastin time (PTT), and international normalized ratio (INR) are other tests of liver function. The measurement of liver enzymes may be used to indicate the degree of liver damage.

Significance of Changes

The greater the liver dysfunction, the longer the half-life of medications that are metabolized by the liver. Liver dysfunction is also associated with an increase in ammonia levels within the blood. Increased ammonia levels may result in a change in the level of consciousness. In a heavily sedated patient, these changes may not be apparent until sedation is weaned.

Nutrition

Nutritional assessment is important because poor nutrition can affect a patient's ability to wean from mechanical

TABLE 6-7
Liver Function Tests

Test	Normal	Critically Increased	Significance of Abnormal Values
ALT	7–56 units/L	Not established	Medications may not metabolize as expected
AST	10–50 units/L	Not established	Medications may not metabolize as expected
ALK	40–125 units/L	Not established	Medications may not metabolize as expected
Lactate	0.7–2.1 mEq/L	> 4 mEq/L	May indicate the presence of anaerobic metabolism
Albumin	3.3–5.2 g/dL	Not established	Decreases with critical illness, increasing the likelihood for pulmonary edema due to low oncotic pressure
PT	12–15 seconds	> 30 seconds	Increases indicate increased bleeding time and increased risk of bleeding with suctioning and ABG draws
PTT	25–39 seconds	> 50 seconds	Increases indicate increased bleeding time and increased risk of bleeding with suctioning and ABG draws
INR	0.8–1.2 seconds	> 5 seconds	Increased likelihood of bleeding (suctioning and ABG draws) when elevated and clotting (disseminated intravascular coagulation [DIC]) when reduced

ABG, arterial blood gas; ALK, alkaline phosphatase; ALT, alanine transaminase; AST, aspartate aminotransferase; INR, international normalized ratio; PT, prothrombin time; PTT, partial thromboplastin time.

ventilation. Muscle weakness that accompanies malnutrition makes it difficult for the patient to assume the work of spontaneous breathing. It is for this reason that nutritional assessment is performed so that the caloric load of the patient can be titrated to meet nutritional needs.

Harris-Benedict Equation

The Harris-Benedict equation can be used to estimate a patient's caloric requirements to determine tube feeding mixtures. It is based on height, weight, age, and gender. It may seriously underestimate the calories needed by a critically ill patient because it does not take the disease state into account, as shown by Picolo et al. (2016). **Box 6-5** shows the Harris-Benedict equation.

Calorimetry

Calorimetry measures the amount of heat released by the body to determine metabolism. Because direct calorimetry is not a practical way to determine a patient's metabolic rate, indirect calorimetry is an alternative for this purpose.

Indirect Calorimetry

With indirect calorimetry, the patient's oxygen consumption and carbon dioxide production during steady state are measured to determine the metabolic rate. The most difficult part of indirect calorimetry is reaching a steady state (a stable rate of oxygen consumption and CO_2 production) in the face of rapidly altering physiology. Knowing the metabolic rate of a patient allows the caloric requirement to be accurately determined. This allows the caloric needs to be met. If the caloric

BOX 6-5 Harris-Benedict Equation

Men: $BMR = 66.5 + (13.75 \times \text{weight in kg}) + (5.003 \times \text{height in cm}) - (6.755 \times \text{age in years})$
Women: $BMR = 655.1 + (9.563 \times \text{weight in kg}) + (1.850 \times \text{height in cm}) - (4.676 \times \text{age in years})$

The number obtained is multiplied by a factor that estimates the physical activity level to estimate the total energy expenditure.

BMR, basal metabolic rate.

needs are not met, skeletal muscle, including the diaphragm, can be broken down to meet the body's protein requirements. If caloric needs are exceeded, the oxygen requirement and CO_2 production are increased. Both consequences increase the load on the lungs to maintain a minute ventilation that maintains homeostasis.

Meeting the Nutritional Needs of the Intensive Care Unit Patient

Nutritional replacement can be either enteric, through the gastrointestinal (GI) tract, or parenteral, through the bloodstream. Enteral is the preferred route, as it maintains the function of the GI tract and allows for delivery of a greater diversity of nutrients. Tube feedings designed for the enteral route are comprised of proteins, fats, and sugars in a balance percentage to support the body's requirements. Parenteral mixtures also contain proteins, fats, and sugars, but they are all in digested form as they are being infused directly into the bloodstream. Micronutrients, vitamins, and minerals needed by the body must also be included in feeding mixes. Calcium is especially important in muscle contraction, as it forms the cross-bridge between actin and myosin in the muscle myofibril, allowing contraction to occur. Decreased muscle strength is also observed in patients with inadequate magnesium and phosphate levels, which can lead to increased time on mechanical ventilation as weaning is impaired by muscle weakness.

Level of Consciousness

The patient's level of consciousness should be routinely assessed. Some level of sedation is expected for a patient on mechanical ventilation to decrease the patient's awareness of the situation. However, weaning cannot commence if the sedation is excessive. A reduction in sedation (or break, or sedation holiday), with a subsequent change in the level of consciousness, is routine before a weaning trial.

How It Is Determined

In a nonintubated patient, level of consciousness is assessed by the patient's alertness and ability to answer questions. This is a more difficult assessment in a patient who is sedated or in whom an ET tube has been placed. In this setting, the patient's ability to open the eyes and follow other simple commands assesses the level of consciousness. (See also ABCDEF Bundle in Chapter 15.)

Significance of Changes

An acute reduction in the level of consciousness signals both an acute change in body physiology and the need for immediate assessment. Level of consciousness deteriorates with liver failure as ammonia levels in the blood increase. Level of consciousness also alters with hypoxemia and hypercapnia. The use of sedative medications is expected to be accompanied by a change in the level of consciousness.

Critical Care Monitoring

Intracranial Pressure

Intracranial pressure (ICP) is the pressure within the cerebrum. It may be altered by mechanical ventilation if elevated thoracic pressure impedes venous return from the head. It is measured by placement of a catheter into a ventricle within the brain, a procedure called a ventriculostomy.

Normal ICP

The ICP is normally <10 mm Hg. Increases may decrease cerebral perfusion pressure (CPP), which can lead to brain anoxia if severely reduced. CPP, which equals mean arterial pressure (MAP) minus ICP, may be monitored in critically injured patients. It is normally 80 to 85 mm Hg. Any condition that elevates the ICP or reduces the MAP will reduce the CPP. A reduction in CPP may reduce cerebral blood flow, leading to anoxia in the brain.

Significance of Changes

Mechanical ventilation can both decrease the MAP and increase the ICP, potentially causing a reduction in CPP. The effect of a reduction in CPP is a potential increase in brain anoxia. Monitoring of ICP is especially crucial in patients already at risk for elevations (e.g., those with head injuries). When the ICP becomes elevated, it can be reduced back to more normal levels by draining fluid through the ventriculostomy catheter.

Apnea Test

The **apnea test** is used to monitor a patient to determine if brain death is present. The CO_2 is allowed to rise above 60 mm Hg while monitoring for respiratory movement. No respiratory movement implies brain death is present.

How It Is Performed

There are a variety of ways to perform the test. One method involves using a transtracheal catheter set at 4 to 10 L/min to provide oxygen to the patient during the test. Another method uses the ventilator in continuous positive airway pressure (CPAP) mode with a pressure support of 0 cm H_2O, FIO_2 1.0, and backup apnea disabled. The ventilator may also be set in SIMV with a very low set minute ventilation or an SIMV set at 0. An ABG is drawn before the test is begun and again after 10 minutes.

Before performing an apnea test, the patient should be assessed. During the assessment, the FIO_2 should be set to 1.0 to preoxygenate the patient. The patient should be assessed to determine if he or she is stable, with a temperature above 32°C and a stable blood pressure with a systolic pressure of at least 90 mm Hg. The initial ABG should show a normal or slightly alkalotic pH with a $Paco_2$ of about 40 mm Hg. The patient should also be euvolemic, and paralytic medications should be stopped.

There is no clear consensus on how long the test should last, but 10 minutes is the most common time frame used. If the systolic blood pressure drops below 90 mm Hg, the oxygen saturation drops below 85%, or more than 10 minutes have passed, the test is terminated.

Significance of Results

The test is positive if there is no respiratory effort despite an increase in the $Paco_2$, which implies that the patient's brain stem is no longer responsive to carbon dioxide (i.e., brain dead). Complications of the apnea test include hypotension, pneumothorax, acidosis, hypoxia, and cardiac dysrhythmia. If complications occur, or if the patient assessment contraindicates the test, there are several alternatives. Cerebral blood flow can be determined by a Doppler study or computed tomography (CT) angiography. An evoked potential study can also be performed to determine electrical activity in the brain.

Doll's Eyes Test

Another test to monitor the extent of injury in patients with head trauma is the test of the **vestibulo-ocular reflex**, commonly called the **doll's eyes test**. Normally, when the head is moved from side to side, the eyes deviate to the opposite side of the head and then gradually move midline. When the head is move upward, the eyes deviate down and vice versa (**Figure 6-8**).

How It Is Performed

To perform the doll's eyes test, the eyes are opened and the head is turned from side to side and up and down. During this process, the direction of deviation of the eyes is noted.

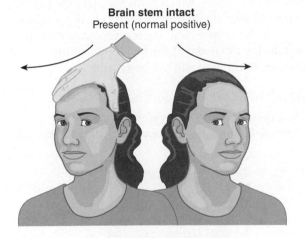

Brain stem intact
Present (normal positive)

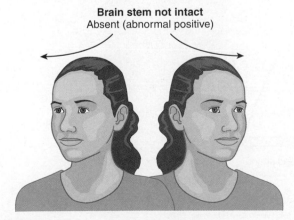

Brain stem not intact
Absent (abnormal positive)

FIGURE 6-8 Normal and abnormal doll's eyes test.

Significance of Results

Lack of deviation may occur in patients with head trauma to their brain stem. They may exhibit what is termed doll's eyes, when the eyes remain midline with head movement. This patient may have acute trauma, which could reverse with time as swelling and inflammation within the brain reduce. If the doll's eyes persist, this may signal a chronic lack of reflexes, which is an ominous sign.

Caloric Test

Another method to test the vestibulo-ocular reflex, as discussed under "Doll's Eyes Test," is to perform a **caloric test**. Like the doll's eyes test, it is used to assess the level of trauma to the brain stem.

How It Is Performed

During this test, cold or warm water is injected into the ear and the patient's response is noted. If the reflexive mechanisms are intact, cold water irrigation should deviate the eyes toward the opposite side of irrigation and warm water should deviate the eyes toward the side of irrigation.

Significance of Results

Brain injury is indicated when the eyes deviate to the side of irrigation if cold water is used or to the opposite side if warm water is used. Lack of response would also imply brain injury with a poor prognosis.

Glasgow Coma Scale

The Glasgow Coma Scale (GCS) is a simple patient assessment procedure to evaluate the severity of head or brain injury. The minimum score is a 3 (deep coma or vegetative state) and the maximum score is 15 (normal fully awake). When GCS scoring is done to evaluate patients with traumatic brain injury (TBI), the severity of TBI is classified into mild, moderate, and severe.

The three components that make up the GCS are eye opening (E), verbal responses (V), and motor responses (M). These individual scores are added (E + V + M) to come up with a composite score. The severity of brain injury is classified as mild (score 13 to 15), moderate (score 9 to 12), and severe (score = 3 to 8). (See also Chapter 14, Trauma Critical Care Issues.)

Cuff Leak Test

The **cuff leak test** monitors for the presence or absence of airway swelling in a patient with an ET tube. Prior to removal of the tube, it is important to determine that an intact, open airway is present. If the airway has swelled, removing the tube may cause complete airway closure if swelling continues or a very narrowed airway that would offer great resistance to airflow.

How It Is Performed

The cuff of the ET tube is deflated to perform the test. While the cuff is deflated, exhaled volumes and breath sounds around the cuff are monitored. Exhaled volumes should be less than inhaled volumes by more than 15%, and a leak should be heard around the area of the ET tube cuff.

Significance of Results

If a leak is observed, as evidenced by decreased exhaled volume and breath sounds, the airway has not swelled up to the diameter of the ET tube, and airway problems after extubation are unlikely. If no leak is observed, the airway has swollen around the ET tube and removal of the tube is likely to be accompanied by airway closure or restriction.

Bubble Study

During echocardiography, a sound wave is bounced off the heart to produce a picture of the heart. It can be used to determine the cardiac output. Blood flow through the heart can also be monitored using echocardiography with a technique known as a **bubble study**.

How It Is Performed

Normal saline with small bubbles in it is injected via a peripheral intravenous (IV) line. The blood containing the bubble travels to the right side of the heart. Blood flow through the heart is monitored via echocardiography to track the path of the bubbles through the heart.

Significance of Results

If a cardiac defect is present, such as an atrial septal defect, the bubbles can be seen moving from the right side of the heart to the left side through the defect. If no

defect is present, the bubbles are filtered out by the lungs. This same bubble study can also be used to detect a ventricular septal defect or a patent ductus arteriosus.

Hemodynamic Monitoring

Arterial Catheters

Arterial catheters are placed to provide continuous assessment of blood pressure and serve as a route to draw arterial blood from a patient. Mechanical ventilation may decrease the blood pressure if venous return is decreased, so careful monitoring is indicated.

Parts of the Catheter

The arterial catheter setup includes an indwelling catheter, noncompliant tubing, a transducer, and a monitor. The catheter can be placed in any artery, but the radial is preferred since it is the most superficial and collateral circulation to the hand is provided by the ulnar artery. Once placed, the catheter is connected to a transducer, which converts the pressure signal from the artery to an electrical signal. The electrical signal is then displayed on a monitor. The tubing used to connect the catheter must be able to withstand pressure without altering it, so low compliance tubing is used. A pressurized bag, containing a heparin solution, provides a continuous flow into the artery, which helps maintain the patency of the catheter. It also provides for a continuous fluid between the catheter and the transducer so pressure monitoring can occur. If the fluid is not continuous, the pressure monitored will not be accurate.

Waveforms and Their Significance

The expected arterial waveform is shown in **Figure 6-9**. The peak of the waveform is the systolic

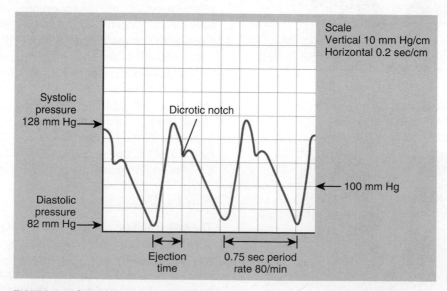

FIGURE 6-9 Arterial blood pressure waveform.

Hess, D. *Respiratory Care: Principles and Practice*, 3rd ed. Burlington, MA: Jones & Bartlett Learning, 2016.

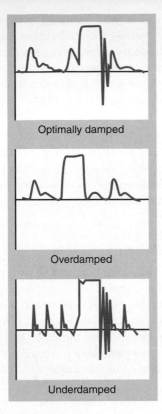

Optimally damped

Overdamped

Underdamped

FIGURE 6-10 The square wave test.

blood pressure, and the lowest point is the diastolic blood pressure. The notch in the descending limb (dicrotic notch), occurs with closure of the aortic semilunar valve. The square wave test (**Figure 6-10**) is used to ensure proper functioning of the system. The flush valve is compressed and released, allowing fluid from the pressurized bag to be released. The transducer should produce a square waveform that oscillates or bounces before returning to the baseline. No more than two oscillations should occur. If the system is overdamped (see Figure 6-10), there will be no more than one oscillation and the dicrotic notch will become indistinct. Air in the tubing or a clot in the catheter can cause this. The systolic blood pressure will be underestimated, and the diastolic blood pressure is overestimated when the system is overdamped. An underdamped system (see Figure 6-10) does the opposite and overestimates the systolic and underestimates the diastolic. When the square wave test is done to an underdamped system, there are more than two oscillations at the end of the square wave. Underdamping can occur with tachycardia rhythms, catheter whip, and hypothermia. It may also occur if the tubing used is too stiff and uncompliant according to Ortega et al. (2017).

The transducer should be placed at the level of the phlebostatic axis, which is at the midaxillary line of the fourth intercostal space. If the transducer is above this level, the measured blood pressure will be lower than actual. If the transducer is below this level, the measured blood pressure will be higher than actual. The transducer should also routinely be calibrated by exposing it to atmospheric pressure and zeroing it to this pressure.

Normal arterial blood pressure is <120 mm Hg systolic and <80 mm Hg diastolic. It is affected by the cardiac output and the vascular tone of the systemic arterioles. Increases in cardiac output or vascular tone (vasoconstriction) increase the blood pressure, while decreases in either decrease the blood pressure. The difference between the systolic and diastolic blood pressure (pulse pressure) can be used to assess the cardiac output. Larger pulse pressure is associated with greater cardiac output and vice versa. Many noninvasive ways to assess cardiac output, discussed in more detail later in this chapter, capitalize on this association.

Central Venous Pressure Catheter

These are catheters placed in a central vein to monitor the pressure. Central venous pressure (CVP) may be monitored to trend fluid balance, preload of the heart, and the influences of mechanical ventilation on the cardiac system.

Parts of the Catheter

The parts of the CVP catheter are similar to those of an arterial catheter. An indwelling catheter is placed and connected to a monitor via tubing. In this way, the pressure within the central veins can be monitored.

Placement

The catheter is introduced into a large central vein, such as the subclavian or internal jugular vein, and threaded so the tip lies in the superior vena cava or right atrium. These catheters can be used to deliver a medication into a large vein that will quickly dilute it and rapidly distribute it because of the proximity to the heart. CVP can also be monitored. The CVP is normally the lowest pressure in the cardiovascular system at approximately 2 to 6 mm Hg. This low pressure facilitates blood return to the heart. Increases in CVP occur when blood volume increases, the right side of the heart fails, or when intrathoracic pressure increases. As CVP increases, the pressure gradient for blood to return to the heart is decreased, which decreases venous return to the heart. CVP will decrease with hypovolemia or when intrathoracic pressure is very negative, as seen with a high work of breathing. CVP may be used to determine fluid status, especially when giving a fluid bolus.

Waveforms and Their Significance

The CVP waveform (**Figure 6-11**) consists of an a wave, a c wave, and a v wave. The a wave occurs with atrial contraction, and the apex of this wave is equivalent to the right ventricular end-diastolic pressure because the tricuspid valve opens with atrial contraction. Loss of the a wave is seen with atrial fibrillation as there is no coordinated atrial contraction. The c wave represents closure of the tricuspid valve. The v wave occurs as the right atrium fills with blood. A huge v wave can signal tricuspid regurgitation. Blood from the right ventricle flowing up into the right atrium increases the right atrial pressure during this filling phase.

Pulmonary Artery Catheter

The pulmonary artery (PA) catheter, also known as the Swan-Ganz catheter, is inserted via a large vein and allowed to float through the right side of the heart, coming to rest within the pulmonary artery system.

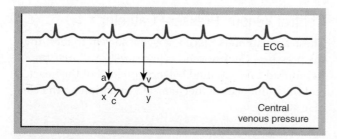

FIGURE 6-11 The central venous pressure waveform. ECG, electrocardiogram.

Hess, D. *Respiratory Care: Principles and Practice*, 3rd ed. Burlington, MA: Jones & Bartlett Learning, 2016.

This catheter allows for monitoring of the right atrial pressure or CVP along with pulmonary artery pressure (PAP) and pulmonary artery occlusion pressure (also called pulmonary artery wedge pressure, pulmonary capillary wedge pressure). It may also be used to deliver fluids and medications to the patient.

Parts of the Catheter

The catheter has four channels (**Figure 6-12**). It can be used to continuously measure pulmonary artery pressure, draw mixed venous blood samples, measure cardiac output, and measure left ventricular end-diastolic pressure.

Ports and Their Use

The right atrial injectate port will be within the right atrium when the catheter has been placed in the pulmonary artery. This port is used to administer fluid when measuring the cardiac output. It can also be used for medication delivery and monitoring of right atrial pressure. There may also be a proximal port in the right ventricle that is used to administer fluid or medication infusions.

A thermistor, which is temperature sensitive, is found near the tip of the catheter. It is used to monitor the temperature of the blood when cardiac output is measured by the thermodilution method.

The distal port, which lies in the pulmonary artery, is used for continuous measurement of mixed venous oxygen saturation and pulmonary artery pressure. It can also be used to draw blood to determine other mixed venous values.

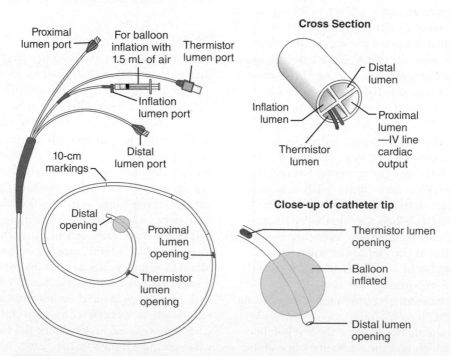

FIGURE 6-12 The pulmonary artery catheter. IV, intravenous.

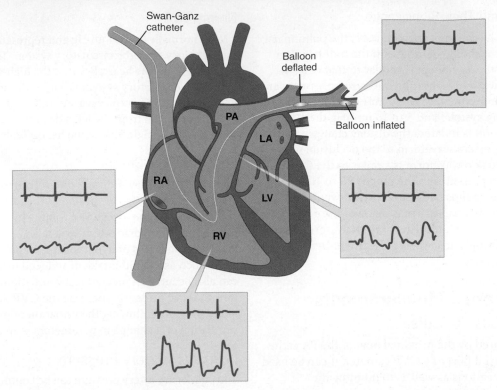

FIGURE 6-13 Insertion of the pulmonary artery catheter. LA, left atrium; LV, left ventricle; PA, pulmonary artery; RA, right atrium; RV, right ventricle.

Reproduced from Longnecker D, Brown D, Newman M, Zapol, W. *Anesthesiology*. New York, NY: McGraw-Hill, 2012. (© McGraw-Hill Education)

A balloon port allows inflation and deflation of a balloon near the tip of the catheter. When this balloon is inflated, the tip of the catheter is isolated. Because the pulmonary veins have no valves, the pressure of the left atrium can then be estimated. This pulmonary artery occlusion pressure. approximates the left ventricular end-diastolic pressure as the bicuspid valve is open throughout most of the left atrial filling phase as noted by Gidwani et al. (2013).

Placement

During insertion, the waveforms seen on the monitor indicate the position of the catheter (**Figure 6-13**). It is placed into a large central vein, such as the subclavian or internal jugular, so the first waveform seen will be the CVP waveform. At this point, the balloon is inflated and the catheter is carried along with the blood flow, floating through the right side of the heart. As it enters the right ventricle, the waveform display changes from the CVP waveform to the right ventricular waveform, with a corresponding pressure of 25/0. The catheter continues to float through the pulmonary semilunar valve into the pulmonary artery. The waveform will change from the right ventricular waveform to that of the pulmonary artery. The catheter will stop when the balloon circumference no longer allows it to float any further. The pulmonary artery occlusion waveform will then be seen. At this point, the balloon

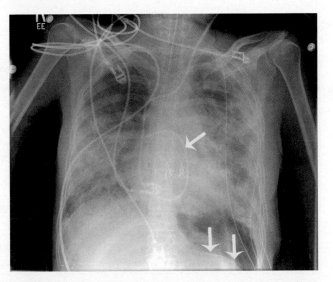

FIGURE 6-14 Chest x-ray of a pulmonary artery (PA) catheter. Single arrow points to the PA catheter placed in the right PA.

is deflated and the catheter secured. The insertion distance should be noted so catheter position can be confirmed routinely. The actual insertion distance depends on the entry point used, varying from 40 to 45 cm. On the chest x-ray (**Figure 6-14**), the catheter can be seen entering the right side of the heart and looping around to enter the right pulmonary artery. On the rare occasion in which it enters the left pulmonary artery, it does not loop around in the right ventricle.

Waveforms and Their Significance

If the catheter has been properly placed, the pulmonary artery waveform should be noted on the monitor. The appearance of the waveform is similar to that of a systemic arterial waveform, but the measured pressures are much lower, approximately 25/10 mm Hg (ranging from 20 to 35 mm Hg systolic and 5 to 15 mm Hg diastolic). When the balloon is inflated, the display changes from the pulmonary artery waveform to the occlusion waveform. The occlusion waveform is similar to the CVP waveform, with pressures in the range of 5 to 10 mm Hg. If the catheter slips back into the right ventricle, the right ventricular waveform is seen with pressures of approximately 25/0. Monitoring of the waveforms can help ensure appropriate catheter placement before measurements are recorded.

Hemodynamic Measurements

Central Venous Pressure

CVP is monitored by the proximal port of the PA catheter or by the distal port of a CVP catheter. It can be used to deliver medications as well as to monitor the CVP. CVP monitoring is assessed to indicate a patient's fluid balance and track the effects of mechanical ventilation on cardiac physiology.

Normal CVP

CVP is normally 2 to 6 mm Hg and represents the lowest pressure within the circulatory system. This facilitates blood return to the heart. Because the highest pressure within the circulatory system is within the aorta and the lowest is within the vena cava and right atrium, blood flow is in the direction from the left side of the heart, through the body, to the right side of the heart (**Table 6-8**).

Significance of Changes

Increased CVP may reduce blood return to the heart and therefore the stroke volume. If the heart cannot compensate for the low stroke volume by increasing the heart rate, the cardiac output will fall. Elevated CVP may occur in states of hypervolemia in patients with either increased fluid intake or reduced urine output. It can also occur with mechanical ventilation, as increased intrathoracic pressures increase the CVP. A drop in the blood pressure following the initiation of mechanical ventilation or a change in parameters is an ominous sign.

Pulmonary Artery Pressure

The pulmonary artery pressure can be continuously measured with a pulmonary artery catheter with the balloon deflated. The normal PA waveform resembles that obtained from an arterial catheter, but the pressures are lower.

TABLE 6-8
Hemodynamic Monitoring Measurements

Measurement	Normal Range	Significance of Abnormal Changes
HR	60–100/min	Tachycardia associated with hypoxemia, fever, anxiety, stress, medications
BP	90–140/60–80 mm Hg	May decrease with mechanical ventilation if venous return is disrupted by high intrathoracic pressure
CVP	2–6 mm Hg	Increases with fluid overload/right-sided heart failure, pulmonary embolism; decreases with hypovolemia
PAP	20–35/5–15 mm Hg	Increases with left-sided heart failure and fluid overload; decreases with hypovolemia and cardiovascular collapse
PAOP	5–10 mm Hg	Increases with left-sided heart failure and fluid overload; decreases with hypovolemia and cardiovascular collapse
CO	4–8 L/min	Increases with stress, sepsis, fever, hypervolemia, medications; decreases with pulmonary embolism, high PEEP levels, blood loss/hypovolemia, high intrathoracic pressures from mechanical ventilation
PVR	110–250 dyne·sec/cm^5	Increases with hypoxemia, pulmonary emboli, emphysema, pneumothorax; decreases with oxygen, nitric oxide/pulmonary vasodilators, calcium channel blockers
SVR	900–1400 dyne·sec/cm^5	Increases with vasoconstrictors, hypovolemia, late septic shock; decreases with vasodilators and early septic shock

BP, blood pressure; CO, cardiac output; CVP, central venous pressure; HR, heart rate; PAOP, pulmonary artery occlusion pressure; PAP, pulmonary artery pressure; PEEP, positive end-expiratory pressure; PVR, pulmonary vascular resistance; SVR, systemic vascular resistance.

Normal PAP

The pulmonary artery pressure is approximately 25/10 mm Hg (20 to 35 mm Hg systolic and 5 to 15 mm Hg diastolic). The mean pulmonary artery pressure is normally about 15 mm Hg (10 to 20 mm Hg) and its continuous reading is available on the hemodynamic monitor. The mean pressure can also be estimated by adding the systolic pressure to twice the diastolic pressure and dividing the resulting answer by 3 (i.e., systolic + 2(diastolic)/3) (see Table 6-8).

Significance of Changes

The pulmonary artery pressure will increase with left-sided heart failure, hypervolemia, and pulmonary vasoconstriction, associated with acidemia and hypoxemia. It decreases with hypovolemia and pulmonary vasodilation. Nitric oxide, epoprostenol (Flolan/Veletri) and other pulmonary vasodilating agents used to improve $\dot{V}/\dot{Q}$ matching can all lower the pulmonary artery pressure. Nitroglycerin and morphine, as well as many sedative medications, may also cause vasodilation and lower the pulmonary artery pressure.

Mechanical ventilation also may affect the PA pressures. High intrathoracic pressures with applied PEEP may increase pulmonary vascular resistance (PVR) and PA pressure. However, the resulting decrease in venous return and right sided heart output may decrease PA pressures. The reversal of hypoxemia with mechanical ventilation may also reduce the PA pressures. The ultimate effect of mechanical ventilation on PA pressure is a complex process that is based on the individual patient and his or her cardiopulmonary status prior to mechanical ventilation.

Pulmonary Artery Occlusion Pressure

Pulmonary artery occlusion pressure (PAOP) is measured when the balloon at the tip of the pulmonary artery catheter is inflated to occlude a branch of the pulmonary artery. The lack of valves in the pulmonary veins allows pressure equilibration with the left atrium. When the bicuspid valve is open during diastole, the pressure obtained via wedging the balloon also approximates the left ventricular end-diastolic pressure. For this reason, the pulmonary artery wedge pressure is sometimes substituted for left atrial pressure and left ventricular end-diastolic pressure.

How It Is Performed

The balloon on the tip of the pulmonary artery catheter is inflated with air. Usually only about 1.5 mL of air is required to inflate the balloon and obtain the occlusion measurement. If more air is injected and the balloon ruptures, an air embolism may result.

Normal PAOP

The PAOP is normally between 5 and 10 mm Hg. The waveform on the monitor should change from the pulmonary artery waveform to that of the occlusion waveform (see **Figure 6-13**). Once the measurement is obtained, the air should be removed from the balloon, and the pulmonary artery waveform should reappear on the monitor.

Significance of Changes

The PAOP increases with left-sided heart failure and mitral (bicuspid) valve stenosis. As left atrial pressure increases, the pulmonary artery pressure also increases. This increase in pulmonary blood pressure, or pulmonary hydrostatic pressure, can lead to pulmonary edema. Cardiogenic pulmonary edema is characterized by an enlarged heart and an elevated pulmonary capillary wedge pressure above 18 mm Hg.

The PAOP is influenced by intrathoracic pressure; the measurement is routinely taken at end expiration to reduce this influence. It has been suggested that at PEEP levels greater than 15, one-half of the PEEP level should be subtracted from the measured occlusion pressure. If the balloon ruptures or malfunctions, the occlusion pressure can be approximated to be equal to the pulmonary artery diastolic blood pressure.

Cardiac Output (CO) Measurement

Invasive Methods

Cardiac output is the amount of blood ejected by the ventricle per minute. It is equal to the stroke volume (amount ejected per beat) times the heart rate. Because the stroke volume cannot be directly measured, the cardiac output cannot be directly measured. A thermodilution technique can be done using a pulmonary artery catheter to estimate the cardiac output. Chilled or room temperature liquid is rapidly injected via the right atrial injectate port of the pulmonary artery catheter. The blood this liquid is diluted in will cool slightly, and this change in blood temperature, as well as how long it takes the cooled blood to reach the thermistor, is measured by the thermistor. From this information, the cardiac output can be estimated. Normally, the cardiac output is 4 to 8 L/min.

Some pulmonary artery catheters allow continuous monitoring of cardiac output. They work by intermittently heating the blood via a filament in the right atrium and then measuring the change in temperature at the thermistor.

The Fick equation for oxygen consumption can be rearranged to solve for cardiac output. This requires the measurement of oxygen consumption, which can be difficult in an intensive care unit (ICU) patient. **Box 6-6** shows the Fick equation.

BOX 6-6 Fick Equation

$$V_{O_2} = CO \times C(a - v)O_2$$

V_{O_2}, oxygen consumption; CO, cardiac output; C(a-v)O_2, arterial-mixed venous oxygen content difference.

Pulse power analysis is based on the concept that pulse pressure varies with changes in the stroke volume. Using a central venous catheter and an arterial line, a bolus of lithium chloride is given through the central venous catheter and then measured in the arterial line. Pulse pressure analysis compares favorably with measurements taken from a pulmonary artery catheter.

Pulse contour analysis measures the area under the systolic part of an arterial pressure waveform. This area is proportional to the stroke volume. To perform pulse contour analysis, both a central venous catheter and an arterial line must be placed. A solution is injected into the central venous catheter and a thermistor in the artery measures temperature changes. An alternate device requires only an arterial line. The arterial waveform is analyzed every 20 seconds, and the standard deviation of the data point reflects the pulse pressure. The pressure recording analytic method analyzes the area under the entire arterial waveform to determine stroke volume and subsequently cardiac output.

Noninvasive Methods

The value or accuracy of noninvasive methods of measuring the cardiac output are related to how closely they correlate with the gold standard, which is thermodilution. (Box 6-8 later in this section indicates how well each method compares to thermodilution.)

An esophageal Doppler device measures stroke volume using ultrasound technology. Flow in the descending aorta is measured and the velocity of the flow determined. This information is used to determine the stroke volume. This will not measure the total stroke volume, however, since the coronary arteries, the carotid arteries, and the brachiocephalic artery have received some blood flow prior to it reaching the descending aorta.

Transesophageal echocardiography is widely used to assess the cardiac status of a patient. The difference between this method and the esophageal Doppler is in the placement of the transducer. The transesophageal measurement is done at the level of the aortic valve, so it captures the entire stroke volume.

The NICO system (Novametrix, Wallingford, CT) (**Figure 6-15**) is a partial gas rebreathing method that

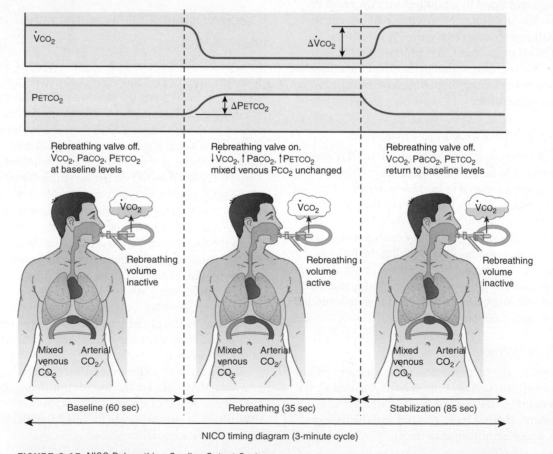

FIGURE 6-15 NICO Rebreathing Cardiac Output System.

Reproduced from Longnecker D, Brown D, Newman M, Zapol, W. *Anesthesiology*. New York, NY: McGraw-Hill, 2012. (© McGraw-Hill Education)

can be used on mechanically ventilated patients to determine the cardiac output. When steady state occurs (oxygen consumption and carbon dioxide production are steady), the amount of carbon dioxide entering the pulmonary system will equal the amount exhaled. Rebreathing is applied for a short period of time. During this time, the carbon dioxide entering the pulmonary system is unchanged, but the amount exhaled decreases. Cardiac output can be calculated by dividing carbon dioxide production by the difference between venous and arterial carbon dioxide.

Another noninvasive option to measuring cardiac output is thoracic bioimpedance. This method measures the electrical resistance of the thorax when current is applied. This resistance alters with blood flow. The change in impedance with blood flow is used to calculate the cardiac output.

Cardiac output can also be measured noninvasively with impedance plethysmography. This method passes current through electrodes placed on an ET tube, and electrodes placed on the cuff of the tube measure impedance. Impedance changes relate to stroke volume and thus cardiac output.

Portable Doppler devices placed on the chest can measure blood flow, much like the esophageal Doppler. However, this type of Doppler is placed on the chest wall rather than within the body. Blood flow changes reflect the stroke volume. This portable device is easy to use and the results are accurate as long as the Doppler is placed on the chest wall correctly.

A Netherlands-based company has developed an inflatable finger cuff that can measure pulse pressure using plethysmography, working much like a pulse oximeter. It is fairly new and has not yet been validated with more traditional methods of determining cardiac output.

Regardless of the method used to measure the cardiac output, changes in this value indicate the health of the cardiovascular system. Reductions in cardiac output signal a drop in perfusion to the organs and tissues of the body. As the organs and tissues receive less blood flow, they also may not receive enough oxygen to meet their requirements, and dysfunction can occur. Mild dysfunction may be able to be tolerated, but severe dysfunction of any organ will adversely affect the individual.

Hyperdynamic states, in which the cardiac output is elevated, increase the cardiac work. Sepsis, with resulting vasodilation, can cause an increase in cardiac output as can permissive hypercapnia. For this reason, when permissive hypercapnia is instituted, it is applied very slowly, allowing the carbon dioxide to increase over several hours rather than minutes. **Table 6-9** summarizes methods to measure or estimate cardiac output.

TABLE 6-9
Noninvasive Versus Invasive CO Measurements

Method	How It Works	Invasive/Noninvasive	Comparison to Thermodilution
Thermodilution	Cool solution is inserted into the RA and measured by the thermistor in the PA	Invasive	Gold standard against which other methods are compared
Pulse power analysis	Relates changes in pulse pressure to stroke volume	Invasive	Good correlation
Pulse contour analysis	Measures area under the systolic part of the arterial waveform, which is proportional to the stroke volume	Invasive	Good correlation in studies of post–cardiac surgery patients and critically ill patients but errors related to instability and calibration
Esophageal doppler	Measures stroke volume at the level of the descending aorta using ultrasound technology	Invasive	Good correlation but should not be used as the sole method to monitor CO
NICO	Measures end-tidal CO_2 during a period of rebreathing	Noninvasive	Not accurate compared to thermodilution; limited clinical use
Transesophageal Echocardiogra	Measures stroke volume at the level of the aortic valve using ultrasound technology	Invasive	Correlates well but requires a skilled user
Thoracic bioimpedance	Measures the electrical resistance of thorax when current is applied	Noninvasive	Correlates well in cardiac surgical patients but considered more for trending as correlation was not good in critically ill patients
Impedance plethysmography	Measures impedance using electrodes placed on the ET tube and the cuff	Noninvasive	Not yet validated and very expensive
Doppler	Measure blood flow through the chest wall	Noninvasive	Good correlation
Finger cuff	Measures pulse pressure in the finger	Noninvasive	Still not validated

CO, cardiac output; ET, endotracheal; PA, pulmonary artery; RA, right atrium; TEE, transesophageal echocardiography.

Cardiac Index

Dividing the cardiac output by the body surface area determines the cardiac index. This relates the cardiac output to body size. For example, two patients may both have a cardiac output of 5 L/min. For an average size patient, this would be a normal cardiac output. For someone who is 6 ft, 7 in, however, this is not a normal cardiac output. This discrepancy would be obvious if the cardiac index were used. Normal cardiac index is 2.5 to 3.5 $L/min/m^2$. A reduced cardiac index signals that for that patient of that size the cardiac output is inadequate.

Saturation of Venous Blood (S$\bar{v}$O$_2$)

Continuous monitoring of the saturation of oxygen in the mixed venous blood can be done with some pulmonary artery catheters. These catheters are equipped with an oximeter at the tip, which can measure the S$\bar{v}$O$_2$.

Normal S$\bar{v}$O$_2$

Usually, the mixed venous saturation is 75%. This indicates that approximately 25% of the oxygen delivered by the arterial system is consumed by the tissues and 75% returns to the lungs, implying that the body delivers much more oxygen than is actually in demand by the tissues. This means there is a large safety margin in case of an increase in tissue oxygen demand and therefore less chance for hypoxia to occur than if delivery and demand were more perfectly matched.

Significance of Changes

Decreases in mixed venous saturation are seen with arterial desaturation (poorly oxygenated arterial blood) and with sluggish blood flow (low cardiac output). If arterial oxygenation is low, venous oxygenation will also be low. In addition, a lower blood flow allows more time for the tissues to extract oxygen from the blood. The end result is a lower venous oxygen level. Venous levels will also decrease if tissue oxygen demand is increased. Increased demand occurs with excessive movement, such as seizures in a patient, or when the metabolic rate is increased by fever, sepsis, or stress. If the S$\bar{v}$O$_2$ is low because of low arterial oxygenation, then an increase in arterial oxygenation will also increase the S$\bar{v}$O$_2$. If it is low because of a low cardiac output, then increasing the cardiac output will increase the S$\bar{v}$O$_2$. If the S$\bar{v}$O$_2$ is low because

tissue demand is high, reducing the tissue demand will increase it.

High S$\bar{v}$O$_2$ (>75%) levels are not as common as low levels. High levels usually indicate a decrease in tissue utilization of oxygen. This may be seen after administration of a paralytic medication. It is also associated with conditions of histotoxic hypoxia where the tissues are unable to utilize oxygen for metabolism.

Pulmonary Vascular Resistance

PVR reflects the tone in the arterioles in the pulmonary vascular system. There is normally some tone in these vessels, so there is normally some vascular resistance, but it is fairly low.

Normal PVR

Normal PVR is 110 to 250 dyne·sec/cm^5. This value is low because the pulmonary vascular system has low resistance and high compliance compared to the systemic vascular system (Table 6-8).

Calculation

Pulmonary vascular resistance can be calculated if the mean pulmonary artery pressure, PAOP, and cardiac output are known. The calculation is shown in **Box 6-7**.

Significance of Changes

Acidemia and hypoxemia are both pulmonary vasoconstrictors, which increase the pulmonary vascular resistance. In addition, lung diseases (e.g., emphysema) that destroy pulmonary capillaries also increase the pulmonary vascular resistance. Pulmonary vascular resistance can be reduced with the administration of oxygen, if hypoxemia is the cause, or reversal of acidemia. Vasodilators will also reduce the pulmonary vascular resistance and may be used to improve oxygenation by increasing blood flow to ventilated alveoli.

Right Ventricular Stroke Work and Index

Right ventricular stroke work (RVSW) measures how hard the right ventricle must work to cause blood to flow through the pulmonary vascular system, and a higher one indicates high right ventricular workload.

BOX 6-7 Pulmonary Vascular Resistance (PVR) Calculation

$$PVR = \frac{(\text{Mean pulmonary artery pressure} - \text{Left atrial pressure}}{\text{Cardiac output}} \times 80$$

Right ventricular stroke work index (RVSWI) relates the RVSW to the body size.

Normal RVSW

Normal RVSW is 10 to 15 g·m/beat, and normal RVSWI is 7 to 12 g·m/beat/m². These numbers indicate how hard the right ventricle is working to deliver blood to the pulmonary vascular system. In comparison with the systemic system, these numbers are relatively low.

Calculation

If the mean pulmonary artery pressure, right atrial pressure, and stroke volume are known, the RVSW can be calculated. The calculations for RVSW and RVSWI are shown in **Box 6-8**.

Significance of Changes

Increases in pulmonary vascular resistance lead to increases in RVSW and RVSWI. Tachycardia, hypoxemia, increased blood volume, and increased blood viscosity also increase the RVSW and RVSWI. As the RVSW and RVSWI elevate, right ventricular hypertrophy (cor pulmonale) and failure may follow.

Left Ventricular Stroke Work and Index

Left ventricular stroke work (LVSW) measures how hard the left ventricle must work to cause blood flow through the body, and a higher one indicates high left ventricular workload. The left ventricular stroke work index (LVSWI) relates the LVSW to the body size.

Normal LVSW

Normal LVSW is 60 to 80 g·m/beat, and normal LVSWI index is 40 to 60 g·m/beat/m². These numbers are much higher than the RVSW and RVSWI for the, indicating the increased work performed by the left side of the heart against the increased resistance of the systemic vascular system. If the MAPs, PAOP, and stroke volume are known, the LVSW and LVSWI can be calculated (see Box 6-8).

Significance of Changes

Increases in systemic vascular resistance (SVR) lead to increases in LVSW. Tachycardia, hypoxemia, increased blood volume, and increased blood viscosity also increase the LVSW. As the LVSW work elevates, left-sided heart hypertrophy and failure may follow.

Systemic Vascular Resistance

SVR alters with changes in the size of the arterioles within the systemic vascular system. As the arterioles constrict, SVR increases while arteriolar vasodilation decreases SVR.

Normal SVR

Normal SVR is 900 to 1400 dyne·sec/cm⁵. This value is much higher than the normal for pulmonary vascular resistance, indicating the greater resistance in the systemic arteries as compared to the pulmonary arteries. The systemic arteries have a much higher degree of tone.

Calculation

If the MAP, the CVP, and the cardiac output are known, the SVR can be calculated (**Box 6-9**).

Significance of Changes

The higher the SVR, the more work the left ventricle must perform to push blood through the systemic vasculature. In the face of extremely high resistance, the left ventricle may not be able to perform the work, and the cardiac output subsequently falls. The SVR is maintained by output from the CNS, which alters it to help regulate the blood pressure and maintain organ perfusion.

Monitoring the patient is a crucial component of providing safe care to a patient. Through assessment and monitoring, trends in the patient's condition can be recognized and appropriate treatment applied. Ventilator monitoring allows the practitioner to titrate the settings to reduce dyssynchrony and increase patient comfort. Hemodynamic monitoring allows the clinician to identify problems and track the progress of the patient through treatment strategies. It is imperative in today's intensive care environment that clinicians understand and apply appropriate monitoring techniques.

BOX 6-8 RVSW/LVSW Calculations

$$LVSW = (MAP - PCWP) \times SV \times 0.0136$$

$$RVSW = (PA - RAP) \times SV \times 0.0136$$

$$LVSWI = LVSW/BSA$$

$$RVSWI = RVSW/BSA$$

BSA, body surface area; LVSW, left ventricular stroke work; LVSWI, left ventricular stroke work index; MAP, mean arterial pressure; PA, pulmonary artery; PCWP, pulmonary capillary wedge pressure; RAP, right atrial pressure; RVSW, right ventricular stroke work; RVSWI, right ventricular stroke work index; SV, stroke volume.

BOX 6-9 Calculation of SVR

$$SVR = \frac{(MAP - CVP) \times 80}{CO}$$

CO, cardiac output; CVP, central venous pressure; MAP, mean arterial pressure; SVR, systemic vascular resistance.

Summary

Monitoring of the patient on mechanical ventilation is important to ensure safe delivery of mechanical ventilation to the patient. Pulmonary as well as extra-pulmonary side effects must be carefully evaluated for each individual patient. Although multiple patients may have the same diagnosis, each will have his or her own unique physiology and response to interventions. By monitoring the physiologic and hemodynamic responses of the patient, mechanical ventilation can be adjusted and titrated to best meet the needs of each individual patient. This requires a sophisticated level of understanding by the clinician to evaluate the patient as a whole when applying mechanical ventilation.

Bibliography

Monitoring the Ventilator and Patient

Berlin D. Hemodynamic consequences of auto-PEEP. *J Intensive Care Med.* 2014;29(2):81–86.

Case Studies

Case Study 6-1 Mechanical Ventilation

A 5-ft, 2-in female patient on mechanical ventilation has the following information gathered over a 12-hour shift:

Time	PIP (cm H$_2$O)	Plateau (cm H$_2$O)	PEEP (cm H$_2$O)	V$_T$ (mL)
0800	28	24	6	500
1200	34	28	6	500
1600	42	37	6	500
2000	46	40	6	500

PEEP, positive end-expiratory pressure; PIP, peak inspiratory pressure; V$_T$, tidal volume.

1. **What is implied by the data?**

2. **Which x-ray would you most expect to see on this patient at 2000?**

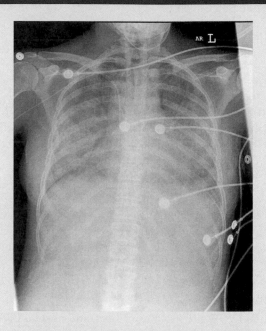

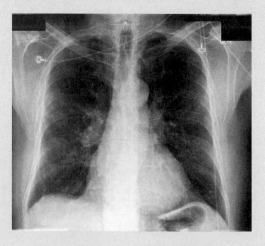

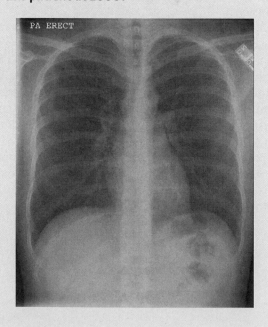

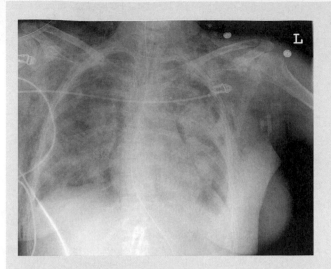

3. What recommendations would be advisable to ventilate a patient with acute respiratory distress syndrome (ARDS)?

Case Study 6-2 Capnography

Following an intubation attempt during cardiopulmonary resuscitation (CPR), a mainstream capnometer is placed on the endotracheal (ET) tube and it shows the following:

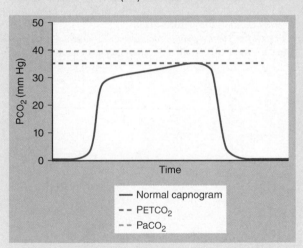

An ABG drawn shortly after measures an arterial CO_2 of 57 mm Hg. The physician questions the placement of the ET tube.

1. How would you verify placement?

2. Following institution of mechanical ventilation with return of spontaneous circulation, what is the expected change in the capnogram?

3. Several hours later, you are called to the patient's bedside by the nurse. The low positive end-expiratory pressure (PEEP) and the low saturation alarm are sounding and the capnometry shows the following:

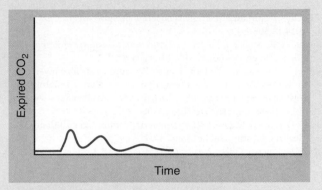

Describe your response to this situation.

Case Study 6-3 Mechanical Ventilation Effects on Other Organ Systems

Mechanical ventilation was initiated 72 hours previously on a patient following cardiopulmonary resuscitation (CPR). The 5-ft, 7-in male patient is in the assist-control (AC) mode with pressure regulated volume control (PRVC) breath type. The target tidal volume is set at 550 mL.

1. How many mL/kg is the target tidal volume?
The physician orders a PEEP increase from 6 cm H_2O to 10 cm H_2O. The patient's blood pressure prior to the PEEP change was 102/68 mm Hg.

2. What is the expected effect on the cardiovascular system if the PEEP of +10 cm H_2O overdistends the alveoli?
About 2 hours after the change, your assessment of the patient reveals crackles bilaterally and the SpO_2 has dropped from 94% to 88% with no change in ventilator settings.

3. What does your assessment suggest?

4. What is the physiologic response expected by the drop in PaO_2? How would you adjust the ventilator settings?

Cairo JM. *Pilbeam's Mechanical Ventilation: Physiological and Clinical Applications.* 6th ed. St. Louis, MO: Elsevier; 2016.

Chan MC, Tseng JS, Chiu JT, et al. Prognostic value of plateau pressure below 30 cm H_2O in septic subjects with acute respiratory failure. *Respir Care.* 2015;60:12–20.

Chang D. *Clinical Application of Mechanical Ventilation.* 4th ed. Clifton Park, NY: Delmar-Cengage Learning; 2014.

El-Baraday GF, El-Shamaa NS. Compliance versus dead space for optimum positive end expiratory pressure determination in acute respiratory distress syndrome. *Indian J Crit Care Med.* 2014;18:508–512.

Kacmarek R, Stoller J, Heuer A. *Egan's Fundamentals of Respiratory Care.* 11th ed. St. Louis, MO: Elsevier; 2017.

Kotani T, Katayama S, Fududa S, et al. Pressure-controlled inverse ratio ventilation as a rescue therapy for severe acute respiratory distress syndrome. *Springerplus.* 2016;5(1):716. Available at www.ncbi.min.nih.gov/pmc/articles/PMC4908089

Oakes D, Jones S. *Oakes' ABG Instructional Guide.* 2nd ed. Orono, ME: Health Education Publications; 2017.

Oakes D, Jones S. *Oakes' Respiratory Care.* 9th ed. Orono, ME: Health Education Publications; 2017.

Pope S. How it works: pulse oximeter. *Flying.* July 5, 2016. Available at www.flyingmag.com/how-it-works-pulse-oximeter

Physiological Monitoring

Cairo JM. *Pilbeam's Mechanical Ventilation: Physiological and Clinical Applications.* 6th ed. St. Louis, MO: Elsevier; 2016.

Chang D. *Clinical Application of Mechanical Ventilation.* 4th ed. Clifton Park, NY: Delmar-Cengage Learning; 2014.

DesJardins T, Burton G. *Clinical Manifestations and Assessment of Respiratory Disease.* 7th ed. St. Louis, MO: Elsevier; 2016:23–25.

Hamm LL, Nakoul N, Hering-Smith KS. Acid-base homeostasis. *Clin J Am Soc Nephrol.* 2015;10:2232–2242.

Hess D, MacIntyre N, Galvin W. *Respiratory Care: Principles and Practice.* 3rd ed. Boston, MA: Jones & Bartlett; 2016.

Kacmarek R, Stoller J, Heuer A. *Egan's Fundamentals of Respiratory Care.* 11th ed. St. Louis, MO: Elsevier; 2017.

Oakes D, Jones S. *Oakes' ABG Instructional Guide.* 2nd ed. Orono, ME: Health Education Publications; 2017.

Picolo M, Lago A, Menequeti M, et al. Harris-Benedict equation and resting energy expenditure estimates in critically ill ventilator patients. *Am J Crit Care.* 2016;25:e21–e29.

Scanlon C, Heuer A, Rodriguez N. *Comprehensive Respiratory Therapy Exam Review.* 3rd ed. Boston, MA: Jones & Bartlett Learning; 2019.

Sun G, Chen J, Uyang B, et al. Liver function is affected by mechanical ventilation after abdominal surgery. *J Am Coll Surg.* 2013;217:556–557.

Hemodynamic Monitoring

Gidwani U, Mohanty B, Chatterjee, K. The pulmonary artery catheter a critical reappraisal. *Cardiol Clin.* 2013;3:545–565.

Hess D, MacIntyre N, Galvin W. *Respiratory Care: Principles and Practice.* 3rd ed. Boston, MA: Jones & Bartlett; 2016.

Kacmarek R, Stoller J, Heuer A. *Egan's Fundamentals of Respiratory Care.* 11th ed. St. Louis, MO: Elsevier; 2017.

Klabunde R. *Normal and Abnormal Blood Pressure.* Philadelphia, PA: Lippincott Williams & Wilkins; 2013.

Oakes D. *Oakes' Hemodynamic Monitoring: An Oakes Pocket Guide.* 6th ed. Orono, ME: Health Education Publications; 2017.

Ortega R, Connor C, Kotova F, et al. Use of pressure transducers. *N Engl J Med.* 2017;376:e26.

Hemodynamic Measurements

Chang D. *Clinical Application of Mechanical Ventilation.* 4th ed. Clifton Park, NY: Delmar-Cengage Learning; 2014.

Hess D, MacIntyre N, Galvin W. *Respiratory Care: Principles and Practice.* 3rd ed. Boston, MA: Jones & Bartlett; 2016.

Kacmarek R, Stoller J, Heuer A. *Egan's Fundamentals of Respiratory Care.* 11th ed. St. Louis, MO: Elsevier; 2017.

Mehta Y, Arora D. Newer methods of cardiac output monitoring. *World J Cardiol.* 2014;6:1022–1029.

Oakes D. *Oakes' Hemodynamic Monitoring: An Oakes Pocket Guide.* 6th ed. Orono, ME: Health Education Publications; 2017.

7

Waveform Analysis and Application

Ruben D. Restrepo, MD, RRT

OUTLINE

OBJECTIVES

1. Identify the variables that make up the scalars and loops.
2. Describe the difference between loops and scalars.
3. Describe air leak in all waveforms that display volume as a variable.
4. Identify airway obstruction and positive bronchodilator response.
5. Describe air trapping and determine level of auto-PEEP.
6. Identify changes in pulmonary mechanics on volume-targeted and pressure-targeted modes.
7. Describe the most common modes of ventilation on scalar graphics.
8. Identify and describe the different types of patient-ventilator asynchronies.

KEY TERMS

air leaks
airway pressure
airway resistance
auto-PEEP
hysteresis
loops
overdistention
patient–ventilator
    asynchrony

patient–ventilator
    interaction
pressure targeted
scalar
spontaneous breath
volume targeted
waveform analysis

Introduction

Ventilator waveforms have become an essential tool in managing patients on mechanical ventilators. They are valuable to the clinician in the intensive care unit (ICU) because they provide important information on the **patient–ventilator interaction**. A significant number of changes in the clinical condition of the patient and the function of the ventilator could be easily confirmed by performing a detailed **waveform analysis**. Patient–ventilator asynchrony is one of the most significant conditions associated with prolonged duration of mechanical ventilation, increased sedation, and even death in the ICU. Interpretation of waveforms has dramatically improved the rate of recognition of asynchrony and its clinical outcomes as it allows the clinician to adjust the ventilator to optimize the patient–ventilator interaction.

This chapter has been designed to provide clinicians with the specific knowledge and interpretive skills necessary to recognize various aspects of patient and ventilator interaction. This section describes the typical tracings and analysis of commonly encountered waveforms during mechanical ventilation.

General Concepts

All modern ventilators display a variety of real-time waveform configurations. Color-coded information, freezing capabilities, scale adjustment for precise measurements, and even tutorials have simplified the interpretation of waveforms. These graphics are displayed in two forms: scalars and loops.

Any single variable displayed against time is known as a **scalar**. The three components that make up the ventilator graphics—flow, volume, and pressure—are plotted against time. These three scalars are generally referred to as pressure-time (P-T), flow-time (F-T), and volume-time (V-T). When viewing scalar graphics, time is conventionally shown on the horizontal (x) axis; flow, volume, and pressure are plotted on the vertical (y) axis (**Figure 7-1**).

Loops are formed by plotting inspiratory and expiratory curves of two of these three variables: pressure, flow, volume. There are two loops available for interpretation: pressure-volume (i.e., compliance) loop (**Figure 7-2**) and flow-volume loop (**Figure 7-3**).

Scalar Graphics

The three time-based scalars (flow-time, volume-time, and pressure-time) are described below.

Flow-Time

Most ventilators allow a clinician to select a flow pattern that is most suitable to the patient. Typically, a descending or constant flow pattern is used with volume-targeted ventilation (**Figure 7-4**). Although the peak flow rate is maintained at the same set value, Ti varies with changes in patient compliance and resistance. Expiration, whether from a mechanical breath or a spontaneous breath, is generally a passive maneuver. An F-T scalar is easily recognized because it is the waveform in which half of the tracing is present above (inspiration) and half is below (expiration) the baseline.

During spontaneous breathing, the inspiratory flow is traced above the baseline, whereas expiratory flow is indicated below the baseline. The F-T curve for the inspiratory portion of a spontaneous breath resembles a sine wave flow pattern (**Figure 7-5**).

Rise Time

Rise time is the time it takes for **airway pressure** to reach a preset maximum value. A rapid rise time value will allow instantaneous delivery of flow at the start of

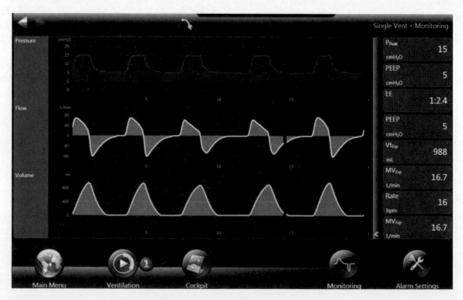

FIGURE 7-1 Pressure-time, flow-time, and volume-time scalars. Paw, airway pressure.
The Bellavista images are © 2019 Vyaire Medical, Inc.; Used with permission.

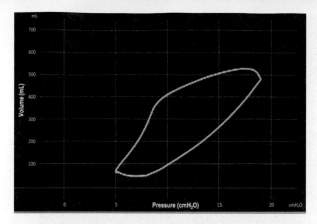

FIGURE 7-2 Pressure-volume loop. Pressure is displayed on the horizontal (x) axis; volume is displayed on the vertical (y) axis.
The Bellavista images are © 2019 Vyaire Medical, Inc.; Used with permission.

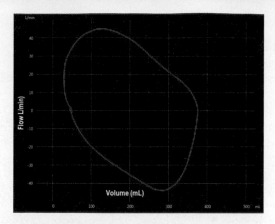

FIGURE 7-3 Flow-volume loop. The horizontal (x) axis is used to indicate volume; flow is displayed on the vertical (y) axis.
The Bellavista images are © 2019 Vyaire Medical, Inc.; Used with permission.

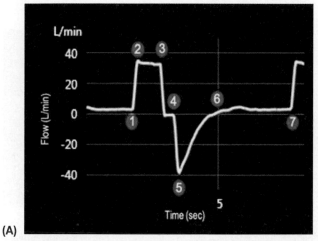

(A)

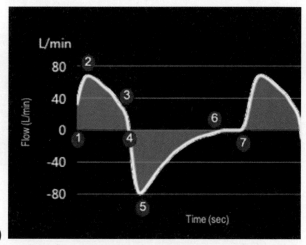

(B)

FIGURE 7-4 Flow-time scalar displaying a square flow pattern, typical of volume-targeted ventilation (A) and pressure-targeted ventilation (B). The inspiratory phase of the F-T scalar displays the initiation of flow at the beginning of inspiration (1). At this time, the exhalation valve closes to permit a mechanical breath to deliver volume to the patient's lungs. The peak inspiratory flow rate (PIFR) can be reached almost instantaneously during a constant flow pattern (2). However, the presence of a rise time or ramp modifies the appearance of this part of tracing as it delays how fast the PIFR is reached. The flow remains at this level (3) until the inspiration is terminated (4), the exhalation valve opens, and passive exhalation begins. The peak expiratory flow rate (PEFR) is reached (5), and expiratory flow reaches baseline (6) before the next breath occurs (7). Notice that the duration of expiratory flow may be shorter than the allocated expiratory time (TE).
The Bellavista images are © 2019 Vyaire Medical, Inc.; Used with permission.

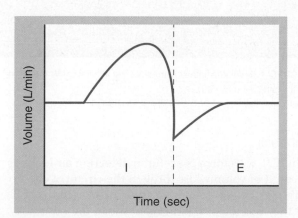

FIGURE 7-5 Flow-time scalar displaying a typical sine wave flow pattern of a spontaneous breath. E, expiration; I, inspiration.

the breath, resulting in an immediate rise in pressure to the preset level. When inspiratory flow is delivered too fast, turbulence can result in a higher than preset airway pressure (Figure 7-6A). Conversely, a slow rise time inhibits initial flow delivery, thus delaying the pressure rise to the preset level (Figure 7-6B).

Airway Obstruction

Exhalation is normally passive. The expiratory flow pattern and peak expiratory flow rate (PEFR) are greatly dependent on the changes in a patient's **airway resistance**. The presence of bronchospasm, airway mucosal edema, or airway inflammation typically results in decreased PEFR and a prolonged expiratory flow. Response to bronchodilator administration will be determined by an increase in

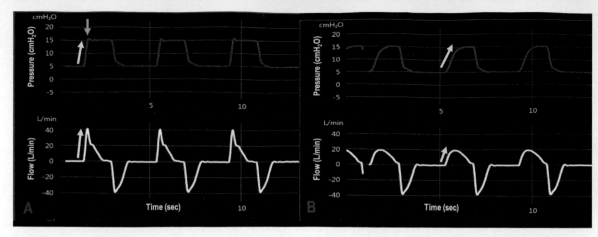

FIGURE 7-6 Flow-time scalar indicating a fast rise time. A sharp rise to peak inspiratory flow rate (PIFR) and airway pressure (yellow arrow) is observed. **(A)** A rapid rise time causes an increase in airway pressure indicated by a "bump" (green arrow). **(B)** A flow-time scalar indicates a slow rise time that delays initial flow delivery, thus slowing the pressure rise to the preset level (yellow arrow).

The Bellavista images are © 2019 Vyaire Medical, Inc.; Used with permission.

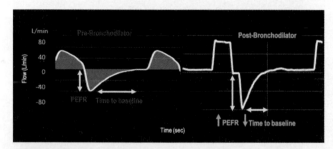

FIGURE 7-7 The presence of airway obstruction typically results in decreased peak expiratory flow rate (PEFR) and a prolonged expiratory flow (left). A positive response to bronchodilator administration (right) increases PEFR and shortens the time it takes for the expiratory flow tracing to return to baseline.

The Bellavista images are © 2019 Vyaire Medical, Inc.; Used with permission.

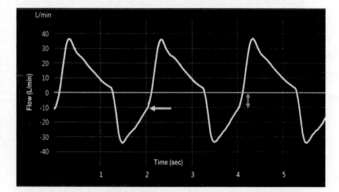

FIGURE 7-8 Flow-time scalar displaying a descending ramp flow pattern. Expiratory flow fails to return to zero before the next breath (yellow arrow) is delivered. The magnitude of trapping is indicated by the blue arrow.

The Bellavista images are © 2019 Vyaire Medical, Inc.; Used with permission.

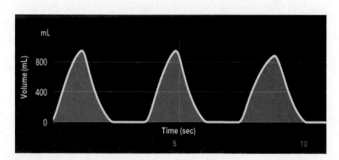

FIGURE 7-9 Volume-time scalar displaying inspiratory V_T (upstroke) and expired V_T (downstroke).

The Bellavista images are © 2019 Vyaire Medical, Inc.; Used with permission.

the PEFR and shortening of the time it takes for the expiratory flow tracing to return to baseline (**Figure 7-7**).

Air Trapping

The presence of **air trapping** should be suspected when the expiratory flow tracing does not return to baseline. Therefore, the next breath starts below the baseline, as seen in **Figure 7-8**.

The presence of air trapping may result from inadequate alveolar emptying as a result of increased airway obstruction. In addition, it could result from short T_E, very high respiratory rate, or excessively long T_I. Even though auto-PEEP could be suspected from the presence of air trapping on the flow-time waveform, its magnitude is directly measured on the pressure-time scalar (discussed in the next section).

Volume-Time

The volume-time scalar is typically displayed as a triangular waveform. It provides a visual representation of the inspiratory tidal volume (V_T) and the expired V_T (**Figure 7-9**).

Air Leak

The V-T waveform is useful in detecting **air leaks** as a result of volume loss through the circuit, a chest tube, bronchopulmonary fistula, or around the cuff of the endotracheal (ET) tube. When the expiratory tracing smoothly descends, and then plateaus but does not reach baseline, it indicates the presence of a leak in the system. It should be noted that in air leaks, the expiratory tidal volume does not reach baseline for *every* mechanical breath. (Note: In air trapping, the expiratory tidal volume does not reach baseline only for two or three consecutive breaths. The expiratory tidal volume for the next subsequent breath will exceed the inspiratory tidal volume and the tracing will go below the baseline.) The volume of the leak can be easily estimated by measuring the distance from the plateau to the end of the expiratory tracing (**Figure 7-10**).

Changes in Pulmonary Mechanics

If the ventilator is set on any pressure-controlled mode of ventilation, the V-T waveform could reveal changes in pulmonary mechanics. Because airway pressure

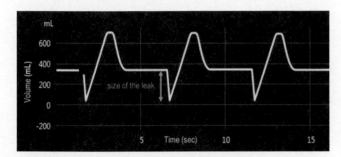

FIGURE 7-10 Volume-time waveform showing the presence of an air leak. The expiratory tracing does not reach baseline (zero) and provides the appearance of a check mark. The volume of the leak can be estimated by measuring the distance from the plateau to the end of the expiratory tracing (arrow).

is preset, VT decreases if either airway resistance increases or lung compliance decreases, and vice versa (**Figure 7-11**).

Pressure-Time

Unlike the F-T waveform, the P-T scalar of a **spontaneous breath** (unassisted) indicates inspiration below the baseline and expiration is traced above. A mechanical breath provides visual representations of the peak inspiratory pressure (PIP) and positive end-expiratory pressure (PEEP). In the presence of PEEP, the entire mechanical breath will start and end at that preset PEEP level (**Figure 7-12**).

Controlled Versus Assisted Breath

A P-T scalar is used to verify the trigger mechanism of the mechanical breath. If the breaths are initiated at the baseline (without negative pressure) at fixed intervals, the breath is time triggered (control mode). In assist mode (patient trigger), the patient initiates the breath by generating a negative pressure and associated flow. The ventilator sensor recognizes the patient's effort and delivers a mechanical breath. This event can be observed on the P-T scalar where a small negative deflection below the baseline precedes a mechanical breath (**Figure 7-13**). This negative pressure deflection may not be visible if flow compensation or flow trigger is active.

Plateau Pressure

Although dynamic lung mechanics can be observed from a P-T waveform, the addition of an end-inspiratory pause or inflation hold creates the plateau pressure

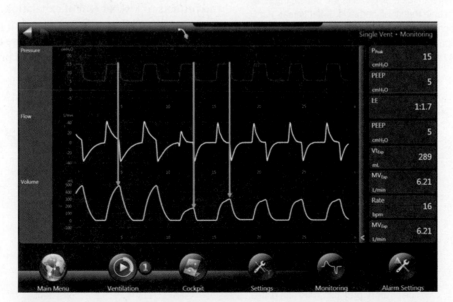

FIGURE 7-11 Scalars demonstrating how on a pressure-controlled mode, changes in VT (arrows) indicate worsening or improvement of pulmonary mechanics. Paw, airway pressure.

(Pplat) and provides information to calculate static (lung) mechanics. During this maneuver, the exhalation valve is kept in a closed position at end-inspiration of a mechanical breath, and the static volume is held in the lungs. For clinical purposes, the plateau pressure is often used as a surrogate of the alveolar pressure to calculate static lung compliance.

The difference between PIP and Pplat typically reflects the pressure required to overcome airway resistance. Bronchospasm, main stem intubation, airway secretions, and other types of airway obstructions are verified from an increase in this PIP-Pplat gradient (**Figure 7-14**).

Auto-PEEP

Incomplete expiration prior to the initiation of the next breath causes progressive air trapping, which is easily recognized from the F-T waveform. This accumulation of air increases alveolar pressure at the end of expiration, which is referred to as **auto-PEEP**. Its magnitude is directly measured from the P-T scalar after performing an end-expiratory hold (**Figure 7-15**).

Loops

Loops are the two-dimensional graphic displays of two scalar values. The most commonly used for analysis and interpretation are the pressure-volume loop (PVL) and the flow-volume loop (FVL). These will be discussed in detail.

Pressure-Volume Loop

When the tracing of a dynamic breath is displayed counterclockwise, the breath delivered is a mechanical breath. On the other hand, a clockwise tracing indicates a spontaneous breath. The angle, shape, and size of the loop impart pertinent information to the clinician. In an assisted mechanical breath, the tracing can begin clockwise indicating patient's effort but resumes in counterclockwise fashion for the mechanical delivery. A PVL traces changes in pressures and corresponding changes in volume. Inspiration begins from the functional residual capacity (FRC) level and terminates when the preset parameter (volume or pressure) is achieved. The tracing continues during expiration and returns to FRC at end of exhalation. When PEEP is applied, the PVL shifts to the level of PEEP on the horizontal scale (**Figure 7-16**). Because changes in pressure and volume during a mechanical breath reflect the

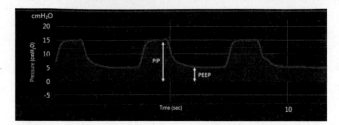

FIGURE 7-12 Pressure-time waveform of a mechanical breath displaying the peak inspiratory pressure (PIP) and positive end-expiratory pressure (PEEP).

The Bellavista images are © 2019 Vyaire Medical, Inc.; Used with permission.

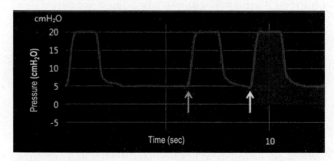

FIGURE 7-13 Pressure-time scalar shows the difference between a controlled time-triggered breath (blue arrow) and the patient-triggered breath (yellow arrow). Observe the small negative deflection at the beginning of the last breath, which indicates patient's effort as observed in an assisted breath.

The Bellavista images are © 2019 Vyaire Medical, Inc.; Used with permission.

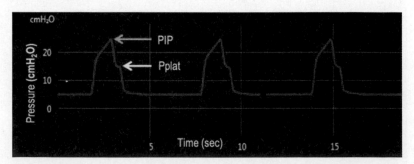

FIGURE 7-14 Pressure-time waveform indicating a pressure gradient between peak inspiratory pressure (PIP) and plateau pressure (Pplat) (10 cm H_2O) that is consistent with the presence of increased airway resistance. Observe that the Pplat (15 cm H_2O) is consistent with a normal lung static compliance.

The Bellavista images are © 2019 Vyaire Medical, Inc.; Used with permission.

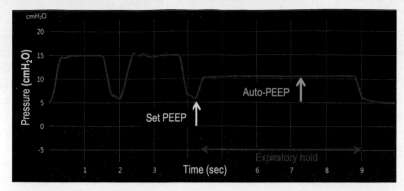

FIGURE 7-15 Pressure-time waveform showing a set/machine positive end-expiratory pressure (PEEP) of 5 cm H_2O (yellow arrow). After performing an end-expiratory hold maneuver, the set PEEP raises because of air trapping to 10 cm H_2O (auto-PEEP).

The Bellavista images are © 2019 Vyaire Medical, Inc.; Used with permission.

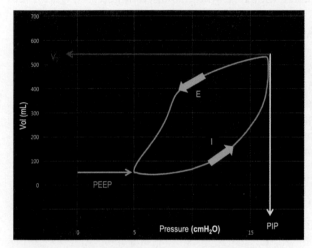

FIGURE 7-16 This pressure-volume loop shows a mechanical breath that occurs in a counterclockwise fashion. Inspiration (I) starts at a preset level of positive end-expiratory pressure (PEEP) (blue arrow) and exhalation (E) begins after either a preset peak inspiratory pressure (PIP) (yellow arrow) or VT (red arrow) has been reached.

The Bellavista images are © 2019 Vyaire Medical, Inc.; Used with permission.

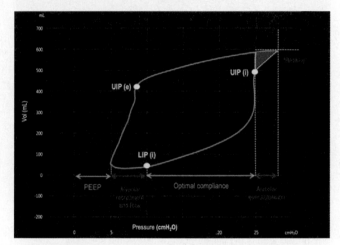

FIGURE 7-17 Pressure-volume loop (PVL) showing inflection points (IPs). The lower inflection point (LIP) represents the opening pressure, whereas the upper inflection points (UIPs) represent either the presence of alveolar overdistention [UIP (i)] or lung recoil and airway resistance characteristics [UIP (e)]. The beak-shaped part of the PVL at end of inspiration (red-shadowed area) is the region of pressure where rising pressure does not lead to increasing volume and indicates the presence of alveolar overdistention. PEEP, positive end-expiratory pressure; Raw, airway resistance.

The Bellavista images are © 2019 Vyaire Medical, Inc.; Used with permission.

compliance, PVL is essentially a compliance loop. When the PVL shifts toward the pressure axis (right), the compliance is decreased. On the other hand, shifting of the PVL toward the volume axis (left) indicates increase in compliance.

Inflection Points and Alveolar Overdistention

An inflection point is a mathematical term that refers to a point of a curve at which a change in the direction of curvature occurs. Inflection points in a PVL can represent changes in alveolar opening and closing, and are also termed P_{flex}. The lower inflection point is of questionable clinical value in a dynamic curve because of limited accuracy, but the lower inflection point roughly corresponds to the pressure at which alveoli open/fill at a faster rate, whereas the upper inflection points represent either the presence of alveolar **overdistention** (during inspiration) or lung recoil and airway resistance

characteristics (during exhalation). Many ventilators are programmed to perform quasi-static PVL maneuvers to provide more useful graphics. Because a dynamic PVL is affected by airway resistance as well as respiratory system compliance, a static or quasi-static PVL is used to determine the inflection points more accurately (especially when used to set PEEP on a ventilator). Plotting transpulmonary pressure helps guide the setting of PEEP when pleural pressure is unusually high (such as chest wall rigidity and conditions that increase abdominal pressure on the diaphragm). The beak-shaped part of the PVL at end of inspiration, which lends it its penguin-like shape, is the region of pressure where rising pressure does not lead to increasing volume. The lung is simply overstretched (**Figure 7-17**).

Changes in Pulmonary Mechanics

A shift to the right of the inspiratory limb of the PVL in a volume-controlled mode indicates that a higher pressure is required to overcome either airway resistance (decreased dynamic compliance) or lung recoil (static compliance). Observe the pressure required to deliver the same tidal volume in the two graphs in **Figure 7-18**.

A similar shift to the right of the inspiratory limb of the PVL will be observed in a pressure-controlled mode. However, a preset pressure will be associated with a lower V_T as a result of decreased lung compliance (**Figure 7-19**).

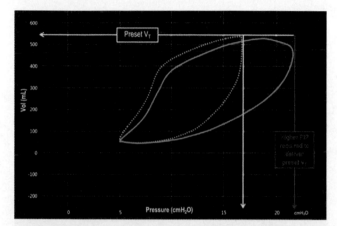

FIGURE 7-18 Pressure-volume loop (PVL) changes observed with alterations of pulmonary mechanics. Two PVLs are depicted. The dotted loop is the initial tracing, whereas the solid loop shows a typical shift to the right of a PVL indicating that a higher peak inspiratory pressure (PIP) is required to deliver the same tidal volume (decreased compliance).

The Bellavista images are © 2019 Vyaire Medical, Inc.; Used with permission.

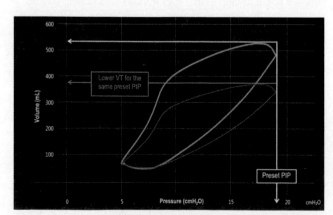

FIGURE 7-19 A similar shift to the right of the inspiratory limb of the pressure-volume loop is observed in a pressure-controlled mode. However, a preset peak inspiratory pressure (PIP) will be associated with a lower V_T as a result of decreased lung compliance.

The Bellavista images are © 2019 Vyaire Medical, Inc.; Used with permission.

Increased Hysteresis

Surface tension and frictional forces contribute to differences in the shape of the PVL during expansion and deflation. This difference results from one measured variable changing at a faster rate than another plotted against it, referred to as **hysteresis.** The presence of increased airway resistance with air trapping will result in a shift to the right of the inspiratory limb of the PVL (to overcome resistance) and also in a shift of the expiratory upper inflection point to the left. Pressure increases faster than volume, causing the horizontal distance of the loop to expand. As the exhalation valve opens, airway pressure drops but expiratory volume does not decrease at the same rate because of air trapping. Patients with obstructive disorders and air trapping typically exhibit a wide PVL with increased hysteresis (**Figure 7-20**).

Air Leak

When the expiratory limb of the PVL does not return to zero volume, an air leak is present (**Figure 7-21**). As discussed earlier under the topic of volume-time scalar and air leaks, failure of expiratory volume to return to baseline zero occurs for every mechanical breath. Air trapping can produce a similar tracing but only for two or three mechanical breaths.

Flow-Volume Loop

Although there is no set convention in assigning the inspiratory and expiratory to a specific side of the horizontal axis on an FVL, most ventilators display inspiration above it and exhalation below it. Traditional spirometry displays the FVL completely opposite to ventilators. A flow-volume

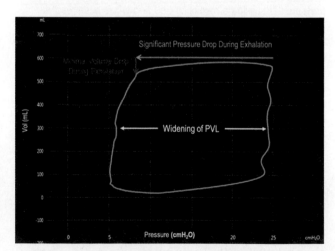

FIGURE 7-20 Pressure-volume loop (PVL) waveform widening of the loop (increased hysteresis). As the exhalation valve opens, airway pressure drops (blue arrow), but expiratory volume does not decrease at the same rate (red arrow) due to air trapping.

The Bellavista images are © 2019 Vyaire Medical, Inc.; Used with permission.

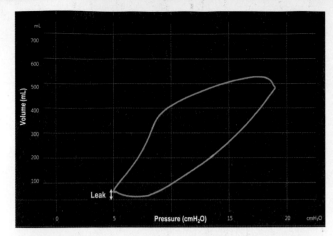

FIGURE 7-21 Waveform displaying how the expiratory limb of the pressure-volume loop fails to return fully to the starting point. The gap between the two points indicates the magnitude of the leak.
The Bellavista images are © 2019 Vyaire Medical, Inc.; Used with permission.

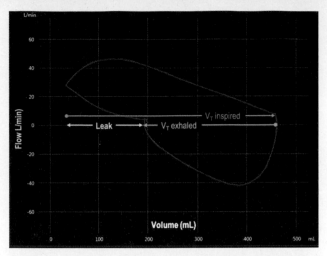

FIGURE 7-23 Flow-volume loop displaying an expired limb of the waveform not fully returning to zero. The gap indicates the magnitude (in mL) of the leak.
The Bellavista images are © 2019 Vyaire Medical, Inc.; Used with permission.

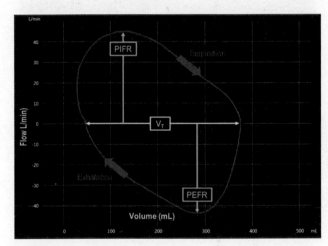

FIGURE 7-22 Waveform showing a typical configuration of the flow-volume loop. Peak inspiratory flow rate (PIFR), peak expiratory flow rate (PEFR), and V$_T$ are labeled.
The Bellavista images are © 2019 Vyaire Medical, Inc.; Used with permission.

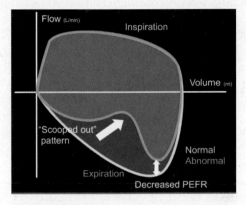

FIGURE 7-24 Typical scooping of the expiratory tracing of the flow-volume loop and decreased peak expiratory flow rate (PEFR) observed on patients with airway obstruction.

loop displays the following information: peak inspiratory flow rate (PIFR), PEFR, and V$_T$ (**Figure 7-22**).

Air Leak

Under ideal conditions, expired volume should be equal to inspired volume. When this occurs, the loop closes where it originally started. In case a leak is present, the loop never closes, and the gap indicates the magnitude (in mL) of the leak (**Figure 7-23**).

Increased Airway Resistance

Increased airway resistance, such as in asthma and chronic obstructive pulmonary disease (COPD), is commonly associated with a "scooping" of the expiratory

tracing of the FVL and a decreased PEFR. A positive response to bronchodilator will show an improvement on both the configuration of the expiratory tracing and the PEFR (**Figure 7-24**).

Airway Secretions/Accumulation of Condensate

The presence of secretions in the large airways, as well as excessive fluid condensation in the ventilator circuit, appear as a distinctive pattern in the FVL known as a "sawtooth" pattern, which can be present on both inspiration and expiration (**Figure 7-25**).

Ventilator Mode Recognition

Every mechanical breath is classified according to three important parameters: trigger (initiation), limit, and

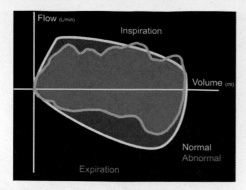

FIGURE 7-25 Flow-volume loop showing a typical "sawtooth" appearance consistent with the presence of secretions in the large airways or excessive condensate in the ventilator circuit.

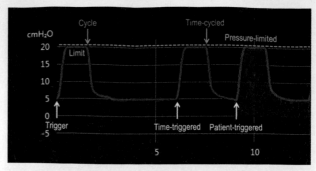

FIGURE 7-26 Pressure-time scalar showing the variables that define a mechanical breath (trigger limit cycle) and the difference between a patient-triggered (assisted) and time-triggered (controlled) breath, and pressure-limited and time-cycled breath.

The Bellavista images are © 2019 Vyaire Medical, Inc.; Used with permission.

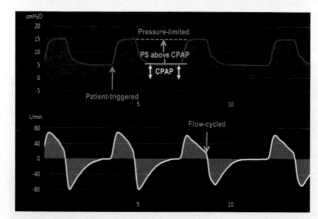

FIGURE 7-27 Pressure-time and flow-time (F-T) waveforms consistent with the use of continuous positive airway pressure (CPAP) set at 5 cm H_2O plus pressure support (PS) set at 10 cm H_2O above CPAP. F-T waveform indicates the breath cycles when flow decreases to 25% of peak inspiratory flow rate (PIFR). Paw, airway pressure.

The Bellavista images are © 2019 Vyaire Medical, Inc.; Used with permission.

cycle (termination), as shown in **Figure 7-26**. Despite the increasing number of acronyms associated with modes of ventilation, a mechanical breath is either **volume targeted** [by controlling either (a) inspiratory flow and inspiratory time or (b) volume] or **pressure targeted** (by limiting the inspiratory pressure). When the clinician sets the VT or inspiratory pressure, the mechanical breath is either volume limited or pressure limited. Volume and pressure "controlled" modes of ventilation simply refer to the control variable for each breath. Cycling occurs when the exhalation valve opens and thus terminates the breath delivery. The variables used to end the breath are either the set time or a predetermined expiratory flow.

Continuous Positive Airway Pressure Plus Pressure Support

Continuous positive airway pressure (CPAP) displays a spontaneous breath on a P-T waveform that starts at the preset pressure level. Pressure support (PS) augments spontaneous breaths with positive pressure to provide a higher volume for all spontaneous breaths. A pressure-supported breath is by definition patient triggered, pressure limited, and flow cycled. Inspiration ends when a preset expiratory flow reaches a predetermined value (typically 25% of the peak flow). The delivered volume is dependent on the patient's lung compliance, airway resistance, and inspiratory demand (**Figure 7-27**).

Volume Control–Continuous Mandatory Ventilation

Volume control–continuous mandatory ventilation (VC-CMV) is the most frequently used mode in ICUs. It is a ventilator mode in which the machine delivers the set VT during every inspiration, whether machine triggered (controlled) or patient triggered (assisted) (**Figure 7-28**).

Pressure Control–Continuous Mandatory Ventilation

Pressure control–continuous mandatory ventilation (PC-CMV) is a ventilator mode in which the machine delivers the set inspiratory pressure during every inspiration, whether machine triggered (controlled) or patient triggered (assisted) (**Figure 7-29**).

Synchronized Intermittent Mandatory Ventilation

Synchronized intermittent mandatory ventilation (SIMV) can provide full ventilatory support, but it is primarily used to provide partial mechanical support. With SIMV, breaths can be either mandatory (ventilator controlled) or spontaneous. The mandatory breaths are synchronized with patient effort (patient triggered). The mandatory breaths can be either volume controlled or pressure controlled. The remaining inspiratory efforts of the patient produce spontaneous breaths that may be pressure supported (**Figure 7-30**).

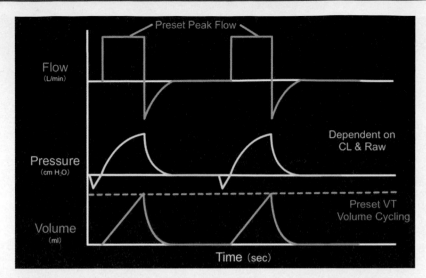

FIGURE 7-28 Scalars showing typical appearance of a volume control–continuous mandatory ventilation (VC-CMV) mode. The machine delivers the set VT during every inspiration, whether machine triggered (controlled) or patient triggered (assisted). Paw, airway pressure; Raw, airway resistance.

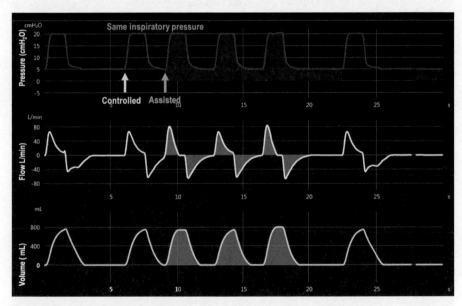

FIGURE 7-29 Scalars showing typical appearance of a pressure control–continuous mandatory ventilation (PC–CMV) mode. The machine delivers the set inspiratory pressure, whether machine triggered (controlled) or patient triggered (assisted). Paw, airway pressure.

The Bellavista images are © 2019 Vyaire Medical, Inc.; Used with permission.

Airway Pressure Release Ventilation

Airway pressure release ventilation (APRV) is a time-controlled adaptive ventilation strategy that incorporates CPAP with an intermittent release phase. APRV applies CPAP (P high) for a prolonged time (T high) to maintain adequate lung volume and alveolar recruitment, with a time-cycled release phase to a lower set of pressure (P low) for a short period of time (T low, or release time) where most of ventilation and CO_2 removal occurs (**Figure 7-31**). Spontaneous breathing can occur during the P high duration, as observed in **Figure 7-32**.

Patient–Ventilator Asynchrony

Patient–ventilator asynchrony (PVA) is a condition in which a mismatching between neural (patient) and mechanically (ventilator) assisted breaths occurs. PVA may be in the form of ineffective or missed triggering, also known as trigger asynchrony, or ineffective termination of mechanical breath, also known as cycle asynchrony. Both conditions refer essentially to "phase asynchrony." Included in PVA, however, is flow asynchrony, in which the ventilator flow delivery is inadequate to match the patient's ventilatory flow demand despite a matched inspiratory time.

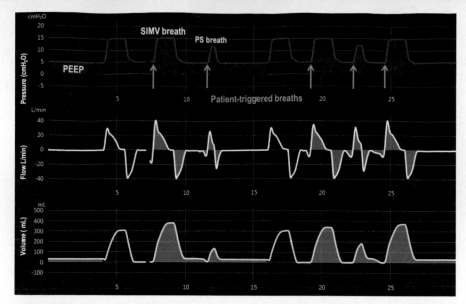

FIGURE 7-30 Example of scalar waveforms showing synchronized intermittent mandatory ventilation (SIMV; pressure controlled) plus pressure support (PS). Some mandatory breaths are synchronized with patient efforts. The remaining inspiratory efforts of the patient produce spontaneous breaths that are pressure supported. Paw, airway pressure.

The Bellavista images are © 2019 Vyaire Medical, Inc.; Used with permission.

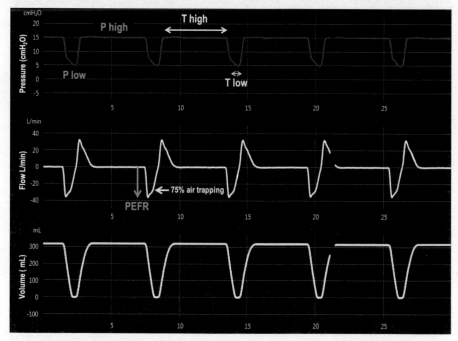

FIGURE 7-31 Pressure-time waveform for airway pressure release ventilation (APRV). "P high" is the high continuous positive airway pressure (CPAP), "P low" is the low CPAP (or low positive end-expiratory pressure [PEEP] if no spontaneous breathing), "T high" is the duration of "P high," and "T low" is the release period or the duration of "P low." Observe that in APRV, generating air trapping at 50% to 75% in the flow-time waveform is recommended. Paw, airway pressure.

The Bellavista images are © 2019 Vyaire Medical, Inc.; Used with permission.

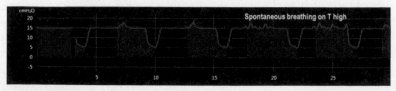

FIGURE 7-32 Pressure-time waveform for airway pressure release ventilation (APRV) showing spontaneous breathing on the "P high."

The Bellavista images are © 2019 Vyaire Medical, Inc.; Used with permission.

Trigger Asynchrony

When inspiratory efforts are excessive, patient's work of breathing increases. Sometimes, those efforts are wasted and do not result in a triggered breath at all (**Figure 7-33**). Both types of asynchrony are usually resolved by increasing trigger pressure or flow sensitivity. The presence of auto-PEEP is associated with missed-trigger asynchrony. Auto-PEEP also increases the work of breathing due to increase of required trigger pressure (auto-PEEP + sensitivity trigger pressure).

As previously indicated, a normal PVL traces in a counterclockwise direction. A clockwise tracing prior to the initiation of a mechanical breath indicates patient effort. Adjusting the sensitivity can minimize this effort (**Figure 7-34**).

Auto-trigger

Auto-triggering, which happens when a ventilator breath occurs without patient effort, is associated with low respiratory drive, prolonged exhalation time in the absence of PEEPi (auto-PEEP), cardiogenic oscillation, hiccup, low triggering threshold (high sensitivity), water in the circuit, or circuit leak (**Figure 7-35**).

Flow Asynchrony

Flow asynchrony, also known as "flow starvation," is a form of PVA that occurs when a patient is demanding more flow than the ventilator provides. This type of PVA can be observed on scalars (**Figure 7-36**) and loops (**Figure 7-37**).

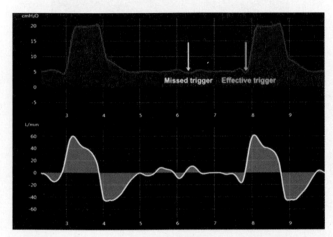

FIGURE 7-33 Pressure-time and flow-time (F-T) scalars showing trigger asynchrony. An inspiratory effort (yellow arrow) is not followed by delivery of a mechanical breath (missed trigger). The F-T displays small spontaneous fluctuations of flow compared to flow characteristics of two mechanical breaths. Paw, airway pressure.

The Bellavista images are © 2019 Vyaire Medical, Inc.; Used with permission.

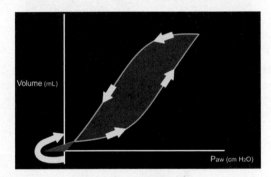

FIGURE 7-34 Pressure-volume loop showing a patient-triggered breath. The curved arrow indicates patient effort, and the size of the red-shaded area is reflective of the degree of patient effort required to trigger the mechanical breath. Paw, airway pressure.

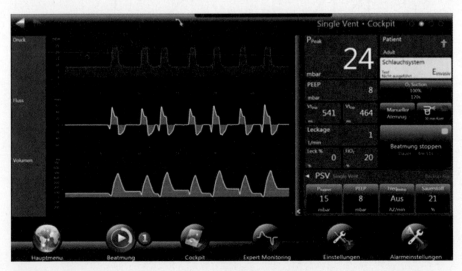

FIGURE 7-35 Scalar waveforms showing how an air leak causes the circuit pressure to drop below the set positive end-expiratory pressure and trigger the ventilator. Paw, airway pressure.

The Bellavista images are © 2019 Vyaire Medical, Inc.; Used with permission.

Cycle Asynchrony

Patient–ventilator asynchrony may occur if the flow at which the ventilator cycles to exhalation does not coincide with the termination of neural inspiration. Ideally, the ventilator terminates inspiratory flow in synchrony with the patient's neural timing, but frequently the ventilator terminates inspiration either early (premature cycling) or late (delayed cycling). Most current mechanical ventilators include adjustable cycling features that, when used in conjunction with waveform graphics, can enhance patient–ventilator synchrony.

Premature Cycling (Double Trigger)

During premature cycling, inspiratory muscles continue to contract after the ventilator has switched to exhalation phase, causing the mechanical ventilator to sense a second effort, and possibly resulting in a second breath, commonly referred to as "stacking of breaths" or "double triggering" (**Figure 7-38**).

Delayed Cycling

If a patient wants to terminate inspiration before the ventilator does, this asynchrony is called delayed cycling. The patient actively exhales, causing a rise in airway pressure at the end of the mechanical breath before termination of inspiration (**Figure 7-39**).

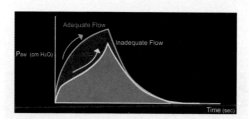

FIGURE 7-36 A pressure vs. time diagram shows a significant drop in pressure during inspiration and a scooped-out pattern due to patient effort demanding more flow than delivered. Paw, airway pressure.

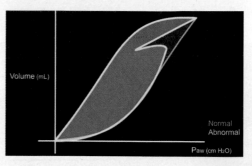

FIGURE 7-37 Pressure-volume loop and pressure-volume loop with either a deflection or a scooped-out pattern of the inspiratory limb indicating patient effort in the middle of the breath in an effort to match flow demands. Paw, airway pressure.

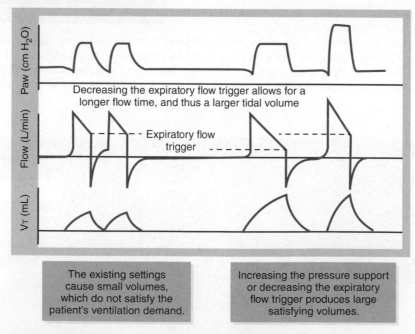

Decreasing the expiratory flow trigger allows for a longer flow time, and thus a larger tidal volume

Expiratory flow trigger

The existing settings cause small volumes, which do not satisfy the patient's ventilation demand.

Increasing the pressure support or decreasing the expiratory flow trigger produces large satisfying volumes.

FIGURE 7-38 Scalar graphics showing double triggering, defined as two consecutive ventilator cycles separated by an expiratory time less than one-half the mean inspiratory time. Double triggering occurs when the ventilator inspiratory time is shorter than the patient's inspiratory time. Patient effort is not completed at the end of the first ventilator cycle and triggers a second ventilator cycle. Paw, airway pressure.
© Alex Yartsev.

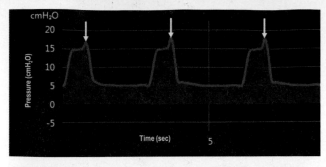

FIGURE 7-39 Delayed cycling leads to a spike (arrows) in airway pressure in late inspiration on the pressure-time waveform.

Summary

Ventilator waveforms provide extremely important information about the patient–ventilator interaction. Just monitoring ventilator parameters on screen is no longer enough to assess patients undergoing mechanical ventilation. Scalars and loops offer a variety of configurations to appreciate the most significant changes that occur while a patient is placed on any ventilatory mode.

While mode recognition is important, detecting changes in pulmonary mechanics, determining response to bronchodilators, and identifying patient–ventilator asynchronies could significantly affect patient outcomes in the ICU.

Case Study

Case Study 7-1 Patient-Ventilator Asynchrony

1. The clinician is called to the intensive care unit (ICU) for an assessment of a patient with chronic obstructive pulmonary disease (COPD) who is mechanically ventilated. The ICU clinician is looking at the P-T and F-T waveforms to determine why the patient has increased work of breathing. On first look at the F-T scalar, what would be the most significant change observed to explain the patient's condition?

   a. Fast rise time

   b. Flow starvation

   c. Air trapping

   d. Air leak

2. What would suggest the P-T waveform to explain the increased work of breathing?

   a. Trigger asynchrony

   b. Flow asynchrony

   c. Cycle asynchrony

   d. a and c

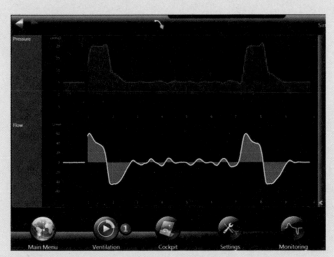

Bibliography

Introduction

Branson RD. Patient-ventilator interaction: the last 40 years. *Respir Care.* 2011;56:15–24.

Dhand R. Ventilator graphics and respiratory mechanics in the patient with obstructive lung disease. *Respir Care.* 2005;50:246–261.

Natalini G, Tuzzo D, Rosano A, et al. Assessment of factors related to auto-PEEP. *Respir Care.* 2016;61:134–141.

Natalini G, Tuzzo D, Rosano A, et al. Effect of external PEEP in patients under controlled mechanical ventilation with an auto-PEEP of 5 cm H_2O or higher. *Ann Intensive Care.* 2016;6:53.

Pierson D. Patient-ventilator interaction. *Respir Care.* 2011;56:214–228.

Prabhakaran P, Sasser WC, Kalra Y, et al. Ventilator graphics. *Minerva Pediatr.* 2016;68:456–469.

Ventilator Mode Recognition

MacIntyre NR. Patient-ventilator interactions: optimizing conventional ventilation modes. *Respir Care.* 2011;56:73–84.

Ventilator Asynchrony

Blokpoel RG, Burgerhof JG, Markhorst DG. Patient ventilator asynchrony during assisted ventilation in children. *Pediatr Crit Care Med.* 2016;17:e204–e211.

Epstein SK. How often does patient-ventilator asynchrony occur and what are the consequences? *Respir Care.* 2011;56:25–38.

Gentile MA. Cycling of the mechanical ventilator breath. *Respir Care.* 2011;56:52–60.

Kacmarek RM, Pirrone M, Berra L. Assisted mechanical ventilation: the future is now! *BMC Anesthesiol.* 2015;29:110.

Piquilloud L, Jolliet P, Revelly JP. Automated detection of patient-ventilator asynchrony: new tool or new toy? *Crit Care.* 2013;17:1015. doi:10.1186 /cc13122

Ramirez II, Arellano DH, Adasme RS, et al. Ability of ICU health-care professionals to identify patient-ventilator asynchrony using waveform analysis. *Respir Care.* 2017;62:144–149.

Sassoon CS. Triggering of the ventilator in patient-ventilator interactions. *Respir Care.* 2011;56:39–51.

Subirà C, de Haro C, Magrans R. Minimizing asynchronies in mechanical ventilation: current and future trends. *Respir Care.* 2018;63:464–478.

CHAPTER

8

Management of Mechanical Ventilation

David W. Chang, EdD, RRT

OUTLINE

OBJECTIVES

1. List and describe the strategies to improve ventilation.
2. List and describe the strategies to improve oxygenation.
3. Describe the initial ventilator alarm settings.
4. Explain how prone positioning, tracheal gas insufflation, and mechanical insufflation-exsufflation improve ventilation or oxygenation.
5. List the initial ventilator settings for ARDS and decompensated heart failure.
6. Differentiate the ventilator settings between noninvasive and mechanical ventilation for severe asthma and acute exacerbation of COPD.
7. Describe the unique ventilator settings for patients injured in mass casualty incidents.
8. Differentiate between START and SOFA triage systems.
9. List the initial ventilator settings for mass casualty incidents.

KEY TERMS

absolute shunt
acute exacerbation
  of COPD
acute respiratory
  distress syndrome
air trapping
ARDSNet
auto-PEEP
decompensated
  heart failure
decremental recruitment
  maneuver
mass casualty

mechanical insufflation-
  exsufflation
noninvasive ventilation
permissive hypercapnia
prone positioning
pressure support
SOFA
START
tracheal gas insufflation
triage
tromethamine (THAM)
venous admixture

Introduction

Mechanical ventilation supports an individual's ventilation and oxygenation needs. It is a frequently used life-support procedure in acute and subacute patient care settings. In critical care, different modes and ventilator settings are available to manage a wide range of pathological conditions. Outside the acute setting, patients with chronic or irreversible pulmonary conditions can benefit from mechanical ventilation at home or other subacute care settings. This chapter provides the fundamental management techniques and special strategies for unique patient conditions during mechanical ventilation.

During mechanical ventilation, the patient must be the primary focus at all times. Errors can occur with the ventilator, monitoring devices, lab test analysis, recording of data, reporting, and interpretation of data. These errors can be avoided by providing patient-focused care. In other words, the clinical data and data interpretation must match the patient's condition.

Fundamental Ventilator Management Strategies

Two basic premises of effective mechanical ventilation are to provide (1) sufficient ventilation and (2) oxygenation to a patient during a period of critical illness. For management of ventilation, use of respiratory frequency (f), tidal volume (VT), and pressure support ventilation on the ventilator are three common methods. Fraction of inspired oxygen (FIO$_2$), continuous positive airway pressure (CPAP), and positive end-expiratory pressure (PEEP) are three basic tools for management of oxygenation.

Since ventilation and oxygenation are closely related to each other, changing a setting to regulate ventilation will affect oxygenation. By the same logic, changing a setting on the ventilator to regulate oxygenation may affect ventilation, to a lesser degree. These interactions are reliable in most instances when the patients do not have significant ventilation-perfusion mismatch or intrapulmonary shunting. **Table 8-1** shows how changing a setting on the ventilator may affect ventilation and oxygenation. For example, an increase in ventilation lowers the PaCO$_2$ and increases the PaO$_2$ and related oxygenation indices (e.g., SpO$_2$). During weaning from mechanical ventilation, a decrease in ventilation (e.g., ↓f) typically results in an increase in PaCO$_2$ and a decrease in PaO$_2$ and related indices.

Strategies to Improve Ventilation

Hypoventilation is defined as an abnormally high PaCO$_2$ (>45 mm Hg). Spontaneous respiratory frequency and tidal volume only describe a patient's breathing pattern; they do not reflect the degree of carbon dioxide exchange at the alveolar-capillary level. An arterial PaCO$_2$ above the upper normal range (45 mm Hg) indicates hypoventilation. Patients with chronic obstructive

TABLE 8-1
Ventilator Setting Change and Its Effects on Ventilation and Oxygenation

Ventilator Setting Change	Ventilation	Oxygenation
↑ f	↑↑	↑
↑ VT	↑↑	↑
↑ PSV	↑↑	↑
↑ ΔP (Bilevel PAP, APRV)	↑↑	↑
↑ FIO$_2$	nl or ↓	↑↑
↑ CPAP	nl or ↓	↑*
↑ PEEP	nl or ↓	↑*

*Intrapulmonary shunting responding to CPAP or PEEP
APRV, airway pressure release ventilation; CPAP, continuous positive airway pressure; PAP, positive airway pressure; PEEP, positive end-expiratory pressure; PSV, pressure support ventilation; VT, tidal volume.

pulmonary disease (COPD) and chronic CO$_2$ retention have a higher baseline PaCO$_2$, often about 50 mm Hg. It is essential to note that when using PaCO$_2$ as a target for weaning from mechanical ventilation, the patient's baseline blood gases (i.e., PaCO$_2$ and PaO$_2$) should be used. Using a patient's "optimal" PaCO$_2$ as a target for mechanical ventilation and weaning offers a more appropriate physiologic goal. The following sections describe strategies to improve ventilation.

Respiratory Frequency

Alveolar ventilation (V̇A) reflects the effectiveness of gas exchange at the alveolar level. The minute alveolar ventilation is determined by the frequency, tidal volume, and dead space volume (VD). V̇A has an inverse relationship with the PaCO$_2$. Under normal conditions, a higher level of alveolar ventilation results in a lower PaCO$_2$, and vice versa.

As shown in the following equation, V̇A can be increased by either increasing the frequency or tidal volume. It can also be increased by reducing the anatomic dead space volume (e.g., tracheostomy) or the mechanical dead space volume (e.g., a shorter endotracheal [ET] tube). V̇A can also be increased by reducing the physiologic dead space (i.e., improving pulmonary perfusion).

$$\dot{V}A = f \times (V_T - V_D)$$

Spontaneous Breathing

Because anatomic dead space volume remains rather constant, the alveolar ventilation for a spontaneously breathing patient can be improved by increasing the spontaneous frequency or tidal volume. Increase in spontaneous breathing frequency is often a compensatory response to hypoxia, especially for patients with restrictive lung diseases (e.g., atelectasis). Patients with chronic airflow obstruction (e.g., COPD) tend to breathe deeper and slower due to high lung compliance, low elastic recoil, and air trapping. During mechanical ventilation, a patient's spontaneous breathing effort (frequency and tidal volume) are negatively affected by excessive use of analgesic or sedative.

Mechanical Ventilation

The mandatory or controlled frequency on a ventilator is predetermined. Depending on the mode, spontaneous breathing between mandatory breaths may or may not be allowed. In modes in which spontaneous breathing is allowed between mandatory breaths (e.g., synchronized intermittent mandatory ventilation [SIMV]), the minute ventilation is the sum of mechanical frequency and tidal volume, as well as the spontaneous frequency and tidal volume. Proper frequency setting on the ventilator primarily relies on a patient's spontaneous breathing effort.

Assist/Control and SIMV

When the frequency is changed during mechanical ventilation, the minute ventilation will vary based on the modes of ventilation. In assist/control (A/C) or similar modes, each patient-assisted (triggered) breath will result in a mechanical tidal volume. In SIMV mode, each spontaneous breath will be the patient's spontaneous tidal volume. By comparing the same number of patient-assisted breaths between A/C and SIMV, the minute ventilation in A/C mode usually provides a larger minute ventilation.

There are many methods for weaning from mechanical ventilation. If the frequency control is used for a weaning purpose, the A/C mode must first be changed to a mode that allows spontaneous breathing (e.g., SIMV).

Air Trapping and Auto-PEEP

Air trapping and **auto-PEEP** occur during mechanical ventilation under various conditions, including lung disease (e.g., emphysema) and inappropriate ventilator settings (e.g., insufficient expiratory time, excessive frequency, or tidal volume). Excessive mechanical frequency reduces the respiratory time cycle (i.e., time for each mechanical breath), and it does not allow complete or near-complete exhalation. Depending on the degree of incomplete exhalation, it may lead to air trapping or auto-PEEP. Air trapping or auto-PEEP may be managed initially by reducing the frequency or tidal volume (or bronchodilator therapy if indicated). Applying therapeutic (extrinsic) PEEP equivalent to up to 85% of the measured auto-PEEP is the remaining option to reduce auto-PEEP (most applicable to gas trapping caused by early small airway collapse, as with emphysema).

It should be noted that presence of air trapping is evident at the end-exhalation point on the flow-time waveform (i.e., end flow does not reach baseline). Auto-PEEP is evaluated by reviewing the pressure-time waveform (i.e., excessive pressure above end-expiratory pressure at end-exhalation during airway occlusion). Air trapping implies the *likelihood* of auto-PEEP, and this correlation is not absolute. Reviewing the pressure-time waveform by means of an end-expiratory occlusion maneuver is more clinically relevant because it confirms the presence of auto-PEEP *and* shows the severity of auto-PEEP.

Tidal Volume

In addition to frequency, tidal volume is another component of minute ventilation. The mechanical tidal volume is set on the ventilator based on a patient's predicted body weight (PBW) and the target plateau pressure. One of the ideal tidal volume ranges is from 6 to 8 mL/kg PBW, and the recommended plateau pressure threshold is <30 cm H_2O. When the plateau exceeds 30 cm H_2O, the tidal volume should be set at the lower range (e.g., 6 mL/kg). In some conditions (e.g., acute respiratory distress syndrome [ARDS]) that require lung protection from pressure-induced or volume-induced lung injuries, the tidal volume may be set as low as 4 mL/kg.

The tidal volume range is based on the Acute Respiratory Distress Syndrome Network (**ARDSNet**) recommendations. It is noteworthy to respiratory therapy students that this range from 6 to 8 mL/kg has been adopted by the National Board for Respiratory Care (NBRC) for its credentialing examinations.

Pressure Support

Pressure support ventilation (PSV) augments a patient's spontaneous tidal volume. PSV is not active and cannot be used if a patient does not have spontaneous breathing efforts or the mode of ventilation (e.g., assist/control) does not allow spontaneous breaths.

For spontaneous breathing without mechanical support (e.g., during spontaneous breathing trial), the initial pressure support (PS) is titrated upward to a target of spontaneous tidal volume from 6 to 8 mL/kg or a spontaneous frequency of ≤25/min. The tidal volume titration endpoint correlates with the low tidal volume lung protection recommendations. Once a spontaneous breath is detected, the ventilator delivers a constant peak flow to reach and maintain the preset PS. This continuous flow fills the lungs and increases the airway and alveolar pressures. Near the end of a PS breath, the inspiratory flow stops when the end flow reaches a ventilator-specific threshold (e.g., 5 L/min or 25% of peak flow). PSV is a form of pressure ventilation and, as such, it responds to changing lung compliance. As the lung compliance improves, the spontaneous tidal volume will increase. To prevent hyperinflation and volume-induced lung injuries, it is important to monitor a patient's spontaneous tidal volume during PSV. The PS level should be adjusted accordingly for an appropriate tidal volume.

Other Strategies to Improve or Sustain Ventilation

In addition to frequency, tidal volume, and pressure support, other strategies to improve or sustain adequate ventilation include improvement of airway patency and reduction (bypass) of anatomic and physiologic dead space.

Airway Patency and Airflow Resistance

Airway patency for effective ventilation can be achieved by increasing the airway caliber or decreasing the airflow resistance. Common methods to increase the airway caliber include use of a largest ET tube as appropriate for patient, use of bronchodilators to reverse bronchospasm, reduction of airway inflammation with inhaled corticosteroids, and removal of secretions by chest physiotherapy, secretions clearance techniques, or suctioning.

As described, the airflow resistance is reduced with a larger airway caliber. During mechanical ventilation, improvement of airflow resistance becomes evident when the pressure gradient between peak inspiratory pressure (PIP) and plateau pressure (Pplat) is decreased. The Pplat can be obtained by a brief end-inspiratory pause that produces a pressures plateau. Helium/oxygen mixture has been used as an alternative method to reduce the airflow resistance during mechanical ventilation.

Reduction of Mechanical and Physiologic Dead Space

Other methods to reduce work of breathing or increase ventilation efficiency include reduction of mechanical and physiologic dead space. Mechanical dead space can be reduced by shortening the length of an ET tube or reducing the size of add-ons connected to the ET tube. A shorter ET tube also enhances the removal of secretions during ET suctioning. When a tracheotomy is indicated, the tracheostomy tube offers a lower mechanical dead space.

Physiologic dead space is increased when alveolar ventilation exceeds pulmonary perfusion. Under this high ventilation-perfusion ($\dot{V}/\dot{Q}$) mismatch condition, a portion of alveolar ventilation cannot take part in gas exchange due to lack of pulmonary perfusion. Causes of reduced pulmonary perfusion include hypoxic vasoconstriction, pulmonary hypertension, and pulmonary embolism. Physiologic dead space can be reduced by identifying and resolving the respective causes of inadequate pulmonary perfusion (a therapeutic example is placing a patient in prone position, as with a RotoProne® bed).

Permissive Hypercapnia

Permissive hypercapnia is a strategy to reduce the likelihood of lung injury due to excessive volume or pressure during mechanical ventilation. This procedure produces intentional hypercapnia ($\uparrow Paco_2$ >50 mm Hg) by using a low ventilator tidal volume in the range of 4 to 8 mL/kg. In volume-controlled ventilation, a low tidal volume reduces the peak inspiratory pressure, plateau pressure, and mean airway pressure. Low lung volume and airway pressures reduce the likelihood of lung injuries. Since plateau pressure approximates the average alveolar pressure, it is used as a titration endpoint for the low-volume strategy. ARDSNet guidelines recommend a plateau pressure of <30 cm H_2O, and it should be used as the initial titration target. In pressure-controlled ventilation, the peak inspiratory pressure should be set initially the same as the plateau pressure during volume-controlled ventilation. This initial pressure may subsequently be titrated for a target tidal volume in the range of 4 to 8 mL/kg.

Negative complications for permissive hypercapnia include hypoventilation, CO_2 retention, hypoxemia, and combined acidosis (due to hypoventilation and anaerobic metabolism). If uncorrected, persistence acidosis may lead to neurological confusion, increased intracranial pressure, neuromuscular weakness, cardiovascular impairments, and increased pulmonary vascular resistance. These potential complications may be reduced by keeping the pH within the patient's normal range. For induced hypercapnia, the pH may be normalized by administering bicarbonate or tromethamine (discontinued in the United States as of May 2016). Bicarbonate is an alkalizing agent, and its usefulness for acute and severe acidosis is well known. However, bicarbonate may not be useful in pH regulation during permissive hypercapnia because it adds CO_2 during the formation and dissociation of carbonic acid ($H_2CO_3 \rightarrow CO_2 + H_2O$). **Tromethamine (THAM)** is a non-bicarbonate buffer that directly reduces the H^+ ion concentration and indirectly reduces the CO_2 level. These two actions of THAM work in tandem and result in an increased bicarbonate level. Its action on CO_2 reduction is an added benefit to patients undergoing permissive hypercapnia procedure. The initial amount of 0.3 M THAM needed is calculated by: Body weight in kg $\times$ Base deficit in mEq/L. Side effects of THAM include hypoglycemia, respiratory depression, and hemorrhagic hepatic necrosis. The management strategies during permissive hypercapnia are outlined in **Figure 8-1**.

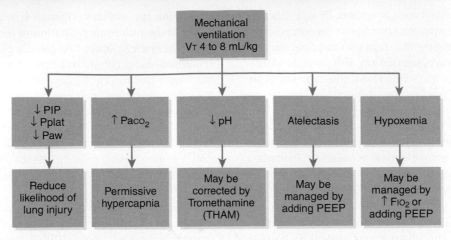

FIGURE 8-1 Management strategies during permissive hypercapnia. Paw, airway pressure; PEEP, positive end-expiratory pressure; PIP, peak inspiratory pressure; VT, tidal volume.

Strategies to Improve Oxygenation

During mechanical ventilation, the patient's oxygenation status is monitored continuously by SpO_2 and periodically by PaO_2. Under some conditions (e.g., carbon monoxide poisoning, presence of dysfunctional hemoglobins), SpO_2 and PaO_2 cannot be used to assess this type of hypoxemia because they do not measure the oxygen bound to the hemoglobin. Arterial oxygen content (CaO_2) by CO-oximetry measures the total amount of oxygen in arterial blood (oxygen bound to hemoglobin and oxygen dissolved in plasma). For this reason, CaO_2 should be used to evaluate the oxygenation status of patients with CO poisoning and dysfunctional hemoglobins.

Ventilation, FIO_2, CPAP, PEEP, prone positioning, recruitment maneuver, high-frequency oscillatory ventilation (HFOV), and airway pressure release ventilation (APRV) are procedures that can improve a patient's oxygenation status. HFOV and APRV are discussed in other chapters of this book. Some of these topics are discussed under different sections in this chapter.

Ventilation, FIO_2, CPAP, and PEEP

Depending on the underlying pathophysiology, uncomplicated hypoxemia can be corrected by providing or increasing ventilation, oxygen, CPAP, or PEEP. Ventilation is the treatment of choice for hypoventilation (e.g., postanesthesia recovery). Oxygen therapy is ideal for mild hypoxemia due to simple ventilation-perfusion mismatch (e.g., segmental consolidation). For moderate and severe hypoxemia due to absolute (true) shunt (**absolute shunt** = anatomic shunt + capillary shunt), CPAP or PEEP is usually necessary. CPAP is used when the patient's ventilatory status is adequate and sustainable as documented by $PaCO_2$ measurements. PEEP is needed to manage absolute shunt during mechanical

ventilation. **Figure 8-2** summarizes the methods to improve oxygenation based on different causes of hypoxemia.

Hypoxemia Due to Hypoventilation

Hypoxemia due to acute hypoventilation (acute respiratory acidosis) is evident when the $PaCO_2$ is increased

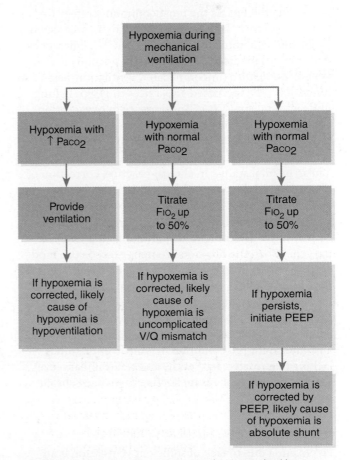

FIGURE 8-2 Methods to improve oxygenation categorized by different causes of hypoxemia. PEEP, positive end-expiratory pressure.

without complete renal compensation. In this case, the HCO_3^- is near normal. Postanesthesia recovery is an example of acute hypoventilation that requires only short-term mechanical ventilation. For patients with normal cardiopulmonary functions, this type of hypoxemia can be easily resolved by supplemental oxygen and ventilation.

Hypoxemia due to chronic hypoventilation (compensated respiratory acidosis) may require continuing supplemental oxygen or mechanical ventilation. Patients with COPD may only require a low level of supplemental oxygen, noninvasive ventilation. Occasionally, exacerbation of COPD with acute-on-chronic hypercapnic respiratory failure (severe respiratory acidosis) may require intubation and invasive mechanical ventilation. For patients with high cervical spinal cord injuries, continuous supplemental oxygen *and* invasive mechanical ventilation are required.

Increasing the FIO_2 on ventilator is the most common method to correct hypoxemia. This method works well in most clinical conditions, with the exception of hypoxemia due to absolute shunt (refractory hypoxemia).

Hypoxemia Due to Venous Admixture

Increasing the FIO_2 is the most common strategy to treat hypoxemia. This is done frequently in areas such as the neonatal intensive care unit (NICU), emergency department, medical, and ICUs. In hypoxemia due to **venous admixture** (uncomplicated ventilation-perfusion mismatch), the increased FIO_2 raises the PaO_2 in lung units with normal $\dot{V}/\dot{Q}$. This increase in oxygenation compensates for the decrease in oxygenation in lung units with abnormal $\dot{V}/\dot{Q}$ mismatch. In venous admixture, oxygen therapy often returns the PaO_2 and CaO_2 to a near-normal status. In clinical practice, correction of hypoxemia in simple $\dot{V}/\dot{Q}$ mismatch typically requires an FIO_2 of below 0.4. Refractory hypoxemia describes a pathological process in which hypoxemia does not respond well to a moderate amount of supplemental oxygen. When the FIO_2 requirement exceeds 0.5, moderate to severe absolute shunt should be suspected. Two indices of absolute shunt are decreasing P/F ratio (PaO_2/FIO_2) and increasing pulmonary shunt fraction ($\dot{Q}sp$/$\dot{Q}T$). ARDS is an example in which bilateral pulmonary edema and atelectasis cause absolute shunting. Because absolute shunt is a condition in which ventilation is lacking (e.g., atelectasis) at the alveolar-capillary level, oxygen therapy alone is ineffective to manage absolute shunting.

Hypoxemia Due to Absolute Shunt

Hypoxemia due to lack of sufficient ventilation is an important clinical condition during mechanical ventilation. Lack of ventilation leads to low $\dot{V}/\dot{Q}$ mismatch—perfusion in excess of ventilation. Absolute shunt is a type of intrapulmonary (right-to-left) shunt because the blood in the pulmonary circulation (from right ventricle to left ventricle) cannot take part in gas exchange and it remains deoxygenated. This type of hypoxemia typically has a near-normal $PaCO_2$ because of rapid CO_2 clearance during invasive mechanical ventilation. Absolute shunting leads to refractory hypoxemia because deoxygenated blood in the pulmonary artery cannot receive sufficient oxygen from the poorly ventilated alveoli. ARDS is a condition causing refractory hypoxemia, and this condition does not readily respond to a moderate to high concentration of oxygen.

A combination of oxygen therapy and PEEP are often used to correct refractory hypoxemia. PEEP increases the functional residual capacity (FRC) and residual volume (RV). Since normal gas exchange occurs at the FRC level, PEEP improves ventilation by overcoming the shunt-producing conditions (e.g., atelectasis, pulmonary edema) that reduce FRC. Another advantage of PEEP is its ability to reverse absolute shunt and refractory hypoxemia when applied with a lung recruitment maneuver.

PEEP is an airway pressure modality during invasive mechanical ventilation. For patients with adequate and sustainable spontaneous breathing efforts (as documented by serial $PaCO_2$), CPAP may be used. It should be emphasized that CPAP, as a stand-alone mode, may increase the work of breathing. It should not be used if the patient has inadequate respiratory reserve as documented by low maximal inspiratory pressure or increasing $PaCO_2$. For patients with ARDS, the ARDSNet recommends the *initial* ventilation settings and FIO_2/PEEP combinations for reaching an oxygenation target of ≥88% oxygen saturation (**Table 8-2**).

TABLE 8-2
ARDSNet Initial Settings for ARDS

Parameter	Recommended Initial Setting or Target
Mode of ventilation	Volume controlled ventilation Assist/control mode
Frequency	12–14/min Titrate to patient's baseline pH or $PaCO_2$ Reduce frequency with signs of air trapping
Tidal volume	6–8 mL/kg
Plateau pressure	<30 cm H_2O (use VT as low as 4 mL/kg PBW to reach target)
SaO_2 or SpO_2	88–95%
FIO_2 and PEEP	Use following combination to keep SaO_2 ≥88%:

FIO_2	0.3	0.4	0.5	0.6	0.7	0.8	0.9	1.0
PEEP	5	5–8	8–10	10	10–14	14	16–18	20–24

ARDS, acute respiratory distress syndrome; ARDSNet, Acute Respiratory Distress Syndrome Network; PBW, predicted body weight; PEEP, positive end-expiratory pressure; VT, tidal volume.

Perfusion

Hypoxemia due to lack of pulmonary perfusion is another important clinical condition during mechanical ventilation. Lack of pulmonary perfusion leads to high $\dot{V}/\dot{Q}$ mismatch (i.e., ventilation in excess of perfusion). This condition is also called dead space ventilation or wasted ventilation. Decrease in pulmonary perfusion may be caused by conditions such as bradycardia, tachycardia (low ventricular refill time and volume), hypovolemia, congestive heart failure, pulmonary hypertension, congenital heart defects, and medications that reduce heart rate or pulmonary perfusion. These perfusion related conditions should be investigated when a properly ventilated patient develops sudden or persistent hypoxemia.

Arterial Oxygen Content

For patients with appropriate mechanical ventilation and sufficient pulmonary perfusion, hypoxemia may develop when the oxygen-carrying capacity of the blood is diminished. This can occur in anemia or presence of dysfunctional hemoglobin.

As shown in the following equation, arterial oxygen content (CaO_2) is determined by the hemoglobin, oxygen saturation, and arterial PO_2. In a patient with 15 gm% of hemoglobin and normal O_2 saturation and PaO_2, about 98% of oxygen is carried by the functional hemoglobin in blood. Insufficient amount of blood (e.g., hypovolemia) and hemoglobin (e.g., anemia), or presence of dysfunctional hemoglobin (e.g., carbon monoxide poisoning, sickle cell disease, methemoglobinemia), can lead to a significant reduction in CaO_2. A low CaO_2 cannot sustain the patient's oxygenation needs, especially in critical illnesses where the oxygen demand is greatly increased.

$$CaO_2 = (Hb \times 1.34 \times O_2\ Sat) + (PaO_2 \times 0.003)$$

Ventilator Alarms and Events

Ventilator alarms provide safety for critically ill patients who are often unable to speak or communicate effectively. These audible or visual alarms are triggered when the ventilator/patient condition exceeds the preset alarm limits. This alert system prompts the clinicians to attend to the patient without delay. In critical events, such as power failure, the alarms cannot be paused or turned off until the cause of the alert has been rectified. In noncritical events, such as high-pressure limit alarm triggered by coughing, it can auto-reset once the coughing has stopped. These noncritical alarms may also be paused briefly to allow a short procedure (e.g., endotracheal suctioning).

Ventilator alarms have different classifications. The European Committee for Standardization established the priority systems (high priority, medium priority, and low priority) to alert clinicians with patient safety concerns. The American Association for Respiratory Care published a consensus statement recommending three levels of alerts (Level 1: immediately life threatening, Level 2: potentially life threatening, Level 3: nonventilator events not likely to be life threatening). In addition to these ventilator alarms, external alerts are also available to monitor the patient's changing physiologic status (SpO_2, heart rate, etc.). These external alarms provide an added level of safety for conditions that may not be detected by ventilator alarms (e.g., severe internal bleed leading to increased heart rate and arterial desaturation). It is important to note that persistent or continuous alarms must be investigated, and the conditions causing these alarms must be rectified promptly. The alarm limits must not be adjusted to accommodate (silence) these persistent alarms without valid justifications. This unjust action can cause grave harm to the patient. **Table 8-3** provides the suggested initial ventilator alarm settings. A discussion on each alarm setting follows.

High-Pressure Alarm

High-pressure alarm is triggered when the peak inspiratory pressure exceeds the preset high-pressure limit. The most common causes are conditions leading to airflow obstructions or decrease in compliance. Examples of airflow obstruction include mucus plugs, bronchospasm, ET tube obstruction due to secretions, kinking or biting, and water condensation in the ventilator circuit. Examples of decreased compliance include tension pneumothorax (sudden change) and atelectasis (gradual change). This high-pressure alarm usually coincides with simultaneous triggering of the low volume alarm because the inspiratory flow (inspiratory volume) is stopped immediately when the high-pressure limit is breached. The high-pressure alarm limit may be set at 10 cm H_2O above the current peak inspiratory pressure.

TABLE 8-3
Initial Ventilator Alarm Settings

Alarm	Initial Setting
High-pressure	10 cm H_2O *above* peak inspiratory pressure
Low-pressure	10 cm H_2O *below* peak inspiratory pressure
Low tidal volume/ minute volume	25% *below* current tidal volume or minute ventilation
High-frequency	10–20% *above* current total frequency
Low-frequency/ apnea	2–6/min *below* current total frequency
High PEEP	2 cm H_2O *above* current PEEP
Low PEEP	2 cm H_2O *below* current PEEP

PEEP, positive end-expiratory pressure.

The high-pressure alarm limit must never be raised to "silence" the alarm without a valid reason. For example, a newly developed tension pneumothorax will trigger the high-pressure alarm immediately. Cardiovascular collapse can occur if the high-pressure alarm limit is repeatedly raised to "silence" the alarm without a thorough investigation of the underlying reason for alarm trigger.

Low-Pressure and Low-Volume Alarms

The most common triggers for low-pressure and low-volume alarms are circuit disconnection and air leaks in the ventilator/patient system (e.g., cuff leak, chest tube leak). Low-pressure alarm limit may be set at 10 cm H_2O below the current peak inspiratory pressure. Low tidal volume and minute ventilation alarm limits may be set at 25% below the current values. If these alarms do not auto-reset, the clinician must assess the patient and ventilator to determine and rectify the cause of alarm. Sometimes the alarm limits are breached as a result of changing patient condition. For example, the low-pressure alarm during volume-controlled ventilation may be triggered when the patient's compliance has improved significantly. Likewise, during pressure-controlled ventilation, the low-volume alarm may be triggered when the patient's compliance has decreased significantly.

High-Frequency Alarm

Rapid shallow breathing is a clinical sign of respiratory distress as it increases dead space ventilation, metabolism, and CO_2 production. High-frequency alarm is triggered when the total frequency (mandatory and spontaneous) exceeds the preset high-frequency limit. Common causes of this alarm include hypoxia, inappropriate ventilator setting, and patient experiencing pain and anxiety. The high-frequency alarm may be set at 10% to 20% above the current total frequency. The high-frequency alarm limit should be lowered accordingly during the weaning process.

Low-Frequency/Apnea Alarms

Low-frequency and apnea alarms are triggered when the total frequency falls below the preset frequency limit. These alarms are also triggered in circuit disconnection or similar conditions. The low-frequency limit should be adjusted accordingly when the patient's spontaneous frequency is increased (e.g., awakening from anesthesia, hypoxia, anxiety) or decreased (e.g., sleeping, under sedation, during weaning). The initial low-frequency/apnea alarm should be set at 2 to 6 breaths/min below the current total frequency if the alarm is used to monitor patient's spontaneous breathing effort. For patients with a high spontaneous breathing frequency, the high value from the range should be used.

High/Low PEEP Alarms

Many critically ill patients receive mechanical ventilation with PEEP for treatment of refractory hypoxemia. High PEEP alarm is used to alert presence of auto-PEEP that may occur in severe air trapping. The high PEEP alarm may be set at 2 cm H_2O above the current PEEP. Low PEEP alarm is triggered in conditions of losing airway pressure. Examples include cuff leak and circuit leak. Low PEEP alarm may also be triggered when the inspiratory flow delivered by the ventilator is insufficient to meet the patient's inspiratory demand. The patient may show signs of air hunger, chest retraction, tachypnea, and tachycardia. On the flow-time waveform, the peak inspiratory flow may drop slightly because the positive inspiratory flow by the ventilator is partially overcome by the negative inspiratory flow by the patient. The low PEEP alarm may be set at 2 cm H_2O below the current PEEP. The low PEEP alarm can be problematic in the presence of a persistent leak.

Adjunctive Ventilator Management Strategies

When the traditional ventilator settings fail to provide adequate ventilation or oxygenate, other management strategies may be considered. The following sections provide a discussion on these adjunctive methods—prone positioning, tracheal gas insufflation, and mechanical insufflation-exsufflation.

Prone Positioning

In a supine position, the posterior lobes receive the majority of pulmonary perfusion due to gravity-dependent blood flow. **Prone positioning** (PP) provides more ventilation to the posterior lobes and better $\dot{V}/\dot{Q}$ matching. For patients with severe $\dot{V}/\dot{Q}$ mismatch, PP provides short-term improvement to ventilation, oxygenation, and hypoxemia. PP also improves $\dot{V}/\dot{Q}$ matching and gas exchange while the patient is in a prone position.

For prone patients, the rapid rise in oxygenation is not sustainable once the patient is returned to a supine position and previous mode of ventilation. For this reason, PP is primarily used to manage critically ill patients with acute hypoxia on a short-term basis. Compared to the traditional supine positioning, PP does not improve the survival rate of patients with acute respiratory failure and mild to moderate ARDS.

Indications and Contraindications

The primary indications for PP are persistent refractory hypoxemia and ARDS with a PaO_2/FIO_2 of <150 mm Hg. During mechanical ventilation, patients under consideration for PP should be receiving FIO_2 >0.6, PEEP >5 cm H_2O, and V_T near 6 mL/kg PBW.

Contraindications for PP include increased intracranial pressure, hemodynamic instability, unstable spinal cord injury, recent abdominal or thoracic surgery, flail chest, and inability to tolerate PP.

Duration and Beneficial Response to PP

If no contraindication for PP exists, a team of clinicians is assembled to prone the patient. Turning a critically ill patient from supine to prone requires a coordinated effort to avoid mishaps, such as inadvertent line disconnection. There is no recommended timing or duration for proning patients with ARDS. Duration of PP ranges from short duration (4 hours prone and 2 hours supine during the day) to long duration (20 hours of continuous prone and 4 hours of supine). According to the Proning Severe ARDS Patients (PROSEVA) study, PP was maintained for up to 28 days.

The duration of PP should be individualized based on tolerance and stability of clinical signs. If the patient tolerates the prone trial and the P/F ratio, mPaw (mean airway pressure), and oxygenation index (OI) are within normal limits, prone positioning may continue for 12 hours or longer each day. A *reduction* of OI by ≥20% from baseline indicates a beneficial response to PP.

Risk and Complications of PP

Endotracheal tube obstruction (kinking, secretions), accidental extubation, pressure sores on dependent areas, arrhythmias, hypotension, vomiting, and intravenous (IV) line disconnection are potential risks and complications of PP. To mitigate these conditions, rotating beds (e.g., RotoProne) may be used to minimize the potential harms during physical turning of the patients.

Tracheal Gas Insufflation

Tracheal gas insufflation (TGI) can be used as an adjunctive method for lung protection in ARDS since it allows use of lower tidal volume and frequency during mechanical ventilation. TGI can also reduce the respiratory work in intubated patients with neuromuscular weakness. TGI provides a continuous or phasic gas flow during mechanical ventilation. A controller is used to regulate and deliver air or oxygen (usually 5 L/min) via a small catheter into the distal end of the ET tube. The gas exits the ET tube and reaches above the carina. The TGI gas flow supplements the inspiratory flow provided by the ventilator. The combined flow (ventilator and TGI) facilitates elimination of CO_2 and lowers the work of breathing.

Continuous or Phasic Flow

The insufflation may be continuous or phasic (intermittent). In continuous flow TGI, the gas flow goes to the airway during inspiration and expiration. Since the flow is continuous, undesirable effects include drying of airway and secretions, increased tidal volume delivery, development of auto-PEEP, and increased triggering effort.

In phasic flow TGI, the gas flow goes to the airway during the last half of a tidal expiration. This phasic timing helps to flush out the ET tube (about 4% exhaled CO_2) with fresh gas during expiration and prefills the ET tube with fresh gas (0% CO_2) for the next tidal inspiration.

Forward and Reverse Thrust Catheters

In one research study using animal models, the efficacy of CO_2 elimination by TGI was evaluated by combining TGI with HFOV. Two different TGI catheters were used. The *forward* thrust TGI catheter (**Figure 8-3A**) adds air and flushes the CO_2 in the airway. The *reverse* thrust catheter (**Figure 8-3B**) removes air from the airway and flushes the CO_2 in the ET tube.

Both TGI catheters significantly increased the P/F ratio and decreased the $Paco_2$. These data show that TGI is capable of improving oxygenation and ventilation when combined with HFOV.

The *forward* thrust catheter increased the carinal pressure by 30%, whereas the reverse thrust catheter decreased the carinal pressure by 44%. Since the carinal pressure reflects closely to the airway pressure, TGI is capable of altering the distal airway pressure. A lower distal airway pressure (reverse thrust catheter) may lead to atelectasis, whereas a higher distal airway pressure (forward thrust catheter) may create an auto-PEEP effect.

Potential Uses of TGI

The potential applications of TGI include reduction of dead space, reduction of CO_2 rebreathing, and decrease of airway pressure and tidal volume requirements. The $Paco_2$ may be reduced with no change in minute ventilation (tidal volume and frequency). With a lower tidal volume requirement, TGI has reduced secondary lung injury and chronic lung disease in newborns. It has also reduced the work of breathing during weaning from mechanical ventilation. Although this technique is not popular due to lack of research and development, it has the potential to be a useful adjunct in mechanical ventilation.

Mechanical Insufflation-Exsufflation

Mechanical insufflation-exsufflation (MI-E) is a noninvasive mechanical ventilation technique that uses adjustable positive and negative pressures during a respiratory cycle. During spontaneous inspiration, the positive pressure provides an assisted deep breath. During spontaneous expiration, the negative pressure generates a high velocity (300 to 600 L/min) expiratory gas flow, mimicking a cough maneuver.

Indications

Indications for MI-E include lung hyperinflation and secretion clearance for patients with weak respiratory muscles or coughs (e.g., spinal cord injury, spinal muscular atrophy, motor neuron disease, Duchenne and other muscular dystrophies).

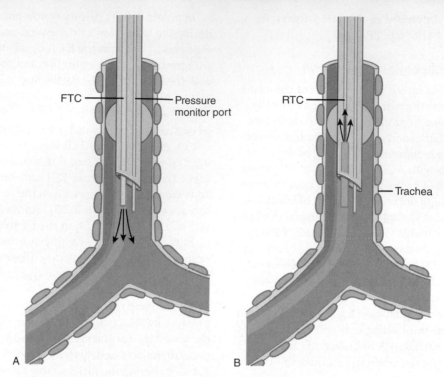

FIGURE 8-3 (**A**) A *forward* thrust tracheal gas insufflation catheter. (**B**) A *reverse* thrust tracheal gas insufflation catheter. FTC, forward thrust catheter; RTC, reverse thrust catheter.

Procedure

MI-E is administered via a large-bore aerosol tubing and a mask. For patients with an artificial airway, MI-E can be delivered via the endotracheal or tracheostomy tube with the cuff fully inflated. The recommended treatment pressures for MI-E are +40 cm H_2O for inspiration and −40 cm H_2O for expiration. The minimal pressures of +30 and −30 cm H_2O may be used as the starting point and they may be adjusted according to patient tolerance and therapeutic goals. Some cough assist MI-E devices can provide oscillation to further facilitate an effective cough.

Each MI-E treatment session lasts about 5 minutes. The patient should be allowed to rest for a brief period after each coughing episode. Patient tolerance and vital signs are evaluated accordingly for treatment continuance. The effectiveness of MI-E may be documented by presence of productive coughs and improvement of breath sounds from clearance of retained secretions.

Acute Respiratory Distress Syndrome

The key pulmonary features of **acute respiratory distress syndrome** (ARDS) include severe reduction in lung compliance and bilateral infiltrates. These conditions result in increased work of breathing, ventilatory failure, and refractory hypoxemia. The heterogeneous nature of lung impairment in ARDS makes positive pressure ventilation difficult. In areas of collapsed alveoli (low compliance), a higher driving pressure is needed to provide adequate alveoli opening and ventilation. This repetitive opening and closing of these atelectatic alveoli may lead to a condition called atelectrauma. At the same time, an increased driving pressure may lead to overdistention of alveoli with normal or high compliance. This condition is called volutrauma. Finding an ideal driving pressure for patients with ARDS is difficult because of the variability of lung compliance and opening pressure requirement. The ARDSNet study recommends keeping the plateau pressure ≤30 cm H_2O under volume-controlled ventilation. Even at this recommended plateau pressure, overdistention can still occur. The plateau pressure should be kept as low as possible while keeping the compliance or oxygenation indices at a safe level.

Adjustment of Ventilator Settings for ARDS

When a patient presents the signs of ARDS (P/F ≤300 mm Hg, bilateral infiltrates consistent with pulmonary edema, no clinical evidence of left atrial hypertension), the adjustment of ventilator settings should focus on providing lung protection and oxygenation. **Table 8-4** summarizes the adjustment of ventilator settings for patients with ARDS.

Potential for Lung Recruitment

The potential for successful recruitment of collapsed alveoli is greater in patients with a lower P/F (Pao_2/Fio_2) ratio, lower compliance, and a higher V_D/V_T (dead space to tidal volume) ratio. A low P/F ratio is defined as <150 mm Hg at a PEEP of 5 cm H_2O. A lower compliance is identified by an improvement of measured compliance when the PEEP is titrated from 5 to 15 cm H_2O. A higher V_D/V_T ratio correlates with a lower $Paco_2$ because ventilation exceeds perfusion in dead space ventilation. A high $\dot{V}/\dot{Q}$ enhances elimination of CO_2 and produces a lower $Paco_2$. In ARDS, not all lung units respond similarly to recruitment maneuver. At 5 cm H_2O of PEEP, severe ARDS (P/F ≤100 mm Hg) has the greatest lung recruitability while mild ARDS (P/F >200 mm Hg) has the lowest recruitability. The P/F ratio in the Berlin definition assessed at 5 cm H_2O PEEP may be used to evaluate and identify patients for lung recruitment.

Patients with a low potential for alveolar recruitment (mild ARDS), a lower PEEP should be set to provide lung protection. For patients with a high potential for recruitment (moderate to severe ARDS), a higher PEEP setting should be used as it stabilizes alveoli and offers better alveolar homogeneity in the lungs.

Methods for Lung Recruitment

Lung recruitment is defined as a systemic technique using sustained increase in airway pressure (i.e., CPAP,

---

TABLE 8-4
Adjustment of Ventilator Settings for ARDS

Setting	Note
Ventilator mode	Volume controlled or pressure controlled
Tidal volume	Adjust volume or pressure to reach initial V_T 8 mL/kg PBW PBW for male = 50 + 2.3 [height in inches − 60] PBW for female = 45.5 + 2.3 [height in inches − 60]
Tidal volume reduction	Lower V_T to 6 mL/kg PBW Reduce V_T by 1 mL/kg at intervals ≤2 hours until V_T = 6 mL/kg PBW
Frequency	Keep frequency ≤35/min Set initial frequency to reach baseline minute ventilation before low tidal volume strategy
pH	Keep pH 7.30–7.45 If pH 7.15–7.30, increase frequency until pH >7.30 or $Paco_2$ <25 (maximum set frequency 35/min) If pH <7.15, increase frequency to 35/min (may increase V_T in 1-mL/kg steps) until pH >7.15 (plateau pressure target of 30 cm H_2O may be exceeded) If pH >7.45, frequency may be reduced
Plateau pressure	Keep Pplat ≤30 cm H_2O If Pplat >30 cm H_2O, decrease V_T by 1-mL/kg steps If Pplat <25 cm H_2O and V_T <6 mL/kg, increase V_T by 1-mL/kg steps until Pplat >25 cm H_2O or V_T = 6 mL/kg If Pplat <30 cm H_2O and breath stacking or dyssynchrony occurs, correct cause of dyssynchrony or increase V_T in 1-mL/kg steps to 7–8 mL/kg if Pplat remains ≤30 cm H_2O
Fio_2	Keep Pao_2 55–80 mm Hg or Spo_2 88–95% Use a minimum PEEP of 5 cm H_2O *If necessary, use the following PEEP/Fio_2 combination to reach Pao_2/Spo_2 target

Lower PEEP (*lower* potential for recruitment)

*For mild ARDS (P/F 200–300 mm Hg)

Fio_2	0.3	0.4	0.4	0.5	0.5	0.6	0.7	0.7	0.7	0.8	0.9	0.9	0.9	1.0
PEEP	5	5	8	8	10	10	10	12	14	14	14	16	18	18–24

Higher PEEP (*higher* potential for recruitment)

*For moderate and severe ARDS (P/F < 200 mm Hg)

Fio_2	0.3	0.3	0.3	0.3	0.3	0.4	0.4	0.5	0.5	0.5–0.8	0.8	0.9	1.0	1.0
PEEP	5	8	10	12	14	14	16	16	18	20	22	22	22	24

ARDS, acute respiratory distress syndrome; PBW, predicted body weight; PEEP, positive end-expiratory pressure; Pplat, plateau pressure; V_T, tidal volume.
Table data from National Institutes of Health, National Heart, Lung, and Blood Institute. ARDS Clinical Network mechanical ventilation protocol summary. March 6, 2019. Available at http://www.ardsnet.org/files/ventilator_protocol_2008-07.pdf

plateau pressure) to open collapsed alveoli and applying sufficient PEEP to keep the lungs open. An ideal recruitment maneuver protects the lungs and improves oxygenation. Many methods have been described and used for lung recruitment. They include sustained alveoli inflation followed by decremental PEEP titration, stepwise recruitment by using incremental PEEP titration, APRV, HFOV, periodic sigh breaths during mechanical ventilation, and prone positioning. These methods all have their own merits and limitations. The following sections describe a recruitment maneuver followed by a decremental PEEP titration (open lung approach).

Decremental Recruitment Maneuver

In this example of **decremental recruitment maneuver,** there are four key elements: sedation, initial recruitment, determination of optimal PEEP, and final recruitment. The steps for decremental recruitment maneuver using oxygenation as an indicator are summarized in **Table 8-5**.

Decompensated Heart Failure

Mechanical ventilation offers many benefits to patients with **decompensated heart failure.** When patients are in respiratory distress due to acute or progressing hypoxia, the work of breathing often consumes as much as 16% of the cardiac output. Utilization of available cardiac output is greatly increased in heart failure. This is because patients with heart failure often have less than 50% of the maximal cardiac output normally achieved by healthy individuals. Mechanical ventilation can shift the work of breathing from patient to ventilator, allowing the limited cardiac output to meet the metabolic needs of other major organs. Study has shown that pressure support as low as 5 cm H_2O results in a decrease of 46% to 60% in the work of breathing. This means a sizable reduction in the utilization of cardiac output to support work of breathing.

Initial Ventilator Settings for Heart Failure

The recommended initial ventilator settings in **Table 8-6** are intended for patients with heart failure and reduced

---

TABLE 8-5
Decremental Recruitment Maneuver Using Oxygenation as an Indicator

Step	Note
1. Sedation	Patient is mechanically ventilated Patient is sedated until no spontaneous breathing effort Vital signs are monitored and supported accordingly
2. Continue sedation	Apply FIO_2 of 1.0 for 20 min Use closed suction system for removal of secretions
3. *Initial* RM	Apply FIO_2 of 1.0 and CPAP of 40 cm H_2O for up to 40 sec Discontinue RM if one of the following conditions occurs: SpO_2 <88% HR >140/min or <60/min MAP <60 mm Hg or >20 mm Hg from baseline Cardiac arrhythmia
4. After *initial* RM	Resume mechanical ventilation with PCV A/C mode, FIO_2 1.0, PIP 15 cm H_2O, and PEEP 20 cm H_2O (total 35 cm H_2O) After 5 min, hemodynamic and gas exchange data are evaluated If P/F has <20% increase from baseline, repeat RM (up to three times)
5. Following *initial* RM	If P/F has >20% increase, FIO_2 is reduced in 5–20% increments until SpO_2 stabilizes between 90% and 94%
6. Following SpO_2 stabilization	PEEP is reduced by 2 cm H_2O every 15–20 min until SpO_2 drops below 90%
7. Optimal PEEP	PEEP immediately before SpO_2 drops below 90%
8. *Final* RM	Apply FIO_2 of 100% and CPAP 40 cm H_2O for 40 sec
9. After *final* RM	Initiate mechanical ventilation with settings from step 4 Use FIO_2 from step 5 Use PEEP from step 7* *If compliance is used as an indicator (lower inflection point of pressure-volume waveform), add 2 cm H_2O to PEEP from step 7.

A/C, assist/control; CPAP, continuous positive airway pressure; HR, heart rate; MAP, mean arterial pressure; PCV, pressure-controlled ventilation; PEEP, positive end-expiratory pressure; PIP, peak inspiratory pressure; RM, recruitment maneuver.
Table data from Borges JB, Okamoto VN, Matos GF, et al. Reversibility of lung collapse and hypoxemia in early acute respiratory distress syndrome. *Am J Respir Crit Care Med.* 2006;174:268–278; Girgis K, Hamed H, Khater Y, et al. A decremental PEEP trial identifies the PEEP level that maintains oxygenation after lung recruitment. *Respir Care.* 2006;51:1132–1139; Toth I, Leiner T, Mikor A, et al. Hemodynamic and respiratory changes during lung recruitment and descending optimal positive end-expiratory pressure titration in patients with acute respiratory distress syndrome. *Crit Care Med.* 2007;35:787–793.

ejection fraction. These recommendations are based on achievement of outcomes that yield the most benefits and least adverse effects.

Mode

Cardiogenic pulmonary edema can occur when the hydrostatic pressure gradient increases between the pulmonary capillaries and surrounding interstitial space. In the early phase, fluid accumulates in the extravascular space (interstitial edema). If uncorrected, the elevated interstitial hydrostatic pressure causes movement of fluid into the alveoli (pulmonary edema). The resulting pulmonary edema leads to decrease in lung compliance, refractory hypoxemia, and increase in work of breathing. Kuhn et al. (2016) recommend an assist/control mode (vs. SIMV) in the early phase of mechanical ventilation to guarantee maximal respiratory support and reduce the work of breathing. This mode and early intervention also help to preserve the pulmonary mechanics and minimize the strain imposed on the heart.

TABLE 8-6
Initial Ventilator Settings for Patients with Heart Failure and Reduced Ejection Fraction

Parameter	Recommended Setting
Mode	Assist/control mode initially to guarantee adequate respiratory support
Frequency	Titrate to normal pH (7.35–7.45) or $PaCO_2$ (35–45 mm Hg)
Tidal volume	6–8 mL/kg PBW* PBW for male = 50 + 2.3 [height in inches – 60] PBW for female = 45.5 + 2.3 [height in inches – 60] *Evaluate patient for lung protection when Pplat is >30 cm H_2O.
FIO_2	Titrate to SpO_2 92–96%. Rapid reduction of FIO_2 following initiation of mechanical ventilation
Pressure support	(Spontaneously breathing only) 5 cm H_2O of PS to overcome airflow resistance Titrate PS for an appropriate spontaneous V_T based on the patient's PBW
PEEP	(For patients with decompensated HF) 5 cm H_2O and titrate upward in 2–3 cm H_2O steps every 15–30 min to reach SpO_2 ≥92%, guided by hemodynamic changes and indices of end-organ perfusion (e.g., ICP)
Plateau pressure	Keep <30 cm H_2O Consider alternative diagnosis (e.g., pulmonary) if PPplat >30 cm H_2O

HF, heart failure; ICP, intracranial pressure; PBW, predicted body weight; Pplat, plateau pressure; PS, pressure support; V_T, tidal volume.
Data from Kuhn BT, Bradley LA, Dempsey TM, Puro AC, Adams JY. Management of mechanical ventilation in decompensated heart failure. *J Cardiovasc Dev Dis.* 2016;3(4):33.

Frequency

The frequency should be set and adjusted in tandem with the tidal volume setting. The initial tidal volume (6 to 8 mL/kg PBW) and subsequent adjustments are mainly for alveolar ventilation and lung protection. The frequency, in conjunction with tidal volume and flow rate, plays a major role in the determination of minute ventilation, inspiratory time, I:E ratio, air trapping, and auto-PEEP. Frequency is also the main parameter used in the weaning process. The initial frequency should be set and titrated to a pH of 7.35 to 7.45 or a $PaCO_2$ of 35 to 45 mm Hg.

Tidal Volume

During spontaneous breathing, respiratory muscles can utilize as much as 16% of the cardiac output. The cardiac output of patients with decompensating heart failure may be as low as 50% of the maximal cardiac output for healthy individuals. Respiratory support for patients with heart failure becomes a necessity for two reasons. It helps to reduce both the work of breathing and myocardial work. By providing respiratory support with mechanical ventilation, the conserved cardiac output would become available for perfusion to other vital organs.

The recommended ventilator tidal volume is 6 to 8 mL/kg PBW unless contraindicated for conditions that require a higher tidal volume setting (e.g., severe respiratory acidosis, increased intracranial pressure).

FIO_2

Localized deficiency of oxygen in the lung parenchyma often leads to hypoxic vasoconstriction in the pulmonary circulation. Constriction of these pulmonary vessels in areas of poor ventilation (and oxygenation) helps to shunt the blood to areas with adequate ventilation. The consequences of prolonged hypoxic vasoconstriction include increased pulmonary vascular resistance, increased right ventricular afterload, and increased work of right ventricle. If uncorrected and over time, right-sided heart failure (cor pulmonale) may develop.

Excessive oxygen can also be detrimental to the patient. FIO_2 greater than 0.5 can lead to oxidative stress and formation of harmful oxygen free radicals. Free radicals of oxygen occur when an oxygen molecule is split into two single atoms with unpaired electrons. These single oxygen atoms (free radicals) scavenge the body to seek out other electrons so they can become a pair. This process can damage the cells, proteins, and DNA.

Oxygen toxicity can also occur when the patient is exposed to an FIO_2 >0.5. The severity of toxicity is also a function of the duration of exposure. In oxygen toxicity, the free radicals form superoxide anion $[O_2^-]$, hydroxyl radical (•OH), and hydrogen peroxide (H_2O_2). The hydroxyl radicals are the neutral form of hydroxide ion (OH^-), and they are highly reactive and can easily form other hydroxyl groups. Some hydroxyl radicals can cause damage to macromolecules such as proteins, lipids, and DNA.

Clinically, oxygen toxicity can cause complications such as tracheobronchitis, absorptive atelectasis (due to washout of inert nitrogen gas), hypoxemia, and diffuse alveolar damage, which has a radiographic image similar to that for ARDS.

No consensus has been established for the level of F_{IO_2} or the length of exposure required to cause oxygen toxicity. The general guideline is to keep the F_{IO_2} ≤0.5. If the F_{IO_2} is >0.5, CPAP or PEEP should be used to lower the F_{IO_2} requirement. The critical care clinician should use the lowest F_{IO_2} for a SpO_2 range of 92% to 96%. The F_{IO_2} should also be titrated down to a safe level as soon as feasible following initiation of mechanical ventilation.

Pressure Support

Pressure support (PS) augments a patient's spontaneous tidal volume. The addition of 5 cm H_2O of PS can reduce the work of spontaneous breathing by 46% to 60%. For patients with decompensating heart failure, pressure support plays a vital role in reducing the work of breathing and myocardial work. In addition to tidal volume and frequency on the ventilator, PS should be part of the overall strategy for ventilatory support. The patient must have spontaneous breathing efforts to use PS because it is only active during the inspiratory phase of spontaneous breaths. A minimum 5 cm H_2O of PS should be used to overcome the airflow resistance imposed by the ventilator circuit and artificial airway. Additional PS may be titrated for an appropriate spontaneous tidal volume based on the patient's PBW.

PEEP

Positive pressure ventilation (PPV) increases the intrathoracic pressure. This change is more profound when PEEP is added to PPV. The PEEP-mediated increase in intrathoracic pressure is passed on to the right atrium. Elevation of right atrial pressure leads to a decrease of venous return (due to a lower pressure gradient between vena cava and right atrium). A decrease of venous return results in a decrease in cardiac output. This may be beneficial to patients with congestive heart failure, but this benefit must be weighed against any potential adverse effects (e.g., inadequate preload and end-organ hypoperfusion).

In healthy individuals, the effects of therapeutic PEEP on reducing the afterload and cardiac output are minimal. For patients with left ventricular systolic dysfunction (dilated cardiomyopathy in particular), PEEP provides beneficial effects by optimizing the left heart function and related parameters (e.g., cardiac output). Study has shown PEEP increases the cardiac output in patients with elevated pulmonary artery occlusion pressure (i.e., >18 mm Hg). PEEP also improves right atrial pressure, pulmonary artery occlusion pressure, and cardiac index in mechanically ventilated post-coronary artery bypass graft patients with left ventricular dysfunction.

For mechanically ventilated patients with decompensated heart failure, Kuhn et al. (2016) recommend an initial PEEP of 5 cm H_2O with stepwise increases of 2 to 3 cm H_2O every 15 to 30 min as needed. The optimal noninjurious PEEP should be guided by the patient's hemodynamic measurements and end-organ perfusion indices (e.g., intracranial pressure). PEEP must be applied with caution, however. Excessive PEEP can negatively affect the patients with low end-diastolic volume. Potential adverse effects of PEEP for this patient population include decrease in venous return, preload, and afterload (i.e., cardiac output). Insufficient cardiac output causes hypoperfusion of major organs that rely on high perfusion (e.g., brain, kidneys).

Before weaning of patients without decompensating heart failure, the spontaneous breathing trial typically uses a combination of 5 cm H_2O of PEEP and ≤8 cm H_2O of PSV. For patients with decompensating heart failure, Kuhn et al. (2016) recommend a minimal level of PEEP (or no PEEP) for the spontaneous breathing trial. The rationale of no PEEP is its ability to reveal the degree of patient optimization of the underlying cardiac conditions.

Plateau Pressure

As described in a previous section, the recommended tidal volume should be 6 to 8 mL/kg PBW. Adjustment of tidal volume setting is partly dependent on Pplat. A lower tidal volume should be considered for conditions of low lung compliance, as indicated by an elevated alveolar distending pressure or plateau pressure >30 cm H_2O.

In most ICUs, the Pplat is used to estimate the alveolar distending pressure. This measurement is a good indicator of lung compliance when the intrapleural pressure is not available. Measuring the intrapleural pressure (or its substitute, esophageal pressure) requires the placement of an esophageal balloon—a procedure not tolerated by many patients, especially those being mechanically ventilated. A special design of some nasogastric tubes does not require a balloon, so tolerance is less of an issue.

Transpulmonary pressure = Alveolar pressure (or Pplat) − Intrapleural pressure (or esophageal pressure)

Severe Asthma

The onset of acute asthma symptoms may be grouped by slow onset and rapid onset. Type I acute asthma (slow onset) shows a gradual worsening of airflow obstruction along with a history of chronic and poorly controlled asthma. Type II acute asthma (rapid onset) typically has a presentation of sudden narrowing of the airways and other associated clinical signs and symptoms. Fulminant (sudden and severe) asthma is another term to describe type II acute asthma.

About 2% to 4% of patients admitted to hospital for acute exacerbation of asthma require mechanical ventilation. On admission, most of these patients display severe airflow obstruction, air trapping, use of accessory respiratory muscles, tachycardia, hypercapnia, and hypoxemia. Patients who have respiratory arrest, altered sensorium, and extreme physical exhaustion are intubated immediately and placed on mechanical ventilation. This section describes the initial ventilator settings and respiratory care strategies for these patients.

Initial Noninvasive Ventilation Settings for Acute Asthma

Noninvasive ventilation (NIV) has been used successfully to manage asthma in adults and children. However, in patients with acute respiratory failure due to exacerbation of asthma, NIV does not offer any benefits over traditional mechanical ventilation. To be considered for NIV, patients with acute asthma must be conscious and cooperative. They should also have stable hemodynamic status. Since the interface for NIV cannot protect the airway, patients should have an intact gag reflex and without excessive secretions.

The basic initial settings for NIV are similar to that used for mechanical ventilation with a frequency from 10/min to 14/min. The tidal volume is determined by the ΔP—the pressure gradient between inspiratory positive airway pressure (IPAP) and expiratory positive airway pressure (EPAP). The IPAP is used to change the tidal volume. A higher IPAP provides a larger tidal volume, and vice versa. To reach a target tidal volume, the EPAP is set at ≤5 cm and then the IPAP is adjusted to reach a tidal volume from 7 to 9 mL/kg.

The frequency and tidal volume may be adjusted lower if there are signs of air trapping. Air trapping or auto-PEEP may be assessed by evaluating the irregular exhaled tidal volumes (volume-time waveform). The exhaled tidal volume may be less than the set tidal volume for two to three cycles followed by a much larger exhaled tidal volume on the next cycle. Presence of air trapping is also evident when the expiratory flow fails to return to baseline (flow-time waveform). Presence of auto-PEEP can be documented by the excessive PEEP at end-exhalation (pressure-time waveform).

It should be noted here that air trapping responds more favorably by decreasing the frequency or tidal volume than increasing the inspiratory flow. In one study using constant V_T 600 mL and f 14/min (respiratory time cycle = 4.3 seconds), changing the flow rate and flow pattern from 60 L/min (decelerating) to 120 L/min (constant) yielded a *significant* increase in I:E ratio (from 1:3 to 1:13) but only a *slight* increase in expiratory time (from 3.2 seconds to 4.0 seconds). The 0.8 second gain in expiratory time does not greatly increase the exhaled volume (or

TABLE 8-7
Initial Noninvasive Ventilation Settings for Acute Asthma

Parameter	Recommended Setting
Mode	NIV
Frequency	10–14/min (↓ with signs of air trapping)
EPAP	≤5 cm H_2O
IPAP	Adjust IPAP for a target tidal volume
Tidal volume	7–9 mL/kg (↓ with signs of air trapping but may ↑ anatomic dead space)
Minute ventilation	Keep <10 L/min
Fio_2	Titrate to Spo_2 ≥90%

EPAP, expiratory positive airway pressure; IPAP, inspiratory positive airway pressure; NIV, noninvasive ventilation.
Table data from Brenner B, Corbridge T, Kazzi A. Intubation and mechanical ventilation of the asthmatic patient in respiratory failure. *Proc Am Thorac Soc.* 2009;6:371–379. doi:10.1513/pats.P09ST4; Leatherman J. Mechanical ventilation for severe asthma. *Chest.* 2015;147:1671–1680. doi:10.1378/chest.14-1733.

reduce air trapping). This is because the 0.8 second gain occurs at the end of the expiratory cycle when the flow (volume/time) is slowest due to expiratory flow decay.

In summary, air trapping should initially be managed by decreasing the frequency or tidal volume. While increasing the inspiratory flow significantly changes the I:E ratio, this change has a minimal effect on increasing the expiratory time or exhaled volume. **Table 8-7** provides the initial NIV settings for acute asthma.

Initial Ventilator Settings for Acute Asthma

Airflow obstruction, hyperinflation, air trapping, and auto-PEEP are the key features of severe asthma. Mechanical ventilation may be necessary if NIV and interventions by medications do not promptly reverse the deteriorating clinical conditions.

Minute ventilation (tidal volume × frequency) is the primary determinant of air trapping and lung hyperinflation. Reducing the frequency has a modest impact on the Pplat and auto-PEEP. As previously described, prolongation of expiratory time contributes little to the exhaled volume (i.e., trapped gas) due to flow decay toward the end of exhalation. In addition, air trapped behind occluded airways in asthma does not respond well to decreasing the frequency or tidal volume.

The recommended frequency and tidal volume for asthma are 10 to 14/min and 7 to 9 mL/kg, respectively. A minute ventilation of <10 L/min offers the most beneficial effect because a high minute ventilation worsens air trapping in patients with severe asthma. An auto-PEEP of up to 15 cm H_2O should be tolerated, and applied PEEP is not recommended for auto-PEEP in

TABLE 8-8
Initial Ventilator Settings for Severe Asthma

Parameter	Recommended Setting
Mode	SIMV
Frequency	10–14/min ($\downarrow$ with signs of air trapping or Pplat >30 cm H_2O)
Tidal volume	7–9 mL/kg ($\downarrow$ with signs of air trapping or Pplat >30 cm H_2O but may $\uparrow$ anatomic dead space)
Minute ventilation	Keep <10 L/min
F_{IO_2}	Titrate to SpO_2 ≥90%
PEEP	≤5 cm H_2O
Auto-PEEP	Keep <15 cm H_2O (applied PEEP is not recommended for auto-PEEP)
Plateau pressure	Keep <30 cm H_2O

PEEP, positive end-expiratory pressure; Pplat, plateau pressure; SIMV, synchronized intermittent mandatory ventilation.
Table data from Brenner B, Corbridge T, Kazzi A. Intubation and mechanical ventilation of the asthmatic patient in respiratory failure. *Proc Am Thorac Soc.* 2009;6:371–379. doi:10.1513/pats.P09ST4; Leatherman J. Mechanical ventilation for severe asthma. *Chest.* 2015;147:1671–1680. doi:10.1378/chest.14-1733.

TABLE 8-9
Medications for Mechanically Ventilated Patients with Severe Asthma

Medication	Recommendation
Short-acting beta agonist (albuterol)	4 to 6 puffs of MDI or 2.5 mg by intermittent nebulizer or equal dose via MDI Combination therapy with ipratropium should be considered
Methylprednisolone	2 mg/kg/day
Combination of fentanyl (Duragesic) *and* propofol (Diprivan) or benzodiazepine	Deep sedation may be required to prevent patient-ventilator dyssynchrony Select drug combination and titrate dosage for desired level of sedation
Neuromuscular blocking agent	May be needed to augment sedation Intermittent bolus doses are preferred over continuous infusion

MDI, metered dose inhaler.

patients with severe asthma and ongoing air trapping. **Table 8-8** provides the initial ventilator settings for severe asthma.

Hypercapnia

In acute asthma, hypercapnia is common during mechanical ventilation. Airflow obstruction, air trapping, and increase in physiologic dead space are factors that contribute to the retention of $PaCO_2$. Hypercapnia causes dilation of cerebral vessels, increase of intracranial pressure, constriction of pulmonary vessels, and decrease of myocardial contractility. Even with these adverse effects, hypercapnia should not be fully corrected by increasing the minute ventilation ($\uparrow$ frequency or $\uparrow$ tidal volume). The reason is that a higher minute ventilation may further increase the physiologic dead space and air trapping.

The most serious consequences of severe hypercapnia are increased cerebral perfusion and increased intracranial pressure. These changes in the brain can lead to cerebral anoxia. Development of cerebral anoxia in patients with severe asthma is most likely when cardiorespiratory arrest occurs at home or in a vehicle en route to the hospital. Once in the hospital, prompt intubation and mechanical ventilation greatly reduce the incidence of cerebral anoxia due to severe hypercapnia.

Other rare consequences of severe hypercapnia are those that affect the brain (cerebral edema and subarachnoid hemorrhage), the lungs (constriction of pulmonary vessels), and the heart (decrease in contractility and arrhythmias). Sodium bicarbonate is not recommended as an alkalinizing agent for persistent acidosis (pH 7.15 to 7.20). If an alkalinizing agent is necessary for persistent acidosis, tromethamine should be considered. Since many patients with severe hypercapnia show improvement within 12 hours of intubation and mechanical ventilation, alkalinizing agents, such as tromethamine (not available in U.S.), should be withheld unless there is an urgent need to correct acidosis-induced myocardial depression (e.g., arrhythmia, hemodynamic instability).

Other Management Techniques for Severe Asthma

In addition to intubation and mechanical ventilation, patients with severe asthma should receive one or more of the following medications: bronchodilators, corticosteroids, sedatives, and neuromuscular blocking agents. Bronchodilators are used to reverse airflow obstruction. Corticosteroids are used to reduce or suppress inflammation and mucus production. Sedatives and neuromuscular blocking agents are used to prevent patient–ventilator dyssynchrony in patients with severe asthma, air trapping, and auto-PEEP. Their uses are summarized in **Table 8-9**.

Heliox, inhalational anesthetics (e.g., isoflurane), ketamine (an IV anesthetic with bronchodilator property), bronchoscopy, and extracorporeal life support are some nontraditional tools for the management of severe asthma. They may have some benefits to the overall patient care plan. If the patient is not responding to the traditional management strategies, these methods may be tried on a short-term basis.

Acute Exacerbation of COPD

COPD accounts for over 100,000 deaths and 500,000 hospitalizations in the United States annually. Most of these patients with stable COPD have compensated respiratory acidosis and receive their medical care at home or in an outpatient setting. Exacerbation of COPD may occur under unfavorable conditions (e.g., tracheobronchial infection, environmental exposures, heart failure) leading to acute-on-chronic hypercapnic respiratory failure. **Acute exacerbation of COPD** is characterized by chronic airflow obstruction, dyspnea, coughs, and sputum production. Arterial blood gases will show worsening $Paco_2$, decompensating pH, and severe hypoxemia. Using clinical presentations as a guide, a range of COPD severity (severe, moderate, mild) may be observed in these patients (**Table 8-10**).

This condition is generally managed by inhaled long-acting anticholinergic (or β-agonist bronchodilator) plus a short-acting β-agonist. Systemic corticosteroids are preferred over inhaled steroids. Antibiotics and oxygen therapy are used as indicated for this patient population. In cases of acute exacerbation with hypercapnic or oxygenation failure, these patients with COPD typically require noninvasive or invasive ventilation. The following sections describe the recommended settings for these patients.

Initial Noninvasive Ventilation Settings for Acute Exacerbation of COPD

Noninvasive ventilation is a technique of ventilation without using an artificial airway. Instead of an ET tube or similar device, an interface is used to provide ventilation and oxygenation. The European Respiratory Society and American Thoracic Society (ERS/ATS) strongly recommend that NIV be used for hospitalized patients with acute or acute-on-chronic hypercapnic respiratory failure due to COPD exacerbation. These patients benefit from NIV as it reduces the need for intubation, mortality, complications of therapy, and length of hospital and ICU stays.

The results of a Cochrane review on the use of NIV in patients with COPD report similar benefits of NIV (Osadnik et al., 2017). They include reduction of mortality risk, need for endotracheal intubation, length of hospital stay, and incidence of complications not related to NIV.

During NIV, the tidal volume is determined by the ΔP—the pressure gradient between IPAP and EPAP. As mentioned earlier, the IPAP is used to change the tidal volume. A higher IPAP provides a larger tidal volume, and vice versa. The EPAP functions as PEEP, and it usually remains between 4 and 7 cm H_2O. **Table 8-11** outlines the initial NIV settings for patients with exacerbation of COPD.

NIV Intolerance or Failure

Patient may show intolerance to NIV due to incorrect settings (e.g., insufficiency flow, excessive or

TABLE 8-10
Types 1, 2, and 3 of Acute Exacerbations of COPD

Clinical Finding	Type 1 (Severe)	Type 2 (Moderate)	Type 3 (Mild)
Worsening dyspnea	X		
Increase in sputum purulence	X		
Increase in sputum volume	X		
	All three	Any two	Any one above plus one of the following: Upper respiratory tract infection in past 5 days; Fever without apparent cause; Increased wheezing; Increased cough; 20% increase in respiratory rate or baseline heart rate

COPD, chronic obstructive pulmonary disease.
Table data from Snow V, Lascher S, Mottur-Pilson C. Evidence base for management of acute exacerbations of chronic obstructive pulmonary disease. *Ann Intern Med.* 2001;134(7):595–599. doi:10.7326/0003-4819-134-7-200104030-00015

TABLE 8-11
Initial *Noninvasive* Ventilation Settings for Patients with Exacerbation of COPD

Parameter	Recommended Setting
Ventilator	Ventilators designed specifically to deliver NIV should be used
Mode	Bilevel positive airway pressure (or similar) CPAP should not be used as a stand-alone mode as it does not provide ventilation
Interface for NIV	Full face mask is preferred (should have an integral exhalation port on the mask or in circuit)
Humidification	Recommended to prevent mucosal dryness or development of tenacious secretions
Frequency	Titrate to pH >7.35 or $Paco_2$ <50 mm Hg Reduce frequency to keep extrinsic PEEP <12 cm H_2O
Tidal volume	6–8 mL/kg PBW by adjusting the ΔP (IPAP − EPAP) PBW for male = 50 + 2.3 [height in inches − 60] PBW for female = 45.5 + 2.3 [height in inches − 60]
IPAP	12–15 cm H_2O
EPAP	4–7 cm H_2O
Fio_2	Keep <60% Following stabilization, titrate Fio_2 to Spo_2 of 88–92% or patient's baseline Pao_2

COPD, chronic obstructive pulmonary disease; CPAP, continuous positive airway pressure; EPAP, expiratory positive airway pressure; IPAP, inspiratory positive airway pressure; NIV, noninvasive ventilation; PBW, predicted body weight; PEEP, positive end-expiratory pressure.

inadequate IPAP). The clinician should evaluate the patient and ensure the settings are based on the patient's current condition. Clinical signs of NIV intolerance or failure include tachycardia, tachypnea, desaturation, decrease in sensorium, diaphoresis, and patient–ventilator dyssynchrony. On occasion, the patient will remove the interface due to air hunger, insufficient flow, or inappropriate settings. Recognition of these signs is important because prolonged NIV failure can lead to depletion of oxygen store and pulmonary reserve.

Discontinuance of NIV

The 2016 British Thoracic Society (BTS)/Intensive Care Society (ICS) guidelines suggest that NIV can be discontinued once the acidosis and hypercapnia have returned to baseline during sustainable spontaneous breathing. Greater than 30 minutes of unassisted breathing can be used as the threshold for sustained spontaneous breathing. The acceptable pH and $Paco_2$ for NIV discontinuance are >7.35 and <50 mm Hg, respectively.

Initial Ventilator Settings for Acute Exacerbation of COPD

NIV is the initial management of choice for patients with exacerbation of COPD. When NIV fails to maintain ventilation or oxygenation, the patient should be intubated and mechanically ventilated. **Table 8-12** outlines the initial ventilator settings for acute exacerbation of COPD.

TABLE 8-12
Initial Ventilator Settings for Acute Exacerbation of COPD

Parameter	Recommended Setting
Mode	SIMV or A/C Pressure-controlled ventilation
Flow pattern	Decelerating
Frequency	6–8/min
Tidal volume	Titrate pressure to reach 8–12 mL/kg PBW PBW for male = 50 + 2.3 [height in inches − 60] PBW for female = 45.5 + 2.3 [height in inches − 60]
Fio_2	Keep ≤0.50 Following stabilization, titrate Fio_2 to Spo_2 of 90% or patient's baseline Pao_2
Pressure support	(Spontaneously breathing only) 5 cm H_2O of PS to overcome airflow resistance Titrate PS for an appropriate spontaneous VT (SIMV)
PEEP	≤5 cm H_2O to counter auto-PEEP
Plateau pressure	Keep <30 cm H_2O

A/C, assist/control; COPD, chronic obstructive pulmonary disease; PEEP, positive end-expiratory pressure; PS, pressure support; SIMV, synchronized intermittent mandatory ventilation; VT, tidal volume.

Following a period of stabilization, the patient's nutritional status, muscle strength, and endurance should be evaluated prior to weaning attempt. For a successful weaning outcome, the $Paco_2$ and Pao_2 should be titrated and maintained at patient's normal values. $Paco_2$ and Pao_2 values near 50 mm Hg are more physiologic to patient's needs for appropriate spontaneous breathing efforts.

Mass Casualty

A **mass casualty** condition can be defined as an unexpected situation in which the large number of severely injured or deaths exceeds the capacity of acute care centers to respond in a timely manner. Mechanical ventilation is frequently required in mass casualty situations because these injuries often involve injuries to the major organs or systems.

Some injuries in mass casualty are related to natural causes. Examples include the SARS epidemic of 2002 and 2003, influenza pandemic in 1918, and disasters such as earthquakes and hurricanes. Other injuries are man-made events, including catastrophes due to terrorism, detonation of nuclear fission devices, biological agents, or toxic chemicals. For example, individuals exposed to nerve agents often require immediate mechanical ventilation. Nerve agents are acetylcholinesterase inhibitors that lead to an accumulation of large amounts of acetylcholine at the muscarinic and nicotinic receptors throughout the body. Sudden exposure to these nerve agents causes a sudden surge of acetylcholine and leads to unconsciousness, seizures, flaccid paralysis, and apnea. This action mimics the effects of depolarizing neuromuscular blocking agents.

Triage Systems for Mass Casualty Incidents

In mass casualty incidents, the injured must be assessed quickly to determine the level of care needed. **Triage** uses predetermined criteria to assign individuals from a large pool of injured for grouping and making medical care decisions. The principles of triage were used as early as during Napoleon's wars from 1799 to 1815. Unlike the current medical triage system, early military triage gave the *less* wounded a high priority to receive care so that they may return to the battlefield. In today's triage system, highest priority for medical care is given to those critically injured who are most likely to *survive*.

Prehospitalization Triage Systems

The most common prehospitalization triage system in the United States is **START** (simple triage and rapid treatment) (**Figure 8-4**). It is used by first responders on site, and the individuals are transported to acute care facilities based on the prioritized triage results. The pediatric version is JumpSTART. SALT (Sort, Assess, Lifesaving interventions, Treatment/transport) is another prehospitalization triage system that includes lifesaving interventions (LSI), including control of hemorrhage, opening of airway, chest decompression (for tension pneumothorax), and autoinjector antidotes.

Triage System for Hospitalized Patients

The Sequential Organ Failure Assessment (SOFA) score was created in a consensus meeting of the European Society of Intensive Care Medicine in 1994, and it was refined in 1996. SOFA uses six major criteria (respiration, cardiovascular, renal, coagulation, liver, and central nervous system) to evaluate and predict the outcomes of critically ill hospitalized patients. The primary use of SOFA is to determine and allocate the limited resources available in the hospital to those who are most likely to survive. For example, a high score (e.g., ≥11) suggests palliation care only as it correlates with a mortality rate of 95%. A SOFA score from 10 to 8 calls for the highest priority of care. Intermediate critical care is provided to those with a SOFA score of ≤7. **Figure 8-5** shows the SOFA scoring method.

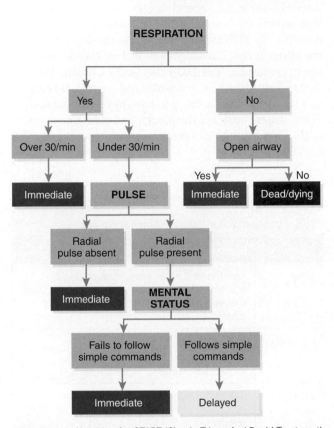

FIGURE 8-4 Algorithm for START (Simple Triage And Rapid Treatment).
Available at https://www.slideserve.com/remington/start-triage

Stockpiled Surge Mechanical Ventilators

Since mass casualty is an unexpected event, planning is frequency lacking in terms of physical space, number of clinicians trained in critical care, and types and number of critical care equipment. For physical space other than ICUs, additional space that is appropriately equipped with oxygen source may include postanesthesia units, emergency department triage areas, and hospital rooms. Medical professionals may be recruited from surrounding communities or regions. In terms of the types and number of critical care equipment, portable mechanical ventilators are probably the most difficult to stockpile. This is because portable ventilators have unique characteristics and operational requirements. Training of staff, storage, and distribution of ventilators also impose additional challenges. **Table 8-13** summarizes the unique characteristics and requirements for stockpiled surge ventilators.

Initial Ventilator Settings for Mass Casualty

The initial ventilator settings for mass casualty should follow the basic protocol for normal lungs (**Table 8-14**). During the course of mechanical ventilation, the

Organ dysfunction	0 point	1 point	2 points	3 points	4 points
Respiration P_aO_2/ FIO_2	>400 mm Hg (>53.3 kPa)	<400 mm Hg (<53.3 kPa)	<300 mm Hg (<40 kPa)	<200 mm Hg (<26.7 kPa) with respiratory support	<100 mm Hg (<13.3 kPa) with respiratory support
Cardiovascular MAP or vasoactive treatment	MAP ≥70 mm Hg	MAP <70 mm Hg	Dopamine ≤5 µg/kg/min or dobutamine any dose	Dopamine >5 µg/kg/min or norepinephrine or epinephrine ≤0.1 µg/kg/min	Dopamine 15 µg/kg/min or norepinephrine or epinephrine >0.1 µg/kg/min
Renal Creatinine or urine output/24 h	<110 µmol/L	110–170 µmol/L	171–299 µmol/L	300–440 µmol/L or urine output <500 mL/24 h	>440 µmol/L or urine output <200 mL/24 h
Coagulation Platelets	≥150 x 10⁹/L	<150 x 10⁹/L	<100 x 10⁹/L	<50 x 10⁹/L	<20 x 10⁹/L
Liver Bilirubin	<20 µmol/L	20–32 µmol/L	33–101 µmol/L	102–204 µmol/L	>204 µmol/L
Central nervous system (GCS)	15	13–14	10–12	6–9	<6

FIGURE 8-5 The Sequential Organ Failure Assessment (SOFA) scoring method. MAP, mean arterial pressure; GCS, Glasgow Coma Scale.
Karlsson S, Varpula M, Ruokonen E, et al. Incidence, treatment, and outcome of severe sepsis in ICU-treated adults in Finland: the Finnsepsis Study. *Intensive Care Med.* 2007;33(3):435–443.

patient should be monitored and evaluated frequently for signs of increase in airflow resistance and decrease in lung compliance. For patients with inhalational lung injuries, the airflow resistance may show a significant increase due to acute bronchospasm and mucosal edema. The PIP and Pplat gradient for these patients is increased. For patients with parenchymal lung injuries, the static compliance typically shows a gradual and steady decrease with a concurrent increase in Pplat. The PIP and Pplat gradient remains unchanged, however.

The subsequent ventilator settings may be adjusted according to the changing clinical conditions. For increase in airflow resistance with air trapping, the ventilator settings should focus on a steady reduction of frequency or tidal volume. For decrease in lung compliance, the ARDS lung protection strategy should be started as early as possible. For patient–ventilator dyssynchrony, sedatives and analgesics may be used for patient comfort and delivery of ventilation and oxygenation.

Burns and Smoke Inhalation

Burns and smoke inhalation are common in building fires and industrial or chemical explosions. Depending on the severity, severe burns and smoking inhalation often require systemic management, airway care, and mechanical ventilation.

Burn Terminology

First-degree burn is defined as epidermal burn that shows only reddening of the skin surface. It heals within days without scars. Second-degree burn is subdivided into superficial dermal burn (SDB) and deep dermal burn (DDB). SDB forms a blister and the dermis below the blister is red. It usually heals in 1 to 2 weeks without hypertrophic scar. DDB also forms a blister. The dermis below the blister is white and anemic. It heals in 3 to 4 weeks and is likely to have hypertrophic scar. Third-degree burn is a deep burn and causes necrosis of the entire skin thickness. It has a white or brown

TABLE 8-13
The Unique Characteristics and Requirements for Stockpiled Surge Ventilators

Characteristic	Requirement
Cost and usefulness	Low cost; easy to learn, operate, and maintain
Power source	A/C with long-lasting battery backup
Age group	Adult, pediatric, and neonate
Mode of ventilation	Volume- or pressure-controlled ventilation with assist/control or SIMV
Basic settings	Frequency, tidal volume, Fio₂, flow or I:E ratio, PEEP
Operational oxygen source	High- or low-flow oxygen source
Display	Exhaled volume or peak inspiratory pressure
Alarms	Audible and visual alarms for disconnection, apnea, high pressure, low source gas pressure

A/C, assist/control; PEEP, positive end-expiratory pressure; SIMV, synchronized intermittent mandatory ventilation.
Data from Daugherty EL, Talmor DS, Rubinson L. Sustained mechanical ventilation outside of traditional intensive care units. Available at https://www.sccm.org/getattachment/a9deba0e-406f-4506-87c6-9568b15dd333/Sustained-Mechanical-Ventilation-Outside-of-Tradit

TABLE 8-14
Initial Ventilator Settings for Mass Casualty

Parameter	Recommended Setting
Mode	Assist/control mode initially to guarantee adequate respiratory support, especially those using analgesic and sedative for control of pain and anxiety
Frequency	≥12/min Titrate to normal pH (7.35–7.45) or Paco₂ (35–45 mm Hg)
Tidal volume	6–8 mL/kg PBW* PBW for male = 50 + 2.3 [height in inches – 60] PBW for female = 45.5 + 2.3 [height in inches – 60] *Evaluate patient for lung protection when Pplat is >30 cm H₂O. Use low tidal volumes for patients with reduced chest wall compliance due to severe burns and formation of scar tissues on chest wall.
Fio₂	<0.60** Titrate to Spo₂ 92–96% **Use 1.0 Fio₂ for patients with smoke inhalation. The half-life of carboxyhemoglobin is 5 h, 60 min, and 30 min for breathing room air, Fio₂ of 1.0, and Fio₂ of 1.0 at 3 atm hyperbaric condition, respectively.
Pressure support	(Spontaneously breathing only) 5 cm H₂O of PS to overcome airflow resistance Titrate PS for an appropriate spontaneous V$_T$ based on patient's PBW
PEEP	5 cm H₂O Increase PEEP with refractory hypoxemia
Plateau pressure	Keep <30 cm H₂O Consider lung protection if Pplat >30 cm H₂O and signs of ARDS

ARDS, acute respiratory distress syndrome; PBW, predicted body weight; PEEP, positive end-expiratory pressure; PS, pressure support; V$_T$, tidal volume.

leatherlike appearance or completely charred skin. It takes up to 3 months to heal and produces hypertrophic scar. Characteristics and recovery time for first-, second-, and third-degree burns are summarized in **Table 8-15**.

Estimation of Burn Area

The area of skin burn may be estimated by the Rule of Nines or Rule of Fives. The Rule of Fives is more precise for different patient populations (infant, child, and adult). These two methods of estimation are shown in **Figure 8-6**.

Respiratory Implications of Burns

The most severe complication of burns is infection. This is because the protective layer of skin no longer exists. Pathogens enter the subdermal layer easily, and they thrive in a moist, warm, and nutrient-rich environment. Other complications that affect the respiratory

TABLE 8-15
Characteristics and Recovery Time for First-, Second-, and Third-Degree Burns

Degree of Burn	Characteristic	Recovery
First-degree burn	Reddening of the skin surface Patient feels pain	Within days
Second-degree superficial dermal burn	Blister; dermis below blister is red Patient feels pain	1–2 weeks
Second-degree deep dermal burn	Blister; dermis below blister is white and anemic Patient may not feel pain	3–4 weeks
Third-degree burn	Necrosis through the dermis; white or brown leatherlike appearance or completely charred skin Patient does not feel pain	Up to 3 months

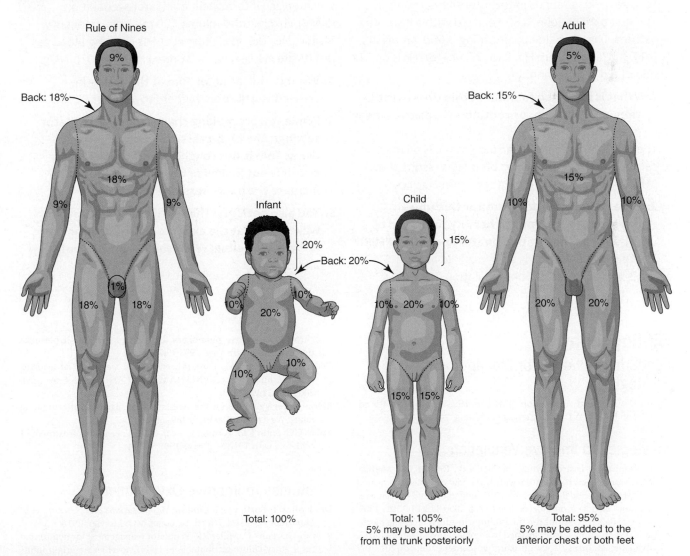

FIGURE 8-6 Rule of Nines (adult on far left); Rule of Fives (infant, child, and adult on right).

Reproduced with permission from Yoshino Y, Ohtsuka M, Kawaguchi M, et al. The wound/burn guidelines-6: guidelines for the management of burns. *J Dermatol.* 2016;43(9):989–1010. doi: 10.1111/1346-8138.13288 mechanics include loss of airway due to facial burn; atelectasis due to severe pain; hypoventilation due to use of opioid and sedative for control of pain and agitation; and increase in work of breathing due to reduced chest wall compliance. These events, plus those related to inhalation injury to the lung parenchyma, often put the patient at high risk of respiratory failure.

Smoke inhalation is the leading cause of death due to fires. The upper airway is affected by the extreme direct heat from fire and it causes thermal injury. Smoke that contains soot and particulate matters can cause irritation or chemical injury to the airways. Carbon monoxide (CO) and gases, such as cyanide (CN), can cause asphyxiation and toxicity. In severe cases, mechanical ventilation or hyperbaric oxygen therapy may become necessary.

Summary

This chapter provides the fundamental and adjunctive strategies to manage ventilation and oxygenation during mechanical ventilation. Setting of ventilator alarms under different patient conditions is also included. For clinical conditions that often require unique management strategies, individual sections are created for mechanically ventilated patients with ARDS, decompensated heart failure, severe asthma, acute exacerbation of COPD, and mass casualty injuries.

Case Study

You are making rounds in the intensive care unit (ICU). The first patient, John, a 50-year-old with a history of asthma, has the following morning blood gas results: pH 7.30, $Paco_2$ 51 mm Hg, Pao_2 72 mm Hg. He is on 5 L/min of oxygen via cannula.

1. **What is indicated for John at this time—ventilation, more oxygen, or continuous positive airway pressure (CPAP)?**

The second patient, 30-year-old Emma, is on mechanical ventilation. Her morning blood gas results show pH 7.42, $Paco_2$ 38 mm Hg, Pao_2 65 mm Hg, Fio_2 0.3.

2. **What is indicated for Emma at this time—increased ventilation, higher Fio_2, initiation of CPAP, or positive end-expiratory pressure (PEEP)?**

The third patient, Tom, is a 40-year-old admitted 2 days earlier for smoke inhalation. He is on synchronized intermittent mandatory ventilation (SIMV) 14/min, tidal volume 600 mL, total frequency 14/min, Fio_2 0.6, PEEP 3 cm H_2O. His morning blood gas results are pH 7.44, $Paco_2$ 36 mm Hg, Pao_2 50 mm Hg.

3. **What is indicated for Tom at this time—increased ventilation, higher Fio_2, higher PEEP?**

4. **While you are making changes to the ventilator settings, the high-pressure alarm goes off suddenly. Tom is not coughing, and the ventilator circuit is not kinked or obstructed. Should you increase the high-pressure limit?**

5. **You also notice on the ventilator flow-time waveform that the expiratory flow does not return to baseline. What should you evaluate and do next?**

Bibliography

Fundamental Ventilator Management Strategies

Chang DW. *Clinical Application of Mechanical Ventilations.* 4th ed. Clifton Park, NY: Delmar Cengage Learning; 2014.

Strategies to Improve Ventilation

Acute Respiratory Distress Syndrome Network, Brower RG, Matthay MA, Morris A, et al. Ventilation with lower tidal volumes as compared with traditional tidal volumes for acute lung injury and the acute respiratory distress syndrome. *N Engl J Med.* 2000;342(18):1301–1308.

Bocklage T, Balk RA. Setting the tidal volume in adults receiving mechanical ventilation: lessons learned from recent investigations. 2017. Available at https://www.nbrc.org/wp-content/uploads/2017/07/Setting-the-Tidal-Volume.pdf

Georgopoulos D, Giannouli E, Patakas D. Effects of extrinsic positive end-expiratory pressure on mechanically ventilated patients with chronic obstructive pulmonary disease and dynamic hyperinflation. *Intensive Care Med.* 1993;19:197–203.

Keller RH, Jasmer RM, Luce JM, et al. The treatment of acidosis in acute lung injury with THAM. *Am J Respir Crit Care Med.* 2000;161:1149–1153.

Marini JJ. New options for the ventilatory management of acute lung injury. *New Horiz.* 1993;1(4):489–503.

Nahas GG, Sutin KM, Fermon C, et al. Guidelines for the treatment of acidemia with THAM. *Drugs.* 1998;55:191.

Strategies to Improve Oxygenation

Des Jardins T, Burton GG. *Clinical Manifestations and Assessment of Respiratory Disease.* 7th ed. St. Louis, MO: Elsevier; 2016.

Ramsey CD, Funk D, Miller RR. Ventilator management for hypoxemic respiratory failure attributable to H1N1 novel swine origin influenza virus. *Crit Care Med.* 2010;38(4 Suppl):e58–e65.

Ventilator Alarms and Events

Chang DW. *Clinical Application of Mechanical Ventilations.* 4th ed. Clifton Park, NY: Delmar Cengage Learning; 2014.

IngMar Medical. Ventilator alarm settings guide. Available at https://www.ingmarmed.com/wp-content/uploads/2015/06/Ventilator-Alarm -Settings-Guide.pdf

Adjunctive Ventilator Management Strategies

Ballard E, Puthussery R, Pattani H, et al. Mechanical insufflation-exsufflation (MIE): current UK practice. *Eur Respir J.* 2017;50:PA2176. doi:10.1183/1393003.congress-2017.PA2176

Blanch LL. Clinical studies of tracheal gas insufflation. *Respir Care.* 2001;46:158–166.

Fan E, Del Sorbo L, Goligher EC, et al. An official American Thoracic Society/European Society of Intensive Care Medicine/Society of Critical Care Medicine clinical practice guideline: mechanical ventilation in adult patients with acute respiratory distress syndrome. *Am J Respir Crit Care Med.* 2017;195:1253–1263. doi:10.1164 / rccm.201703-0548ST

Guérin C, Reignier J, Richard JC, et al. Prone positioning in severe acute respiratory distress syndrome. *N Engl J Med.* 2013;368:2159–2168. doi:10.1056/NEJMoa1214103

Homnick DN. Mechanical insufflation-exsufflation for airway mucus clearance. *Respir Care.* 2007;52:1296–1305.

Kacmarek RM. Complications of tracheal gas insufflation. *Respir Care.* 2001;46:167–176.

Oliver RE, Rozycki HJ, Greenspan JS, et al. Tracheal gas insufflation as a lung-protective strategy: physiologic, histologic, and biochemical markers. *Pediatr Crit Care Med.* 2005;6:64–69.

Ortiz AC, Muneshika M, Martins FA. Influence of tracheal gas insufflation during capnography in anesthetized patients. *Rev Bras de Anestesiol.* 2008;58:440–446. https://dx.doi.org/10.1590/S0034-70942008000500002

Stephen D, Stephen D, Solomon D, et al. Tracheal gas insufflation combined with high-frequency oscillatory ventilation. *Crit Care Med.* 1996;24:458–465.

Acute Respiratory Distress Syndrome

Borges JB, Okamoto VN, Matos GF, et al. Reversibility of lung collapse and hypoxemia in early acute respiratory distress syndrome. *Am J Respir Crit Care Med.* 2006;174:268–278.

Chiumello D, Cressoni M, Carlesso E, et al. Bedside selection of positive end-expiratory pressure in mild, moderate, and severe acute respiratory distress syndrome. *Crit Care Med.* 2014;42:252–264.

Girgis K, Hamed H, Khater Y, et al. A decremental PEEP trial identifies the PEEP level that maintains oxygenation after lung recruitment. *Respir Care.* 2006;51:1132–1139.

Hess DR. Recruitment maneuvers and PEEP titration. *Respir Care.* 2015;60:1688–1704.

National Institutes of Health, National Heart, Lung, and Blood Institute. ARDS Clinical Network mechanical ventilation protocol summary. March 6, 2019. Available at http://www.ardsnet.org/files/ventilator_protocol_2008-07.pdf

Toth I, Leiner T, Mikor A, et al. Hemodynamic and respiratory changes during lung recruitment and descending optimal positive end-expiratory pressure titration in patients with acute respiratory distress syndrome. *Crit Care Med.* 2007;35:787–793.

Villar J, Pérez-Méndez L, López J, et al. An early PEEP/F$_{IO_2}$ trial identifies different degrees of lung injury in patients with acute respiratory distress syndrome. *Am J Respir Crit Care Med.* 2007;176:795–804.

Decompensated Heart Failure

Grace MP, Greenbaum DM. Cardiac performance in response to PEEP in patients with cardiac dysfunction. *Crit Care Med.* 1982;10:358–360.

Kuhn BT, Bradley LA, Dempsey TM, et al. Management of mechanical ventilation in decompensated heart failure. *J Cardiovasc Dev Dis.* 2016;3:33.

Miller JD, Smith CA, Hemauer SJ, et al. The effects of inspiratory intrathoracic pressure production on the cardiovascular response to submaximal exercise in health and chronic heart failure. *Am J Physiol Heart Circ Physiol.* 2007;292:H580–H592.

Tobin MJ. Extubation and the myth of "minimal ventilator settings." *Am J Respir Care Med.* 2012;185:349–350.

Severe Asthma

Brenner B, Corbridge T, Kazzi A. Intubation and mechanical ventilation of the asthmatic patient in respiratory failure. *Proc Am Thorac Soc.* 2009;6:371–379. doi:10.1513/pats.P09ST4

Leatherman J. Mechanical ventilation for severe asthma. *Chest.* 2015;147:1671–1680. doi:10.1378/chest.14-1733

Rochwerg B, Brochard L, Elliott MW, et al. Official ERS/ATS clinical practice guidelines: noninvasive ventilation for acute respiratory failure. *Eur Respir J.* 2017;50:1602426. doi.org/10.1183/13993003.02426-2016

Stefan MS, Nathanson BH, Lagu T, et al. Outcomes of noninvasive and invasive ventilation in patients hospitalized with asthma exacerbation. *Ann Am Thorac Soc.* 2016;13:1096–1104. doi:10.1513 / AnnalsATS.201510-701OC

Williams AM, Abramo TJ, Shah MV, et al. Safety and clinical findings of BiPAP utilization in children 20 kg or less for asthma exacerbations. *Intensive Care Med.* 2011;37:1338–1343. doi:10.1007/s00134-011-2238-9

Acute Exacerbation of COPD

Davidson AC, Banham S, Elliott M, et al. BTS/ICS guideline for the ventilatory management of acute hypercapnic respiratory failure in adults. *Thorax.* 2016;71:ii1–ii35.

Guthrie K. Noninvasive ventilation and the critically ill. Available at https://lifeinthefastlane.com/non-invasive-ventilation

Hess DR, Kacmarek RM. *Essentials of Mechanical Ventilation.* 3rd ed. New York, NY: McGraw-Hill Education/Medical; 2014.

Osadnik CR, Tee VS, Carson-Chahhoud KV, et al. Non-invasive ventilation for the management of acute hypercapnic respiratory failure due to exacerbation of chronic obstructive pulmonary disease. *Cochrane Database Syst Rev.* 2017;7:CD004104. doi:10.1002/14651858.CD004104.pub4

Snow V, Lascher S, Mottur-Pilson C. Evidence base for management of acute exacerbations of chronic obstructive pulmonary disease. *Ann Intern Med.* 2001;134(7):595–599. doi:10.7326/0003-4819-134-7 -200104030-00015

Wedzicha JA, Miravitlles M, Hurst JR, et al. Management of COPD exacerbations: a European Respiratory Society/American Thoracic Society guideline. *Eur Respir J.* 2017;49:1600791. doi:10.1183/13993003.00791-2016

Mass Casualty

Daugherty EL, Talmor DS, Rubinson L. Sustained mechanical ventilation outside of traditional intensive care units. Available at https://www.sccm.org/getattachment/a9deba0e-406f-4506-87c6-9568b15dd333/Sustained-Mechanical-Ventilation-Outside-of-Tradit

McCafferty RR, Lennarson, PJ. Common chemical agent threats. *Neurosurg Focus.* 2002;12:e3.

SOFA score. Available at https://www.researchgate.net/figure/The-SOFA-score_ tbl1_47934086

START triage system. Available at https://www.slideserve.com/remington/start-triage

Yoshino Y, Ohtsuka M, Kawaguchi M, et al. The wound/burn guidelines 6: guidelines for the management of burns. *J Dermatol.* 2016;43:989–1010. doi:10.1111/1346-8138.13288

9

Critical Care Procedures

David W. Chang, EdD, RRT

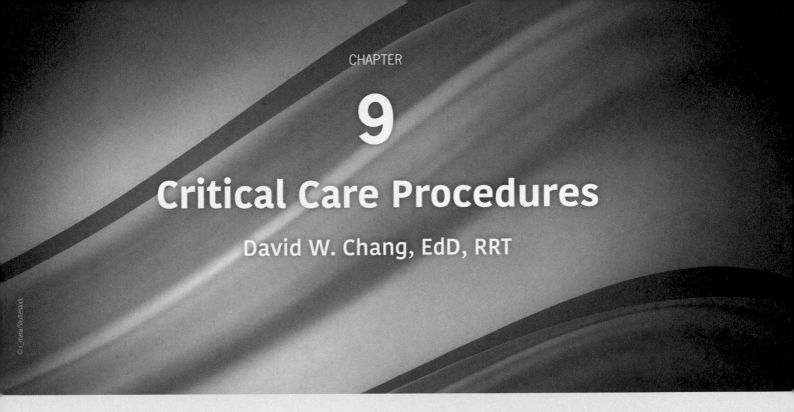

OUTLINE

OBJECTIVES

1. Describe the five-wire and three-wire setups for cardiac monitoring.
2. Differentiate between arterial catheter, pulmonary artery catheter, central venous catheter, and peripheral venous catheter.
3. Describe the technique and devices to create an intraosseous access.
4. Describe the procedure and application of intraosseous infusion.
5. Differentiate the following samples obtained by flexible bronchoscopy: forceps biopsy, transbronchial lung biopsy, transbronchial needle aspiration biopsy, bronchial brushing.
6. Name a topical anesthetic, sedative, and analgesic used in flexible bronchoscopy.
7. Describe the procedure and application of mini-BAL.
8. Differentiate between operative tube thoracostomy and trocar tube thoracostomy.
9. Describe the operative functions of the following chest tube drainage systems: single-chamber, two-chamber, and three-chamber.
10. Select the appropriate mode of patient transport.
11. Differentiate between MRI safe and MRI conditional.

KEY TERMS

arterial catheter
asystole
biopsy
bronchial alveolar lavage
brushing

central venous catheter
colony-forming units
cytology
fentanyl (Duragesic)
flexible bronchoscopy

forceps
Heimlich valve
intraosseous infusion
midazolam (Versed)
mini-bronchoalveolar
  lavage

MRI conditional
MRI safe
operative tube
  thoracostomy
peripherally inserted
  central catheter

propofol (Diprivan)
pulmonary artery catheter
suction control chamber
transbronchial lung biopsy
transbronchial needle
  aspiration

trocar tube thoracostomy
ventricular fibrillation
ventricular tachycardia
water seal chamber

Introduction

This chapter includes seven key procedures commonly performed in the critical care settings. These procedures are cardiac monitoring, arterial and venous access lines, intraosseous infusion, assisting in bronchoscopy, mini-bronchoalveolar lavage, chest tube and drainage system, and transport of critically ill patients. Depending on the hospital protocols and policies, these procedures may be done by physicians, respiratory therapists, nurses, emergency medical technicians, or paramedics. As a member on the critical care team, each clinician should be knowledgeable in these procedures.

Cardiac Monitoring

Cardiac monitoring is one of the most common assessment tools used in critical care settings. It allows continuous monitoring of the heart rate and rhythms in stable patients. For patients with cardiac abnormalities, cardiac monitoring may be used to titrate dosage and document response to medications, evaluate heart rate changes with exercise and sleep, and adjust the dose of QT-prolonging medications. In addition to these functions, cardiac monitoring also provides instant alerts when dangerous arrhythmias develop. Unlike the traditional 12-lead (10-wire) electrocardiogram (ECG), a common cardiac monitor uses three or five wires.

Types of Cardiac Monitoring

Cardiac monitoring is performed by using multiple-lead or single-lead placement. Multiple-lead monitoring provides more information. The type of cardiac monitoring selected is based on the clinical indications. For example, lead V1 can be used to monitor premature atrial contraction, premature ventricular contraction, wide complex ventricular tachycardia, and ventricular pacing activity. Because some of these arrhythmias are life threatening, V1 lead is often the choice for this patient population.

Five-Wire and Three-Wire Setups

The five-wire setup (**Figure 9-1**) provides information on three bipolar leads (I, II, and III) and six chest leads. It uses four limb electrodes (RA, LA, RL, and LL) plus the chest electrode. The single unipolar chest electrode may be moved and placed at any one of the chest lead positions (i.e., V1–V6), as in a traditional 12-lead ECG. A five-wire setup using the V1 lead is commonly done for telemetry monitoring.

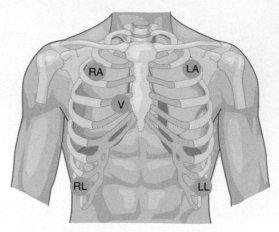

FIGURE 9-1 A five-wire lead placement with V1 chest lead.

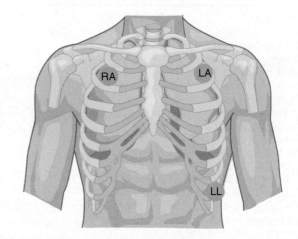

FIGURE 9-2 A typical three-wire lead placement.

If cardiac rhythm information on the chest leads is not indicated, a simpler three-wire setup may be used (**Figure 9-2**). This setup uses the RA, LA, and LL electrodes and it monitors the bipolar leads (I, II, and III). If possible, these three electrodes on the chest should be placed at equal distance from the heart for optimal display of cardiac rhythms.

Dangerous Arrhythmias

Dangerous arrhythmias can be life threatening without immediate intervention because they may lead to a severe deficit of cardiac output. A wide range of reduction in cardiac output may be due to absence of heart beat (**asystole**), poor contractility (**ventricular fibrillation**),

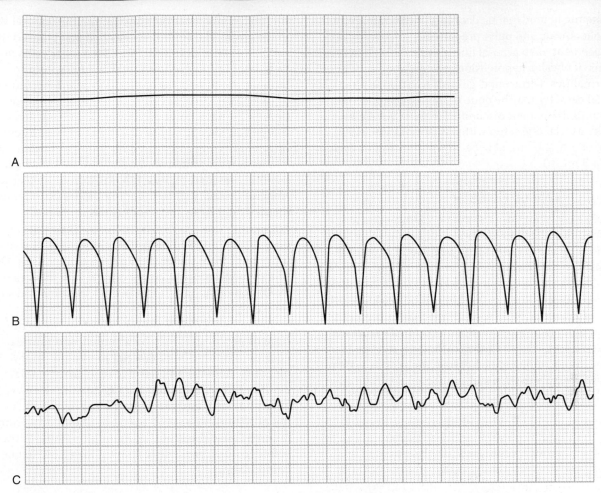

FIGURE 9-3 Three common life-threatening arrhythmias. (**A**) Asystole. (**B**) Ventricular tachycardia (with or without pulse).
(**C**) Ventricular fibrillation.

poor ventricular filling due to limited refill time (tachycardia), and dysfunction of heart muscles (myocardial infarction and ischemia). Life-threatening arrhythmias are shown in **Figure 9-3**. Among these arrhythmias, only ventricular fibrillation and *pulseless* **ventricular tachycardia** are shockable rhythms.

Arterial and Venous Access Lines

Arterial and venous access lines provide many critical care support functions. On the arterial side of circulation (blood vessels leading blood *away* from their respective ventricles), there are systemic and pulmonary arteries. On the venous side of circulation (blood vessels leading blood *toward* their respective ventricles), there are systemic and pulmonary veins. This section focuses on three types of access lines in blood vessels: systemic arterial catheter, systemic venous catheter (central and peripheral), and pulmonary artery catheter.

Systemic Arterial Catheter

Systemic arteries receive oxygenated blood from the left heart. This oxygenated blood supports the metabolic

functions of major organs and body systems. In a critical care setting, systemic arterial access lines allow arterial blood sampling for blood gases and monitoring of hemodynamic data in the systemic circulation. Contraindications for arterial catheterization include lack of adequate collateral circulation (e.g., radial and ulnar arteries), infection of soft tissue or skin at puncture site, vascular disease of intended artery, and severe coagulopathy.

The systemic arterial line is commonly inserted at the radial (first choice) or brachial artery. Occasionally the femoral artery is used. Insertion of an arterial catheter follows the traditional arterial puncture technique. The **arterial catheter** has a catheter-over-needle design. Once the artery is successfully punctured, the needle/catheter assembly is held steady and the guide wire is advanced into the artery followed by the catheter. The needle and guide wire are then removed, leaving the catheter inside the artery. An arterial line setup is attached to the catheter to complete the procedure. The finished arterial line setup uses a slow continuous infusion drip to keep the artery and catheter from clotting. The setup also has transducers for measurement of systemic hemodynamic data (e.g., heart rate; systolic, diastolic, mean, and pulse pressures).

Placement of an arterial line may be difficult in conditions of obesity, hypotension, edema, and vascular abnormalities. Ultrasound-guided insertion of a radial arterial catheter may be done to improve success rate and minimize patient discomfort. **Figure 9-4** shows a typical arterial line setup with a flush solution (0.9% saline or 1 to 2 U/mL of heparin solution at an infusion rate of 3 mL/h).

Systemic Venous Catheter

The primary functions of systemic venous catheterization include collection of blood samples for laboratory studies (e.g., complete blood count, blood chemistry, coagulation panel, culture and sensitivity), infusion of blood, and administration of fluid or parenteral nutrition. Venous blood is not used for blood gas analysis because of inconsistent levels of oxygen consumption and carbon dioxide production due to regional variations in metabolism. Also, a venous catheter is not used for hemodynamic monitoring because the venous system is a low-pressure system and has regional variations in blood volume and pressure.

Central and Peripheral Venous Catheter

The most common veins used for placement of a central line are the internal jugular in the neck, the subclavian vein near the clavicle, and the femoral vein in the groin. The **central venous catheter** is inserted and placed in a large systemic vein. Larger veins provide three functions: infusion of a large volume of solution or multiple intravenous (IV) solutions, infusion of parenteral nutrients with high osmotic concentration, and dilution of medications. Rapid infusion of a large volume of IV fluid may be necessary in acute hypotension (e.g., sepsis, severe blood loss). Parenteral nutrients with protein and carbohydrate have high osmotic pressure, making it hazardous to smaller peripheral vessels and surrounding tissues. Rapid movement of fluid from surrounding tissues to peripheral vessels may damage both structures. Shrinkage or destruction of tissues may occur as a result of water movement from the tissues to peripheral vessels. Dilution of medication in a large central vein reduces the likelihood of damage to the peripheral veins and surrounding tissues.

Immediate complications, which occur at the time of procedure, may be grouped into four categories: vascular (e.g., arterial or venous injury, bleeding, hematoma), cardiac (e.g., arrhythmia, cardiac arrest), pulmonary (e.g., pneumothorax, air embolism), and placement (e.g., incorrect resting position). Repeated attempts due to procedural failures cause most of these complications. Ultrasound-guided procedures have a lower incidence of complication.

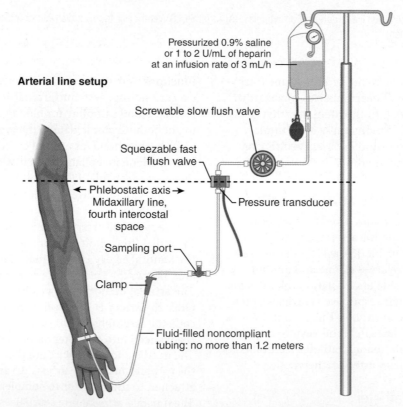

FIGURE 9-4 A typical systemic arterial line setup. The sampling port (as shown) is for illustration only. The sampling port is proximal to the puncture site to reduce the amount of flush solution for blood draws.

Peripherally Inserted Central Catheter

A **peripherally inserted central catheter** (PICC) line is a catheter inserted into a peripheral vein in the arm (e.g., cephalic vein, basilic vein, or brachial vein). It is advanced proximally toward the heart until the tip rests in the distal superior vena cava or cavoatrial junction.

Immediate complications of PICC line during insertion include injury to local structures and phlebitis at insertion site. Air embolism, hematoma, and catheter malposition may also occur. After insertion and a period of use, common complications include infection (due to poor sterile technique), blood clot, and malposition of the catheter. To minimize late complications, aseptic and sterile techniques, good security of catheter, and periodic evaluation of the entire setup are required.

Pulmonary Artery Catheter

The pulmonary artery carries mixed venous blood (deoxygenated and CO_2-rich blood) from the right heart to the alveolar-capillary membrane for oxygen loading and CO_2 unloading. Because the pulmonary circulation is between the right and left heart, it is under considerable influence by the pressures in the right ventricle, lung parenchyma, and left ventricle.

The primary functions of **pulmonary artery catheter** (PAC) include collection of mixed venous blood sample and measurement of hemodynamic and cardiac output values. Mixed venous blood sample is collected via the PAC with the catheter balloon deflated. This sample is used to calculate cardiac parameters, such as mixed venous oxygen content and physiologic shunt. For hemodynamic measurements, a four-lumen PAC may be used to measure the pressures in the vena cava or right atrium and pulmonary artery.

The location of the measurement port and balloon inflation/deflation are used to designate preload or afterload. For example, the pressure measured in the right atrium is at a point *before* the right ventricle. The right atrial pressure is therefore called right ventricular *preload*. See **Table 9-1** for the parameters in hemodynamic monitoring.

Many variables can affect a correct interpretation of hemodynamic data. It is essential to gather all pertinent clinical information before an interpretation is made. In general, blood flow obstruction *downstream* (e.g., left heart) causes an increase of volume/pressure at a point *upstream* (e.g., pulmonary artery). Using this example, obstruction in left heart (e.g., left ventricular failure, mitral valve stenosis) may lead to an increase of pulmonary artery pressure (PAP) and pulmonary artery occlusion pressure (PAOP). However, hypoxic vasoconstriction and pulmonary edema may also increase the PAP, but not the PAOP. Correct interpretation of hemodynamic data requires more than the hemodynamic data alone.

Intraosseous Infusion

Administration of fluids and drugs typically involves a central or peripheral venous access line. These traditional IV access lines may not be available during cardiac arrest or in conditions with severe hypotension and collapsed veins. **Intraosseous (IO) infusion** via the bone marrow channel is an alternative to fast venous access. This section covers the advantages of an IO route, technique and devices to create an IO access, and drug delivery via IO route. In 1986, the American Heart Association approved use of IO access during pediatric resuscitation. In 2003, the International Liaison Committee on Resuscitation (ILCOR) recognized the use of IO access as a valuable alternative when IV access is not readily available.

Advantages of an IO Route

In animal models, fluids and drugs go from the bone marrow channel to the systemic circulation very quickly (within 20 seconds). In humans, the fluid infused inside the bone marrow cavity enters the medullary venous sinusoids into the central venous sinus. The fluid is then drained into the central venous circulation via the nutrient or emissary veins.

Fast access is the major advantage of an IO access line. The entire procedure can be completed in 1 to 2

TABLE 9-1
Hemodynamic Monitoring Parameters

Location of PAC Tip	Preload/Afterload	Example	Normal Range (mm Hg)
Vena cava or right atrium	Right ventricular preload	Systemic hypervolemia (↑ CVP), hypovolemia (↓ CVP)	CVP (2–6)
Pulmonary artery	Right ventricular afterload	Pulmonary hypertension (↑ PAP, normal PAOP)	$PAP_{systolic/diastolic}$ (20–35/5–15) PAOP (5–10)
Pulmonary artery occlusion pressure (pulmonary capillary wedge pressure)	Left ventricular preload	Left heart failure or obstruction (↑ PAP, ↑ PAOP)	$PAP_{systolic/diastolic}$ (20–35/5–15) PAOP (5–10)
Systemic artery	Left ventricular afterload	Systemic hypertension or hypotension	SBP (120/80)

CVP, central venous pressure; PAP, pulmonary artery pressure; PAOP, pulmonary artery occlusion pressure; SBP, systolic blood pressure.

minutes. IO puncture is relatively easy to perform, and it has a success rate of about 80%, even in hypotensive conditions. Fluids and a wide range of drugs can be administered via the IO route. Venous blood sample can also be drawn for laboratory studies (chemistry, venous blood gases, blood type, and cross-match). The advantages of an IO access line are summarized in **Table 9-2**.

Technique and Devices to Create an IO Access

There are several puncture sites for obtaining IO access (**Table 9-3**). After finding an appropriate puncture site (e.g., proximal tibia [**Figure 9-5**]), it is prepped with an antiseptic wipe, such as betadine. The skin of an adult is manually penetrated with a 13- to 16-gauge short-shaft IO needle (neonates to 5-year-olds, 18- or 20-gauge spinal needle) until it meets the bone. At this point, the drill is started until resistance disappears—a sign of penetration into the hollow bone marrow cavity. Control of the drill is crucial to prevent overpenetration and puncture of the posterior aspect of the bone structure. Once in the proper position, the drill is replaced with 10-mL syringe filled with 5 mL 0.9% saline solution. Slow aspiration of the syringe from the IO access adaptor should yield blood from the bone marrow cavity. Two to 3 mL of normal saline may be used to flush the IO needle if aspiration does not yield blood from the bone cavity. Swelling of the tissues around the puncture is a sign of incorrect needle placement. If this occurs, the needle must be removed. Once the IO access line is correctly placed, dressing is applied, and an IV line is attached to the needle adaptor for fluid or drug administration. For needles with a stylet, the stylet is removed before aspiration of blood for verification of correct needle placement.

For conscious patients and in nonemergency situations, topical anesthesia should be given subcutaneously to the puncture site by using 2 mL of a 2% lidocaine solution administered slowly over 2 minutes. It may be repeated once for a total of 80 mg (4 mL) lidocaine. The IO access is for short-term use only (<24 hours). Another permanent IV access line should be prepared once the patient is stabilized. This IO procedure should be done only *once* at each puncture location. If an attempt is unsuccessful, another location must be used.

Assisting in Bronchoscopy

A bronchoscope is an instrument that goes into the airways to perform diagnostic and therapeutic procedures. It may be "rigid" or "flexible." Because of its larger size, rigid bronchoscopy is used to manage obstruction of the trachea or *proximal* bronchus. It may also be used to insert airway stents. The **flexible bronchoscope** uses a light source and glass fibers to transmit live visuals (termed *fiberoptic* bronchoscope). A number of years ago a new flexible bronchoscope technology (termed *video* bronchoscopy) was introduced that represents the majority of flexible bronchoscopes in current use. It provides superior, high-definition video and an improved light source, and is more durable than fiberoptic technology. The instruments can investigate tumors or obstructions in the airways and lungs, provide lavage and suction, and obtain specimens using lavage fluid, cytology brushes, transbronchial needle aspiration, or biopsy forceps. Bronchoscopic devices are also available for retrieving foreign objects, performing electrocautery tasks, and aiding in performing difficult intubations or percutaneous tracheostomies.

TABLE 9-2
Advantages of Intraosseous Access

Advantage	Notes
Patient type	Adult, pediatric, and neonatal population
Easy access	Suitable in conditions of hypotension and collapsed veins
Fast access	1 to 2 minutes
High success rate	About 80%
Blood sample	Suitable for laboratory studies, blood type, and cross-match
Fluid and drug	Suitable for fluids, resuscitation drugs, analgesics, anesthetics, sedatives, antibiotics, opioid antagonist, neuromuscular blockers, and others

TABLE 9-3
Needles and Sites for Intraosseous (IO) Access

Patient Population	Needle for IO Access	Site
Neonates and children up to 5 years	18- or 20-gauge spinal needle	Proximal tibia (first choice) Distal tibia (medial aspect of ankle) Distal femur (2 fingerwidths above knee) Anterior-superior iliac spine
Adults	13- to 16-gauge short-shaft IO needle	Proximal tibia Distal tibia Distal femur Sternum Greater tuberosity of humeral head* (below shoulder) Distal radius Distal ulna Iliac crest

*Avoid the biceps tendon that is located in a groove between the greater and lesser tuberosity.

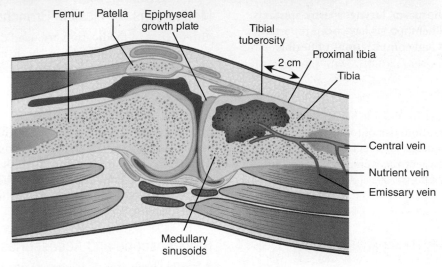

FIGURE 9-5 Intraosseous puncture site on the proximal tibia.

Indications for Flexible Bronchoscopy

In general, diagnostic bronchoscopy is indicated for the evaluation of tumors, persistent atelectasis, persistent or unexplained cough, localized or fixed wheeze, unexplained airway obstruction, hemoptysis, inflammation and infection, interstitial pulmonary disease, staging of lung cancer before surgery, and unexplained hoarseness or vocal cord paralysis. The indications also include investigation and confirmation of preliminary diagnosis based on patient history, physical exam, and other laboratory data. **Biopsy** (tissues) and **cytology** (cells) are two broad categories of diagnostic application of **flexible bronchoscopy** (Table 9-4).

Therapeutic applications of bronchoscopy include removal of foreign bodies (e.g., small objects aspirated by children); removal of excessive secretions, mucus plugs, polyps, or endobronchial tissues; bronchopulmonary lavage for pulmonary alveolar proteinosis; laser resection of tumor; placement of airway stent; and placement of endotracheal (ET) tube with head in neutral position (i.e., high cervical injury). Drainage of a lung abscess may also be done if flooding the airway with purulent material can be avoided.

Contraindications for Flexible Bronchoscopy

The absolute contraindications for bronchoscopy include unstable hemodynamic status, persistent life-threatening arrhythmias, refractory hypoxemia before or during the procedure, acute ventilatory failure with hypercapnia during spontaneous breathing, coagulopathy or bleeding condition, and tracheal obstruction. Relative contraindications include uncooperative patient, recent (within 6 weeks) myocardial infarction, partial tracheal obstruction, moderate to severe hypoxemia, hypercapnia, and lung abscess (danger of flooding the airway with purulent material). Transbronchial biopsy should be done with caution in

TABLE 9-4
Selected Diagnostic Application of Flexible Bronchoscopy

Procedure		Application
Biopsy	**Transbronchial lung biopsy** (TBLB)	A **forceps** is used to collect lung tissue samples for the diagnosis of diffuse interstitial lung diseases, primary and metastatic peripheral lung cancers
	Transbronchial needle aspiration biopsy (TBNAB)	A sheathed needle is used to collect lung tissue samples for the diagnosis of primary and metastatic peripheral lung cancers as well as submucosal, peribronchial, and mediastinal tumors
Cytology	Endobronchial toilet	Removal and examination of retained secretions in lung parenchyma as in ventilator-associated pneumonia or ventilator-related event
	Brushing	Collection of cytology samples at sites where biopsy samples cannot be obtained
	Bronchial alveolar lavage (BAL)	A distal lung segment is wedged by the insertion tube and lavaged with up to 10 mL of fluid. The fluid is aspirated for cytology exam

patients with uremia, superior vena cava obstruction, or pulmonary hypertension because of increased risk of bleeding.

Hazards and Complications

Adverse effects of medications used before and during bronchoscopy are the main hazards. Hypoxemia, hypercapnia, bronchospasm, laryngospasm, epistaxis, pneumothorax, and hemoptysis have been reported as potential hazards and complications of flexible bronchoscopy.

Procedure

The general procedure for flexible bronchoscopy involves patient preparation, use of topical anesthesia, use of sedative and analgesic, selection of appropriate sampling tool, and patient recovery. **Figure 9-6** outlines the essential steps for conscious sedation during flexible bronchoscopy.

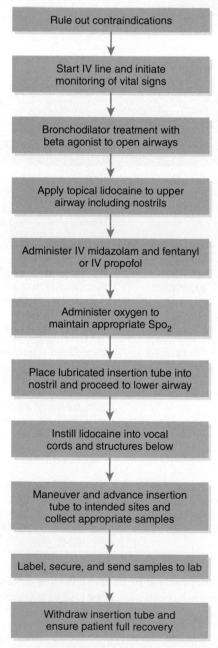

Rule out contraindications

Start IV line and initiate monitoring of vital signs

Bronchodilator treatment with beta agonist to open airways

Apply topical lidocaine to upper airway including nostrils

Administer IV midazolam and fentanyl or IV propofol

Administer oxygen to maintain appropriate Spo_2

Place lubricated insertion tube into nostril and proceed to lower airway

Instill lidocaine into vocal cords and structures below

Maneuver and advance insertion tube to intended sites and collect appropriate samples

Label, secure, and send samples to lab

Withdraw insertion tube and ensure patient full recovery

FIGURE 9-6 Essential steps for conscious sedation during flexible bronchoscopy. IV, intravenous.

Medications for Flexible Bronchoscopy

Three types of medication are used during flexible bronchoscopy. A topical anesthetic is used to desensitize the sensory receptors along the upper airway, vocal cords, and conducting airways. A combination of sedative and analgesic is used to provide patient comfort and to reduce sensation of anxiety and pain. The analgesic also reduces the coughing reflex. The recommended sedative/analgesic combination is **midazolam (Versed)** and **fentanyl (Duragesic)**. As an alternative, **propofol (Diprivan)** may be used. **Table 9-5** outlines the use of medications during flexible bronchoscopy.

Bronchoscope and Accessories

A flexible bronchoscope consists of a handle and an insertion tube. The handle has an eyepiece and hand-control mechanisms. The typical flexible insertion tube is 400 to 600 mm in length. The angle of motion for the tip is 120° to 180° up and 60° to 130° down. The diameter of the working channel is up to 3.2 mm. The bending mechanism allows the clinician to direct and advance the insertion tube to intended structures. At the distal end of the insertion tube, a light source and video scope provide live visuals at the eyepiece and a monitor. The channel outlets at the distal end are used for installation of saline or topical anesthetics, suction, or passage of cytology brush, aspiration needle, or biopsy forceps. **Figure 9-7** shows a flexible bronchoscope with handle and insertion tube. **Figure 9-8** shows collection of a lavage cytology sample. **Figure 9-9** shows a cytology brush, biopsy needle, and biopsy forceps.

Placement of Insertion Tube

After patient preparation (including adequate topical anesthetic), the distal end of the insertion tube is coated with a water-soluble lubricant and inserted via the nostril, mouth (with bite block), ET tube, or tracheostomy tube. The insertion tube is advanced through the vocal cords, trachea, left or right main stem bronchus, and to the intended branches of bronchi and segments. For spontaneously breathing patients, oxygen therapy is provided to maintain an appropriate Spo_2. If the patient has an artificial airway, an aerosol setup is used to provide supplemental oxygen and humidity. Supplemental oxygen is required because the insertion tube increases the airflow resistance and work of breathing during the procedure.

For mechanically ventilated patients, an adaptor is used to maintain ventilation and airway pressures during the procedure. Minor air leaks may occur and the lost volume can be compensated by increasing the tidal volume (in volume-controlled ventilation) or peak inspiratory pressure (in pressure-controlled ventilation). The high-pressure limit needs to be increased because

TABLE 9-5
Recommended Medications During Flexible Bronchoscopy*

Purpose	Medication	Notes
Topical anesthesia	Lidocaine	Lidocaine is preferred over other topical anesthetics The recommended total topical lidocaine dose is 4–8 mg/kg (often lower) with 2 to 5 mL of 2% solution in the nares and variable amount below the vocal cords. Use minimal effective dose *before and during* bronchoscopy to decrease cough and reduce sedative dose during procedure Use caution in patients with advanced age, impaired liver function, and congestive heart failure
Sedative and opioid (use A *or* B)	(A) Midazolam *and* fentanyl	This benzodiazepine and opioid combination provide synergistic effects on patient outcome and tolerance Both drugs have quick onset, rapid peak effect, short duration of effect (fast recovery) Fentanyl provides antitussive effect and is preferred over other opioids Recommended dose: midazolam 0.01–0.1 mg/kg; fentanyl: initial dose of 25–50 µg with supplemental doses of 25 µg (total dose of 200 µg)
	(B) Propofol	Produces similar sedation, amnesia, and patient outcome and tolerance compared with other combinations of benzodiazepine and opioid Short duration of effect (fast recovery time) Recommended dose: 20 mg bolus (1–2 mg/kg total dose)

*Atropine sulfate, an anticholinergic, is *no longer* recommended as a pretreatment as it does not increase lung function or decrease bronchial secretions.
Modified from Pearson D, McLaughlin C, Shutak D, et al. Reduction in lidocaine dose administration for flexible bronchoscopy following order set implementation. *Chest.* 2015;148:808A; Wahidi MM, Jain P, Jantz M, et al. American College of Chest Physicians consensus statement on the use of topical anesthesia, analgesia, and sedation during flexible bronchoscopy in adult patients. *Chest.* 2011;140:1342–1350.

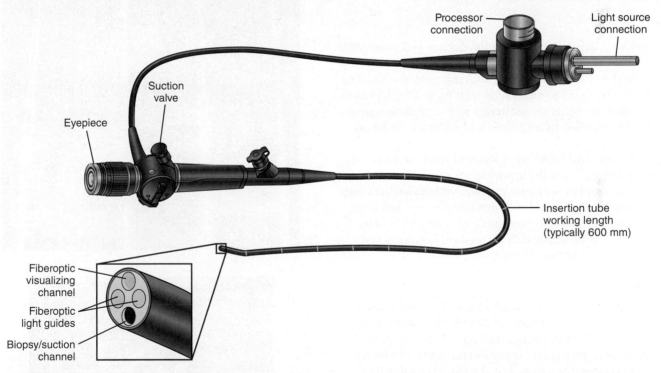

FIGURE 9-7 A flexible bronchoscope with handle and insertion tube.
Courtesy of Olympus Corporation of the Americas, Center Valley, Pennsylvania.

of the increase in airflow resistance imposed by the insertion tube.

Collection of Samples

In addition to suction and removal of secretions, a flexible bronchoscope can collect different types of specimens. These specimens include cytology (brush or lavage) and tissue biopsy (forceps biopsy, transbronchial lung biopsy, and transbronchial needle aspiration biopsy).

Cytology Lavage and Bronchial Brushing

Cytology examination may be necessary when pathologic change is seen during a flexible bronchoscopy procedure. Cytology samples from alveolar lavage or

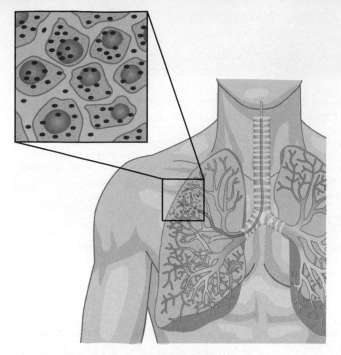

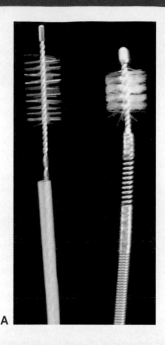

FIGURE 9-8 Collection of a lavage cytology sample.

brushing are used in Gram stain, culture and sensitivity, or examination of cell characteristics.

In alveolar lavage, a distal lung segment is wedged by the insertion tube and lavaged with up to 10 mL of fluid. The fluid and cells are suctioned with a vacuum source via the insertion tube channel and collected for laboratory study.

In bronchial brushing, a shielded small brush is used for brushing along the bronchial mucosa. The loosened cells adhered to the brush are then withdrawn back into the shield. The entire brush assembly is removed from the channel. A microscopic slide may be prepared by fixing the cells with a suitable method (e.g., acid-fast stain with Ziehl-Nielsen method).

Forceps Biopsy

Forceps biopsy is performed within the visual range of the insertion tube. Tissue specimens are collected by passing the biopsy forceps through the biopsy channel outlet. Once reaching the intended site, the forceps is then opened and closed by the clinician using the control handle. The tissues collected by the forceps is retrieved for laboratory study.

Transbronchial Lung Biopsy

In transbronchial lung biopsy (TBLB), the procedure is similar to forceps sampling except that the sample is collected during a forced exhalation maneuver. The patient is instructed to inhale maximally, and the opened forceps is advanced to the distal airway near the target site. The patient then exhales maximally, pressing the lung tissues against the biopsy forceps. The opened forceps is closed forcefully to collect the sample for laboratory study.

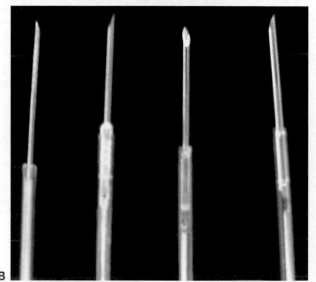

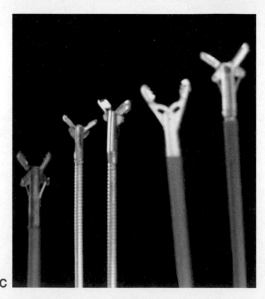

FIGURE 9-9 (**A**) Cytology brush. (**B**) Biopsy needle. (**C**) Biopsy forceps.

Transbronchial Needle Aspiration Biopsy

Transbronchial needle aspiration biopsy (TBNAB) collects tissue samples by applying aspiration while moving the needle at the sampling site. This technique is used when the lesion is beyond the bronchial wall and there is no lesion in the bronchial lumen. The distal end of the insertion tube is pressed gently against the target puncture site. The tip of the needle is then firmly projected through the mucosal wall. Aspiration (suction) is applied while moving the tip of the insertion tube back and forth and from side to side. The specimen (inside the needle) and the needle are retrieved from the bronchoscope. A syringe is used to expel the specimen from the needle for laboratory study.

Complications of Flexible Bronchoscopy

Flexible bronchoscopy is a safe procedure, but complications can occur. They may be acute complications (e.g., pneumothorax, hypoxemia, hemorrhage) or late complications (e.g., infections).

Pneumothorax

Biopsy instruments are sharp and far reaching. In extremely rare instances, pneumothorax may develop when the punctured lung parenchyma leaks air into the pleural cavity. Development of tension pneumothorax during positive pressure ventilation is an acute event. The signs and symptoms often include sudden increase in peak inspiratory pressure, diaphoresis, tachypnea, tachycardia, hypotension, and oxygen desaturation. Chest tube is required for large tension pneumothorax and it should be readily available during bronchoscopy procedure.

Hypoxemia

Hypoxemia is a common complication during and after the procedure. This may be due to increase in airflow resistance caused by the insertion tube, prolonged suctioning of lavage fluid, ventilation-perfusion ($\dot{V}/\dot{Q}$) mismatch from residual lavage fluid in the lungs, and hypoventilation induced by sedative and analgesic. Supplemental oxygen may be needed for up to 4 hours after bronchoscopy.

Hemorrhage

In bronchoscopy, collection of samples involves use of sharp instruments (e.g., needle to puncture structure) or traumatic procedures (e.g., forceps to extract tissues). Hemorrhage is often an unavoidable complication. Minor bleeding may be stopped by hypertonic saline lavage. For substantial bleeding, vasopressor such as epinephrine (e.g., 1 mL of 1:1000 epinephrine with 9 mL normal saline given in 2-mL portions) often stops bleeding from the biopsy site. Bleeding may also be stopped by wedging the bleeding site with the distal end of the insertion tube. In larger airways, wedging may be possible by inflating the balloon of a 6-Fr Fogarty embolectomy catheter inserted through a channel. Bronchoscope with a built-in coagulation electrode can also be used to stop hemorrhaging by using the heat-induced coagulation mode.

Infection

Infection is a late complication of bronchoscopy. In severe cases, infections by *Mycobacterium tuberculosis* and *Pseudomonas aeruginosa* have been reported. These adverse conditions validated the importance of infection control for reusable bronchoscope insertion tubes. Cross-contamination of healthy lung segments by infected ones may occur as the insertion tube goes from one location to another. Bronchoalveolar lavage fluid also poses a similar risk for cross-contamination.

Post-bronchoscopy Complications

Hypoxemia and arrhythmias are the most common complications during and after bronchoscopy. Continuous pulse oximetry and appropriate oxygen therapy should be used as indicated during the recovery period. Serious complications, such as hemorrhage and pneumothorax, are rare (0.08%). If a patient's condition deteriorates suddenly, physical assessment and chest radiography should be done immediately to rule out development of pneumothorax.

Post-bronchoscopy Care

Following bronchoscopy, the patient's vital signs are monitored until they are stable. Presence of wheezing and bronchospasm should be treated with a β-agonist bronchodilator. Uncomplicated arterial desaturation can be managed by titrating supplemental oxygen for a goal of > 90% SpO_2. Food and drink are withheld until the gag reflex has returned.

Cleaning and Care of Equipment

To prevent nosocomial infection, equipment and supplies used in bronchoscopy must be cleaned, disinfected, or sterilized as indicated. The insertion tube or portion of bronchoscope that makes contact with the mucosal membrane or infectious diseases (e.g., tuberculosis or hepatitis B) must be sterilized. Completion of sterilization procedures and restocking of disposables and consumables should be documented according to hospital protocol.

Mini-bronchoalveolar Lavage

Mini-bronchoalveolar lavage (mini-BAL) is a non-bronchoscopic procedure to obtain a lavage sample from the lungs. The most common application of mini-BAL is to diagnose presence of pneumonia. In a 2014 study by Meyer et al. mini-BAL diagnosed a significantly higher percentage of bacterial pneumonias than did nasotracheal suctioning. In addition, expectorated sputum commonly collected at bedside yielded no diagnoses.

Pneumonia presents many clinical signs and symptoms, including productive cough, fever, dyspnea, fatigue, and chest pain. To make a diagnosis, sputum samples are needed for laboratory studies, either by Gram stain, direct microscopic identification, or culture and sensitivity. The quality of sputum samples is dependent on the method of sampling. The least desirable sample is the sputum obtained by productive or induced coughs. These samples are "contaminated" with microbes in the mouth and upper airway. The most desirable sample is one obtained by bronchoalveolar lavage via a bronchoscope. This bronchoscope-directed sampling can target the suspected lung region, and the sample represents the microbial environment in the targeted location.

Mini-BAL Catheter

Traditional flexible bronchoscopy is an invasive and costly procedure. As an alternative, blind- or mini-BAL is a simpler and quicker procedure. This catheter may be inserted by a clinician with appropriate training and experience.

The results from min-BAL samples have a good correlation with the results from a traditional flexible bronchoscopy. The mini-BAL catheter is a telescoping catheter (**Figure 9-10**) with a suction adaptor, supplemental oxygen port, directional outer catheter, protected inner catheter, and a distal soft radiopaque tip. Laboratory data from this sample provide the clinicians the data they need to make an accurate diagnosis for initiation of appropriate antibiotic treatments.

Insertion of Mini-BAL Catheter

Mini-BAL catheters come in two sizes: 16-French and 13-French outside diameter. This mini-BAL catheter is inserted "blindly" without the guidance of a bronchoscope. For this reason, the precise sampling site is not known. However, the directional tip may guide the catheter to the left or right lung.

The catheter is not completely sterile, but a small dissoluble plug (or a soft cushioned radiopaque tip) at the distal end of the catheter reduces airway injury and contamination during insertion. Once the catheter tip is in a wedged position, up to 10 mL of lavage fluid is instilled. After lavage, the solution is withdrawn with

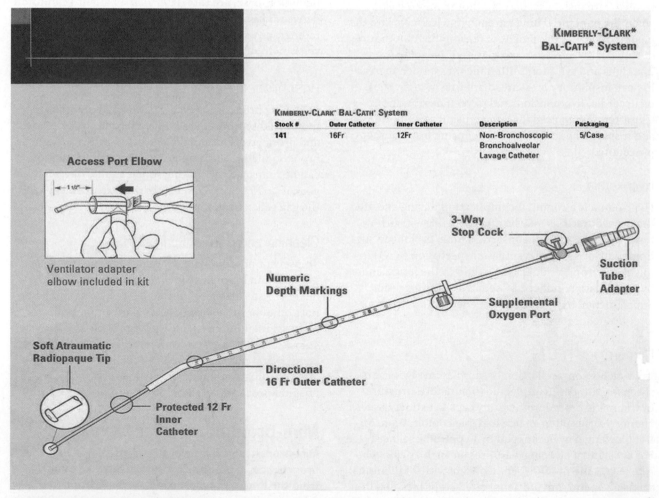

FIGURE 9-10 Kimberly Clark BAL-CATH System with a 16-Fr outer catheter.
Courtesy of Kimberly Clark.

a large syringe. The sample is placed in a sputum container for laboratory study. If residual lavage fluid is found at the distal end of the catheter, it is cut and sent for laboratory study as well.

Thresholds for Diagnosis of Pneumonia

The number of **colony-forming units** (CFUs) in a mini-BAL sample is used to diagnose pneumonia. CFU is a count of viable bacterial cells in a given volume of sample. For BAL samples, a colony count of $>10^4$ CFU/mL indicates pneumonia. At this threshold, the diagnostic sensitivity and specificity are 91% and 78%, respectively. It has a positive predictive value of 83%. The CFU count should be used in conjunction with other clinical signs and symptoms of pneumonia (e.g., fever, purulent sputum, lung consolidation).

Complications of Mini-BAL

During the mini-BAL procedure, the airways and lungs are subjected to vagal stimulation and suctioning of lavage fluid (and air), and accumulation of residual lavage fluid in the lungs. Oxygen desaturation is the most frequent complication. Other complications include bradycardia, arrhythmias, changing vital signs, and increased intracranial pressure. Occurrence of these complications may be reduced by preoxygenating the patient, using closed-circuit technique, and shortening the duration of lavage and suctioning.

Chest Tube and Drainage System

Tube thoracostomy is the insertion of a chest tube into the pleural cavity to drain air (pneumothorax) or fluid (e.g., pleural effusion, hemothorax, and empyema). These pleural conditions can afflict patients who are breathing spontaneously or receiving mechanical ventilation. Because chest tube and vacuum drainage system are commonly used in acute care settings, clinicians should have a good working knowledge of these devices.

Indications for Chest Tube

The chest tube provides continuous drainage of air or fluid until the underlying cause is resolved. A functional chest tube also relieves pressure buildup due to trapped air (tension pneumothorax) or excessive fluid in the pleural cavity (e.g., large pleural effusion). Indications for chest tube include tension pneumothorax, persistent or recurrent pneumothorax, hemothorax, malignant pleural effusion, empyema, traumatic hemopneumothorax, and postoperative care (e.g., thoracotomy, cardiac surgery). Chest tube is also indicated for pleurodesis, a procedure for instillation of sclerosing agents into the pleural space for the treatment of refractory effusion. Development of tension pneumothorax during mechanical ventilation is an acute and severe condition. If left untreated, it may lead to severe hypoxemia, hypotension, and circulatory collapse.

Pneumothorax (spontaneous or tension) may be caused by puncture of the lung parenchyma in chest trauma, excessive volume or pressure during positive pressure ventilation, rupture of bleb in emphysema, air leaks in bronchopleural fistula, and subpleural cyst. Iatrogenic (healthcare-related) pneumothoraces may occur during performance of thoracentesis or placement of central venous lines. Biopsy procedures during bronchoscopy may also lead to unintended pneumothorax.

Pleural fluid buildup may be caused by chest trauma (hemothorax), heart failure (pleural effusion), intra-abdominal infection (empyema), and blockage of lymphatic system (chylothorax).

Contraindications for Chest Tube

There are no absolute contraindications for use of chest tube. Relative contraindications include infection, unstable rib cage (e.g., flail chest), and persistent bleeding at the insertion site. Postinsertion bleeding, hematoma, and laceration of lung parenchyma or intra-abdominal organs are potential complications. Benefits of chest tube must be weighed against the potential complications.

Chest Tube Selection and Placement

Chest tubes ranging in size from 36 to 40 Fr are recommended for adults. Sizes from 28 to 32 Fr are suitable for teens and small adults. Chest tube size for children is 18 Fr and for neonates 12 to 14 Fr. These sizes are suitable for drainage of fluid, including blood (hemothorax) and pus (empyema). For pneumothorax, a size from 16 to 20 Fr is sufficient because air has a much lower flow resistance than fluid. In addition, air does not form clots in the chest tube as would blood or pus. **Table 9-6** shows the suggested chest tube sizes.

Because the pleural cavity is a sterile environment, the entire chest tube procedure should be done under sterile condition. To treat pneumothorax, the chest

TABLE 9-6
Selection of Chest Tube Size Based on Patient and Purpose

Patient	Size (French)	Purpose
Adult	36 to 40 16 to 20	Fluid Air
Teen and small adult	28 to 32 16 to 20	Fluid Air
Child	18	Fluid or air
Neonate	12 to 14	Fluid or air

tube is placed at the second or third intercostal space along the midclavicular or midaxillary line. For drainage of fluid (blood, pus), the chest tube is placed from the fourth to sixth intercostal space along the midaxillary line (**Figure 9-11**). With the patient in supine position most of the time, the midclavicular line is not suitable for drainage of gravity-dependent fluids.

During chest tube insertion (with or without trocar), the point of entry is directly over the body of the rib to avoid puncture of the arteries, veins, and intercostal nerves as these structures are below each rib. **Figure 9-12** shows the placement of a chest tube entering the mid-axillary line directly over a rib.

Operative Tube Thoracostomy

In **operative tube thoracostomy,** an incision is made parallel to and above the intended rib along the midcla-vicular line or midaxillary line. It is followed by dissec-tion into the pleural cavity. Digital inspection is used to locate the pleural cavity between the parietal and visceral pleurae. This technique avoids placement of the chest tube between the parietal pleura and the chest wall. Once the pleural cavity is located, the chest tube is guided into the pleural cavity by the finger and a hemo-stat (or Kelly clamp).

The operative method using a finger is more in-volved, but it is safer than the trocar method because the trocar is a sharp instrument. The operative method requires a larger incision than the trocar method be-cause the chest tube, finger, and hemostat must enter the pleural cavity simultaneously (**Figure 9-13**).

Trocar Tube Thoracostomy

In **trocar tube thoracostomy,** an incision is also made parallel to and above the intended rib. The chest tube with trocar inside is inserted through the incision. The chest tube/trocar setup should not enter the chest wall

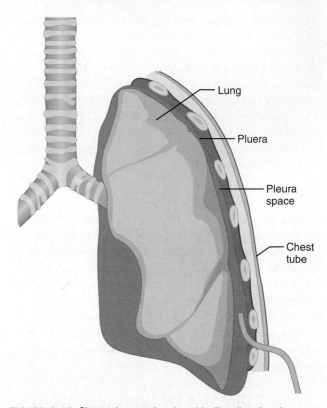

FIGURE 9-12 Chest tube entering the midaxillary line directly over a rib to avoid puncture of the arteries, veins, and intercostal nerves that lie below each rib.

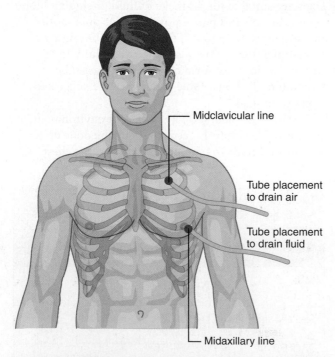

FIGURE 9-11 Chest tube insertion sites showing second intercostal space along midclavicular line for pneumothorax; fifth intercostal space along the midaxillary line for pleural fluid.

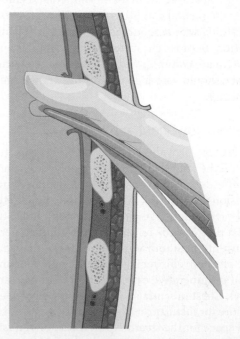

FIGURE 9-13 Operative tube thoracostomy. Note the chest tube, finger, and hemostat enter the pleural cavity simultaneously.

more than 1 to 2 cm, depending on the chest wall thickness. Deep entry may puncture the lung parenchyma. Correct placement of the chest tube/trocar setup in the pleural cavity may produce a gush of air (tension pneumothorax) or fluid (e.g., pleural effusion). Careful patient evaluation is crucial at this point because puncture of the lung parenchyma may also produce a gush of air.

Once inside the pleural cavity, the chest tube is advanced over the trocar into the pleural cavity. This process is similar to the catheter-over-needle setup in arterial line placement. The chest tube is clamped with a forceps before withdrawing the trocar completely. This method is faster than the operative method because it requires a smaller incision. Trocar method produces less tissue trauma and patient discomfort with adequate local anesthesia.

Following placement, the rigid chest tube is connected to the flexible tubing with a connector flange. Kinking and clotting of the flexible tubing must be avoided because these conditions will lower or stop the vacuum suction, hinder lung re-expansion, and may cause the air or fluid to enter the pleural cavity. Stale fluid from the drainage system should not be allowed to re-enter the pleural cavity due to infection concerns. Fluid contamination may occur during patient transport when the chest tube drainage system is placed next to the patient.

Chest Tube Drainage System

Immediately after correct placement of a chest tube, it is connected to a drainage system. Since fluid is gravity dependent, the chest tube drainage system must be kept below the pleural cavity at all times. The primary functions of a chest tube drainage system are to free the trapped air or fluid in the pleural cavity and to keep air or fluid from re-entering the pleural cavity. The most common chest tube drainage system in the hospital consists of three chambers.

There are also single-chamber and two-chamber systems. These two systems do not require a continuous vacuum source because they drain fluid by gravity. If suction is needed, a three-column system should be used. The single-chamber and two-chamber systems are easy to improvise. They can be a useful substitute in a mass casualty situation where three-chamber drainage systems are not readily available.

Single-Chamber Drainage System

In emergency situations when a traditional three-chamber drainage system is not available, a single-chamber system may be improvised by using common supplies. The single-chamber drainage system (**Figure 9-14**) works as a combined collection chamber and water seal chamber. It consists of a long tube and a short tube in a single unit. One end of the long tube is connected to the chest tube, and the other end is submerged in 2 cm of water. The short tube allows air and

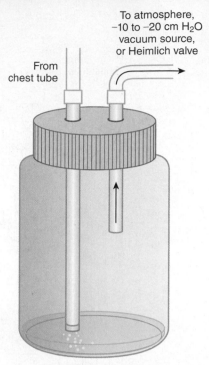

FIGURE 9-14 Single-chamber chest tube drainage system with tube submerged 2 cm H_2O.

Chest drain: FAQ. Available at http://www.medicine-on-line.com/html/skills/s0001en.htm

pressure to vent outside the chamber. A one-way valve (e.g., **Heimlich valve**) may be added onto this short tubing to prevent air from entering the pleural cavity. The 2 cm of water in the chamber works as a water seal that allows air to vent out but not return to the pleural cavity. The work of spontaneous breathing is proportional to the submersion depth of the long tube.

Since the long tube collects pleural fluid, the submersion depth of this long tube may exceed 2 cm over time. This means that the patient's work of breathing will increase as the pleural fluid accumulates in the column, increasing the submersion depth of the long tube. If the patient is on volume-controlled ventilation, the airway pressures will gradually *increase*. If the patient is on pressure-controlled ventilation, the delivery volume will gradually *decrease*. For this reason, the fluid level in a single-chamber system must be checked and maintained at 2 cm to avoid increase in work of breathing.

Some bubbling from the long tube is normal as long as air is leaving the pleural cavity. If bubbling stops, either the pleural cavity is void of air or an obstruction has developed in the system. A careful patient/device assessment should be done to identify the cause of air stoppage.

Two-Chamber Drainage System

The two-chamber drainage system (**Figure 9-15**) is similar to the single-chamber drainage system with one exception. The collection chamber collects the fluid drainage and the water seal function is separated in

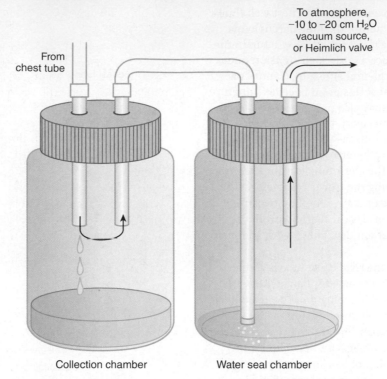

From
chest tube

To atmosphere,
−10 to −20 cm H₂O
vacuum source,
or Heimlich valve

Collection chamber   Water seal chamber

FIGURE 9-15 Two-chamber chest tube drainage system with tube submerged 2 cm H₂O.

Chest drain: FAQ. Available at http://www.medicine-on-line.com/html/skills/s0001en.htm

another chamber. The volume of pleural drainage can be measured from the collection chamber. The work of breathing is not affected by the drainage fluid because the submersion depth of the long tube remains unchanged at 2 cm.

Three-Chamber Drainage System

The three-chamber drainage system may be with water (wet) or without water (dry). This system requires a continuous vacuum source, and it is very versatile. It can drain fluid (or air), provide water seal, regulate vacuum level to the pleural cavity, and monitor air leak. The collection chamber collects fluid drainage from the pleural cavity. The **water seal chamber** has 2 cm of water and prevents air from re-entering the chest cavity. In some drainage systems, the cap for the water seal column has a pressure relief valve. It opens in case of excessive pressure due to a blocked suction source or obstructed suction tubing. This feature prevents excessive pressure in the system and pleural cavity. The **suction control chamber** regulates the amount of vacuum (suction) to the pleural cavity. In a "wet" three-chamber system, 10 to 20 cm H₂O is the recommended level in the suction control chamber. This will produce from −10 to −20 cm of vacuum to the pleural cavity (**Figure 9-16**). In a "dry" three-chamber system, the level of vacuum is set by a dial. Some dry systems have a preset −20 cm H₂O of vacuum (**Figure 9-17**).

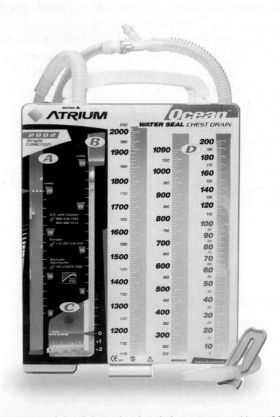

FIGURE 9-16 A "wet" three-chamber drainage system with 10–20 cm H₂O in the suction control chamber.

Under normal working condition, the vacuum draws air (if any, from the pleural cavity) into the water column in the suction control chamber creating a constant slow bubbling presentation. Too much bubbling in the suction control chamber means the wall vacuum is set too high. The amount of bubbling does not reflect the level of suction applied to the pleural cavity. The suction to the pleural cavity is determined by the water level and submersion depth of the venting tube in the suction control chamber.

The water level in the suction control chamber must be monitored and kept at a desired level (from −10 to −20 cm). Evaporative water loss in the suction control chamber will decrease the suction level to the pleural cavity. **Table 9-7** summarizes the operating features of chest tube drainage systems.

With a three-chamber drainage system, the fluid collection chamber should be inspected to note the volume and characteristics of the fluid drainage. When the drainage system is used to collect fluid, the volume from the pleural cavity should decrease over time.

Care and Removal of Chest Tube

Under normal operating conditions, the fluid will drain into the collection chamber. The volume, duration of collection, color, and consistency of the fluid collected in this chamber should be noted. This information is needed to monitor the progress of the patient and functions of the chest tube.

Drainage System Issues

The water level in the water seal chamber normally fluctuates with respiration. If no bubbling is seen and the water level does not move with respiration, this suggests the lungs have been fully expanded from compression or a kink in the tubing has developed. In pneumothorax, a slow bubbling in the water seal chamber is normal as the trapped air is gradually leaving the pleural cavity. If the bubbling is intermittent along with mild fluid movement, it suggests an intermittent air leak from the lungs or drainage system. If bubbling is excessive, air leak in the pleural cavity or drainage system should be investigated. This excessive leak is a serious problem and must be corrected immediately.

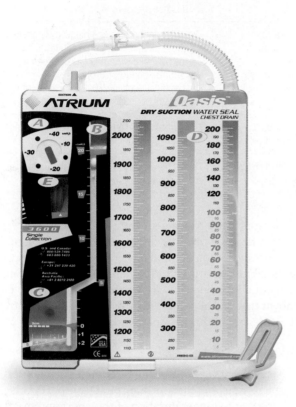

FIGURE 9-17 A "dry" three-chamber drainage system with a dial to adjust the vacuum level to the pleural cavity.

TABLE 9-7
Operating Features of Chest Tube Drainage Systems

System	Operating Feature	Caution
Single-column	Simple to improvise when three-column drainage system is not readily available Single chamber combines drainage collection and water seal functions	Work of breathing increases as pleural fluid accumulates in chamber No vacuum to pleural cavity; drainage by gravity Keep chamber upright and below thorax at all times
Two-column	Simple to improvise when three-column drainage system is not readily available Separate drainage collection and water seal chambers Accumulation of pleural drainage does not increase work of breathing	Open water seal chamber (may add Heimlich one-way valve or vacuum source) Keep chamber upright and below thorax at all times
Three-column	Require vacuum source Separate drainage collection, water seal, and suction control chambers	Maintain continuous vacuum from −10 to −20 cm H_2O Overfill of water in suction control chamber will increase suction level to pleural cavity (underfill of water or evaporative water loss will decrease suction level)

Chest Tube Issues

If the drainage holes on the distal end of chest tube become visible outside the chest wall, the chest tube has migrated outside the pleural cavity. Repositioning or reinsertion of the chest tube should be done as soon as possible by a physician. Should the chest tube be disconnected from the chest, an occlusive dressing (e.g., Vaseline gauze) must be applied over the incision opening. The dressing is taped on three sides to allow venting of excessive pressure from the pleural cavity.

Disconnection of chest tube from the drainage system is another urgent issue. When this occurs, clamp the chest tube and reconnect it with a new drainage system. Clamping of the chest tube should not exceed 1 minute. If a new drainage system is not available, the distal end of the chest tube should be submerged in 2 cm of water to keep air from entering the pleural cavity during inspiration. The physician should be notified for any of these mishaps. The patient should be monitored closely for signs of respiratory distress. Milking or clamping of the chest tube should not be done routinely unless it is done to clear visible clots in tubing or immediately before discontinuation and removal of the chest tube.

Removal of Chest Tube

The chest tube can be removed when the pleural drainage has stopped or slowed to <100 mL in 24 hours, or when the pneumothorax has resolved and there is no further air leak. The suture is first removed, and the patient is instructed to perform a Valsalva maneuver right before removal of the chest tube. The Valsalva maneuver builds up and maintains the pressure in the pleural cavity to keep air from entering. A petroleum gauze and dressing are applied to the opening immediately. Chest radiography is done in 4 hours to confirm proper lung re-expansion and to rule out recurring pneumothorax.

Transport with Chest Tube

On occasion, patients with a chest tube may need to be moved to another location for testing (e.g., MRI). In addition to an oxygen source, primary emergency drugs and airway equipment should be available during transport. The transport team must properly maintain the chest tube and drainage system by keeping the drainage system upright and lower than the patient's chest at all times. The chest tube and patient's vital signs are monitored during transport. Emergency supplies such as petroleum gauze, dressing, and Heimlich valve should be available for inadvertent chest tube disconnection at the chest or at the drainage system. **Table 9-8** summarizes the key points during transport of patient with chest tube.

Transport of Critically Ill Patients

Critically ill patients often have impaired organs or systems, and they may need special tests and treatments.

TABLE 9-8
Key Points During Transport of Patient with Chest Tube

Item	Note
Chest tube	Must be connected to a functional drainage system Must not be clamped or occluded (this action may prevent re-expansion of lungs or induce tension pneumothorax during positive pressure ventilation)
Drainage system	Must be kept upright and below the patient's chest (drainage of contaminated fluid into the pleural cavity may cause infection) Must not be tipped or dropped Must apply a continuous −10 to −20 cm H_2O vacuum source
Petroleum jelly and dressing	Should be available for chest tube disconnect at the chest
Heimlich valve	Should be available for chest tube disconnect at the drainage system

If the tests or treatments are only offered at another site (within hospital or another hospital), the patient and supporting equipment and devices must be moved together. Transport of critically ill patients should be carried out with a dedicated transport team. Evidence has shown that use of dedicated transport teams improves the outcome of this patient population.

Adverse Events

Adverse events (AEs) are more frequent during interhospital transport than intrahospital transport. This may be due to longer duration of transport and more unexpected intervening factors during interhospital transport. The patients undergoing interhospital transport typically have more acute and severe conditions.

Interhospital Transport

Depending on the patient population, severity of illness, degree of injury due to trauma, and mode of transport, the reported AEs during interhospital transport include hypothermia, drug and procedure errors, hypoxia, cyanosis, tachycardia, hypertension, hypotension, loss of intravenous access, unplanned extubation, and cardiopulmonary arrest. Some of these AEs could be prevented or minimized by allowing hemodynamic stabilization before transport. **Table 9-9** lists the potential complications during interhospital transport of a patient requiring ventilation.

Intrahospital Transport

For intrahospital transport, AEs include issues related to management, ventilation, circulation, monitor, and patient identification. **Table 9-10** summarizes the incidents reported during intrahospital transport.

TABLE 9-9
Complications During Interhospital Transport of Patient Requiring Ventilation

Complications	Remedy
Hyperventilation or variable tidal volume during manual ventilation	Use transport ventilator
Loss of positive end-expiratory pressure (PEEP)	Use transport ventilator with PEEP capability Use PEEP valve during manual ventilation
Unstable hemodynamic status	Provide a higher F_{IO_2}, determine and resolve cause
Loss of power or equipment failure	Begin manual ventilation
Hypoxemia due to extreme high altitude	Use pressurized aircraft Use higher F_{IO_2} Monitor expired tidal volume and increase volume delivery in hypobaric condition at high altitude (decrease volume on descent to low altitude)

Modified from Beckmann U, Gillies DM, Berenholtz SM, et al. Incidents relating to the intra-hospital transfer of critically ill patients—an analysis of the reports submitted to the Australian Incident Monitoring Study in Intensive Care. *Intensive Care Med.* 2004;30:1579–1585; Dockery, WK, Futterman C, Keller SR, et al. A comparison of manual and mechanical ventilation during pediatric transport. Crit Care Med. 1999;27(4):802–806; Farmer JC. Respiratory issues in aeromedical patient transport. *Respir Care Clin North Am.* 1996;2:391–400; Waydhas C, Schneck G, Duswald KH. Deterioration of respiratory function after intra-hospital transport of critically ill surgical patients. *Intensive Care Med.* 1995;21:784–789.

TABLE 9-10
Incidents Reported During Intrahospital Transport

Type of Incident	Example
Management	Poor communication Inadequate or inappropriate staffing Inadequate notice of arrival
Ventilation	Malposition of artificial airway Unsecured airway Unplanned or accidental extubation Incorrect portable ventilator setup
Circulation	Disconnection of vascular line Disconnection of connector
Monitor	Inadequate or inappropriate monitoring Incorrect alarm setting or setup
Patient identification	Wrong patient transported

Indications and Contraindications

Interhospital transports are typically done when the receiving facility offers a different (usually higher) level of patient care. Indications for interhospital transport include heart transplant, burn care, and hyperbaric medicine. Intrahospital transports are commonly done when the test or procedure (e.g., CT scan and MRI) cannot be done at the patient location. The following sections discuss the key elements in the transport of critically ill patients.

Contraindications for transport of critically ill patients include acute ventilatory failure, untreated refractory hypoxemia, unstable hemodynamic status, lack of secured airway control, lack of cardiopulmonary monitoring, and lack of qualified transport team members. Unstable patients (hemodynamic or neurologic) must not undergo a prolonged transport because the required resources for patient management are often not readily available during the transport. The patients must be stabilized before any transport attempt.

In regard to safety concerns, there is no oversight for transport teams. The Joint Commission does not have a set of mandated standards for patient transport. The Commission on Accreditation of Medical Transport Systems is the only accrediting agency and about 20% of the transport teams are accredited by this commission.

Equipment and Supplies

The availability of medical equipment and supplies during patient transport is limited because of time or space constraints. For this reason, the list of equipment and supplies is somewhat dictated by the type of transport (i.e., ground or air) and the purpose of transport (i.e., intrahospital or interhospital, duration of transport). **Table 9-11** outlines the basic respiratory care equipment and supplies for patient transport.

Types of Transport

Transport of mechanically ventilated patients imposes unique challenges because of the special needs: transport ventilator, emergency supplies, and experienced transport team. The type of transport is mainly dictated by the distance between the departing and destination facilities. Traffic pattern and urgency of patient condition are additional considerations. Five modes of transportation are available for patient transport: ground by ambulance; air by rotary wing aircraft (helicopter), propeller-drive aircraft, and jet; and sea by boat or ship. Transport by sea is seldom performed unless the location is isolated by a body of water and air transport is not available. There are advantages and disadvantages associated with each mode of transportation (**Table 9-12**).

Procedures for Interhospital Transport

Prior authorization between the transport sites must be obtained. Before departure, the patient is stabilized and all necessary equipment, supplies, and monitoring devices are gathered. Devices requiring batteries are fully charged. New batteries are installed for devices such as

TABLE 9-11
Basic Respiratory Care Equipment and Supplies for Patient Transport

Type of Equipment or Supply	Example
Patient assessment and monitors*	Stethoscope (different types and sizes) Pulse oximeter (Spo_2) Capnography ($Etco_2$) for prolonged transport or patients with head injury that require close control of $Paco_2$ ECG monitor Noninvasive blood pressure monitor Temperature
Ventilation	Manual resuscitation device** (different types and sizes) Intubation supplies Suction devices Chest tube decompression device (e.g., Heimlich valve)
Mechanical ventilator	Transport ventilator with at minimum these features: Battery Volume or pressure controlled High pressure and disconnection alarms Frequency, AC, SIMV, PSV, Fio_2, CPAP, PEEP Examples: Crossvent 4+ (Bio-Med Devices), EMV (Impact Instrument), Avian, LTV1000 and LTV 1200 (Carefusion), HT70 (Newport Medical), T1 (Hamilton Medical) Respirometer to adjust delivered V_T at different altitudes
Oxygenation	Oxygen source (cylinder) Oxygen devices appropriate to patient's condition
Medications	ACLS drugs for resuscitation and stabilization

*Because of the noise level during transport, all monitors should have visual and audible alarms.
**Not recommended for longer term transport due to inconsistent volume delivery.
AC, assist/control; ACLS, advanced cardiac life support; CPAP, continuous positive airway pressure; ECG, electrocardiogram; PEEP, positive end-expiratory pressure; PSV, pressure support ventilation; SIMV, synchronized intermittent mandatory ventilation.

TABLE 9-12
Modes of Patient Transportation

Mode	Advantage	Disadvantage
Ground	Distance <150 miles Low cost Safe	Traffic pattern Not suitable for long distance
Rotary wing (helicopter)	Distance <150 miles Not limited by traffic pattern on ground May land on rough terrain	Higher cost than ground transport Must have landing pad at both facilities Not suitable for long distance Noise and confined space
Propeller	Distance 100–200 miles Not limited by traffic pattern on ground	Require ground transportation between airport and both facilities Not suitable for long distance Noise and confined space
Jet	Distance >200 miles or intercontinental transport	High cost May affect delivered tidal volume with changing altitude Require advanced planning Require ground transportation between airport and both facilities
Sea	For locations isolated by body of water and air transport is not available	Require advanced planning Require ground transportation between dock and medical facility

laryngoscope handle and pulse oximeter. Spare batteries and size "E" oxygen cylinders are obtained. For safety concerns, the combined oxygen content should be at least twice the volume needed for a one-way transport. Monitors are calibrated, and appropriate alarm limits are set based on the patient's condition. All tubes and lines are secured prior to departure. Patient's vital signs, ET tube position, ventilator settings, and any adverse events are recorded in a log. This information is verbally reported to the staff at the destination facility.

Magnetic Resonance Imaging

Magnetic resonance imaging (MRI) is probably the most challenging and hazardous transport in terms of preparation, specialized equipment, and patient/staff safety. The strong magnetic field produced by the MRI scanner may draw metal objects to the scanner or render some medical devices inoperable. The objects include equipment with ferrous (iron-containing) materials (e.g., ventilator, oxygen cylinders) and implantable devices (e.g., pacemakers, defibrillators). Other devices that contain metal wires (e.g., reinforced ET tubes, pulmonary and central venous catheters) have the potential to cause burns on patients as the wires heat up near a strong magnetic source. All transport equipment in the MRI suite must be resistant to the magnetic source produced by the scanner.

MRI safe is a term to describe the equipment or device that poses no hazards in an MRI environment. **MRI conditional** describes the equipment or device that is safe under certain specified conditions (i.e., distance from magnet source, magnet strength). Occasionally, the ventilator may be placed outside the MRI suite while the mechanically ventilated patient undergoes the MRI procedure. Drawbacks with this strategy include an increased work of breathing due to airflow resistance of long tubing, an increased triggering pressure requirement, and loss of delivered tidal volume due to effects of tubing compressible volume.

MRI-Compatible Ventilators

Among transport ventilators, several are capable of providing mechanical ventilation safely in an MRI environment. Examples of these MRI-compatible ventilators include Hamilton-MR1, pNeuton (Models A, mini, S), Pneupac ParaPAC, Pneupac VR1, ParaPAC 200DMRI, CAREvent MRI, iVent201, and Servo-i (nonportable). Due to the special design of MRI-compatible ventilators, the type and number of alerts or alarms are limited. Critical care clinicians should become familiar with the available alarms for these MRI-compatible ventilators.

Summary

This chapter provides a synopsis of procedures commonly performed in critical care settings. The procedures and devices covered in preceding sections include arterial and venous access lines, intraosseous infusion, bronchoscopy, mini-BAL lavage, chest tube and drainage system, and transport of critically ill patients. Though the procedures are typically performed by different individuals with specialized training and background, all clinicians should have a sound knowledge of what is being done. Knowledgeable clinicians and a cohesive team approach should enhance patient care and provide better patient outcomes.

Case Studies

A patient in the intensive care unit (ICU) with bilateral pneumonia is undergoing a flexible bronchoscopy procedure to obtain bronchoalveolar lavage (BAL) samples.

1. **List the recommended medications for this procedure and describe the rationale for using these medications.**

2. **Should atropine sulfate be used before flexible bronchoscopy?**

3. **Define CFU and describe its threshold for a diagnosis of pneumonia.**

4. **What is a simpler method to obtain BAL samples without a traditional flexible bronchoscopy?**

   During rounds in the surgical ICU, the clinician is checking the chest tube and drainage system of a mechanically ventilated patient. A chest tube was inserted 30 minutes ago for a 40% right-sided tension pneumothorax.

1. **The suction control chamber is bubbling vigorously. Is this observation normal? If not, what should be done?**

2. **The water seal chamber does not show any bubbling. Is this observation normal? If not, what should be done?**

3. **What should be done if the chest tube is inadvertently disconnected from the chest?**

4. **What is the purpose of performing a Valsalva maneuver during removal of chest tube?**

Bibliography

Cardiac Monitoring

Epstein AE, DiMarco JP, Ellenbogen KA, et al. Guidelines for device-based therapy of cardiac rhythm abnormalities. *Circulation.* 2008;117:e350–e408. doi:10.1161/CIRCUALTIONAHA.108.189742

Jacobson C. Optimum bedside cardiac monitoring. *Prog Cardiovasc Nurs.* 2007. Available at https://doi.org/10.1111/j.0889-7204.2000.080402.x

Sandau KE, Funk M, Auerbach A, et al. Update to practice standards for electrocardiographic monitoring in hospital settings. A scientific statement from the American Heart Association. *Circulation.* 2017;136:e273–e344. doi:10.1161/CIR.0000000000000527

Arterial and Venous Access Lines

Ailon J, Mourad O, Chien V, et al. Ultrasound-guided insertion of a radial arterial catheter. *N Engl J Med.* 2014;371:e21. doi:10.1056/NEJMvcm1213181

Kornbau C, Lee KC, Hughes GD, Firstenberg MS. Central line complications. *Int J Crit Illn Inj Sci.* 2015;5:170–178. doi:10.4103/2229-5151.164940

Pittiruti M, Hamilton H, Biffi R, et al. ESPEN guidelines on parenteral nutrition: central venous catheters. *Clin Nutr.* 2009;28:365–377.

Robertson-Malt S, Malt GN, Farquhar V, et al. Heparin versus normal saline for patency of arterial lines. *Cochrane Database Syst Rev.* 2014;5:CD007364. doi:10.1002/14651858.CD007364.pub2

Intraosseous Infusion

Buck ML, Wiggins BS, Sesler JM. Intraosseous drug administration in children and adults during cardiopulmonary resuscitation. *Ann Pharmacother.* 2007;41:1679–1686.

Mason J. Easy IO placement (video). EM:RAP Productions. Available at https://www.youtube.com/watch?v=KHXSfh2ZRDM

Sá RA, Melo CL, Dantas RB, Delfim LV. Vascular access through the intraosseous route in pediatric emergencies. *Rev Bras Ter Intensiva.* 2012;24:407–414.

Wang HE. Intraosseous infusion. *Prehosp Emerg Care.* 2002;7:280–285.

Assisting in Flexible Bronchoscopy

American Association for Respiratory Care. Clinical practice guideline: bronchoscopy assisting—2007 revision & update. *Respir Care.* 2007;52:74–80.

Aderaye G, Egziabher H, Aseffa A, et al. Comparison of acid-fast stain and culture for Mycobacterium tuberculosis in pre- and post-bronchoscopy sputum and bronchoalveolar lavage in HIV-infected patients with atypical chest X-ray in Ethiopia. *Ann Thorac Med.* 2007;2:154–157. doi:10.4103/1817-1737.36549

Agerton T, Valway S, Gore B. Transmission of a highly drug resistant strain (strain W1) of *Mycobacterium tuberculosis*: community outbreak and nosocomial transmission via a contaminated bronchoscope. *JAMA.* 1997;278:1073–1077.

Alvarado CJ, Reichelderfer M. APIC guideline for infection prevention and control in flexible endoscopy. *Am J Infect Control.* 2000;28:138–155.

Culver DA, Gordon SM, Mehta A. Infection control in the bronchoscopy suite: a review of outbreaks and guidelines for prevention. *Am J Respir Crit Care Med.* 2003;167:1050.

Geraci G, Pisello F, Sciume C, et al. Complication of flexible fiber-optic bronchoscopy. Literature review. *Ann Ital Chir.* 2007;78:183 192.

Merck Manuals. Contraindications for flexible fiberoptic bronchoscopy. Available at https://www.merckmanuals.com/professional/pulmonary -disorders/diagnostic-and-therapeutic-pulmonary-procedures /bronchoscopy#v913167

Merck Manuals. Indications for flexible fiberoptic bronchoscopy. Available at https://www.merckmanuals.com/professional/Search Results?quer y=bronchoscopy

Michele TM, Cronin WA, Graham NM, et al. Transmission of *Mycobacterium tuberculosis* by a fiberoptic bronchoscope: identification by DNA fingerprinting. *JAMA.* 1997;278:1093–1095.

Pearson D, McLaughlin C, Shutak D, et al. Reduction in lidocaine dose administration for flexible bronchoscopy following order set implementation. *Chest.* 2015;148:808A. Available at https://journal.chestnet.org /article/S0012-3692(16)36707-1/fulltext

Pue CA, Pacht ER. Complications of fiberoptic bronchoscopy at a university hospital. *Chest.* 1995;107:430–432.

Srinivasan A, Wolfenden LL, Song X, et al. An outbreak of *Pseudomonas aeruginosa* infections associated with flexible bronchoscopes. *N Engl J Med.* 2003;348:221–227.

Wahidi MM, Jain P, Jantz M, et al. American College of Chest Physicians consensus statement on the use of topical anesthesia, analgesia, and sedation during flexible bronchoscopy in adult patients. *Chest.* 2011;140:1342–1350.

Weber DJ, Rutala WA. Lessons from outbreaks associated with bronchoscopy. *Infect Control Hosp Epidemiol.* 2001;22:403–407.

Yildiz P, Özgül A, Yilmaz V. Changes in oxygen saturation in patients undergoing fiberoptic bronchoscopy. *Chest.* 2002;121:1007–1008.

Mini-Bronchoalveolar Lavage

American Thoracic Society. Guidelines for the management of adults with hospital-acquired, ventilator-associated, and healthcare-associated pneumonia. *Am J Respir Crit Care Med.* 2005;171:388–416.

Mayhall CG. Ventilator-associated pneumonia or not? Contemporary diagnosis. *Emerg Infect Dis.* 2001;7(2):200–204.

Meyer P, Rousseau H, Maillet JM, et al. Evaluation of blind nasotracheal suctioning and non-bronchoscopic mini-bronchoalveolar lavage in critically ill patients with infectious pneumonia: a preliminary study. *Respir Care.* 2014;59:345–352. doi.org/10.4187/respcare.02356

Chest Tube and Drainage System

Chang DW. *Clinical Application of Mechanical Ventilation.* 4th ed. Clifton Park, NY: Delmar Cengage Learning; 2014.

Laws D, Neville E, Duffy J. BTS guidelines for the insertion of a chest drain. *Thorax.* 2003;58:ii53–ii59.

Transport of Critically Ill Patients

Beckmann U, Gillies DM, Berenholtz SM, et al. Incidents relating to the intra-hospital transfer of critically ill patients—an analysis of the reports submitted to the Australian Incident Monitoring Study in Intensive Care. *Intensive Care Med.* 2004;30: 1579–1585.

Blakeman TC, Branson RD. Inter- and intra-hospital transport of the critically ill. *Respir Care.* 2013;58:1008–1023.

Dockery WK, Futterman C, Keller SR, et al. A comparison of manual and mechanical ventilation during pediatric transport. *Crit Care Med.* 1999;27:802–806.

Farmer JC. Respiratory issues in aeromedical patient transport. *Respir Care Clin North Am.* 1996;2:391–400.

Livy K. "On the road again...." The transport of a critically ill patient. Canadian Association of Critical Care Nurses. Available at https://www.caccn.ca/files/7C%20On%20The%20Road%20Again%20(K%20 Livy).pdf

Waydhas C, Schneck G, Duswald KH. Deterioration of respiratory function after intra-hospital transport of critically ill surgical patients. *Intensive Care Med.* 1995;21:784–789.

Whiteley S, Macartney I, Mark J, et al. *Guidelines for the Transport of the Critically Ill Adult.* 3rd ed. London, UK: The Intensive Care Society; 2011.

©s_maria/Shutterstock

OUTLINE

OBJECTIVES

1. Describe the four components of pharmacokinetics.
2. Explain the principle of pharmacodynamics.
3. Describe the pharmacotherapy for aerosolized vasodilators and antimicrobials.
4. Differentiate between aerosols delivered via mechanical ventilator, noninvasive positive pressure ventilation, and high-flow nasal cannula.
5. Discuss the pharmacotherapy of medications that are instilled directly into the airway.
6. Explain the mechanism of action, indications, contraindications, and adverse effects of sedative/hypnotic agents.
7. Discuss dosage and delivery options for analgesics.
8. Explain the mechanism of action, indications, contraindications, and adverse effects of depolarizing and nondepolarizing neuromuscular blocking agents.
9. Describe the indications and mechanism of action for reversal agents.
10. Explain the mechanism of action, indications, contraindications, and adverse effects of vasopressors and inotropic drugs.
11. Discuss the pharmacotherapy of medications that may lead to methemoglobinemia and the treatment for methemoglobinemia.
12. Describe the pharmacology of drugs used to prevent deep vein thrombosis, ulcers, and delirium.
13. Describe the mechanism of action, indications, contraindications, and adverse effects of diuretics.

KEY TERMS

absorption	deep vein thrombosis	ketamine	opioids
agonists	(DVT)	metabolism	peptic ulcers
analgesia	distribution	methemoglobinemia	reversal agent
antagonists	diuretics	neuromuscular	tolerance
antimicrobials	elimination	blocking agents	vasodilator
benzodiazepines	inotropic		

Introduction

Since smoking stramonium cigarettes to treat asthma, pharmacotherapy for respiratory illnesses has come a long way. Clinicians deliver medication across a wide range of settings. This chapter will focus on pharmacotherapy delivered in the critical care setting. The focus of pharmacotherapy is always the patient. Clinicians need to prescribe the correct medication at the correct dose; pharmacists double check that the prescription is safe, effective, and completely correct. While RTs often administer these drugs, they should also be involved in patient education and troubleshooting. Before we begin learning about drugs used in the critical care setting, it is necessary to discuss pharmacokinetics (how the body processes drugs) and pharmacodynamics (how drugs act on the body).

Pharmacokinetics

There are four components to pharmacokinetics:

- **Absorption:** movement of a drug from the site of administration to the bloodstream
- **Distribution:** movement of a drug from the bloodstream to the tissues/cells (site of action)
- **Metabolism:** breaking down the drug (most drugs are metabolized by the liver)
- **Elimination:** removal of drugs or the waste products of drugs that have been metabolized from the body (most drugs are eliminated by the kidneys)

Absorption

The rate at which a drug is absorbed is directly related to the way it is given/administered. Routes of administration include:

- Enteral: direct entry into gastrointestinal (GI) tract via oral, sublingual, buccal (cheek), rectal, or nasogastric (NG) tube administration
- Parenteral: subcutaneous (SC), intramuscular (IM), intravenous (IV); IV medications go directly into the bloodstream (thus the fastest route of administration)
- Percutaneous or mucosal: inhalation, transdermal, topical, vaginal

Drugs are absorbed more quickly in areas where there is a large amount of blood flow, such as the lungs. Once a drug makes it into the bloodstream and can be used by the body, it is called free or unbound drug. The primary sites of absorption are the blood vessels and mucous membranes (located in the mouth, stomach, small intestine, and rectum).

Many factors influence how much drug is absorbed by the body. Drugs with an acidic pH (e.g., aspirin) are better absorbed by the acidic stomach; medications with an alkalotic pH (e.g., Maalox) are better absorbed in the small intestine. Usually an empty stomach increases both the rate of drug absorption and irritation because food slows absorption and decreases irritation. So, if a drug is likely to irritate the stomach, it should be taken with food; if you want it to act quickly, it should be taken on an empty stomach. Certain drugs require food in the stomach for absorption to take place, but this is much less common.

Lipid-soluble drugs are better absorbed through the GI tract. The absorption of topical drugs is affected by how long they are in contact with the skin, the skin's thickness, the size of the area where the medication is administered, and how well the tissue is hydrated. Percutaneous drugs work better on thin skin (infants, elderly). Inhaled medications work better if the patient takes a deeper breath, has lungs that are not diseased, and is well hydrated. Absorption here is rapid because of the lung's large blood supply. High concentrations of drugs are generally absorbed faster, so initial doses may be higher than maintenance doses.

Distribution

The blood level of a drug is the amount of drug circulating in the bloodstream. Protein binding and fat solubility influence drug distribution. For drugs that are bound to protein less free drug is available to act (this is how drugs are sometimes stored—bound to the protein, albumin). Lipid-soluble drugs cross capillary membranes more easily than drugs that are not. For this reason, lipid-soluble drugs reach their site of action faster.

Metabolism

Most drugs are metabolized in the liver. Drugs that are given orally are usually absorbed, in part, in the upper GI tract and exposed to hepatic enzymes (metabolized) before they even get to the bloodstream. This is called the first-pass effect or first-pass metabolism. Drugs that have a high first-pass effect (they are metabolized quickly in the liver) should not be administered orally. A drug's half-life is the amount of time it takes the body to inactivate 50% of the available drug. The longer the half-life of a drug, the longer its effects will last. Individuals who suffer from hepatic impairment will have a more difficult time breaking down drugs for elimination.

Elimination

Most drugs are eliminated via the kidneys, but other ways in which drugs are eliminated include respiration, perspiration, and defecation. Since the kidneys are the primary site of drug excretion, impaired renal function will result in problems eliminating drugs from the system. This is also true of other organs involved in elimination of drugs (lungs, skin, GI tract).

Rate of elimination depends on the chemical composition of the drug, the individual's metabolism, and the medication's route of administration. Because some medications are eliminated through milk glands, they may be passed on to nursing babies. If drugs are not eliminated before new doses are administered, the result is accumulation/cumulation.

Pharmacodynamics

For drugs to work in the body, they must attach to receptor sites on the cell wall. The drug and receptor site fit together like a jigsaw puzzle. You may have heard this explained as the "lock and key" theory.

- **Agonists** are drugs that stimulate the receptor site, mimicking the body's function.
- **Antagonists** are drugs that attach to receptor sites but do not produce a chemical reaction. Instead, an antagonist prevents other drugs from binding to the receptor site (this counteracts the expected effects of other drugs).
- Partial agonists form weak bonds between the drug and receptor sites. An example of a partial agonist is an antidote administered to neutralize a toxic substance.

Dosage forms may be solid or liquid, administered by mouth (per os or PO); percutaneous, applied to the skin or mucous membranes; aerosolized, taken by inhalation; or parenteral, given by injection.

Drug-Drug Interactions

One of three things can happen when two drugs are given together:

1. They produce individual drug effects but have no effect on each other.
2. The drugs increase the overall effect (additive or synergistic effects).
3. The drugs decrease each other's effect (antagonistic effect).

Tolerance is the reaction to a specific drug where its concentration is progressively reduced, requiring increased concentration or amounts of the drug to achieve the desired effect (you have to take more and more of the drug to produce the same effect).

Drug-Diet Interactions

Some medications need to be taken on an empty stomach to be absorbed more quickly. Others are absorbed best when there is food in the stomach.

Drug Actions

Drugs administered locally, such as creams or ointments, work at the site where they are applied. Drugs administered systemically are absorbed into the bloodstream.

Toxic effects of drugs include adverse reactions, which are unintended, undesirable, or unpredicted effects that cause unwanted symptoms. For example, gastric bleeding is an adverse effect associated with nonsteroidal anti-inflammatory drugs (NSAIDs). An allergic reaction, or hypersensitivity to a drug, ranges from mild to life threatening. Anaphylaxis or anaphylactic shock describes a severe, potentially fatal allergic reaction that occurs a short time after drug administration to a patient who is allergic to the drug or one of its components. Signs and symptoms of anaphylaxis include hives/urticaria, bronchospasm, shock (overwhelming vasodilation and hypoperfusion), cyanosis, dyspnea, vascular collapse, loss of consciousness, cardiac dysrhythmias, or cardiac arrest.

For the critical care medications that follow, we will explain the following:

- Generic name: the common name assigned to a drug when it is submitted to the Food and Drug Administration (FDA) for approval; typically, lowercase
- Available dosage forms
- Mechanism of action: how the drug works
- Indications: when/under what circumstances/conditions the drug should be prescribed
- Contraindications: when/under what circumstances/conditions the drug should not be prescribed
- Adverse effects/side effects

Drug Delivery

Dosage for selected drugs are provided in this section. Since the drug dosages are dependent on the patient's condition and characteristics, drug interaction and other factors, clinicians must exercise extreme caution during drug administration.

Aerosolized Agents (Other Than Bronchodilators)

Although certainly the most common medication, bronchodilators are not the only drugs that are delivered via aerosol. In critical care, clinicians also deliver aerosolized vasodilators and antimicrobials to their patients.

Vasodilators

Inhaled nitric oxide (iNO) (a **vasodilator**) works by relaxing smooth muscle of the vasculature to cause vasodilation. It is typically administered to patients in acute respiratory failure and pulmonary hypertension in all age groups. In a systematic review of 17 randomized controlled trials (RCTs) of iNO on preterm infants with pulmonary disease, the authors reported that iNO did not improve survival. Perhaps more importantly, the review concluded that infants with severe lung disease who were treated in the first few days of life experienced a 20% increase in severe bleeding into the brain. The quality of evidence was moderate to high in concluding that iNO does not improve the outcomes for preterm infants with pulmonary disease, and for the sickest neonates, iNO may contribute to increased risk of intracranial hemorrhage.

In another review, the objective was to determine whether iNO improved outcomes in children and/or adults with acute respiratory failure. After examining 14 trials with 1,275 subjects, the authors concluded that there was insufficient evidence to support iNO to treat either of these groups. Despite initial improvements in oxygenation after 24 hours, iNO was not shown to improve survival, and may be detrimental because it may lead to renal impairment (there was a statistically significant increase in renal failure in the iNO groups).

Aerosolized prostacyclin can be administered to adults and children with acute respiratory distress syndrome (ARDS). Prostacyclin is a naturally occurring prostaglandin (similar to iNO) that relaxes blood vessels, stops platelets from clotting, and has anti-inflammatory properties. Although the quality of evidence was low and only two studies met the standard for inclusion, the only systematic review of inhaled prostacyclin as treatment for ARDS concluded that there was not a clear improvement in outcomes (i.e., oxygenation or survival rates). On a positive note, these trials did not show adverse events such as bleeding or organ dysfunction. The authors concluded that more RCTs are needed before a definitive conclusion on its efficacy can be made.

Antimicrobials

Certain antibiotics (**antimicrobials**) can be nebulized for patients with chronic infections (e.g., ventilator-associated pneumonia or VAP), or as long-term preventive treatment in patients with colonization, as occurs in patients with cystic fibrosis (CF), those with bronchiectasis, and those on mechanical ventilators.

The medical literature to date does not demonstrate a clinical benefit to the use of aerosolized antibiotics in the treatment of VAP. Although aerosolized antibiotics used in combination with IV antibiotics appears to offer bactericidal advantages compared to IV antibiotics alone.

A systematic review of inhaled antibiotics to treat pulmonary infections in people with CF included 18 trials with more than 3,000 people, ages 5 to 56. The authors concluded that, when compared to a placebo, inhaled antibiotics both improved lung function and reduced the number of exacerbations. Nebulized antibiotics evaluated in the studies included tobramycin, amikacin, gentamycin, colistin, ceftazidime (a β-lactam), and vancomycin. Although adverse effects were uncommon with any of the antibiotics, tobramycin showed the fewest side effects. Current guidelines recommend inhaled tobramycin for individuals (≥6 years old) with CF and persistent *Pseudomonas aeruginosa* infection.

Along with systemic corticosteroids, aerosolized amphotericin B has been used to prevent aspergillosis (a fungal infection) in asthmatic patients and those with CF. Allergic bronchopulmonary aspergillosis (ABPA) occurs in nearly 10% of patients with CF, and recent studies suggest that antifungal agents may reduce the number of ABPA exacerbations in this population.

Aerosolized pentamidine (an antifungal agent) is indicated for prevention of *Pneumocystis jiroveci* pneumonia (PJP) in HIV-positive patients. It is most often used as a second-line medication, with trimethoprim-sulfamethoxazole as the first choice for PJP prophylaxis due to its efficacy, low cost, and potential benefit to prevent other opportunistic infections.

Because outbreaks of PJP have been described in renal transplant recipients, and aerosolized pentamidine is frequently used for prophylaxis in these patients, Macesic and colleagues examined use of the drug among patients who received kidney transplants. The authors reported that renal transplant recipients with a history of respiratory disease were at greater risk of developing bronchospasm when treated with aerosolized pentamidine.

Ribavirin is an antiviral medication that has been historically used to treat respiratory syncytial virus (RSV) and delivered through a small-particle aerosol generator (SPAG). Since its approval by the FDA in 1986, ribavirin has failed to make a significant impact on either mortality or length of hospitalization in this patient population. More recently, studies have shown that ribavirin is an effective treatment option for adult and pediatric patients who are immunocompromised as a result of organ or stem cell transplantation. In addition to broadening the indications for ribavirin, advances in aerosol technology warrant an evaluation of delivery devices. A study by Walsh and colleagues (2016) concluded that a vibrating mesh micropump nebulizer may provide an effective alternative to the SPAG in administering ribavirin.

Airway Instillation (Other Than for Advanced Cardiac Life Support [ACLS] Application)

Epinephrine is typically used to manage minor airway bleeding during bronchoscopy, but recommended doses and dilutions of epinephrine for endobronchial administration vary widely because of its unpredictable effects on the airways. Current guidelines contraindicate its use in elderly patients and patients with dysrhythmias and/or coronary artery disease since epinephrine may worsen the catecholamine response. It is further recommended that endobronchial instillation should be used with caution, especially when routine continuous electrocardiographic monitoring is not available or recommended in patients undergoing bronchoscopy.

Endotracheal instillation of local anesthetics, such as lidocaine, is commonly used to suppress the patient's cough during bronchoscopy. Lidocaine may be administered in aerosolized form through a spray catheter so that it is better distributed in the airways. Dreher et al. compared this method to administration via syringe through the bronchoscope. The study revealed that there was no difference between the two methods with regard to patient tolerance or safety. However, the aerosolized delivery method was associated with reduced dosages of both lidocaine and IV fentanyl (an opioid sedative).

It is common practice to instill normal saline solution (NSS) into a patient's endotracheal or tracheostomy tube before suctioning, even though evidence shows that it is unlikely to be effective in mobilizing secretions. The most recent American Association for Respiratory Care (AARC) Clinical Practice Guideline does not recommend direct instillation of NSS prior to suctioning.

Airway bleeding may occur either during or as a complication of bronchoscopy. Peralta and colleagues evaluated direct instillation of an absorbable gelatin and thrombin slurry (semiliquid mixture) as treatment for spontaneous and procedure-related bleeding. The study examined 13 cases in which standard procedures using cold saline and epinephrine were unsuccessful at hemostasis. The gelatin thrombin slurry (GTS) was administered through the working channel of the bronchoscope. Hemostasis was achieved in 77% of cases. Although more studies are necessary to determine its safety and efficacy, GTS may be a promising therapy to control bleeding during bronchoscopy.

Aerosol Delivery in Special Circumstances

In critical care settings, aerosols may not always be administered in the conventional way. They may be delivered via mechanical ventilation, noninvasive positive pressure ventilation (NPPV), or high-flow nasal cannula (HFNC). A systematic review of the medical literature comparing metered-dose inhaler (MDI) and nebulizer bronchodilator administration reported that there is not enough high-quality evidence to support the use of any particular delivery method via mechanical ventilation.

NPPV and HFNC are increasingly used in the treatment of patients suffering acute respiratory failure. These same patients may also be prescribed aerosolized medications. According to Hess, evidence supports both use of aerosol therapy in patients receiving NPPV and administration of aerosol therapy without discontinuing NPPV. More research is needed on aerosol administration during HFNC to make a recommendation on this therapy.

Sedatives/Hypnotics

Sedative/hypnotic drugs are central nervous system (CNS) depressants, reducing both physical and mental activity levels. The effects of sedatives and hypnotics are dosage dependent. Sedatives produce relaxation and a calming effect; hypnotics produce sleep.

Benzodiazepines

Benzodiazepines are a commonly used, fairly safe group of drugs that treat anxiety and insomnia. The prototype (first or typical version of a drug) is diazepam (Valium). Note all of the generic names end in -*pam* or -*lam*, which is much easier to remember than all of the names. Common drugs in this class include alprazolam (Xanax), lorazepam (Ativan), midazolam (Versed), and temazepam (Restoril).

These drugs are highly lipid-soluble (because they need to cross the blood-brain barrier to be effective). Their dosage should be the lowest to produce the desired effect without daytime somnolence/drowsiness. They are available PO and by IM or IV injection.

The benzodiazepines bind to benzodiazepine receptors in the brain and enhance the inhibitory effects of gamma-aminobutyric acid (GABA), the major inhibitory neurotransmitter in the CNS. They are given to treat anxiety disorders, such as generalized anxiety disorder (GAD), panic disorder, phobias, social anxieties, obsessive-compulsive disorder (OCD), and post-traumatic stress disorder (PTSD). They may also be given preoperatively to relax patients before surgery. They are sometimes used to produce sleep in patients in critical care areas—if these patients are able to relax, both work of breathing and myocardial work decrease, and patients use less oxygen and energy on vital functions that can instead be used in the healing process.

Although benzodiazepines are relatively safe compared to other CNS depressants, they should be used with caution in patients with respiratory impairment, in elderly patients (their metabolism is slower, so drugs may remain in their system longer), and patients with hypersensitivity (allergies to the drug or its components), renal, or hepatic impairment. Because most drugs are metabolized in the liver and eliminated through the kidneys, disorders of either organ impair its ability to break down and/or clear drugs from the body.

When the drug is discontinued, the dose should be tapered to avoid withdrawal symptoms. The most common side effects include dizziness, weakness, confusion, irritability, and memory impairment. The most dangerous adverse effect is toxicity—too much of these drugs can lead to respiratory depression or failure, coma, or death.

Hypnotics used to treat insomnia are usually prescribed for up to 4 weeks. These drugs should be used intermittently to treat insomnia because patients develop tolerance, reducing the effectiveness of the drug. Alcohol should never be used with a hypnotic. The elderly population consumes one-third to one-half of all sedatives and hypnotics prescribed because of the sleep disturbances that accompany aging. Also, chronic conditions associated with aging (arthritis, cardiac dysrhythmias, or dyspnea) tend to interrupt sleep.

Opioids

Most **opioids** are schedule II drugs because of the danger of addiction. The most commonly used drugs in the intensive care setting are morphine, fentanyl, and hydromorphone; they are used to treat moderate to severe pain. Opioids are available through nearly every route of administration, but the most common routes used in critical care include IM, IV, epidural, or transdermal. Opioids bind to opioid receptors in the CNS, activating the endogenous analgesia system. Transmission of pain from peripheral nerves is blocked, and the release of substance p (which causes pain) is inhibited in central and peripheral nerves. The result is analgesia, sedation, euphoria, and decreased GI motility. All patients may not experience all of these effects, or they may experience them to varying degrees.

In addition to treatment of moderate to severe pain, opioids are used to treat pain that often occurs during invasive diagnostic procedures (e.g., colonoscopy, labor and delivery, and postoperative pain). Other critical care patients who may be prescribed an opioid agent include those suffering from chronic pain (e.g., cancer; spasm associated with GI or renal system disorders).

Contraindications include hypersensitivity to the drug or its components, renal or hepatic impairment, respiratory depression, chronic obstructive pulmonary disease (COPD), and neurological impairment. Opioids should be used with caution in elderly patients because they are especially sensitive to respiratory depression and confusion. Meperidine (Demerol) and morphine are physically incompatible, so they cannot be delivered in the same syringe. They also should not be used together because of potentiation (one drug increasing the effects of another drug).

Adverse effects of opioids may include decreased GI motility (opioid-induced constipation [OIC]); nausea and vomiting (N/V); urinary retention (this may be problematic for men with benign prostatic hypertrophy [BPH]); physical dependence; respiratory depression, ranging from lethargy to coma (includes impaired cough reflex); confusion; and dizziness, lightheadedness, or orthostatic hypotension.

Ketamine

Ketamine is an anesthesia drug used in surgery and during certain medical tests and procedures that may not be well tolerated by the patients. It is delivered either IM or IV. The mechanism of action for ketamine is unknown. However, it is known to affect certain CNS pathways to rapidly produce a general state of anesthesia (loss of sensation and awareness) and analgesia.

Contraindications for ketamine include hypersensitivity, uncontrolled hypertension, heart disease, or alcoholism. Side effects may include bradycardia, shallow breathing, lightheadedness, dizziness, drowsiness, N/V, and blurred vision. Patients who are receiving CNS depressants may require more time to recover from anesthesia with ketamine.

Propofol

Propofol is the most commonly used parenteral (IV) anesthetic in the US. It is also used to sedate patients requiring mechanical ventilation in critical care settings or to maintain induced coma. It has a rapid onset of action and rapid reversal once administration is stopped. The mechanism of action for propofol is similar to benzodiazepines—it binds to GABA receptors in the CNS. It is delivered via IV.

The FDA recommends against propofol use in patients who are allergic to eggs, egg products, soybeans, or soy products. As with ketamine, if propofol is used for 3 hours or longer, it may affect brain development of a child under the age of 3 years or an unborn baby whose mother receives the drug. Propofol should be used with caution in patients who suffer from seizure disorder, renal or hepatic impairment. Possible side effects of propofol include shallow breathing, dizziness, or bradycardia. Long-term use can lead to Propofol Infusion Syndrome, which may result in death.

Dexmedetomidine

Dexmedetomidine is a sedative used in the critical care setting to sedate mechanically ventilated patients. It may also be used as an anesthetic. Dexmedetomidine is a centrally acting α_2 receptor agonist approved by the FDA in 1999 for short-term sedation (<24 hours) in intubated and mechanically ventilated patients. Because it does not work by the GABA-mimetic system, a mechanism common with other sedatives (e.g., benzodiazepines and propofol), it is free from respiratory suppressive effects. In a retrospective analysis of a multicenter, randomized, double-blind, placebo-controlled study of 33 postsurgical patients after extubation, Venn et al. found that no differences existed in respiratory rates, arterial partial carbon dioxide tension, or oxygen saturation in the dexmedetomidine group compared with placebo. Furthermore, the dexmedetomidine group showed significantly higher arterial oxygenation to fractional inspired oxygen (P/F) ratio throughout the 6-hour study period.

Contraindications for dexmedetomidine include hepatic disease, diabetes, hypotension or hypertension, heart block, and dysrhythmias. Possible adverse effects include bradycardia, agitation or anxiety, shallow breathing, muscle weakness, and cough.

Procedural Sedation and Analgesia

Procedural sedation and analgesia (PSA) uses a combination of low-dose sedative and analgesic to achieve mild to moderate sedation. Some of the sedatives mentioned in this chapter are often used in lower doses combined with analgesics to ease patients' pain, discomfort, and anxiety during painful or uncomfortable procedures (e.g., setting fractures, during cardioversion or a transesophageal echocardiogram). These drugs induce decreased levels of consciousness but do not require intubation. Patients are responsive, and their cardiopulmonary status is typically unaffected. The most commonly used sedatives include propofol, midazolam (a benzodiazepine), and dexmedetomidine. The most commonly used analgesics are opioids (discussed in the next section). Ketamine has both sedative and analgesic properties. Minimal and moderate sedation are considered levels of PSA.

Complications that may arise when PSA is used include allergic reactions and oversedation, which may result in cardiac and respiratory depression. Standard monitoring during PSA includes periodic stimulation to quantify the level of consciousness, vital signs, electrocardiography (ECG), and pulse oximetry. A systematic review of studies comparing capnography and standard monitoring to standard monitoring alone concluded that there was no difference in heart, lung, or airway complications with the addition of capnography.

Analgesia

Analgesia is defined as the feeling of no pain. In critical care, this outcome can be achieved by using different drug combinations (analgesics/sedatives) and in different dosages.

Pain

Pain is the most common reason people seek medical attention. An individual's reaction to pain depends on his or her perception of pain, pain threshold (the point at which pain begins to be felt), and tolerance for pain. Patients are generally asked the location of their pain, how long it lasts, and how intense it is on a scale of 1 to 10 (1 being least intense; 10 being most intense).

Acute pain usually does not last long. This type of pain responds well to analgesics when it is caused by actual tissue damage. Chronic pain lasts longer—often patients with chronic pain get used to it over time (their nerve endings become desensitized and a certain level of pain becomes the new normal). Intermittent pain indicates that there are times, positions, or activities when the pain is greater or less. Patients in constant pain do not get relief from their symptom. Local analgesics provide pain relief at the site of administration and in tissues immediately surrounding the administration site. Systemic pain relievers reach the systemic circulation and provide **analgesia** throughout the body.

Nonopioid Analgesics

While opioids and ketamine are used to treat moderate to severe pain, nonopioid analgesics are usually used to control pain that is mild to moderate. Most of the drugs in this category act on the peripheral nervous system (versus the CNS), and most do not cause physical dependency or addiction. They do not alter mental function or cause sedation because of the ceiling effect (once the maximum effect is achieved, increasing the dose does not increase the effects of the drug).

This group of drugs includes the following:

- Aspirin (acetylsalicylic acid [ASA]): This is the most commonly used nonopioid analgesic. ASA is sometimes given with an antacid to minimize irritation to the stomach. Drugs that have an enteric coating also prevent irritation of the stomach (the coating is resistant to the acidic pH of the stomach but is easily absorbed in the small intestine's alkaline environment).
- Acetaminophen can relieve pain and fever, but not inflammation unless the dose is high. It is relatively safe for most individuals except patients with liver disease. Acetaminophen rarely causes GI issues or bleeding, so for patients who take anticoagulants, this is the best nonopioid analgesic.
- NSAIDs include ibuprofen and naproxen. They can reduce fever and inflammation but are less effective than acetaminophen as analgesics. This category is often used to treat inflammatory conditions, such as arthritis.

These drugs described above are collectively known as anti-prostaglandins. Prostaglandins sensitize pain receptors, cause inflammation, increase platelet aggregation, and maintain the mucous lining of the GI tract. ASA and NSAIDs inhibit the synthesis of prostaglandin in both the peripheral and central nervous systems. Since acetaminophen only inhibits synthesis in the CNS, it does not produce adverse side effects on the GI system and platelet function.

Nonopioid analgesics are contraindicated in patients with hypersensitivity to the drug or renal or hepatic impairment. ASA should not be used in children under the age of 15 who have a viral infection, due to the risk of Reye syndrome. ASA should not be taken within 5 days of elective surgery because of its anticoagulative effects. The most common side effects are GI signs/ symptoms.

Neuromuscular Blocking Agents
Depolarizing Agent

Succinylcholine is the only depolarizing neuromuscular blocking agent. It is administered IM or IV with an onset of about 30 seconds to 1 minute, and duration of 5 to 8 minutes. Owing to its quick onset and short duration, it is frequently used for short procedures such as intubation. Succinycholine works by binding to acetylcholine receptors in the neuromuscular junction, causing depolarization and an initial muscle contraction. Since succinylcholine causes sustained depolarization, the muscle cannot repolarize, and the voltage is unable to change for the duration of succinylcholine (no voltage change = no movement). There is no reversal agent for succinycholine. Reversal time depends on the dosage of succinycholine and the amount of acetylcholinestrase (or cholinestrase) present.

Succinylcholine is contraindicated in patients who have a history of malignant hyperthermia, hypersensitivity, neuromuscular disease, or spinal cord injury, or who have had a recent burn or nerve injury. Adverse effects are rare, but may include hypotension, headache, dizziness, transient bradycardia, and muscle pain.

Nondepolarizing Agents

Commonly used nondepolarizing agents are pancuronium (long-acting), atracurium (intermediate-acting), and vecuronium (intermediate-acting). **Neuromuscular blocking agents** are used clinically to facilitate endotracheal intubation and to provide skeletal muscle relaxation during surgery. Available IM or IV, nondepolarizing agents block the transmission of nerve impulses at the neuromuscular junction, causing paralysis of the skeletal muscles (the neuromuscular junction does not depolarize). Tubocurarine/curare is the prototype. Most examples of generic names end in -*curonium* (pancuronium, pipecuronium, rocuronium, vecuronium) or -*curium* (atracurium, cisatracurium, doxacurium, mivacurium). Metocurine is a neuromuscular blocking agent that is secreted entirely through the kidneys and is contraindicated in patients with renal impairment.

Nondepolarizing agents are contraindicated in hypersensitivity, bronchogenic carcinoma, myasthenia gravis, respiratory depression, and hypotension. Side effects may include hypotension, dysrhythmias, dizziness, headache, flushing, and bradycardia.

Reversal and Treatment Agents
Naloxone

Naloxone is a **reversal agent** for treatment of opioid overdose. It is an opioid antagonist and competes for the opioid binding sites. Naloxone can be given through SC, IM, or IV routes. For patients with severe respiratory depression due to opioid overdose, 2 mg of naloxone may be administered via IV injection. For mild respiratory depression, 0.01 mg/kg may be used as the initial dose. Generally a total of 20 mg of naloxone is the upper limit for treatment of opioid overdose. If 20 mg do not show reversal, the patient should be evaluated for other causes of coma. Side effects of naloxone may include N/V, diarrhea, weakness, tremors, tachycardia, hypertension, shivering, and restlessness. Alcohol can increase some of the side effects of naloxone.

Edrophonium

Edrophonium (Tensilon) injection is used to reverse the effects of nondepolarizing neuromuscular blocking agents (e.g., rocuronium and vecuronium). It is an anticholinesterase agent—it slows the activity of cholinesterase (an enzyme that breaks down acetylcholine). By inhibiting this enzyme, a higher level of acetylcholine and return of depolarization at the neuromuscular junction can be achieved. Edrophonium should be used with caution in hypersensitivity, asthma, bradycardia, dysrhythmias, and renal impairment. Side effects may include chest pain, dizziness, fainting, irregular heartbeat, sweating, loss of bladder control, and seizures.

Myasthenic and Cholinergic crises

Myasthenic crisis is a condition in which myasthenia gravis is progressively worsened over a short duration. This rapid deterioration requires immediate treatment with an anticholinesterase agent (e.g., edrophonium).

On the other hand, cholinergic crisis is caused by an excessive amount of acetylcholine (e.g., overdose of anticholinesterase drugs). Atropine and oximes are two antidotes for a cholinergic crisis that include muscarinic and nicotinic effects. Atropine treats the muscarinic effect of acetylcholine. It competitively binds to the postsynaptic muscarinic receptor and prevents the excessive action of acetylcholine. For adults, the atropine dose is 2 mg. It is repeated until signs of atropinization (tachycardia, warm and flushed skin, mydriasis or pupil dilation) are observed. For the nicotinic effect in a cholinergic crisis that is due to nerve gas or organophosphate poisoning, the antidote is a class of drugs called the oximes (e.g., pralidoxime). With timely treatment, oximes are able to separate the bonded nerve gas or organophosphate from acetylcholinesterase. This action prevents or reduces the accumulaiton of excessive acetylcholine. Delayed treatment of a cholinergic crisis due to these types of poisoning may lead to permanent neuromuscular injuries.

In general, anticholinesterase agents (e.g., edrophonium) improve muscle strength in a myasthenia crisis. The same agents worsen muscle strength in a cholinergic crisis.

Flumazenil

Flumazenil reverses the effects of benzodiazepines. It is a GABA antagonist and may be administered intranasally or by injection. Flumazenil should be used with caution in patients with hypersensitivity. Possible side effects are dyspnea, tachypnea, agitation, dizziness, headache, and seizures.

Neostigmine

Neostigmine reverses the effects of nondepolarizing neuromuscular blocking agents. A cholinesterase inhibitor, it is administered by injection. Neostigmine is contraindicated in patients with hypersensitivity, peritonitis, or mechanical obstruction of the urinary or GI tracts. Possible side effects include bradycardia, dysrhythmias, hypotension, dizziness, and cholinergic crisis (if too much is administered).

Sugammadex

Sugammadex is also used to reverse nondepolarizing neuromuscular blocking agents and is administered intravenously. It works by binding the neuromuscular blocking agents, rocuronium and vecuronium, so that they can no longer bind to cholinergic receptor sites. It should be used with caution in patients who have renal or hepatic impairment, hypersensitivity to the drug, a bleeding disorder, low platelet levels, or respiratory impairment. Sugammadex can also diminish the effectiveness or hormonal birth control, so for a week after receiving the drug, alternate methods of birth control should be used. Possible side effects include flushing, itching, eye pain, weakness, bradycardia, N/V, headache, and dizziness.

N-Acetylcysteine

N-Acetylcysteine (NAC) is not a reversal agent but it is effective in treating acetaminophen (Tylenol) overdose. Acetaminophen overdose is one of the most common poisonings because it is found in a variety of over-the-counter (OTC) and prescription pain relievers. NAC prevents the toxic metabolites of acetaminophen from attaching to the protein molecules in the liver. The recommended loading dose of PO (oral) NAC for a 60-kg person is 8,400 mg, followed by 4,200 mg PO every 4 hours for a total of 72 hours (17 maintenance doses). A 10% NAC solution has a concentration of 100 mg/mL.

Vasopressors and Inotropes

Vasopressors are medications that cause vasoconstriction, increasing blood pressure. They are often used in critical care setting to treat hypotension. An **inotropic** drug changes the myocardial strength of contraction (myocardial contractility)—positive inotropes increase it and negative inotropes decrease it. Adrenergic receptors that are related to the list of drugs presented in **Table 10-1** are α_1, β_1, and β_2; dopamine receptors are relevant, too.

- α_1-adrenergic: Located in the walls of blood vessels, these receptors cause vasoconstriction when they are stimulated.
- β_1: The most common receptors in the heart, these receptors result in cardiac stimulation when they are activated (increased heart rate and strength of contraction).
- β_2: Clinicians are accustomed to working with bronchodilators that stimulate β_2 receptors, but they also cause vasodilation in blood vessels.
- Dopamine: These receptors, located in vascular beds in the brain, kidney, mesentery, and heart, lead to vasodilation when stimulated.

Patients receiving monoamine oxidase inhibitors (MAOIs) are extremely sensitive to vasopressors and require much lower doses.

TABLE 10-1
Vasopressors and Inotropic Drugs

Agent	Stimulation	Effect	Primary Use	Contraindications and Side Effects
Norepinephrine	α_1- and β_1-adrenergic	Vasoconstriction modest $\uparrow$ in cardiac output (CO)	Septic shock	Reflex bradycardia in response to $\uparrow$ MAP
Phenylephrine	α_1-adrenergic	Vasoconstriction	Hypotension with SVR <700 dynes/s/cm^5	Contraindicated in SVR >1,200 dynes/s/cm^5
Epinephrine	potent β_1-, moderate α_1-, and β_2-adrenergic	Low doses: $\uparrow$ CO, $\downarrow$ SVR (β_1 effects predominate) High doses: $\uparrow$ CO, $\uparrow$ SVR (α_1 effect predominates)	Anaphylaxis; septic shock (second line after epinephrine); hypotension postoperative CABG	Dysrhythmias; splanchnic (abdominal organs) vasoconstriction
Dopamine	Low doses: dopaminergic; moderate doses: dopaminergic, β_1-adrenergic; high doses: α_1-adrenergic	Low doses: selective vasodilation; moderate doses: $\uparrow$ CO, $\uparrow$ MAP; high doses: vasoconstriction, $\uparrow$ SVR	Cardiac failure; second line alternative to epinephrine	Cardiogenic shock
Dobutamine	β_1-adrenergic	$\uparrow$ HR and strength of contraction (+ chrono- and inotropy); vasodilation	Severe heart failure	Idiopathic hypertrophic subaortic stenosis

CABG, coronary artery bypass graft; CO, cardiac output; HR, heart rate; MAP, mean arterial pressure; SVR, systemic vascular resistance.

Vasopressin (antidiuretic hormone [ADH]) is used in the treatment of diabetes insipidus and esophageal variceal bleeding but may also be beneficial in the treatment of vasodilatory shock. It is mainly used as a second-line medication in the treatment of shock, specifically septic or anaphylactic shock that does not respond to epinephrine. Withdrawal of the drug should be tapered to prevent rebound hypotension. Side effects of vasopressin include hyponatremia and pulmonary vasoconstriction.

Drugs That May Induce Methemoglobinemia

Methemoglobin is an altered state of hemoglobin where in the ferrous irons attached to the heme groups are oxidized to the ferric state, which cannot reversibly bind oxygen. Normal levels of methemoglobin are 1% to 2%. There are two types of **methemoglobinemia**—congenital and acquired. In the congenital version, affected individuals have lifelong cyanosis but are typically asymptomatic. These individuals lack an enzyme that converts methemoglobin (iron in the ferric state) back to functional hemoglobin (iron in the ferrous state). Acquired methemoglobinemia is usually the result of certain drugs that cause excess production of methemoglobin, which shifts the oxyhemoglobin dissociation curve to the left.

The most common drugs that lead to acquired methemoglobinemia are dapsone (an antibacterial) and topical anesthetics benzocaine (e.g., Orajel), lidocaine, and prilocaine. Moderate levels of methemoglobinemia may occur when dapsone is used to treat dermatitis herpetiformis or *Pneumocystis* infection. In a study conducted by Swartzentruber and others involving 138 patients with acquired methemoglobinemia, 42% were the result of dapsone use. Dapsone should be used with caution in patients who carry methemoglobin reductase.

The most severe cases of acquired methemoglobinemia have been associated with the use of benzocaine spray for topical anesthesia or OTC versions (Hurricaine, Anbesol, Topex). In 2011, the FDA included this data in a Safety Announcement. Risk is greatest in infants and patients with significant airway or cardiac disease. The molecular mechanism that causes methemoglobinemia is unknown.

iNO is a pulmonary vasodilator used to treat pulmonary artery hypertension. During the binding and release of NO from hemoglobin, methemoglobinemia is formed at a higher rate than usual. Fortunately, methemoglobinemia during iNO administration is rare when NO is given in the acceptable dose range (5 to 80 ppm).

Nitroprusside (a fast-acting vasodilator) may cause methemoglobinemia in certain patients. Once nitroprusside enters red blood cells following parenteral injection, it receives an electron from ferrous iron (Fe^{2+}), resulting in ferric iron (Fe^{3+}), typical of methemoglobinemia.

Early symptoms of methemoglobinemia include cyanosis, lightheadedness, headache, tachycardia, dyspnea, and lethargy. If levels are high enough, respiratory depression, seizures, coma, and death may occur. Cyanosis is detected with methemoglobin levels between 8% and 12%; levels between 30% and 40% are considered life threatening.

In asymptomatic patients with methemoglobin levels <20%, there is often no other therapy required than discontinuing the drug that caused it. In levels >30%, methylene blue, which reduces methemoglobin to hemoglobin, is the treatment of choice. Dosage is 1 to 2 mg/kg of a 1% solution over 5 minutes. Methylene blue should not be used in patients with G6PD deficiency (congenital methemoglobinemia), because it may result in hemolysis.

Prophylactic Drugs
Deep Vein Thrombosis

Deep vein thrombosis (DVT) occurs when blood clots form in deep veins of the leg or pelvis. These blood clots may form as a result of damage to the veins, not moving for an extended period of time (due to surgery or illness), and pregnancy. Symptoms include erythema (redness), swelling, cramping, and pain at the affected area. DVT is treated with anticoagulant therapy. Most patients who are hemodynamically stable are typically treated with SC low molecular weight heparin (LMW heparin), SC fondaparinux (an anticoagulant chemically similar to LMW heparin), or PO rivaroxaban (an anticoagulant that blocks a clotting factor). IV unfractionated (UF) heparin is typically used in patients who are hemodynamically unstable or suffering from renal failure.

Pharmacologic heparin is the same as the heparin released by mast cells (it combines with antithrombin II to inactivate some of the clotting factors). Many of the generic names have -*arin* in them somewhere (enoxaparin, dalteparin). Heparin mimics endogenous heparin produced by mast cells; it inactivates clotting factors, inhibits conversion of prothrombin to thrombin, and fibrinogen to fibrin. LWM heparin offers the following advantages over UF heparin: greater bioavailability, longer duration of action. Laboratory monitoring is unnecessary because the correlation between clotting factor Xa and recurrent thrombosis is poor, and it can be used as outpatient therapy. Disadvantages include its higher cost and diminished efficacy in obese patients, patients in renal failure, and elderly patients who are underweight. LMW heparin is as effective as fondaparinux.

Patients receiving UF heparin undergo routine monitoring of partial thromboplastin time (PTT) or activated partial thromboplastin time (aPTT), international normalized ratio (INR), and/or prothrombin time (PT), all measures of the amount of time it takes blood to clot. It should be used with caution in the elderly and in patients with renal or hepatic impairment.

Possible side effects include bleeding and irritation at the injection site.

Peptic Ulcers

Peptic ulcers affect the esophagus, stomach, or duodenum. Peptic ulcers that occur in the stomach are called gastric ulcers, which are more common than esophageal ulcers. When patients have a peptic ulcer, there is an imbalance between cell destructive effects (gastric acid, pepsin, *Helicobacter pylori*, NSAIDs) and cell protective effects (mucus, bicarbonate, pancreatic juices, and bile). Seventy percent of gastric/stomach and 85% of duodenal ulcers are caused by *H. pylori* (a gram-negative bacteria). Gastric ulcers take longer to heal than duodenal ulcers, which are often chronic. Stress-related ulcers are more likely to be gastric. Drugs used to treat ulcers include histamine-2 receptor antagonists (H2RAs), proton pump inhibitors (PPIs), and antacids. If the causative agent is *H. pylori*, antibiotics (tetracycline, amoxicillin, clarithromycin) are prescribed along with a PPI or H2RA.

Antacids include OTC oral preparations (Maalox, Tums, Mylanta). These compounds neutralize gastric acid and decrease pepsin production (because they are alkaline, they increase pH, which prevents the conversion of pepsinogen to pepsin). H2RAs are available PO or IV. Generic names end in -*idine* (cimetidine [Tagamet], ranitidine [Zantac]). Histamine causes stimulation of gastric acid secretion by binding to H_2 receptors in gastric mucosa; H2RAs block those receptors so that they do not produce gastric acid.

PPIs are also available for PO or IV administration. Their generic names end in -*azole* (omeprazole [Nexium], lansoprazole [Prevacid], omeprazole [Prilosec]). PPIs inhibit the gastric acid proton pump so that there is no release of acid into lumen. They work better (stronger suppression of gastric acid) and last longer than H2RAs, which leads to faster healing and better symptom relief. Although PPIs tend to work better initially, for maintenance their effects are similar to H2RAs.

This category of drugs should be used with caution in the elderly (except PPIs), those with renal impairment (except PPIs and antacids that contain magnesium), and those with hepatic impairment. Side effects may include the following:

- Antacids bind many drugs and prevent absorption of others.
- H2RAs inhibit hepatic breakdown of many other drugs.
- PPIs may cause GI signs and symptoms or headache.

Delirium

No pharmacologic intervention, used alone or in a group, reliably prevents delirium.

Diuretics

Diuretics block reabsorption of sodium and water in the nephron, which increases urine output (UO) and depletes blood volume (reducing cardiac output (CO) and lowering blood pressure). Loop diuretics act in the ascending limb of the loop of Henle; thiazide and thiazide-type, in the distal convoluted tubule; potassium-sparing in the collecting duct. Loop diuretics are the most effective—furosemide (Lasix) is the most commonly prescribed loop diuretic.

Generic names include the following:

- Loop: most end in -*nide or -mide* (furosemide [Lasix])
- Thiazide and related: most generic names end in -*iazide* (hydrochlorothiazide)
- Potassium-sparing: amiloride

All but loop diuretics are administered PO; loop diuretics are available PO or IV. Loop diuretics are not typically used for maintenance therapy of hypertension, rather in critical care settings when rapid diuresis is desired. Thiazide and related diuretics are the most commonly prescribed and are used for long-term management of heart failure and hypertension. Potassium-sparing diuretics have weak action and they are rarely used alone to treat hypertension and/or heart failure.

Possible adverse effects for potassium-sparing diuretics include N/V and dizziness. For other categories, adverse effects include loss of potassium, dehydration, hyperglycemia (there is more glucose relative to the diminished blood volume, which may aggravate diabetes mellitus), and orthostatic hypotension.

Summary
Pharmacokinetics

The four components of pharmacokinetics are:
- Absorption: movement of a drug from the site of administration to the bloodstream
- Distribution: movement of a drug from the bloodstream to the tissues/cells
- Metabolism: breaking down the drug, mostly by the liver
- Elimination: removal of drugs or the waste products of drugs that have been metabolized from the body, mostly by the kidneys

Pharmacodynamics

- In order for drugs to work in the body, they must attach to receptor sites on the cell wall.
- Agonists stimulate the receptor site, mimicking the body's function.
- Antagonists attach to receptor sites and prevent other drugs from binding to the receptor site.
- Partial agonists form weak bonds between the drug and receptor sites.

Drug Delivery

In addition to bronchodilators, clinicians deliver aerosolized vasodilators (iNO) and antimicrobials to their patients.

- Antimicrobials may be used to treat a variety of infections.
  - Antibiotics are primarily used in patients with CF.
  - Antifungal agents have been used to treat infections in patients with asthma, CF, and PJP in HIV-positive individuals.
  - Antiviral agents are mainly used to treat RSV.
- Epinephrine and lidocaine can be directly instilled into the airway during bronchoscopy to prevent minor bleeding or suppress coughing.
- Aerosol therapy for patients receiving mechanical ventilation or NPPV may be administered via MDI or nebulizer.

Sedatives/Hypnotics

Sedative/hypnotic drugs are CNS depressants. Sedatives produce relaxation and a calming effect; hypnotics produce sleep (effect is largely determined by dosage).

- Pain is the most common reason people seek medical attention.
  - Local analgesics provide pain relief at the site of administration and in tissues immediately surrounding the administration site.
  - Systemic pain relievers reach the systemic circulation and provide analgesia throughout the body.
  - Opioids are used to treat moderate to severe pain; nonopioid analgesics are used to treat mild to moderate pain and include aspirin, acetaminophen, and NSAIDs.

Neuromuscular Blocking Agents

Neuromuscular blocking agents are used clinically to facilitate endotracheal intubation and to provide skeletal muscle relaxation during surgery.

- Succinylcholine (depolarizing agent) is often used during intubation.

- Commonly used nondepolarizing agents are pancuronium (long acting), atracurium (intermediate acting), and vecuronium (intermediate acting).
- Naloxone reverses the effects of opioids in an emergency situation like an overdose. Edrophonium, neostignine, and sugammadex can be used to reverse the effects of nondepolarizing neuromuscular blocking agents.

Vasopressors and Inotropes

- Vasopressors are medications that cause vasoconstriction, increasing blood pressure. They are often used in critical care settings to treat hypotension. An inotropic drug changes the myocardial strength of contraction (myocardial contractility)—positive inotropes increase it, and negative inotropes decrease it.
- Adrenergic receptors that are related to this class of drugs include α_1, β_1, and β_2:
  - Alpha-adrenergic action causes vasoconstriction when stimulated. β_1 receptors in the heart result in cardiac stimulation when they are activated (increased heart rate and strength of contraction).
  - β_2 receptors are commonly used to reverse bronchospasm. They also cause vasodilation in blood vessels.

Drugs That May Induce Methemoglobinemia

Methemoglobin is an altered state of hemoglobin where in the ferrous irons attached to the heme groups are oxidized to the ferric state, which cannot reversibly bind oxygen.

- The most common drugs that lead to acquired methemoglobinemia are dapsone (an antibacterial) and topical anesthetics, benzocaine, lidocaine, and prilocaine.
- Early symptoms of methemoglobinemia include cyanosis, lightheadedness, headache, tachycardia, dyspnea, and lethargy.
- Treatment for low levels (<20%) is discontinuation of the drug that caused it; for levels >30% methylene blue is the treatment of choice.

Case Study

Mr. Jones is a 75-year-old man who suffers from chronic obstructive pulmonary disease (COPD), the primary component of which is emphysema. He also has an enlarged prostate and has been diagnosed with benign prostatic hypertrophy (BPH). He is admitted to the intensive care unit (ICU) on a mechanical ventilator following lung reduction surgery. He has been prescribed morphine for pain. On postoperative day 2, Mr. Jones rates his pain an 8 (on a 1–10 scale) and complains of discomfort as a result of constipation. His urine output has drastically decreased. His wife is concerned that the morphine will cause him to become addicted, and has asked that he be prescribed extra-strength ibuprofen.

1. **What is the likely cause of Mr. Jones's constipation?**

2. **What is the most likely cause of his decreased urine output?**

3. **Is extra-strength ibuprofen an acceptable substitution for morphine?**

4. **Why should the clinicians caring for Mr. Jones be vigilant about monitoring his respiratory status once he is extubated?**

Prophylactic Drugs

- Anticoagulants (mainly heparin) are used to prevent DVT.
- The majority of gastric and duodenal ulcers are caused by *H. pylori* (a gram-negative bacteria). Drugs used to treat ulcers include H2RAs, PPIs, and antacids. If the causative agent is *H. pylori*, antibiotics are prescribed along with a PPI or H2RA.
- No pharmacologic intervention, used alone or in a group, reliably prevents delirium.

Diuretics

Diuretics block reabsorption of sodium and water in the kidney's nephrons, which increases urine output UO and depletes blood volume (reducing CO and lowering blood pressure).

- Loop diuretics are the most effective (furosemide [Lasix] is the most commonly prescribed loop diuretic).

Bibliography

Pharmacokinetics

Brenner GM, Stevens C. Pharmacokinetics. In: *Brenner and Stevens' Pharmacology Textbook*. 5th ed. Philadelphia, PA: Elsevier; 2017:11–26.

Pharmacodynamics

Brenner GM, Stevens C. Pharmacokinetics. In: *Brenner and Stevens' Pharmacology Textbook*. 5th ed. Philadelphia, PA: Elsevier; 2017:27–34.

Drug Delivery

American Association for Respiratory Care. Clinical practice guideline: endotracheal suctioning. *Respir Care*. 2010;55:758–764.

Afshari A, Bastholm BA, Allingstrup M. Aerosolized prostacyclins for acute respiratory distress syndrome (ARDS). *Cochrane Database Syst Rev*. 2017;7:CD007733. doi:10.1002/14651858. CD007733.pub3

Barrington KJ, Finer N, Pennaforte T. Inhaled nitric oxide for respiratory failure in preterm infants. *Cochrane Database Syst Rev*. 2017;1:CD000509. doi:10.1002/14651858.CD000509.pub5

Dreher M, Cornelissen CG, Reddemann MA, et al. Nebulized versus standard local application of lidocaine during flexible bronchoscopy: a randomized controlled trial. *Respiration*. 2016;92:266–273.

Gebistorf F, Karam O, Wetterslev J, et al. Inhaled nitric oxide for acute respiratory distress syndrome (ARDS) in children and adults. *Cochrane Database Syst Rev*. 2016;6:CD002787. doi:10.1002/14651858.CD002787.pub3

Hess DR. Aerosol therapy during noninvasive ventilation or high-flow nasal cannula. *Respir Care*. 2015;60:880–893.

Holland A, Smith F, Penny K, et al. Metered dose inhalers versus nebulizers for aerosol bronchodilator delivery for adult patients receiving mechanical ventilation in critical care areas. *Cochrane Database Syst Rev*. 2013;6:CD008863. doi:10.1002/14651858. CD008863.pub2

Janahi IA, Rehman A, Al-Naimi AR. Allergic bronchopulmonary aspergillosis in patients with cystic fibrosis. *Ann Thorac Med*. 2017;12:74–82.

Khoo KL, Lee P, Mehta AC. Endobronchial epinephrine: confusion is in the air. *Am J Respir Crit Care Med*. 2013;187(10):1137–1138. Available at https://doi.org/10.1164/rccm.201209-1682LE

Le J, Ashley ED, Neubauser MM, et al. Consensus summary of aerosolized antimicrobial agents: application of guideline criteria: insights from the society of infectious disease pharmacists. *Pharmacotherapy*. 2010;30:562–584.

Macesic N, Urbancic K, Ierino F, et al. Is aerosolized pentamidine for *Pneumocystis* pneumonia prophylaxis in renal transplant recipients not as safe as we might think? *Antimicrob Agents Chemother*. 2016;60:2502–2504.

Peralta A, Chawla M, Lee RP. Novel bronchoscopic management of airway bleeding with absorbable gelatin and thrombin slurry. *J Bronchol Intervent Pulmonol*. 2018;25:204–211.

Smith S, Rowbotham NJ, Regan KH. Inhaled anti-pseudomonal antibiotics for long-term therapy in cystic fibrosis. *Cochrane Database Syst Rev*. 2018;3:CD001021. doi:10.1002/14651858 .CD001021.pub3

Walsh BK, Betit P, Fink JB, et al. Characterization of ribavirin aerosol with small particle aerosol generator and vibrating mesh micropump aerosol technologies. *Respir Care*. 2016;61:577–585.

Zhang C, Berra L, Klompas M. Should aerosolized antibiotics be used to treat ventilator-associated pneumonias? *Respir Care*. 2016;61:737–748.

Sedatives/Hyponotics

Benzodiazepines. Drugs.com. Available at https://www.drugs.com/drug-class/ benzodiazepines.html

Juels AN. Procedural sedation. Available at https://emedicine.medscape.com/article/109695-overview

Ketamine. Drugs.com. Available at https://www.drugs.com/mtm/ketamine.html

Lam SW, Alexander E. Drug update: dexmedetomidine use in critical care. *AACN Adv Crit Care*. 2008;19:113–120.

Narcotic analgesics. Drugs.com. Available at https://www.drugs.com/drug-class /narcotic-analgesics.html

Propofol. Drugs.com. Available at https://www.drugs.com/propofol.html

Sjogren P, Elsner F, Kaasa S. Non-opioid analgesics. In: Cherny N, Fallon F, Kaasa S, et al, eds. *Oxford Textbook of Palliative Medicine*. 5th ed. Oxford, UK: Oxford University Press; 2015. doi:10.1093/med/9780199656097 .001.0001

Venn RM, Hell J, Grounds RM. Respiratory effects of dexmedetomidine in the surgical patient requiring intensive care. *Crit Care*. 2000;4:302–308.

Wall BF, Magee K, Campbell SG, et al. Use of capnography in emergency department patients being sedated for procedures. *Cochrane Database Syst Rev*. 2017;3:CD010698. doi:10.1002/14651858. CD010698.pub2

Analgesia

Brenner GM, Stevens C. Pharmacokinetics. In: *Brenner and Stevens' Pharmacology Textbook*. 5th ed. Philadelphia, PA: Elsevier; 2017: 261–272.

Neuromuscular Blocking Agents

Renew JR, Naguuib M. Clinical use of neuromuscular blocking agents in anesthesia. UpToDate. Available at https://www.uptodate .com/contents/clinical-use-of-neuromuscular-blocking-agents-in -anesthesia

Reversal Agents

Edrophonium. Drugs.com. Available at https://www.drugs.com/cons /edrophonium -injection.html

Flumazenil. Drugs.com. Available at https://www.drugs.com/mtm /flumazenil.html

Neostigmine. Drugs.com. Available at https://www.drugs.com/pro /neostigmine -methylsulfate-injection.html

Sugammadex. Drugs.com. Available at https://www.drugs.com/mtm /sugammadex.html

Vasopressors and Inotopes

Manaker S. Use of vasopressors and inotropes. UpToDate. Available at https:// www.uptodate.com/contents/use-of-vasopressors-and-inotropes? search=vasopressors&source=search_result&selectedTitle=1~150 &usage_type=default&display_rank=1

Drugs That May Induce Methemoglobinemia

Prchal JT. Clinical features, diagnosis, and treatment of methemoglobinemia. UpToDate. Available at https://www.uptodate.com/contents/clinical-features-diagnosis-and-treatment-of-methemoglobinemia?search=methemoglobinemia&source=search_result&selectedTitle=1~150&usage_type=default&display_rank=1

Swartzentruber GS, Yanta JH, Pizon. Methemoglobinemia as a complication of topical dapsone. *New England Journal of Medicine.* 2015;372(5):491–492.

FDA. Risk of serious and potentially fatal blood disorder prompts FDA action on oral over-the-counter benzocaine products used for teething and mouth pain and prescription local anesthetics. Available at https://www.fda.gov/drugs/drug-safety-and-availability/risk-serious-and-potentially-fatal-blood-disorder-prompts-fda-action-oral-over-counter-benzocaine.

Prophylactic Drugs

Francis J. Delirium and acute confusional states: prevention, treatment and prognosis. UpToDate. Available at https://www.uptodate.com/contents/delirium-and-acute-confusional-states-prevention-treatment-and-prognosis?search=prevention%20of%20delirium&source= search_result&selectedTitle=1~150&usage_type=default& display_rank=1

Lip GY, Hull RD. Venous thromboembolism: initiation of anticoagulation. UpToDate. Available at https://www.uptodate.com/contents/venous-thromboembolism-initiation-of-anticoagulation-first-10-days?search=heparin&source=search_result&selectedTitle=4~148&usage_type=default&display_rank=3

Medications for stomach ulcer. Drugs.com. Available at https://www.drugs.com /mcd/peptic-ulcer

Diuretics

Brater DC, Ellison DH. Mechanism of action of diuretics. UpToDate. Available at https://www.uptodate.com/contents/mechanism-of-action-of-diuretics?search=diuretics&source=search_result&selectedTitle=1~150&usage_type=default&display_rank=1

Naloxone. Drugs.com. Available at https://www.drugs.com/pro/naloxone.html Zhang C, Berra L, Klompas M: Should aerosolized antibiotics be used to treat ventilator-associated pneumonias? *Respir Care* 61:737–748, 2016.

11

Weaning from Mechanical Ventilation

Jonathan B. Waugh, PhD, RRT, RPFT, FAARC

©s_maria/Shutterstock

OBJECTIVES

1. Define success and failure for discontinuing mechanical ventilation.
2. Contrast simple, difficult, and prolonged weaning from mechanical ventilation.
3. Explain how criteria for assessing ventilation, oxygenation, and pulmonary measurements are used to evaluate patient readiness to start the weaning process.
4. Describe how to prepare patients to increase the likelihood of a successful weaning outcome.
5. Describe the following weaning procedures: spontaneous breathing trial, SIMV, and pressure support ventilation.
6. Describe assessment techniques for determining extubation readiness.
7. List options that can reduce the need for reintubation and the conditions when they would most likely be used.
8. List the causes of weaning failure.
9. Explain when a gradual weaning approach would be considered over a daily diagnostic spontaneous breathing trial.
10. Summarize the key points of referenced national consensus guidelines on weaning and discontinuing ventilator support.
11. Describe the leading causes of failure for attempts to liberate patients from mechanical ventilation and ways to correct them.
12. Differentiate withholding and withdrawing of mechanical ventilation.
13. Differentiate between prolonged mechanical ventilation and chronic ventilator dependence.
14. Explain when a tracheostomy tube is considered in the weaning process and describe its potential benefits.

KEY TERMS

chronic ventilator
  dependence
esophageal pressure
likelihood ratio
pressure support
  ventilation (PSV)
pressure-time index

pressure-time product
prolonged ventilator
  dependence
rapid shallow breathing
  index (RSBI)
respiratory muscle training
shunt fraction

spontaneous breathing
  trial (SBT)
synchronized intermittent
  mandatory
  ventilation (SIMV)
ventilator weaning/
  discontinuance

weaning failure
weaning success
weaning protocol
work of breathing (WOB)

This chapter applies to the following sections of the Advanced Critical Care Specialty Exam:

ACCS I, C, 6, a. Liberation (weaning) from mechanical ventilation

ACCS II, F, 3. Minimizing intubation time, for example, aggressive weaning protocols

ACCS II, H, 3. Withdrawal of life support

Introduction

Mechanical ventilation in its various forms is often a lifesaving intervention but even soon after initiation, the goal is to liberate the patient as soon as possible. The modality is not a treatment or cure but a form of life support until a remedy for the cause of breathing dependence can be accomplished. The longer someone receives mechanical ventilation, the greater the risk of hazards and complications, so the goal is to remove patients from a ventilator as soon as safely possible. This is true even for patients who have **prolonged ventilator dependence** (need for mechanical ventilation for >6 hours/day for >21 days) because the potential for recovery is fluid and can be altered by unseen factors. Proceeding too quickly can also endanger a patient. Reducing time on a ventilator to the shortest period possible is a worthy intermediate goal while waiting for what will allow the final step to liberation. Discontinuing mechanical ventilation should first be safe, and then be conducted as quickly as possible.

Terminology for appropriately discontinuing mechanical ventilation support has expanded to include liberation and discontinuation. However, it is unlikely that the long-standing term *weaning* will diminish in use because of its broad acceptance by clinicians. The majority of patients who receive mechanical ventilation do not require a sophisticated weaning approach. This group is largely composed of postsurgical patients who require breathing support only until anesthesia wears off and hemodynamic stability returns. These otherwise healthy patients will wake up and assume spontaneous breathing even if weaning management is somewhat inept. The remaining patients who have complicated recoveries, comorbidities, and other challenges require clinicians with advanced understanding and expertise to help them resume independent breathing. Failure with this group often means more than just extending the time to wean; it can also have dire and costly consequences for the patients. An interprofessional team

approach to **ventilator weaning/discontinuance** further enhances the ability to help difficult-to-wean patients. Current weaning techniques continue to be refined, and new approaches are being investigated.

Defining Weaning, Weaning Success, and Weaning Failure

More than one meaning has been assigned to the term *weaning* in the literature, so for the sake of clarity we will define a weaning process, weaning success, and weaning failure. A weaning process involves a progressive means of reducing the level of support from artificial ventilation with the goal of transition to independent, spontaneous breathing. It may be rapid or gradual, but it implies a process rather than an event. If a patient is successfully removed from mechanical ventilation in an abrupt fashion, some consider this to be weaning, but the term *ventilator discontinuation* is probably more appropriate. Even if the weaning process does not result in independent ventilation, it may still produce benefit (if not success) by reducing the level of ventilatory support needed (reduction in pressures, frequency, supplemental oxygen, hours per day on a ventilator, etc.).

The medical literature contains multiple definitions of weaning success and failure. The addition of **spontaneous breathing trials (SBTs)** has complicated interpretation of outcomes. This is partly because SBT has meant both a weaning method (alternating periods of spontaneous and supported breathing) and more recently an assessment of the patient's ability to breathe spontaneously at the start of weaning (with or without low levels of pressure support ventilation [PSV] and continuous positive airway pressure [CPAP]). **Weaning success** is defined as persistence of spontaneous breathing for at least 48 hours following extubation. **Weaning failure** is defined as either the failure of an SBT or the need for reintubation within 48 hours following extubation (see **Box 11-1**).

When the healthcare team's assessment of a mechanically ventilated patient determines readiness to begin weaning, a SBT is typically conducted to assess if the patient is ready to discontinue ventilatory support. The patient may undergo several daily SBTs before being able to remain off the ventilator for a sufficient time to be deemed a weaning success. Herein lies some of the difficulty with communicating outcomes clearly in the patient record, to members of the healthcare team,

BOX 11-1 Objective and Subjective Indications of Spontaneous Breathing Trial (SBT) Failure

Failure of SBT is characterized by:

1. Objective indices of failure, such as tachypnea, tachycardia, hypertension, hypotension, hypoxemia or acidosis, arrhythmia; and

2. Subjective indices, such as agitation or distress, depressed mental status, diaphoresis, and evidence of increasing effort.

Failure of an SBT is often related to cardiovascular dysfunction or inability of the respiratory system to support the load of breathing.

and to the patient's family. According to the prevailing definition of weaning failure, not passing an initial SBT assessment would be considered a weaning failure. After several SBT failures, a gradual approach is often employed to condition the patient sufficiently to assume the workload of self-reliant breathing. Difficult-to-wean patients are often moved to special units within the hospital or subacute care facilities that are better equipped for team-based weaning approaches that require more time.

Stages of Weaning

There is a tendency with any multistep process for some aspects to receive less attention than others even though all may be important. Tobin described weaning as seven possible stages to help ensure a thoughtful way of approaching the process and avoid overlooking some part of it (**Figure 11-1**). Stage 1 is "Preweaning," when weaning is not desirable because the patient is not sufficiently recovered or may need conditioning to address atrophied muscles. It may be obvious from clinical signs that even attempting an assessment for weaning readiness would be inappropriate and possibly dangerous to the patient. The clinician uses ingenuity and all resources available to keep this stage as short as possible. While few, some patients remain at this stage and are

termed *chronically ventilator dependent* (i.e., as might occur with a high spinal cord injury).

The transition to Stage 2, "Suspicion of Readiness," occurs when members of the team observe indications that the patient may be ready for weaning and confer for consensus. Awareness of potential patient readiness might seem like it would be somewhat obvious to experienced professionals, but a number of studies do not support this assertion. The large studies conducted by Esteban and Brochard found that many patients are ventilated for a week or more and then successfully discontinued from mechanical ventilation on the first day they are assessed for weaning. That raises the question, Could those patients have tolerated an earlier start on weaning and extubation? This may suggest that clinicians tend to be too conservative when determining when to start the weaning process. If that is the case, a bigger question is, Why do we caregivers have this tendency when we know unnecessary time on a ventilator can be harmful? Some, as chronicled by journalist Malcolm Gladwell, have suggested that when faced with too much information, it predictably hinders decision making. If this is true for identifying when the weaning process ought to start, then we need to work at consistently focusing upon a specific set of most useful measurements and observations. Another influence may be what psychologist and Nobel laureate Daniel Kahneman described as the conflict between the experiencing self and the reflecting self. For example, although the information we observe may indicate a patient is ready for a weaning attempt, our memory of a very bad weaning failure in the past may carry so much influence in decision making that it outweighs what data are clearly indicating in the present. This might also affect decision making on the pace of weaning as well as the starting point. Kahneman also contrasted human thinking as two independent systems, one being fast, intuitive, and requiring little effort but prone to error; the other being slower, using careful thinking and deductive reasoning, and consequently requiring more effort. It is easy to see why the intuitive method would be used more frequently than a reasoned approach, especially if someone feels confident about making quick decisions based upon experience. Following an evidence-based protocol

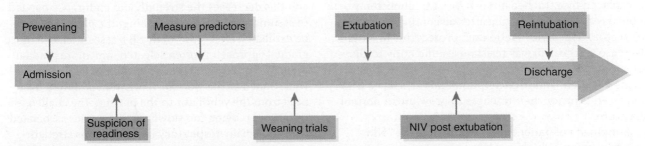

FIGURE 11-1 Stages of weaning. NIV, noninvasive ventilation.

to guide weaning helps protect against being too liberal or conservative in the weaning process.

"Measuring predictors" of weaning readiness in Stage 3 involves obtaining physiologic measurements that serve as predictors and integrating that information with each patient's unique circumstances to arrive at a decision. It is important to realize that most predictor tests produce measurements that can be declared acceptable or unacceptable, but they are no guarantee of outcome. Some people predicted to succeed will in actuality fail weaning, and some predicted to fail would succeed if given an opportunity to discontinue mechanical ventilation. As will be discussed later in this chapter, no one test is strong enough to be used by itself. Even a combination of tests, such as a weaning index, has yet to produce 100% prediction accuracy. Nevertheless, multiple tests interpreted with consideration of each person's particular situation and attributes make for a more confident prediction. Clinicians should consider how close a measurement is to a pass/fail threshold since other factors may require adjusting of the thresholds (e.g., marginally acceptable arterial blood gas values may not really be acceptable if vital signs are at the upper limits of normal).

"Weaning Trials" in Stage 4 involve some form of decreasing ventilator support. Support is either removed abruptly and completely (such as with a successful response to a SBT assessment) or gradually decreased over hours or days using one of many possible methods. While there is evidence that some methods are likely better than others, we cannot say with confidence that the best method has been identified for each type of patient we may have in our care. A goal of this stage is to prevent a patient from reaching the signs of weaning failure. It is preferable to pause the weaning process and allow a patient to stabilize rather than run the risk of failure, which requires considerable time to recover before starting another weaning attempt from the beginning.

A patient who responds to Stage 4 by tolerating removal from mechanical ventilation would advance to Stage 5, "Extubation," which in this case means removal of an endotracheal tube. If an intubated patient has been on mechanical ventilation for an extended period (>3 weeks), it is typical for the endotracheal tube to be replaced by a tracheostomy tube. A tracheostomy tube may remain in use long after discontinuation of a ventilator to facilitate suctioning, protect the airway, or decrease tracheal airway resistance sufficiently to allow for spontaneous breathing. This is particularly true for young children with bronchopulmonary dysplasia who may need time for their tracheas to grow into a normal structure.

A minority of patients may utilize Stage 6, "NIV postextubation," which involves continued ventilator support after extubation using noninvasive ventilation (NIV). Some patients identified to be at greater risk for failure may be supported prophylactically with NIV to help reduce the chance of reintubation. This is most common with older patients who have underlying cardiac or respiratory disease. Having the option to place patients temporarily on noninvasive ventilation postextubation provides a safety net that may give clinicians the confidence to avoid unnecessary delays in extubation for fear of failure.

If a patient reaches Stage 7, "Reintubation," it is usually accompanied by the reinstitution of mechanical ventilation. That is because the additional effort to breathe through an endotracheal tube is often too much for someone with weakened respiratory muscles. Reintubation is often due to multiple reasons that intertwine to weaken a patient's condition, so a thorough evaluation of what led to reintubation should be performed and indicated remedies administered before making another weaning attempt. Even small hindrances should be attended to because cumulatively they can have a significant effect. A fragile patient may require a lengthy period of physical strengthening and building mental self-efficacy (a person's belief in succeeding at accomplishing a task) before attempting weaning again.

Why Are There Different Methods of Weaning?

It would be convenient if there was one best method that could be used to remove all patients from mechanical ventilation, but the broad range of patient conditions requires a variety of techniques. In 2007, weaning from mechanical ventilation was categorized as simple, difficult, or prolonged by an international taskforce of the American Thoracic Society, European Respiratory Society, European Society of Intensive Care Medicine, Society of Critical Care Medicine, and Sóciete de Réanimation de Langue Française (**Figure 11-2**). Recall that we initially categorized patients into two groups (those who easily come off mechanical ventilation and those who do not), and the reality that difficult-to-wean patients usually have multiple attributing factors points to why different methods of weaning/discontinuation exist. The SBT method is generally preferred for a first attempt, especially if the patient has not had a long period of ventilator support. Unfortunately, the diaphragm rapidly loses muscle mass with rest (even partial rest) and this decreases the strength and endurance needed to assume spontaneous breathing. If a patient cannot be extubated after a few daily SBT assessments, a more gradual approach is often selected. The more gradual reduction of ventilatory support allows muscles to be conditioned as the work of ventilation is shifted over time from the ventilator to the patient. The challenge is to avoid moving too slowly as this carries associated risks, especially respiratory infection. This strengthening of a patient should also consider psychological aspects. Someone who has experienced failed weaning attempts may reflexively react with anxiety at the

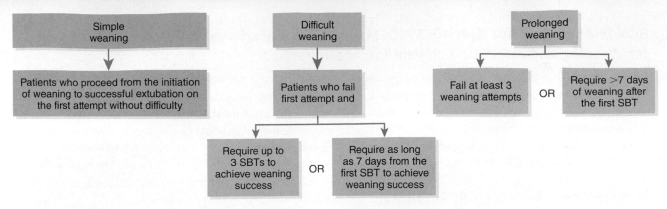

FIGURE 11-2 Classification of patients according to the weaning process. SBT, spontaneous breathing trial.

Modified from Brochard L. Pressure support is the preferred weaning method. Presented at the 5th International Consensus Conference in Intensive Care Medicine: Weaning from Mechanical Ventilation. Hosted by American Thoracic Society (ATS), European Respiratory Society (ERS), European Society of Intensive Care Medicine (ESICM), Society of Critical Care Medicine (SCCM), and Société de Réanimation de Langue Française (SRLF); Budapest, April 28–29, 2005. Available at www.ersnet.org/ers/lr/browse/default.aspx?id52814

mention of another planned attempt to the point that it jeopardizes future success. In such cases, it is helpful to assure the patient that the next attempt will be different in some way from past attempts. This could mean a new ventilator mode will be used, a different schedule or pace, or the addition of a new therapy.

Assessment of Readiness

Determining if a patient is ready to begin the weaning process should be based on evidence-based guidelines. There are many factors to consider but they ultimately reduce to the question of whether a patient has the ability to maintain adequate gas exchange. The primary focus of monitoring ventilation is arterial CO_2 but oxygenation and the function of other organ systems are also concerns. Patients receiving mechanical ventilation for less than 72 hours likely will not require the same detailed assessment as those having longer periods of support.

Regardless of how long a patient has been receiving mechanical ventilation, the assessment of readiness typically has two sequential steps: (1) identify readiness for an SBT, and (2) conduct a diagnostic SBT. First, the patient's overall condition is considered using routine critical care information such as vital signs, adequate oxygenation/acid-base status, hemodynamic stability, pain level, and strength and adequacy of cough to determine if a patient is ready for a formal assessment of discontinuation potential (**Box 11-2**, Recommendations 1 and 2). This might even include a brief SBT of just a few minutes. There are many factors that may impact ventilator dependence but the following items have more important influences: abnormalities of the ventilatory control system, respiratory muscle strength and workload, impaired lung ventilation-perfusion matching, abnormal cardiac function, lung edema, metabolic derangements (e.g., glucose control and adrenal regulation), oxygen delivery to the tissues, and psychological factors. Assessing readiness for discontinuation of ventilatory support typically includes watching for progress in the

aforementioned factors in the form of gas exchange improvement, sufficient cardiovascular function, mental status improvement, adequate neuromuscular and other organ system function, and acceptable radiographic signs. Two Cochrane systematic reviews found no benefit in daily interruption of sedation (aka sedation holidays), but there were conflicting studies noted and one found a COPD (chronic obstructive pulmonary disease) subgroup did have benefit. The 2001 consensus guidelines recommend limited sedation for postsurgical patients based on "Grade A" evidence (see Box 11-2, Recommendations 7 and 8); however, many clinicians have extended this to ventilator patients in general. The American College of Chest Physicians/American Thoracic Society (ACCP-ATS) guidelines update (2017) recommends protocols that attempt to minimize sedation for acutely hospitalized patients ventilated for more than 24 hours but acknowledges the low quality of evidence. No sedation is preferred but satisfactory mental activity is required if on sedation, or a stable neurologic condition if a patient is recovering from central nervous system (CNS) trauma.

The primary consideration when assessing weaning readiness is whether the reason that initially required mechanical ventilation has been sufficiently resolved (it may not require complete resolution). It is important to tailor the use of these criteria to the context of each patient (what is acceptable may vary depending upon an individual's prior typical condition). Many patients can be liberated from a ventilator without meeting all of the criteria. There should be an ongoing vigilance with each shift reporting to the next on a patient's potential readiness for formal assessment.

Once a patient appears to be sufficiently recovered and stable, the second step is to perform a formal assessment in the form of a diagnostic SBT lasting 30 to 120 minutes (see Box 11-2, Recommendation 3). Some clinicians have suggested that there is little or no benefit in extending an SBT beyond 30 minutes. This may be true for most uncomplicated patients who have received mechanical ventilation for less than a week.

BOX 11-2 Summarized 2001 ACCP/SCCM/AARC Evidence-Based Guidelines for Weaning and Discontinuing Ventilatory Support

Recommendation 1: A search for all of the causes that may be contributing to ventilatory dependence should be undertaken if on mechanical ventilation >24 hours (especially for those with failed attempts at withdrawing support). Reversing all possible ventilatory and nonventilatory issues should be integral to the discontinuation process.

Recommendation 2: Patients who are receiving mechanical ventilation for respiratory failure should undergo a formal assessment of discontinuation potential if the following criteria are satisfied:

1. Evidence for some [sufficient] reversal of the underlying cause for respiratory failure;

2. Adequate oxygenation (e.g., PaO_2/FIO_2 ratio >150 to 200; requiring PEEP of no more than 5 to 8 cm H_2O; FIO_2 of no more than 0.4 to 0.5), and pH of more than 7.25;

3. Hemodynamic stability as defined by the absence of active myocardial ischemia and the absence of clinically significant hypotension (i.e., a condition that necessitates no vasopressor therapy or therapy with only low-dose vasopressors such as dopamine or dobutamine); and

4. The capability to initiate an inspiratory effort. The decision to use these criteria must be individualized. Some patients who are not satisfying all of these criteria (e.g., patients with chronic hypoxemia values of less than the thresholds cited) may be ready for attempts at the discontinuation of mechanical ventilation.

Recommendation 3: Formal discontinuation assessments should be performed during spontaneous breathing, not while still receiving substantial ventilatory support. An initial brief period of spontaneous breathing can be used to assess the capability of continuing to a formal SBT. Patient tolerance during SBTs can be assessed by respiratory pattern, adequacy of gas exchange, hemodynamic stability, and subjective comfort. If SBTs are tolerated for 30 to 120 minutes, permanent ventilatory discontinuation should be promptly considered.

Recommendation 4: Removal of a patient's artificial airway should be based on assessments of airway patency and the patient's ability to protect the airway for those who have successfully discontinued ventilatory support.

Recommendation 5: Patients who are receiving mechanical ventilation for respiratory failure who fail an SBT should have the cause of failure determined. After reversible causes of failure are corrected and if the patient still meets the criteria for consideration, subsequent SBTs should be performed every 24 hours.

Recommendation 6: Patients who are receiving mechanical ventilation for respiratory failure who fail an SBT should receive a stable, nonfatiguing, and comfortable form of ventilatory support.

Recommendation 7: Anesthesia and sedation strategies and ventilatory management that are aimed at early extubation should be used for postsurgical patients.

Recommendation 8: Weaning and discontinuation protocols designed for nonclinician healthcare professionals should be developed and implemented by ICUs. Protocols to optimize sedation should also be used.

Recommendation 9: Tracheotomy should be considered after an initial period of stabilization on the ventilator when it becomes apparent that the patient needs prolonged ventilatory assistance. Tracheotomy should then be performed when the patient appears to be likely to gain one or more of the benefits ascribed to the procedure. Patients who may derive particular benefit from early tracheotomy include the following:

- Those who need high levels of sedation to tolerate translaryngeal tubes;

- Those with marginal respiratory mechanics (often manifested as tachypnea) in whom a tracheostomy tube with lower resistance may reduce the risk of muscle overload;

- Those who may derive psychological benefit from the ability to eat orally, communicate by articulated speech, and experience enhanced mobility; and

- Those in whom enhanced mobility may assist with physical therapy efforts.

Recommendation 10: Unless there is evidence for clearly irreversible disease, a patient who requires prolonged mechanical ventilatory support for respiratory failure should not be considered permanently ventilator dependent until 3 months of weaning attempts have failed.

Recommendation 11: Critical care clinicians should familiarize themselves with facilities in their communities or units in hospitals with staff that specialize in managing patients who have prolonged dependence on mechanical ventilation (including published peer-reviewed data from those units, if available). When they are medically stable for transfer, patients who have failed ventilatory discontinuation attempts in the ICU should be transferred to facilities that have demonstrated success and safety with accomplishing ventilator discontinuation.

Recommendation 12: Weaning strategies in the patient who requires prolonged mechanical ventilation should be slow paced and should include gradually lengthening self-breathing trials.

AARP, American Association for Respiratory Care; ACCP, American College of Chest Physicians; ICU, intensive care unit; PEEP, positive end-expiratory pressure; SBT, spontaneous breathing trial; SCCM, Society of Critical Care Medicine.

Reproduced from MacIntyre NR, Cook DJ, Ely EW Jr, et al. Evidence-based guidelines for weaning and discontinuing ventilatory support: a collective task force facilitated by the American College of Chest Physicians, the American Association for Respiratory Care, and the American College of Critical Care Medicine. *Chest* 2001;120(6 Suppl):S375–S395.

Patients with histories of cardiovascular difficulties, COPD, respiratory muscle atrophy, or other complications may need to be monitored for a full 2-hour SBT to confidently decide about readiness. According to a 2012 review by MacIntyre, about 77% of those who tolerated a diagnostic SBTs were able to successfully discontinue mechanical ventilation (it was noted that variations in the SBT conditions among the studies may have diminished the value). Most of the patients who tolerate a diagnostic SBT quickly progress to extubation, so the assessment of weaning readiness also serves as a weaning attempt. Patients who have received prolonged mechanical ventilation often progress from a diagnostic SBT to a more gradual weaning process (see Box 11-2, Recommendation 12). There is controversy as to whether a patient who completes a 2-hour SBT should be allowed to return to ventilatory support for rest. It is possible that borderline passing patients have real potential to benefit from resting and avoiding a failure that would require a significant recovery period. Some studies have shown that respiratory fatigue resulting from low-frequency muscle fatigue (associated with routine activities) takes longer than 24 hours for recovery. Others argue that if a patient has not shown signs of failure by the end of 2 hours of spontaneous breathing, even if indicators are borderline normal, the patient should not be denied an extubation attempt. NIV is recommended for this type of situation to provide a safety net for the patient after extubation while also minimizing unnecessary delays of extubation.

Clinical Measurements as Weaning Predictors

Ventilation

The primary measurement for ventilation status is the partial pressure of carbon dioxide in arterial blood ($Paco_2$). The range for normal $Paco_2$ is 35 to 45 mm Hg, but the upper limit for weaning eligibility is less than 50 mm Hg (with a pH ≥7.35). Patients who have COPD with carbon dioxide retention often live with CO_2 levels greater than 50 mm Hg so the individual's "normal" prior to being placed on mechanical ventilation must be taken into consideration. Alveolar minute ventilation ($\dot{V}A$) and $Paco_2$ are inversely related. Assuming a constant CO_2 production, rising CO_2 levels indicate reduced alveolar ventilation. Noninvasive measures that are similar (but not equivalent) to $Paco_2$ include end-tidal CO_2 pressure ($Petco_2$) and transcutaneous CO_2 pressure ($Ptcco_2$). Although less accurate, the noninvasive measures allow for continuous monitoring, which adds important interpretive value to patient assessment.

Normal minute ventilation ($\dot{V}E$) is approximately 6 L/min (there is normal variation with body size). More than one cutoff value for minute ventilation has been reported in the literature, but a $\dot{V}E$ of less than 10 L/min is the most commonly cited criterion related to weaning readiness and has become one of the standard weaning predictors. Patients who fail a spontaneous breathing attempt typically experience a rapid onset of decreased inspiratory time (T_I). In the brain's respiratory center, expiratory time (T_E) is strongly linked to T_I, so as one shortens, the other follows, inevitably leading to an increase in respiratory frequency (f). A decrease in V_T increases dead space ventilation fraction (V_D/V_T), and this reduced efficiency requires a compensatory increase in $\dot{V}E$ to maintain alveolar ventilation. Tachypnea (>30 to 35 breaths/min in adults) is a sensitive marker of respiratory distress, but it may delay weaning if it is rigidly enforced. Irregular patterns (including rapid shallow breathing, paradoxical breathing, and periods of apnea) during spontaneous breathing indicate a risk for weaning failure. Some adjustment in ventilation during a spontaneous breathing period is expected as the patient assumes the ventilatory load from the ventilator. A decreased ventilatory variability over time (rate, V_T, minute ventilation) is more indicative of failing an SBT because the capacity to increase ventilation is lacking. Combined changes in V_T and f (and therefore $\dot{V}E$) account for most of the increase in $Paco_2$ (the primary indicator of ventilation) observed in the weaning-failure patients. A pH of 7.35 to 7.45 is desirable, and this assumes causes of acid-base disturbances have been sufficiently resolved. Be aware that patients who have been mechanically hyperventilated for an extended period may have a reduced ventilatory drive and many need additional time to resensitize and withdraw from mechanical ventilation.

Patient Effort and Work of Breathing

Increases in airway resistance and decreases in respiratory system compliance lead to increased **work of breathing (WOB)** that may prevent a weaning trial or result in a failed attempt. Pleural pressure is related to the effort the respiratory muscles must expend for ventilation. Since it is not practical to measure pleural pressure in patients, a catheter can be placed in the esophagus near the level of the heart to measure its substitute, **esophageal pressure** (P_{ES}). If P_{ES} is measured during spontaneous breathing, an increase in respiratory work is revealed by greater swings (rise and fall) in esophageal pressure. Several brands of critical care ventilators offer the ability to record esophageal pressure so it is an accessible measurement for patient care.

Increases in resistance or decreases in compliance of the respiratory system lead to an increase of WOB. An increased load due to resistance typically slows respiratory frequency while preserving tidal volume. In contrast, an increased load due to decreased compliance causes a rise in respiratory frequency and a decrease in tidal volume.

Indirect measures of WOB exist because direct measurement is difficult. Calculation of WOB involves measuring the area within the curve created by plotting esophageal pressure against the V_T. It would seem to be a good way to gauge spontaneous ventilatory workload, but it doesn't consider all factors, such as the amount of energy consumed to perform the measured work or the functional condition of the respiratory muscles. WOB appears to be more useful for predicting weaning failure than weaning success. If spontaneous WOB levels are more than 1.6 kg/m/min (16 J/min) or 0.14 kg/m/L (1.4 J/L), success is unlikely. Oxygen cost of breathing (OCB) is a related measurement that assesses how much oxygen is consumed during spontaneous breathing. It is the difference between oxygen consumption during spontaneous breathing and oxygen consumption when the respiratory muscles are at rest during full ventilatory support. The normal OCB is $\leq$5% for healthy individuals. For mechanically ventilated individuals, OCB $\leq$15% suggests a likelihood of weaning success.

Tension-time index (TTI), **pressure-time index (PTI)**, and **pressure-time product (PTP)** are expressions of the respiratory load on the diaphragm and its capacity to handle it. The TTI represents the amount of diaphragm contraction that occurs during the inspiratory portion of the breath cycle and it has been used to predict diaphragm fatigue. The measurement procedure involves measuring pressure changes above and below the diaphragm (transdiaphragmatic pressure) using balloon catheters in the esophagus and stomach as well as inspiratory and total breath times. The TTI value is derived from the contractile force of the diaphragm (esophageal pressures during a tidal breath divided by maximum inhalation effort) multiplied by the T_I divided by total respiratory cycle time. It is like WOB in that it considers the amount of pressure change associated with a breath volume, but it also considers much of the energy expended when no gas is moving and volume is unchanged (when no work is happening—like when a muscle is contracting but no movement is happening). For example, energy is expended to overcome airway resistance prior to gas moving in the airways (overcoming auto-PEEP [positive end-expiratory pressure] is another example). That is why PTI is often compared to oxygen cost of breathing and it helps ascertain respiratory efficiency (WOB accomplished for the amount of oxygen consumed by the respiratory muscles).

The PTI is a simplified, nonivasive version of TTI that is preferred in the clinical setting because it is much less difficult to measure and correlates well to TTI. The PTI substitutes the airway pressure for a tidal breath (Paw) and maximal inspiratory pressure (MIP) for the esophageal pressues used to calculate TTI (PTI = [average Paw/MIP] $\times$ [T_I/T_{TOT}]). Although PTI has been used to predict respiratory fatigue, it is more commonly used as a predictor of successful ventilator discontinuation (PTI $<$0.15 predicts weaning success in adults, children may have a lower threshold). High PTI values can result from increased respiratory load, decreased respiratory muscle strength, or a combination of the two.

The PTP is similar to PTI in that they both measure the efficiency of the respiratory muscles at performing the work of breathing (energy required to handle the respiratory load on the diaphragm) but it is measured differently. The typical method is to calculate the integral of the pressure developed by the respiratory muscles (using esophageal pressure) over the duration of contraction. This method is more complex than the measurement of PTI and therefore less common.

Cardiovascular Sufficiency

Sufficient gas exchange and adequate cardiovascular function are needed to provide satisfactory oxygen delivery and carbon dioxide removal for the tissues. The respiratory muscles carry a large workload and depend on an efficient transport of oxygen by the cardiovascular system. Cardiovascular dysfunction is associated with decreased ventilator discontinuation success. Cardiovascular assessment starts with the basics; heart rate and dysrhythmias should be within acceptable limits and blood pressure should typically be within 90/60 mm Hg to 180/110 mm Hg before considering discontinuation of ventilatory support. Advanced measurements such as central venous pressure (CVP 2 to 6 mm Hg), cardiac output (4 < CO < 8 L/min), and cardiac index (CI >2.5 L/min^{-1}·m^2) are useful for determining cardiovascular stability. In one small study by Lemaire and colleagues, patients with COPD (half had documented ischemic heart disease) developed increases in pulmonary artery occlusion pressure (PAOP), CI, and right and left ventricular end-diastolic volume indexes (increased ventricular preload) after spontaneous breathing for 10 minutes without PEEP. The investigators attributed the increase in left ventricular end-diastolic volume to improved venous return and increased left ventricular afterload. Sixty percent of the patients were weaned after 10 days of diuretic therapy, at which time PAOP had fallen to 9 mm Hg.

There is insufficient evidence to declare a particular PAOP value to be linked with the onset of cardiogenic pulmonary edema, but it is widely held that a PAOP >18 mm Hg during a weaning trial indicates a risk for onset of weaning-induced pulmonary edema. Increases in PAOP during weaning trial failures are not necessarily associated with a decrease in cardiac output. Some have compared resuming spontaneous breathing after a time of rest on a ventilator as similar to the effect of whole-body exercise in that it increases in CO and WOB. Increases in adrenergic tone associated with increased cardiopulmonary effort can produce increases in venous return, left ventricular afterload, cardiac work, and myocardial oxygen demand—all of which may produce myocardial ischemia in susceptible individuals.

When oxygen consumption increases during a weaning trial, it means that a patient who is unable to sufficiently increase CO is susceptible to experiencing a decrease in oxygen delivery to the body. Jubran et al. reported that mixed venous oxygen saturation (Svo_2), an indirect indicator of oxygen delivery and consumption, fell progressively during a 40-minute SBT in weaning failure patients but did not change in successful patients. Oxygen demand ($\dot{V}o_2$) was similar in the two groups during the weaning trial: the successful patients responded with an increase in CI (more oxygen transport) and the failure group simply extracted more oxygen from the blood (causing the fall in Svo_2). The failure patients also had more impaired pulmonary gas exchange (venous admixture [$\dot{Q}va/\dot{Q}t$] of 32%) at the start of the trial.

Mean pulmonary artery pressure (PAP) has been reported to be higher in weaning failure patients than in successful patients. Hypoxemia and acidosis are potent vasoconstrictors and therefore can be factors in increased PAP. If gas trapping occurs in association with deterioration in pulmonary mechanics, this can cause compression of alveolar vessels, resulting in increased PAP. When mean arterial pressure increases but there is no change in CI this indicates an increase in left ventricular afterload (stress on the heart). The function of the heart and lungs is intertwined and must be managed together during the ventilator liberation process.

Pro-brain natriuretic peptide (pro-BNP) is released by heart muscle cells in response to tissue stretching as occurs with increased atrial or ventricular pressure and/or volume overload. Upon release, pro-BNP is immediately converted into the biologically active BNP and inactive BNP (NT-proBNP). "NT-proBNP" resulting from the cleaving of pro-BNP rather than "NT-BNP" may sound odd but the term is correct. Both systolic and diastolic dysfunction of the left ventricle can result in high blood levels of these biomarkers, which are used to screen patients with suspected cardiac disorders. Elevated plasma BNP is typically associated with unsuccessful weaning outcomes, but studies have shown this increase can present differently. An elevated BNP prior to a weaning trial does not necessarily mean that cardiac dysfunction was the cause of weaning failure. Plasma BNP can be elevated for reasons other than cardiac dysfunction, such as advanced age, female gender, renal dysfunction, sepsis, pulmonary hypertension, vigorous fluid management, and extensive use of medications such as diuretics, angiotensin-converting enzyme (ACE) inhibitors, and β-blockers. Some studies report that elevated BNP, values at the beginning of a weaning attempt have the greatest predictive power, whereas others report that an increase during a weaning attempt is more predictive. There is debate on whether NT-proBNP is more reliable than BNP, and consensus on a threshold value to discriminate between weaning-success and weaning-failure patients has yet to be decided (NT-proBNP is inactive and therefore may be a more stable/reliable indicator).

Respiratory Muscle Strength

Respiratory muscle function is a foundational aspect of weaning but the measurements available to assess it are not refined and as reliable as we would like. The most basic measurement is the greatest negative airway pressure achieved during a maximum inspiratory effort against an occluded airway. This is termed *maximum inspiratory pressure* (Pi_{max} or MIP) and it provides a measure of momentary inspiratory muscle strength but not endurance. The literature contains conflicting findings that may be due to multiple factors, such as deliberately excluding patients with the lowest MIP and variability in the testing procedure. The use of Pi_{max} as a weaning predictor originates from a study by Sahn and Lakshminarayan, in which a Pi_{max} value more negative than −30 cm H_2O aligned with successful weaning and a Pi_{max} less negative than −20 cm H_2O encountered failure in a weaning trial. The associated sensitivity, specificity, and predictive values essentially translate as follows: It is very likely that everyone who really can wean from the ventilator will pass the MIP test but a sizable percentage of those who pass the test will not successfully wean. Failing the MIP test is not a reliable predictor of whether someone will actually fail weaning.

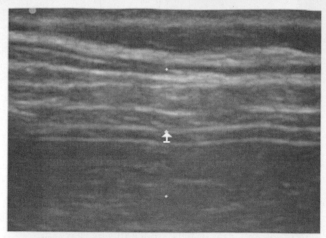

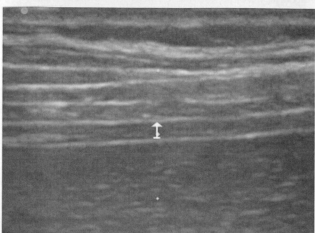

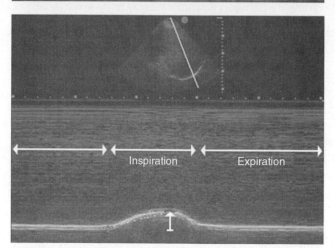

FIGURE 11-3 Diaphragm ultrasonography measurements. The thickness of the diaphragm during exhalation (arrow, top image) increases with contraction during inspiration (arrow, middle image). The duration of contraction and relaxation indicate the inspiratory and expiratory periods, respectively (bottom image).

Reproduced with permission from: Doorduin J, van der Hoeven JG, Heunks LM. The differential diagnosis for failure to wean from mechanical ventilation. *Curr Opin Anaesthesiol.* 2016;29(2):150–157. doi: 10.1097/ACO.0000000000000297

The − 20 to − 30 cm H_2O range of MIP is a gray area that has the least ability to predict an outcome.

Diaphragm ultrasonography is a more recent technique that has been explored as a weaning predictor by way of measuring diaphragm thickness, thickening fraction, and displacement (**Figure 11-3**). It has been used to detect patient-ventilator asynchrony and assessment of respiratory workload. A study by Kim et al. defined diaphragmatic dysfunction as a vertical excursion <1 cm or paradoxical movements and found it in 29% of patients who met criteria for an SBT who showed frequent early and delayed weaning failures.

A diaphragm thickening fraction can be calculated by (thickness [insp] − thickness [exp]) / thickness (exp) (see Figure 11-3). A fraction >30% was found to predict extubation success with a respectable 88% sensitivity and 71% specificity (DiNino et al.). While these measurements may eventually prove to have utility as weaning predictors, their greater value may be for determining the cause of SBT failures when the cause is not revealed by other assessments.

Ventilatory Drive

The pressure generated during the first tenth of a second (0.1 second) of an airway occlusion at the beginning of inspiration ($P_{0.1}$) is a common measurement reflecting the output of the respiratory center. This test is now easily obtained in the clinical setting because most ventilators used in hospitals are programmed to measure the value and it requires no special action by the patient. A normal $P_{0.1}$ is approximately 0.5 to 1.5 cm H_2O during resting breathing. In studies evaluating $P_{0.1}$ as a weaning predictor the thresholds for success and failure ranged from 3.4 to 6.0 cm H_2O, respectively (compiled by Tobin et al). Ventilator-dependent patients with COPD who have a $P_{0.1}$ of more than 6 cm H_2O tend to be difficult to wean. It is possible for the $P_{0.1}$ value to be too high (too much stimulus = air hunger) or low (insufficient stimulus), but assuming the neurological system is functional, high values are the more common abnormality to be remedied. Combining $P_{0.1}$ and MIP in the form of a ratio ($P_{0.1}$/MIP) produces a value that combines ventilatory drive with respiratory muscle strength. It has been described as an early predictor of discontinuation success, and it could be superior to MIP alone, given its previously described limitations.

The **rapid shallow breathing index (RSBI)** or frequency-to-tidal-volume ratio (f/V_T) is arguably the easiest and most powerful single predictor of weaning outcome currently available and arose from research into the causes of weaning failure. Tobin first reported that patients who failed an SBT exhibited a rapid shallow breathing pattern (↑ f and ↓V_T) within the first few minutes of the trial. Yang and Tobin reported a sensitivity of 0.97, a specificity 0.64, positive-predictive value of 0.78, and a negative-predictive value 0.95 and found to be superior when compared to nine other weaning predictors. Because the f/V_T ratio is so easily measured and interpreted, it is often arranged to be frequently checked on a regular basis to detect a patient's readiness to wean at the earliest point possible.

When using f/VT ratio as a predictor of readiness to start an SBT, the originator of the f/VT ratio warns against measuring it while a patient is receiving even low levels of pressure support (PS) or CPAP. A diagnostic SBT allows for the use of low levels of PS or CPAP and clinicians often measure f/VT ratio during the trial without removing PS or CPAP. The use of PS and CPAP have been shown to have a definite effect; f/VT ratio values during unassisted breathing are 23% to 52% higher compared to a PS of 5 cm H_2O and 46% to 82% higher compared to a PS of 10 cm H_2O. It is reasonable to think that low levels of PS simply overcome the resistance associated with an artificial airway. Straus et al. demonstrated that the respiratory work associated with breathing through the supraglottic airway after extubation was almost identical to when breathing through an endotracheal tube before extubation. Likewise, the measurement of f/VT while a patient is receiving CPAP is also significantly altered. Compared to unassisted breathing, a study of healthy subjects on a CPAP 5 cm H_2O had an f/VT ratio 38% less, post–coronary bypass surgery patients on CPAP had an f/VT ratio 49% lower, and ventilated patients on CPAP had an f/VT ratio 21% lower. In the past, some clinicians thought that because an endotracheal tube prevented closure of the glottis, it would result in the loss of "physiologic PEEP," and advised the use of CPAP of 5 cm H_2O as a substitute. Physiologic PEEP does not appear to exist because measured static recoil pressure of the respiratory system is zero at end expiration.

In the original study on f/VT ratio by Yang and Tobin, a value of "105 breaths/min/L" was determined to be the best threshold for discriminating weaning-success patients from weaning-failure patients (for that group). A value less than 105 indicates likelihood of weaning success. This value is often rounded to 100 because it is easier to remember and has essentially the same sensitivity; however, this raises an important consideration. The precision methodology required for a research study does not automatically apply to the clinical setting. A clinician evaluating f/VT ratio values of 107 and 137 would not necessarily act on them in the same way. Neither value is within the desired range that has a high likelihood of successful outcome, but a patient with a value that is close to the threshold and has other predictors that indicate readiness may be allowed a weaning attempt. In fact, Zhang and Qin concluded that a threshold f/VT ratio of 75 while on pressure support ventilation and 100 in T-piece was more accurate for predicting successful weaning. In addition, conditions such as sepsis, fever, supine position, anxiety, and restrictive lung diseases increase the respiratory frequency and hence affect the f/VT ratio. Some other factors such as narrow ET tube, female gender, and suctioning are shown to increase the f/VT ratio. Therefore, clinicians should use multiple types of data, patient characteristics, and context to inform clinical judgment on how to act upon the cutoff value for f/VT ratio.

The f/VT measurement should be taken only after the patient has reached a stable spontaneous breathing pattern (i.e., ≥3 minutes). Since the respiratory drive is affected by factors such as pH, Pa_{CO_2}, and Pa_{O_2}, the initial period of spontaneous breathing does not accurately reflect the patient's gas exchange requirement over time.

Oxygenation

Severe hypoxemia that is not responsive to supplemental oxygen and CPAP is one of the indications for mechanical ventilation. Oxygenation must be adequate before attempting to discontinue mechanical ventilation and a common criterion is a Pa_{O_2} of ≥60 mm Hg (55 mm Hg for COPD patients) with fractional inspired oxygen concentration (FI_{O_2}) greater than 0.4 to 0.5, and PEEP not exceeding 5 to 8 cm H_2O. The Pa_{O_2}/FI_{O_2} ratio, alveoloarterial oxygen tension gradient ($P(A - a)_{O_2}$), and physiologic **shunt fraction** ($\dot{Q}s/\dot{Q}t$) are common computations to evaluate gas exchange and ventilation-perfusion relationships but they are based upon many assumptions. For example, the computations assume a normal hemoglobin level, which may not be the case for many critically ill patients. Related to that is the expectation of a normal arterial oxygen saturation (Sa_{O_2}) and adequate cardiac output. The acceptable levels for weaning are often more lenient than normal ranges, so care must be taken not to violate assumptions for computations and indices, or at least to factor them into interpretation. The Pa_{O_2}/FI_{O_2} ratio is normally above 400 mm Hg but ≥150 to 200 mm Hg is acceptable as a threshold for weaning.

The ratio of physiologic shunt to total perfusion estimates the portion of blood flow that does not take part in gas exchange due to lack of contact with ventilation. The normal range for $\dot{Q}s/\dot{Q}t$ is often listed as ≤10% but it would be more accurate to state it as acceptable, since normal is 5% or less. A $\dot{Q}s/\dot{Q}t$ ≤20% is considered a mild shunt and <15% to 20% shunt is acceptable for weaning purposes. A moderate (20% to 30%) or severe (>30%) shunt should be corrected before weaning is attempted. The $\dot{Q}s/\dot{Q}t$ can be estimated with either the classic or clinical physiologic shunt equation. The clinical equation is easier to calculate because it does not require obtaining a mixed venous blood sample. The estimated shunt equation is not as accurate as the classic physiologic shunt equation as shown here:

$$\frac{\dot{Q}s}{\dot{Q}t} = \frac{(Cc_{O_2} - Ca_{O_2})}{(Cc_{O_2} - C\overline{v}_{O_2})}$$

$\dot{Q}s/\dot{Q}t$: Shunt percent
Cc_{O_2}: End-capillary oxygen content in vol%
Ca_{O_2}: Arterial oxygen content in vol%
$C\overline{v}_{O_2}$: Mixed venous oxygen content in vol%

The $P(A - a)_{O_2}$, or "A-a gradient" as it is often referred to, and increasing values indicate a worsening of hypoxemia and physiologic shunt. Interpretation of the $P(A - a)O_2$ is affected by the age of the patient and inspired oxygen concentration. When breathing room air, every decade of life adds about 4 mm Hg to the expected value for the $P(A - a)O_2$ so a 40-year-old person would be expected to have a value less than 16 mm Hg. If a patient is receiving supplemental oxygen, the expected $P(A - a)O_2$ value would increase 5 to 7 mm Hg for each 10% increase in oxygen. For diagnostic purposes, it is preferred to measure $P(A - a)O_2$ while breathing 100% oxygen if possible. A $P(A - a)O_2$ <350 mm Hg while on 100% oxygen is the criterion for weaning readiness. The $P(A - a)O_2$ on 100% oxygen can also be used to estimate shunt fraction; every 50 mm Hg difference in $P(A - a)O_2$ approximates 2% physiologic shunt. Using this rough approximation, a $P(A - a)O_2$ of 350 mm Hg on 100% oxygen would represent a shunt of about 14%. Keep in mind that although these measurements have been used as predictors of weaning outcome, they have limited evidence to support their use. The $P(A - a)O_2$ is calculated using the following method.

$$P(A - a)O_2 = PAO_2 - PaO_2$$

$P(A - a)O_2$: Alveoloarterial oxygen tension gradient in mm Hg

PAO_2: Alveolar oxygen tension in mm Hg (from the Alveolar Air Equation)

PaO_2: Arterial oxygen tension in mm Hg

Respiratory Mechanics

Physiologic variables for quantifying lung mechanics of interest for weaning from mechanical ventilation can be grouped under three major headings: resistance, elastance, and gas trapping. Increase in resistance, increase in elastance (decrease in compliance), and presence of air trapping (auto-PEEP) are factors that may hinder a successful weaning outcome.

A particularly informative study by Jubran and Tobin reported respiratory mechanics in COPD patients undergoing a weaning trial. Lung inspiratory resistance at the beginning of SBTs was determined to be equivalent for both weaning-failure and weaning-success patients, but by the end of the trial, resistance increased about 60% in the failure patients but it did not change in the success patients. Bronchoconstriction and/or accumulation of secretions were likely explanations for increased resistance in patients with COPD—although both groups (success and failure) had the propensity for airway reactivity and were suctioned before SBTs. Other factors that can contribute to an increase in resistance include an increase in inspiratory flow and a decrease in lung volume.

In the same study, dynamic lung elastance was higher (i.e., the lung compliance was lower) in weaning-failure patients than in weaning-success patients at the start of the trial. At the end of the trial, elastance increased by a percent change of about 60% in the failure patients and

about 41% in the success patients. The increase in elastance may have been caused by dynamic hyperinflation (there was a twofold increase in auto-PEEP), development of pulmonary edema secondary to a diminished left ventricular output, and/or microatelectasis (there was a marked decrease in VT).

The study also reported auto-PEEP, which is an indirect measure of gas trapping. Failure patients had a higher auto-PEEP than the success patients at the beginning of the trial (2.0 vs. 0.7 cm H_2O). The auto-PEEP increased to 4.1 cm H_2O in the failure patients and to 1.1 cm H_2O in the success patients by the end of the trial. After correcting for effect of expiratory-muscle contribution, the portion of total auto-PEEP due to end-expiratory lung volume (gas trapping) was increased in 7 of the 10 patients. This suggests that weaning-failure patients are prone to develop dynamic hyperinflation. Expiratory flow limitation and tachypnea, resulting from a decrease in time available of exhalation, are the most likely determinants of this form of gas trapping. These findings indicate that resistance, elastance, and gas trapping are important to assess when evaluating causes of weaning failure and may be useful as predictors of weaning success.

Vital capacity (VC) is a measurement of pulmonary function that could arguably be an indicator for several of the preceding categories but it is primarily affected by changes in respiratory mechanics. The normal VC is usually between 65 and 75 mL/kg, and a value of 10 mL/kg or more has been suggested to predict a successful weaning outcome. Unfortunately, VC has a mixed record of utility, and its dependence on patient cooperation makes it susceptible to poor effort. A study of patients with Guillain-Barré syndrome reported that VC was helpful in guiding the weaning process. Patients with a vital capacity of less than 7 mL/kg were unable to tolerate as few as 15 minutes of spontaneous breathing, whereas a VC >15 mL/kg (assuming recovery from the illness) saw patients safely extubated. VC is routinely measured as part of spontaneous breathing parameters and it is useful in unique circumstances such as patients with neuromuscular diseases. As a stand-alone parameter, VC is rarely used as a weaning predictor.

Predicting Weaning Outcomes
Success and Failure

There is no predictor of weaning outcome that has been shown to be strong enough to stand on its own. That is why multiple predictors of outcome are evaluated together. No predictor is expected to be perfect at identifying both success and failure, and each one is usually better at predicting one outcome over the other. It is important to understand how prediction of success and failure is interpreted so we can continue to refine weaning approaches and determine the best predictors for specific needs.

Sensitivity and Specificity

Three of the most common measurements used to evaluate weaning predictors are sensitivity, specificity, and likelihood ratio. Sensitivity describes the number of positive test results that are true. It is a measure of the proportion of ventilator patients who are correctly predicted by a test to be successful at weaning and the prediction comes true. For example, the f/V_T ratio has a sensitivity of 0.94 (value compiled by original investigator from studies since the seminal study). This sensitivity could be used to estimate that the proportion (94%) of patients who tested positive for weaning success (f/V_T ≤105) would be removed from the ventilator and be extubated. With this information, the weaning process can be started as soon as possible to avoid potential undesirable consequences that come with prolonged mechanical ventilation. It is desirable to have a weaning readiness test with high sensitivity because we do not want to miss anyone who has the ability to start weaning. This test should be done frequently to identify the patient at the earliest point possible.

Specificity describes the number of negative test results that are true. It is a measure of the proportion of ventilator patients who are correctly predicted by a test to be *unsuccessful* at weaning and the prediction comes true. For example, the f/V_T ratio has a specificity of 0.64. This specificity could be used to estimate that the proportion (64%) of patients who tested positive for weaning failure (f/V_T ≥105) would fail the weaning attempt. Therefore, a test with a high specificity would be very useful for preventing weaning attempts on patients who are not ready.

As good as the f/V_T ratio is as a predictor, the original study reported the test had a relatively low specificity of 0.64. This alone is not sufficient to confirm the presence of weaning failure. A reasonable approach might be to use f/V_T ratio to identify a group of patients who are likely ready to start weaning and then use additional tests to increase specificity for detecting weaning failure during an SBT.

Likelihood Ratio as a Measure of Diagnostic Accuracy

Sensitivity and specificity are common measurements associated with evaluating prediction tests but they have limitations. The positive and negative predictive values are the probabilities that a condition (weaning success or weaning failure) will happen if the test result predicts the outcome.

Likelihood ratios (LRs) are an expression of the odds that a given test result will be present in a patient with a given condition, compared to a patient without the condition. Starting at an LR value of 1 (no difference), as the LR value increases, the probability of success increases and a decreasing LR value indicates that the probability of failure increases. To be of clinical significance, LRs must be at least greater than 2 (success) or less than 0.5 (failure). Even better would be LRs of >10 or <0.1 because they correlate with very large changes in probability. An LR >10 indicates the test result has a large effect on increasing the probability of detecting success if weaning is attempted (10 times greater). The LR value is calculated with the following equation:

$$LR = \frac{\text{Probability of a successful individual having a prediction of success}}{\text{Probability of an unsuccessful individual having a prediction of failure}}$$

The McMaster group (Cook et al.) identified seven parameters to predict successful ventilator discontinuation in several studies ($\dot{V}_E$, MIP, $P_{0.1}$/MIP, CROP, Respiratory f, V_T, f/V_T; MacIntyre, *Respir Care* 2012;57(10):1611–1618). Some of these measurements are made while the patient is still receiving ventilatory support while others require an assessment during a brief period of spontaneous breathing. Unfortunately, despite these parameters showing statistical significance, the clinical applicability of each parameter is low when used alone. Another consideration that must be included when using weaning readiness predictors is that the predictive strength for each parameter changes depending upon whether they are used within the first week of mechanical ventilation or afterward. The primary reason is that only difficult-to-wean patients remain after a week on mechanical ventilation (a more difficult remaining group to wean is harder to predict for success). A list of some of the most common criteria for determining weaning readiness is shown in **Box 11-3**.

Pulmonary Measurements

Spontaneous Breathing Parameters

The spontaneous ventilatory measurements introduced by pulmonologist Thomas Petty have been used for decades as bedside assessments of weaning readiness. Although they have poor predictive strength, they are routinely performed in preparation for weaning attempts because the values are used in the calculation of other measurements. The five spontaneous parameters include the previously described f, V_T, $\dot{V}_E$, VC, and MIP. The patient should be allowed to breathe spontaneously for at least 3 minutes before starting measurement to allow equilibration and obtain representative values for spontaneous breathing. The measurements should be performed in the following order to obtain the best possible results.

Frequency, Minute Ventilation, and Tidal Volume

After several minutes of unsupported ventilation, the frequency of breathing and accumulated $\dot{V}_E$ for a full minute are recorded. If measured manually with a respirometer and watch, the average tidal volume is calculated from these two measurements. Because MIP and

BOX 11-3 Criteria of Readiness for Weaning Trial

Subjective Assessment

Adequate cough

No neuromuscular blocking agents

Absence of excessive secretions

Reversal of the underlying cause for respiratory failure

No continuous sedation infusion or adequate mentation on sedation

Objective Measurements

Stable cardiovascular status, no active myocardial ischemia

No or minimal vasopressor or inotrope (<5 μg/kg/min dopamine or dobutamine)

Heart rate ≤140 beats/min

Systolic BP 90 to 160 mm Hg

Adequate hemoglobin level (≥8 g/dL)

Stable metabolic status (acceptable electrolytes)

Afebrile ($36°$ C $<$ temperature $<38°$ C)

No significant respiratory acidosis ($PaCO_2 <50$ mm Hg with near normal pH)

Spontaneous tidal volume >5 mL/kg

Vital capacity >10 mL/kg

Spontaneous respiratory frequency ≤35/min

Spontaneous minute ventilation <10 L/min

Maximal inspiratory pressure (MIP) ≤-20 to -30 cm H_2O

Rapid shallow breathing index (f/V_T) <105 breaths/min/L

Static compliance (Cst) >30 mL/cm H_2O

$P_{0.1}$/MIP >0.3

CROP >13

Adequate Oxygenation

$PaO_2 >60$ mm Hg or $SaO_2 >90\%$ on $FIO_2 \leq0.4$

$PaO_2/FIO_2 \geq150$ to 200 mm Hg

$P(A - a)O_2 <350$ mm Hg on $FIO_2 \leq1.0$

PEEP ≤8 cm H_2O

BP, blood pressure; CROP, dynamic compliance, respiratory rate, oxygenation, maximum inspiratory pressure; PEEP, positive end-expiratory pressure.

Modified from Boles J. Weaning from mechanical ventilation. *Eur Respir J.* 2007;29:1033–1056; Zein H. Ventilator weaning and spontaneous breathing trials; an educational review. *Emerg.* 2016;4(2): 65–71; MacIntyre N. Evidence-based guidelines for weaning and discontinuing ventilatory support. *Respir Care.* 2002;47:69–90.

VC require maximal patient effort, they should be measured last so that they do not influence the measures obtained during resting breathing.

Vital Capacity

Although the vital capacity maneuver encourages maximal inhalation and exhalation, the patient does not need to forcefully exhale. It is not necessary to tire the patient by requiring three attempts, as with typical spirometry testing.

MIP

The MIP represents the maximal amount of negative pressure a patient can generate with the airway occluded. This test need only be performed once if done correctly, which involves occluding the airway for 20 seconds without leaks. This will be somewhat uncomfortable, so the patient should be forewarned and assured that it will not last longer than the specified period. Normally the measurements will become progressively more negative as the occlusion time increases. It is important not to let the patient take breaths (maintain airway occlusion) during the 20-second period as this affects the accuracy of the measurement. This test can also be performed on unconscious patients using a one-way valve attachment described by Marini et al.

Frequency/Tidal Volume

Martin Tobin, the originator of the f/V_T ratio, advocates the measurement should be accomplished by

disconnecting the patient's endotracheal tube from the ventilator circuit and from supplemental oxygen, so that the patient breathes room air. A handheld spirometer (with a filter) is attached to the end of the endotracheal tube. After the patient has established a regular respiratory rhythm (after 3 minutes), the $\dot{V}E$ is measured for 1 full minute (no shortcuts) while respiratory frequency is simultaneously counted. The values obtained when measuring the spontaneous breathing parameters can also be used for this calculation if performed under the same conditions. The average V_T is calculated as $\dot{V}E$ divided by respiratory frequency. The f/V_T ratio is calculated as respiratory frequency divided by the average tidal volume (must be in liter units). Some clinicians measure f/V_T ratio using ventilator by simulating T-piece conditions (spontaneous mode with continuous flow and zero pressure support ventilation (PSV) and CPAP). Patel et al. reported that the results from the two methods are essentially equivalent.

Static Compliance and Airway Resistance of the Respiratory System

The static compliance (Cst) of the respiratory system is commonly measured as part of routine ventilator management (as discussed in Chapter 1). It is calculated by dividing the exhaled tidal volume (corrected for tubing compliance) by the inspiratory pressure change (plateau pressure – PEEP in cm H_2O). Hess reported that a value of 30 mL/cm H_2O or greater is associated with successful weaning. A rough estimation of the total resistance of the airways can be calculated by dividing the difference in the peak inspiratory pressure and the plateau pressure (cm H_2O) by the inspiratory flow (L/sec, must be a constant flow pattern). This should not be equated to the airway resistance measurement (Raw) obtained in pulmonary function testing and it is affected by many variables, especially ventilator flow rate. No evidence-based threshold for weaning success has been reported for this estimate, but Hess recommends a value less than 10 cm H_2O/L/sec for patients receiving mechanical ventilation. This estimate may be useful to observe the trend of resistance changes and use it to determine if interventions to reduce airway resistance are effective.

Dead Space/Tidal Volume (VD/VT) Ratio

The dead space to tidal volume ratio is a measurement of ventilatory efficiency. It is not a volume but rather the fraction of each breath that does not participate in gas exchange. The recommended threshold for weaning success ranges from 0.55 to 0.60, although it is not well supported. It can be calculated using the following equation:

$$\frac{V_D}{V_T} = \frac{(Pa_{CO_2} - P\bar{E}_{CO_2})}{Pa_{CO_2}}$$

V_D/V_T = Dead space to tidal volume ratio in percentage

Pa_{CO_2} = Arterial carbon dioxide tension in mm Hg

$P\bar{E}_{CO_2}$ = Mixed expired carbon dioxide tension in mm Hg

Traditional Weaning Procedures and Techniques

Spontaneous Breathing Trial

Historically there are two methods of SBT, the diagnostic SBT or the more gradual approach also referred to as T-piece or T-tube trials. The diagnostic SBT is described in the literature as lasting 30 to 120 minutes and allowing 0 to 5 cm H_2O CPAP and 0 to 5 cm H_2O of pressure support (it is preferred that F_{IO_2} not exceed 0.4). The degree of ventilatory support immediately prior to a diagnostic SBT may vary greatly by institution (from full to some degree of partial support). At the beginning of an SBT, the patient either breathes through a T-piece system or remains on the ventilator with the previously stated ranges of little or no PSV and CPAP. Strong opinions exist on whether some or no PSV (or automated tube compensation) and CPAP should be used during an SBT. The American Thoracic Society/American College of Chest Physicians (ATS-ACCP) 2017 (Girard et al.) consensus guidelines update recommends that acutely hospitalized patients ventilated more than 24 hours have the initial SBT conducted with inspiratory pressure augmentation (5 to 8 cm H_2O) rather than without (T-piece or CPAP). A specific duration has not been standardized, only a range from 30 minutes to 2 hours. The clinician must judge how long the SBT should continue using subjective and objective monitoring (Boxes 11-1 and 11-4). The majority of SBT attempts do not require longer than 30 minutes and have a high success rate. Figueroa-Casas et al. reported that patient measurements typically do not change much after the first 20 to 30 minutes of an SBT. Perren et al. randomized ventilator patients to 30-minute and 120-minute SBT durations and found no difference in outcomes. Given the limited evidence available, the consensus guidelines prefer to allow the range of 30 to 120 minutes and allow clinicians to use thoughtful judgment to determine the appropriate duration on an individual patient basis (see Box 11-2, Recommendation 3). The decision process for the most common weaning approach (SBT) is shown in **Figure 11-4**.

Removal of the Artificial Airway

At the end of a diagnostic SBT, the clinician decides whether to extubate the patient or to reinstate ventilator support. The consensus guidelines recommend a separate assessment for determining extubation readiness (see Box 11-2, Recommendation 4). Beyond the

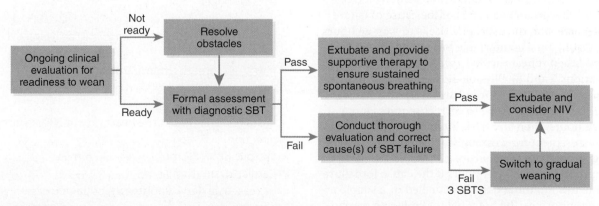

FIGURE 11-4 Example decision steps for the weaning process.
NIV, noninvasive ventilation; SBT, spontaneous breathing trial.

criteria for passing an SBT, additional tests to assess the ability to protect the airway and assure its patency after artificial airway removal have been proposed. Examples include the ability to raise one's head above the pillow, extend the tongue for several seconds or move it to the right or left (cranial nerve function), and an endotracheal tube cuff leak test. The only extubation-specific predictor that has been included in consensus guidelines (ATS-ACCP 2017 update) is the cuff leak test, which can be qualitative or quantitative. A qualitative cuff leak test involves deflating the endotracheal tube cuff and occluding the end with a finger. The patient should be able to breathe around the endotracheal tube if no significant laryngeal edema is present (confirmed by breath sounds or measurement of exhaled carbon dioxide from the airway opening). A quantitative cuff leak test is done by comparing the exhaled tidal volumes with the cuff inflated and deflated. This is done while a patient receives volume-controlled breaths on the ventilator to ensure a consistent volume for comparison. If the difference between the inflated and deflated tidal volumes is at least 10% to 25% or 110 to 130 mL in an adult, this suggests a low probability of laryngeal edema and is supportive of extubation. The supporting evidence for this criterion is low, so caution should be used when considering the results of this test in the decision for extubation. The ATS-ACCP guidelines also recommend that adults who have failed a cuff leak test but are otherwise ready for extubation should receive systemic steroids for at least 4 hours before extubation to help lower the risk of reintubation. The cuff leak test should not be done if the patient has copious amounts of secretions above the cuff.

Failure of SBT

The goal of an SBT is to proceed to extubation, so whether an SBT is discontinued due to patient distress or even if a patient tolerates a diagnostic SBT but was returned to ventilator support, the attempt would be considered a failure (functioning as a diagnostic test). Regardless of the type of SBT failure, the next step is to determine the cause of failure and remedy it (see Box 11-2, Recommendation 5). If the cause of failure can be corrected, the usual practice is to wait 24 hours while resting on a comfortable form of ventilator support and then repeat the SBT (see Box 11-2, Recommendations 5 and 6). Physiologic experiments indicate it takes at least 24 hours to recover from respiratory muscle fatigue. If the time to correct requires more than 24 hours, then an SBT is attempted as soon as the usual assessment for weaning readiness indicates a patient is prepared. Occasionally another SBT might be attempted sooner than 24 hours if the cause for failure was due to something quickly remedied or a simple error in monitoring. The potential for enduring psychological impact from failed weaning attempts should be

considered when deciding when and how to conduct a repeat attempt.

Patients who fail three SBT attempts or who have been on prolonged mechanical ventilation are usually treated with a more gradual weaning approach (see Box 11-2, Recommendation 12). The goal of techniques that involve a gradual reduction in ventilator assistance—whether with **synchronized intermittent mandatory ventilation (SIMV)**, **pressure support ventilation (PSV)**, or T-piece trials of increasing duration. The rationale is to strengthen the respiratory muscles, which may have been weakened during the period of mechanical ventilation. The oldest gradual weaning method is to alternate a patient between periods of spontaneous breathing on T-piece aerosol and full support on a ventilator. There are many variations of this but they all involve increasing time off the ventilator until the patient is spending more time off the ventilator than on it. The highly responsive technology of current ventilators now makes it possible to simulate spontaneous breathing on a T-piece and still retain the monitoring and alarm capabilities of the ventilator. **Box 11-4** summarizes the thresholds that indicate SBT failure (reference **Box 11-5** for application example).

Thus, a series of increasing spontaneous breathing periods alternating with periods of ventilatory support may better be termed "progressive SBT" to differentiate the method from a diagnostic SBT of 30 to 120 minutes. When extubation is attempted with patients who require a gradual weaning approach, noninvasive ventilation or high-flow nasal cannula may be employed to help ensure reintubation is not needed. This approach has been formally recommended by consensus guidelines based upon strong evidence (ATS-ACCP 2017 update).

BOX 11-4 Example Measurement Values That Indicate Spontaneous Breathing Trial Failure

Respiratory frequency >35 breaths/min for 5 minutes or longer
Pao_2 ≤60 mm Hg or Sao_2 <90% on Fio_2 ≥0.5
$Paco_2$ >50 mm Hg (or increase >10 mm Hg); pH <7.32
f/V_T >100 breaths/min/L (rounded from 105)
Heart rate >140 beats/min or increase by ≥20% from baseline
Sustained changes in the heart rate of 20% in either direction
Systolic BP >180 mm Hg or <90 mm Hg
Cardiac dysrhythmias
Increased anxiety, diaphoresis, or paradoxical breathing

Pressure Support

PSV or similar forms of spontaneous breath assist (i.e., proportional pressure support, volume-assured pressure support, volume support) represent another leading weaning technique based upon the findings of several large clinical trials. Besides the previously stated use to counteract gas flow resistance imposed by the artificial airway (5 to 8 cm H_2O) or combining it with another mode such as SIMV, it can be used as a stand-alone mode to augment spontaneous tidal volumes (4 to 8 mL/kg predicted body weight) with higher pressure levels. Typically, the PSV pressure setting is reduced by 2 to 4 cm H_2O increments as tolerated, ideally at least twice a day until the pressure is in the range of 5 to 8 cm H_2O (the level of support during a SBT). Full ventilatory support is desired at night to allow the patient to rest in preparation for SBT and extubation.

Mehta et al. reported that the addition of any level of PS will lead to underestimation of a patient's work of breathing after extubation. Even PSV levels of only 5 cm H_2O before extubation underestimated the WOB performed after extubation by 36% (CPAP of 5 cm H_2O underestimated the WOB after extubation by 23%). PSV-type modes should be carefully monitored when used with COPD patients because prolonged exhalation from increased airway resistance and decreased elastic recoil can lead to patient-ventilator cycling dyssynchrony. In a study by Jubran et al. almost half of patients with COPD who were receiving PSV at 20 cm H_2O were using their expiratory muscles before the ventilator had ended inspiration.

SIMV

The SIMV mode ensures the patient receives periodic positive pressure breaths from the ventilator at a preset rate (either volume or pressure targeted). In addition, the patient can take spontaneous breaths between these mandatory breaths, either assisted with PSV or unassisted. The SIMV mode can be set to deliver full ventilatory support but is considered a weaning mode because of its ability to allow for spontaneous breathing with partial ventilatory support. When used as a weaning method, the mandatory ventilator breath rate is reduced by increments of 1 to 3 breaths/min. An arterial blood gas is obtained about 30 minutes after each change or other monitoring methods are used to confirm tolerance of the reduced level of support. The SIMV weaning method was previously held in high regard because of its theoretical appeal as a gradual respiratory muscle conditioning technique. Unfortunately, studies have revealed the respiratory center in the brain has difficulty adapting to the intermittent nature of the assistance—inspiratory effort is the same for assisted and unassisted breaths. Even more worrisome, at SIMV rates of ≤14 breaths/min, tension-time index (measure of respiratory load and muscle fatigue) for both assisted and unassisted breaths is above the threshold associated with fatigue. The SIMV mode may contribute to respiratory muscle fatigue or hinder recovery from it.

Comparison of Weaning Approaches

In comparisons of SBT, SIMV, and PSV methods of weaning, SIMV is the least effective weaning method based on total duration of mechanical ventilation until weaned. Brochard et al. found the PSV method had fewer weaning failures compared to SIMV or T-piece trials and a shorter weaning time compared to combined T-piece and SIMV patients. Esteban and colleagues studied the same modes and found that T-piece trials of spontaneous breathing were preferable to SIMV and PSV based on time taken to wean from the ventilator. The differences in study protocols for PSV weaning may explain part of the variation in findings. Matić and Majerić-Kogler also found the time of weaning to be shorter for the PSV method. SIMV may be considered a weaning method but it is not recommended as a first choice.

Most patients will be best served using a simple SBT approach (recommended by the consensus guidelines), possibly with repeat attempts. Patients who have been on prolonged mechanical ventilation (i.e., ≥3 weeks) may require a more gradual approach. PSV or T-piece trials would be the first-line choices.

Technology to Assist Weaning
Modes of Ventilation to Support Weaning

Besides the three traditional modes of weaning (spontaneous trials, PSV, and SIMV), there are other closed-loop modes (auto-adjusting based on patient monitoring) that are designed to simplify and perhaps enhance the weaning process. The most common currently available weaning modes are briefly described in **Table 11-1**. While the modes function differently, they all have the goal of adding efficiency to the weaning process while standardizing care to evidence-based practices and hopefully preventing errors. Mandatory minute volume or ventilation (MMV) was first reported in 1977 and has evolved over the decades but its primary function is to ensure that a set target minute volume is achieved (by automatically varying either the frequency of mandatory breaths or level of pressure support as needed). The major concern with MMV is its inability to distinguish if a patient is achieving a target minute volume by an abnormal breathing pattern

(e.g., hypopnea associated with increased respiratory frequency). This can be detected by setting alarm limits appropriately but it still has the weakness of adjusting based upon a single monitored patient variable. In spite of its longevity, it has never generated much interest among clinicians and there is no evidence in the literature to support it being advantageous.

Adaptive pressure ventilation (aka dual control or mode) includes several variations that all attempt to use pressure-targeted breaths (mandatory or spontaneous) to ensure a desired VT. These include pressure-regulated volume control (PRVC), auto flow, volume support ventilation (VSV), volume control plus (VC+), and others. The modes measure patient variables and reduce ventilatory support as patient effort becomes stronger or increases support if patient effort weakens. Oddly, at least two of the modes were introduced commercially without any evidence to support them. These modes may be satisfactory for weaning from a ventilator but there is no evidence to show they are better than other methods of weaning. AutoMode is not so much a stand-alone mode as it is a combination of two modes. It simply switches automatically between VSV (volume-targeted pressure support breaths triggered by the patient) and PRVC (volume-targeted pressure control

TABLE 11-1
Modes of Ventilation to Assist Weaning

Name of Mode	Description
Adaptive support ventilation (ASV)	Closed-loop control of inspiratory pressure and mandatory breath rate on a breath-by-breath basis to maintain preset minimum minute ventilation. Automatically switches to pressure support ventilation (PSV) and adapts pressure support based on respiratory rate and tidal volume.
AutoMode	Switches from a controlled mode (volume-targeted pressure control ventilation) to a support mode (volume-targeted PSV) based on detection of patient triggering of two consecutive breaths.
Intellivent-ASV	Extension of ASV that uses closed-loop control to adjust minute ventilation via modifying PSV level using input from end-tidal carbon dioxide, and fine-tuning oxygenation by adjusting positive end-expiratory pressure and the fraction of inspired oxygen.
Mandatory minute ventilation (MMV)	The first reported automated method for weaning. Closed-loop control of mandatory breath rate or spontaneous breath pressure assist to maintain a preset $\dot{V}_E$. Example: when patient $\dot{V}_E$ meets the set $\dot{V}_E$, no mandatory breaths are given.
Mandatory rate ventilation (MRV)	Closed-loop control to adjust pressure support based on a respiratory rate target.
Neurally adjusted ventilatory assist (NAVA)	Partial ventilatory support proportional to inspiratory diaphragmatic electrical activity measured via an esophageal catheter.
Proportional assist ventilation (PAV)	Adjusts airway pressure based on measurement of compliance and resistance throughout the inspiratory cycle to maintain a clinician selected percentage of degree of support.
Proportional pressure support (PPS)	Similar to PAV, this partial ventilatory support mode overcomes patient respiratory system elastance and resistance by applying pressure proportional to volume and flow needs.
SmartCare/PS	Closed-loop control of pressure support based on monitoring of respiratory rate, tidal volume, and end-tidal carbon dioxide. Tests for extubation readiness using a 1-hour spontaneous breath trial.

Modified from Rose L. Strategies for weaning from mechanical ventilation: a state of the art review. *Intensive Crit Care Nurs.* 2015;31(4):189–195; Branson RD. Modes to facilitate ventilator weaning. *Respir Care.* 2012;57(10):1635–1648.

breaths when there is no patient trigger). There is no published evidence that AutoMode hastens ventilator discontinuation compared to other methods.

Proportional ventilatory support (PVS) is a category of modes of ventilation that provide support that is proportional to the patient's inspiratory effort. A review by Kacmarek concluded research has shown that PVS improves patient–ventilator synchrony. Several ventilators are now available that provide a type of PVS. Proportional assist ventilation (PAV) is a form of PVS designed to synchronize with patient effort and deliver breath support according to patient effort (measured by flow and volume). The greater the patient's effort, the more assistance given by the ventilator (the ventilator amplifies the patient's effort). There is no preselected target volume or pressure, and the patient controls the breathing pattern (all breaths are patient triggered). Neurally adjusted ventilatory assist (NAVA) has a similar goal as PAV but utilizes measurement of the diaphragmatic electromyography (EMG) signal to control breath assistance. A nasogastric tube that has a series of electrodes near its distal end is positioned near the diaphragm to detect nerve activity. The clinician sets how much pressure assist is applied for each millivolt of neural activity. Therefore, both PAV and NAVA sense patient ventilatory effort (differently), which determines how much assistance is provided by the ventilator. Unlike PAV, NAVA greatly improves ventilator triggering because assistance begins as soon as the diaphragm receives nerve stimulation, not as a result of flow in the airway (unaffected by gas trapping or leaks in the circuit). The limited data on PAV and NAVA indicate it may allow better synchrony with patient breathing than PSV. More study is needed to determine the utility of PAV and NAVA for weaning from mechanical ventilation.

Adaptive support ventilation (ASV) is considered to be one of the most sophisticated ventilator modes available and has been studied more than most modes for over 20 years. This mode automatically uses both mandatory and spontaneous pressure-targeted breaths to achieve a desired percentage of the minute ventilation (based on predicted body weight). It uses a well-established equation for ventilation by Otis et al. to determine the optimal combination of tidal volume and frequency for achieving minimal WOB. The ASV mode has been shown to be useful for supporting patients for their entire duration on a ventilator (before as well as during weaning). In most studies, no difference has been shown between weaning with ASV and nonautomated methods.

Intellivent and SmartCare/PS represent a higher level of auto-adjusting modes because they utilize more patient feedback information to adjust. Intellivent is the next generation of ASV, which includes the standard ASV functions plus closed-loop control of PEEP and FIO_2 based on the PEEP/FIO_2 tables from the Acute Respiratory Distress Syndrome Network. The ventilator monitors arterial oxygen saturation by pulse oximetry and allows the clinician to set a desired oximetry saturation value. SmartCare/PS monitors the patient's V_T, f, and exhaled CO_2 and combines the data with patient settings (patient weight, humidifier type, airway type, medical history, and resting at night) to adjust PSV level. It can even be programmed to conduct SBTs automatically and report whether the patient passed or failed.

Research studies adhere to strict care protocols that may create artificially ideal conditions that are often not possible in routine clinical environments. Therefore, the benefit of automated modes may be that they help ensure continuity of care in understaffed environments and enforcement of evidence-based protocols that help ensure consistency in care for all patients.

Automated Artificial Airway Compensation

Many ventilators have the ability to compensate for the added WOB imposed by increased resistance to gas flow from an artificial airway. It is an attempt to simulate spontaneous breathing conditions as if there were no artificial airway present (termed by some as *electronic extubation*). The ventilator continuously calculates the resistive load of the artificial airway with information about the size of the endotracheal tube and measurement of the gas flow rate to precisely counteract the imposed load with a tailored pressure boost throughout inspiration. Some clinicians attempt to achieve this counteracting effect by adding a low level of PSV, but this approach appears to be less responsive to patient needs.

Artificial Intelligence Systems

The term *artificial intelligence* has been associated with some of the closed-loop, auto-adjusting modes of ventilation previously described. However, it is possible to go beyond this self-contained approach by connecting ventilators to a computer network that allows for more expansive data monitoring and more robust decision-making algorithms. Artificial intelligence systems can also be used to prompt clinicians to act or respond accordingly when continuous monitoring data indicate patients are ready for interventions (e.g., initiation of weaning protocols).

Practices to Enhance Weaning Success

Respiratory Muscle Training

Pulmonary specialists have focused on the need to prevent respiratory muscle fatigue during the ventilator weaning process to a degree that may have resulted in ignoring the importance of detecting preexisting respiratory muscle weakness. Many patients who have received prolonged mechanical ventilation have respiratory muscle weakness that becomes the cause of their weaning failure. A 2011 randomized control trial by Martin et al. examined if inspiratory muscle-strength training would improve weaning outcome in patients who had received mechanical ventilation approximately 40 to 50 days before entry into the study. At the end of the study, the strength-training group achieved a significantly more negative MIP with 71% weaned compared to no change in MIP and 47% weaned in the group who received a sham. This study used a simple threshold loader device for training; however, it is possible that other methods of increasing respiratory muscle strength, such as transcutaneous neuromuscular electrical stimulation (TENS), may also expedite weaning.

Interprofessional Collaboration

Regardless of the expected length or difficulty of the weaning process, a team approach to weaning is always advised, with the team size related to the complexity of the patient's condition. Using techniques to restore function to the whole body during a weaning attempt often helps expedite liberation, but these techniques should also be considered earlier, with the hope of hastening when a patient can start a weaning attempt. Besides clinician and nursing colleagues, the weaning team often includes physical and occupational therapists, dietitians, and other specialists as needed. In a study by Schweickert et al. involving patients from two hospitals, a formal program of physical and occupational therapy (exercise and mobilization) was used with patients receiving moderate duration mechanical ventilation (usual care did not include routine physical therapy for ventilated patients). The percentage of patients returning to independent functional status at hospital discharge was 59% for the group with PT+OT and 35% in

the control group, and overall duration of mechanical ventilation was also shorter in the intervention group. Difficult-to-wean patients require greater attention to diet and nutrition, and respiratory therapists often collaborate for metabolic testing of ventilator patients to help maximize respiratory muscle function.

Weaning Protocols

Use of a **weaning protocol** (or more than one based on specific patient groups or unique conditions) is recommended by the ACCP/SCCM/AARC consensus guidelines (see Box 11-2, Recommendation 8). Protocols and clinical practice guidelines should provide a systematic, evidence-based approach to care that requires thoughtful application; they are not just checklists of steps to follow. Of the recent studies that have tested the benefits of weaning protocols, half reported that protocolized weaning is superior to usual care while the others indicated no benefit (no difference compared to usual care). Regardless of whether duration of weaning or ventilator days are reduced with the use of protocols, a patient safety benefit typically comes with enhancing consistency. There are many weaning protocols published in the literature or developed by individual hospitals or departments. The example in **Table 11-2** is a part of what a protocol might look like based upon elements of the ACCP/SCCM/AARC consensus guidelines.

Role of Tracheostomy in Weaning

A tracheostomy is considered when it becomes apparent that a patient will require prolonged ventilator

---

TABLE 11-2
Abbreviated Partial Weaning Protocol Example Using Consensus Guidelines

Strategy	Decision Steps
1. Screening At least once per day the patient should be screened for readiness for weaning. Qualifications: Adequate oxygenation as evidenced by $Pao_2/Fio_2 >150$ or $Pao_2 >60$ mm Hg (or $Sao_2 >0.90$) on $Fio_2 <0.40$–0.50 on PEEP ≤ 5–8 cm H_2O. Hemodynamic stability as evidenced by heart rate ≤ 140 beats/min, systolic BP 90–160 mm Hg, adequate respiratory drive evidenced by $P_{0.1} <6$ cm H_2O, $f/V_T <100$. Disqualifications: Active myocardial ischemia or newly developing significant medical problem.	PASS Evaluation? YES—Proceed to SBT or progressive withdrawal of ventilatory support. NO—Determine cause of failed criteria, remedy, and reassess for readiness in 24 hours. Considerations: There is no clear evidence that fever, anemia (Hb <10 mg/dL), or abnormal mental status should exclude efforts to wean. Patients with active uncontrolled infection; ongoing blood loss/bleeding; or deteriorating mental status should have screening deferred.
2. Weaning Attempt SBT should be conducted on T-piece, PSV ≤ 8 cm H_2O (PEEP ≤ 5 cm H_2O), CPAP 5 cm H_2O or ATC (automatic tube compensation) for 30–120 minutes.	PASS SBT? YES—Proceed to extubation protocol or cases of prolonged duration on mechanical ventilation may consider progressive withdrawal using PSV or T-piece. Consider NIV postextubation for patients at risk for reintubation. NO—Determine cause of failed criteria, remedy, and reassess for readiness in 24 hours. Multiple daily SBTs may be acceptable with some patients as long as there is no clinical evidence for respiratory muscle fatigue.

BP, blood pressure; CPAP, continuous positive airway pressure; NIV, noninvasive ventilation; PEEP, positive end-expiratory pressure; PSV, pressure support ventilation; SBT, spontaneous breathing trial.

assistance. The procedure should be performed as soon as possible after the need for extended intubation has been verified, and it should be based on the patient's wishes. Although some clinicians perform the procedure as early as within 7 days of the onset of respiratory failure, it would certainly be done by the third week of intubation with rare exception. The most important benefits of a tracheostomy are the potential to facilitate discontinuation of mechanical ventilatory support and reduce complications associated with mechanical ventilation. The tracheostomy tube bypasses the upper airway, so it reduces WOB and dead space, and more effective secretion removal is possible. A tracheostomy site typically requires 7 to 10 days to mature; if the tracheostomy tube is displaced in the first 24 to 72 hours, a blind attempt at replacing the tube is highly unlikely to be successful. Removal of a tracheostomy tube is not difficult (typically easier than an endotracheal tube extubation). Surgical closure of the stoma after removal of the tracheostomy tube can be performed so as to leave minimal scarring in most people.

Causes and Correction of Weaning Failure

When a simple weaning approach is not possible (failure of the initial SBT), a more thorough evaluation is often needed, such as described by Heunks and van der Hoeven in **Figure 11-5**. Respiratory muscle weakness is one of the most common reasons for weaning failure, especially among patients receiving prolonged mechanical ventilation. Early mobilization of patients has been promoted for decades, but clinicians are becoming more aggressive with mobilizing patients while on a mechanical ventilation as it appears to have both physical and mental health benefits. **Respiratory muscle training** in the form of inspiratory resistance devices, targeted physical therapy, electrical muscle stimulation, and other methods leads to easily accessible clinical modalities used to overcome muscle weakness. Respiratory muscle weakness can also be related to insufficient levels of magnesium, calcium, or phosphate. Laboratory studies can help determine if mineral supplements are needed, and nutritional assessment can help fine-tune quantity and type of calories in patient feedings to enhance muscle endurance.

If a patient is not able to assume the load of spontaneous breathing because of inefficient functioning of the respiratory system, attempts should be made to reduce dead space volume (COPD patients are particularly susceptible to this). Mechanical dead space can be minimized by shortening the length of the endotracheal tube or converting the patient to a tracheostomy tube. Attachments and add-ons to the patient breathing circuit that add dead space should be removed if possible. An underappreciated form of oxygen delivery inefficiency results from significant anemia. Most hospital policies do not treat anemia until hemoglobin levels fall to 8 g/dL or less. That is about half of the oxygen-carrying capacity of normal hemoglobin levels (and that assumes normal gas exchange). Although the majority of patients do not appear to be significantly hindered during weaning by low hemoglobin levels, it may be a tipping point for those with a complicated clinical condition.

Infectious processes may be hidden to routine screening and require more in-depth probing to locate and treat. Indwelling catheters (vascular, urinary, etc.) are common sources of infection and should be cultured and removed if indicated. Keep in mind that older patients are less likely to exhibit a marked rise in body temperature and have a less robust immune response to infection.

Clinicians often overlook the effect of sleep disturbances on weaning readiness and progress. Patients need to have awareness of night and day cycles for optimal body function. The circadian rhythm of the body influences hormone release, cell regeneration, and important functions. Staff cooperation is needed to help ensure limited interruption of nighttime sleep, a quiet environment, and stress-relieving techniques. Psychological problems also need to be addressed and can be as simple as under- or overstimulation. Positive forms of recreation can be useful, including allowing visitors during daytime hours as much as possible. Patient self-care should be encouraged within safe limits, and a dependable method of communicating with the patient needs to be in place. Moving patients from a critical care unit (if possible) to a less acute environment helps with limiting excessive stimulation from alarms and around-the-clock activity. Medications or trauma may produce reactions requiring a psychiatric consultation.

Chronic Ventilator Dependence

Patients who require mechanical ventilation permanently (i.e., high spinal cord injuries) or for very long periods of time make up a very small proportion of those requiring ventilatory support (<1%). Patients should not be considered permanently ventilator dependent until at least 3 months of ventilator weaning attempts have failed (see Box 11-2, Recommendation 10). These patients are often cared for in subacute or long-term care facilities, an environment that is less intrusive and more like home, or in the home setting if the care requirements can be met. There are specialized weaning centers in some areas that have attained exceptional success with difficult-to-wean patients, including some declared to have **chronic ventilator dependence**. Clinicians should be familiar with local care facilities that specialize in caring for patients receiving prolonged mechanical ventilation (see Box 11-2, Recommendation 11).

	Airway / Lung			Brain		Cardiac	Diaphragm	Endocrine	
	Resistance	Compliance	Gas exchange	Delirium	Other cognitive dysfunction	Cardiac	Diaphragm	Endocrine	Metabolic
ASSESSMENT	Flow-time loops, inspiratory occlusion	Inspiratory/ expiratory occlusion	$P_{(A-aO_2)}$ DO_2	CAM-ICU	Screening: depression, anxiety, sleep pattern	12 lead ECG before / at end of SBT $S\bar{v}O_2$ before / at end of SBT Echocardiography before / after SBT	MIP	Serial physical examination (other neuromuscular disorders)	Electrolytes Blood gas Indirect calorimetry
INTERVENTION	Albuterol, steroids Repeat loops, inspiratory occlusion Auto-PEEP: Modify flow cycle setting in PSV	Radiology: Pleural fluid Atelectasis, ascites Diuretics Chest percussion & drainage		Reorientation Mobilization Haloperidol	Anxiolytics Behavioral therapy Reduce noise & light during sleep	Afterload reduction Inotropes If ischemia: β-blocker optimize hemoglobin	Early mobilization	Early mobilization	Provide adequate energy intake
ADVANCED ASSESSMENT	Diagnostic bronchoscopy during SBT				Psychological consult for depression, anxiety	Pulmonary artery catheter	Examination by neurologist EMG, nerve conduction velocity $P_{0.1}$ Diaphragm fluoroscopy / echography	Plasma cortisol before / after 250 mmol ACTH Plasma thyroid hormone	
ADVANCED INTERVENTION		Thoracentesis				Afterload reduction Inotropes	Reduce analgetics/ hypnotics	Cortisole I.V. Thyroid hormone	
RESCUE ASSESSMENT			Contrast echocardiography: intracardiac shunt			BNP	Phrenic nerve conduction velocity Transdiaphragmatic pressure measurement Diaphragm EMG	Muscle biopsy	
RESCUE INTERVENTION				Dexmedetomidine: Sedative w/o respiratory depression		Inotropic agonists, Pulmonary artery HTN antagonists	Antioxidants (vitamin C & E) Inspiratory muscle training		

FIGURE 11-5 Evaluation of difficult-to-wean patients. For each patient, diagnostics as described in the blue box should be performed to assess the reason(s) for difficult weaning. Endocrine dysfunction is probably relatively rare and therefore is not included in the first line of evaluation. Possible treatment/interventions are mentioned but need to be individualized. If the first-line evaluation does not improve weaning, proceed to the next level (within the affected column). For instance, if airway resistance is elevated but is not affected by albuterol and optimizing ventilator settings, diagnostic bronchoscopy should be performed to visualize the central airways. Risks and benefits should be weighed in each patient. ACTH, adrenocorticotropic hormone; BNP, brain natriuretcic hormone; CAM-ICU, confusion assessment method for the intensive care unit; DO_2, oxygen delivery; ECG, electrocardiogram; EMG, electromyography; HTN, hypertension; I.V., intravenous; $P_{0.1}$, airway occlusion pressure at 100 ms; MIP, maximal inspiratory pressure; PEEP, positive end-expiratory pressure; PSV, pressure support ventilation; SBT, spontaneous breathing trial; $S\bar{v}O_2$, mixed venous oxygen saturation.

Adapted from Heunks LM, van der Hoeven JG. Clinical review: the ABC of weaning failure—a structured approach. Crit Care. 2010;14(6):245. doi: 10.1186/cc9296.

Terminal Weaning

Terminal weaning is the withdrawal of mechanical ventilation with the anticipation that it will result in the death of a patient. This is different from deciding not to place a patient on mechanical ventilation when needed, at the patient's expressed decision (such as end-stage pulmonary fibrosis). Decisions to withdraw life-support measures are difficult even when the patient and family agree. Campbell and Carlson described four concerns to discuss with members of the healthcare team, the patient, and family members: (1) patient's informed request, (2) medical futility, (3) reduction of pain and suffering, and (4) fear and distress.

To give "informed consent" to remove life-sustaining care, a person must adequately comprehend the potential consequences, which include the likelihood of death. The law does not require a particular clinician to initiate the discussion (although an institution may have its own policy). These discussions should ideally occur over a period of time so that the patient has time to think through the issues and be less influenced by transient effects such as pain, medication reactions, and other factors that might interfere with an informed and valid decision.

There is no consensus definition of medical futility, and history provides exceptions to nearly every one suggested. One of the most cited definitions by Schneiderman et al. suggested that medical treatments may be futile if clinicians have concluded that in the last 100 similar cases the treatments were useless. While not perfect, this type of objective assessment can be informed and updated by new advances in medical care and treatment. This may be helpful to patients or family members who have reservations about terminal weaning and uncertainties about the chances of recovery.

It is important to reassure patients and their families that the decision to refuse or discontinue life-support care does not prevent other forms of care, including the relief of pain and promoting comfort. Patients may have misconceptions about what life-support interventions can or cannot do and these need to be sufficiently explored. A patient can choose partial or complete withdrawal or refusal of life-support care. Patients often do not fully hear or comprehend explanations of complex care options the first time, so follow-up is important. It is important for the patient and family members to be adequately informed about what to expect when life support is withdrawn. To the greatest degree possible, family members should be allowed to stay with the patient, and support resources such as a chaplain should be present. Caregivers who are uncomfortable with the process should be given the opportunity to withdraw from the situation.

Summary

Discontinuing mechanical ventilation will be a simple procedure for the majority of patients. One of the greatest responsibilities of caregivers is to work with patients to help them begin the weaning process as soon as possible. The minority of patients who have more difficulty with ventilator liberation depend upon clinicians to keep current in the best evidence-based practices. Current consensus guidelines do not provide a precise, universal method for the weaning process, so careful clinical judgment must be enhanced with input from interprofessional collaboration. The criteria for weaning assessments discussed in this chapter are based on peer-reviewed literature, but there is often minimal evidence to support thresholds and no single weaning assessment has sufficient predictive strength to be used alone. Nevertheless, when multiple assessments are evaluated together, they are very useful as a guide and starting point for weaning trials. The more weaning criteria that are met by a patient, the more likely the weaning process will be successful.

The most common cause of ventilator dependence is a ventilatory workload that exceeds the patient's ventilatory capabilities (others include oxygenation problems, cardiovascular instability, and psychological factors). The first and most important criterion for determining whether a patient is ready for ventilator discontinuation is sufficient resolution of the reason that caused the patient to need ventilatory support. Other factors to address include oxygenation, ventilation, acid-base balance and electrolyte levels, cardiovascular status, kidney function and fluid balance, sleep deprivation, psychological status, nutrition, and overall medical condition.

Of the three traditional weaning techniques, SBT and PSV appear to result in faster discontinuation of ventilatory support when compared to SIMV. Consensus guidelines recommend that weaning for most patients should be guided by a weaning protocol that makes use of an SBT. The use of daily sedation breaks or ensuring minimal sedation is also recommended by current guidelines to hasten weaning. Extubation and removal of ventilatory support often happen in close succession but involve separate assessments or readiness for each. Prior to extubation, patients should be assessed for the ability to maintain and protect their airway and for the presence of upper airway edema.

The most common cause of weaning failure is a ventilatory workload that exceeds the capacity of ventilatory muscles to bear it (often due to weakness or fatigue). Other causes of weaning failure are related to oxygenation problems, cardiovascular instability, the inability to clear secretions, poor mental status, or the presence of an unresolved condition that requires treatment. Long-term ventilator-dependent patients often have goals that focus on enhancing quality of life independent of ventilator removal such as reducing the amount of support, reducing the invasiveness of support, and increasing the patient's level of independent function.

Case Studies

Case Study 11-1 Guillain-Barré Syndrome

A 17-year-old male patient was transferred from a small, rural hospital with a diagnosis of Guillain-Barré syndrome (GBS) (made on the basis of progressive weakness of both upper and lower limbs, autonomic dysfunction, cerebrospinal fluid analysis, and nerve conduction study). His breathing difficulty increased to the point that mechanical ventilation was initiated. The patient received intravenous immunoglobulin and volume control ventilation with other supportive measures. Three weeks after admission, the patient was showing signs of recovery (spontaneous breathing parameters: $\dot{V}E$ 5.2 L/min, f 14 breaths/min, V_T 371 mL, VC 1.8 L, MIP −28 cm H_2O; PBW 160 lb). After 24 days of ventilation, T-piece weaning (with a heated, large volume nebulizer) was used with increasing periods of spontaneous breathing. The patient was extubated successfully on day 30 of ventilation.

Questions:

1. **Was it appropriate to start the weaning process for this patient?**

2. **What evidence supports your position?**

3. **Was this the appropriate method of weaning for this patient?**

Case Study 11-2 End-of-Life Mechanical Ventilation

(Adapted from a case by Paul Rousseau, MD, with permission)

Mr. Benny Williams is a 67-year-old male with a 70 pack-year history of smoking and stage 4 chronic obstructive pulmonary disease (COPD). About 2 years ago, he noted a grayish patch on his tongue but did not immediately seek medical attention. He continued to smoke and use spitless tobacco. About 5 months ago the patient sought medical help after he developed the following symptoms: (1) a feeling that something was caught in the throat, (2) difficulty chewing and swallowing, (3) difficulty pronouncing words, and (4) numbness of the tongue.

Assessment and testing revealed oral squamous carcinoma of parts of the tongue and floor of the mouth, which had unfortunately metastasized to the cervical lymph nodes. He was treated with surgical resection of the tongue with extensive resection of bone and soft tissue.

The malignancy progressed rapidly despite treatment and resulted in extensive tissue necrosis resulting in the following distressing symptoms: (1) strong nasal quality and loss of tongue made speech completely unintelligible, (2) extensive loss of teeth coupled with loss of tongue making it very difficult to swallow, (3) severe facial disfigurement, and (4) necrotic nonhealing oral ulcer causing severe malodor and facial pain.

Initially Mr. Williams's symptoms were relatively well controlled with:

- Methadone (50 mg twice daily)
- Immediate-release morphine sulfate (50 mg every 4 hours or as needed, for breakthrough pain)
- Haloperidol (0.5 mg every 6 hours) for nausea and vomiting
- Lorazepam (0.5 mg every 4 hours) for anxiety

Questions:

1. **Why are four medications needed—what is the justification for each based on the patient information?**

2. **What are potential complications/hazards to monitor?**

This regimen worked well for several weeks, but the pain worsened secondary to extensive local tissue necrosis from progression of the disease, leading to hospital admission for symptom control.

Laboratory Results:

SpO_2 89% on 3 L/min, SpHb 11.8 g/dL, and SpOC 14.5 mL O_2/dL blood via noninvasive oximeter.

Numerous interventions were attempted to relieve Mr. Williams's pain, including:

- Switching from methadone to continuous subcutaneous infusion of morphine (6 mg/h)
- Patient-controlled anesthesia (PCA) of morphine sulfate infusion 2 mg every 15 minutes or as needed
- Lorazepam (0.5 mg every 4 hours)
- Metronidazole gel applied to the ulcerated tissue on the face (to control local infection and thereby the bad odor)
- Nasal cannula at 6 L/min; and a fan gently blowing on his face

Questions:

1. **What is/are the potential benefit(s) from changing how morphine sulfate is administered to the patient?**

2. **In general, what is the primary potential hazard of delivering an opioid drug by this method? What noninvasive device could monitor the patient's "ventilatory" status, especially when the patient is unattended?**

Unfortunately, none of the treatments alleviated or attenuated his sense of severe pain. At this point, a family meeting was held to elicit goals of care and the following was determined:

- Mr. Williams adamantly refused further surgery, chemotherapy, and radiation therapy and received complete support from his wife and adult children.
- Heroic life-prolonging measures (endotracheal intubation with mechanical ventilation, etc.) were discussed with Mr. Williams and his family; however, they elected to forgo artificial ventilatory support and chose to continue with symptomatic treatment, invoking the Russell's do-not-resuscitate election in light of the futility of intubation and assisted ventilation.
- Patient and family refused a feeding tube.
- They elected for comfort care.

Questions:

1. Besides intubation and mechanical ventilation, what does the term "heroic life-prolonging measures" mean in this case?

2. Does this include noninvasive ventilation (justify your answer)?

Over the next week, the patient's pain worsened despite aggressive pain management, and spontaneous ventilation is starting to worsen. The nasal cannula was changed to a high-flow nasal cannula (70% oxygen at 35 L/min BTPS) resulting in an SpO_2 of 93%, SpHb 11.7 g/dL, and SpOC 14.7 mL O_2/dL blood.

Mr. Williams was clearly suffering greatly, and this caused severe distress to his dear wife and loving children who could not bear to see him suffer in this manner. Since his pain was unendurable and refractory to all palliative measures, palliative sedation was proposed as a humane and compassionate approach to allay his suffering.

After explanation of the procedure, both he and his family readily agreed to deep and continuous palliative sedation. An informed consent document was signed and a note describing the indications and plans for palliative sedation was recorded in the patient's chart.

A 4-mg subcutaneous bolus of midazolam was then administered, followed by a continuous subcutaneous infusion of 1.5 mg midazolam per hour. The Ramsay Sedation Scale was utilized to monitor depth of sedation, and the dosage of midazolam was titrated upward to maintain a deep level of sedation (a 4-mg bolus every 30 to 60 minutes, as needed, was utilized, with the continuous infusion increased by 0.5 mg/h after each bolus).

He was sedated within 10 minutes, but after 30 minutes he was still arousable with verbal stimulation and complained of pain. A second bolus of midazolam was then administered and his infusion increased to 2 mg/h.

Questions:

1. Before the second bolus of midazolam was administered, how would you have scored the patient using the Ramsay Scale?

2. What Ramsay Scale score would be desirable for the sedation goal of this patient?

3. Given the difficulty of balancing deep sedation while maintaining spontaneous ventilation, would it be advisable to consider noninvasive ventilation at this point (why or why not)?

Titration continued over the next few hours until he was deeply sedated, with an eventual dose of 5 mg/h required to maintain deep and continuous sedation. He died 4 days later, sedated, peaceful, and with his family at his bedside.

Questions: Choosing a Sedative

1. Given the choice between midazolam, phenobarbital, and propofol, which one would probably have been the best choice for this patient based on the information available?

2. If the midazolam had not been sufficient to facilitate the patient's sedation goal, what else might have been done?

Bibliography

Introduction

Bigatello LM, Stelfox HT, Berra L, et al. Outcome of patients undergoing prolonged mechanical ventilation after critical illness. *Crit Care Med*. 2007;35(11):2491–2497.

Boles JM, Bion J, Connors A, et al. Weaning from mechanical ventilation. *Eur Respir J*. 2007;29(5):1033–1056.

Branson RD. Modes to facilitate ventilator weaning. *Respir Care*. 2012;57(10):1635–1648.

Brochard L, Rauss A, Benito S, et al. Comparison of three methods of gradual withdrawal from ventilatory support during weaning from mechanical ventilation. *Am J Respir Crit Care Med*. 1994; 150(4):896–903.

Esteban A, Frutos F, Tobin MJ, et al. A comparison of four methods of weaning patients from mechanical ventilation. Spanish Lung Failure Collaborative Group. *N Engl J Med*. 1995;332(6):345–350.

Frutos-Vivar F, Esteban A, Apezteguia C, et al. Outcome of reintubated patients after scheduled extubation. *J Crit Care.* 2011;26(5):502–509.

Gladwell M. *Blink: The Power of Thinking Without Thinking.* New York, NY: Little, Brown; 2005.

Kahneman D. *Thinking, Fast and Slow.* New York, NY: Farrar, Straus and Giroux; 2011.

MacIntyre NR, Cook DJ, Ely EW Jr, et al. Evidence-based guidelines for weaning and discontinuing ventilatory support: a collective task force facilitated by the American College of Chest Physicians; the American Association for Respiratory Care; and the American College of Critical Care Medicine. *Chest.* 2001;120(6 Suppl):375S–395S.

MacIntyre NR, Epstein SK, Carson S, et al. Management of patients requiring prolonged mechanical ventilation: report of a NAMDRC consensus conference. *Chest.* 2005;128(6):3937–3954.

Monaco F, Drummond GB, Ramsay P, et al. Do simple ventilation and gas exchange measurements predict early successful weaning from respiratory support in unselected general intensive care patients? *Br J Anaesth.* 2010;105(3):326–333.

Thille AW, Boissier F, Ben-Ghezala H, et al. Easily identified at-risk patients for extubation failure may benefit from noninvasive ventilation: a prospective before-after study. *Crit Care.* 2016;20:48.

Tobin MJ. The new irrationalism in weaning. *J Bras Pneumol.* 2011;37(5):571–573.

Tobin MJ, Laghi F, Jubran A. Narrative review: ventilator-induced respiratory muscle weakness. *Ann Intern Med.* 2010;153(4):240–245.

Tobin MJ, ed. *Principles and Practice of Mechanical Ventilation.* 3rd ed. New York, NY: McGraw-Hill; 2013.

Vallverdu I, Calaf N, Subirana M, et al. Clinical characteristics, respiratory functional parameters, and outcome of a two-hour T-piece trial in patients weaning from mechanical ventilation. *Am J Respir Crit Care Med.* 1998;158(6):1855–1862.

Assessment of Readiness

Aitken LM, Bucknall T, Kent B, et al. Protocol-directed sedation versus non-protocol-directed sedation to reduce duration of mechanical ventilation in mechanically ventilated intensive care patients. *Cochrane Database Syst Rev.* 2015;1:CD009771.

Burry L, Rose L, McCullagh IJ, et al. Daily sedation interruption versus no daily sedation interruption for critically ill adult patients requiring invasive mechanical ventilation. *Cochrane Database Syst Rev.* 2014(7):CD009176.

Laghi F, D'Alfonso N, Tobin MJ. Pattern of recovery from diaphragmatic fatigue over 24 hours. *J Appl Physiol.* 1995;79(2):539–546.

MacIntyre NR. The ventilator discontinuation process: an expanding evidence base. *Respir Care.* 2013;58(6):1074–1086.

Ouellette DR, Patel S, Girard TD, et al. Liberation from mechanical ventilation in critically ill adults: an official American College of Chest Physicians/American Thoracic Society Clinical Practice Guideline: inspiratory pressure augmentation during spontaneous breathing trials, protocols minimizing sedation, and noninvasive ventilation immediately after extubation. *Chest.* 2017;151(1):166–180.

Clinical Measurements as Weaning Predictors

Bellemare F, Grassino A. Effect of pressure and timing of contraction on human diaphragm fatigue. *J Appl Physiol Respir Environ Exerc Physiol.* 1982;53(5):1190–1195.

Bien MY, Shui Lin Y, Shih CH, et al. Comparisons of predictive performance of breathing pattern variability measured during T-piece, automatic tube compensation, and pressure support ventilation for weaning intensive care unit patients from mechanical ventilation. *Crit Care Med.* 2011;39(10):2253–2262.

Brochard L, Pluskwa F, Lemaire F. Improved efficacy of spontaneous breathing with inspiratory pressure support. *Am Rev Respir Dis.* 1987;136(2):411–415.

Chevrolet JC, Deleamont P. Repeated vital capacity measurements as predictive parameters for mechanical ventilation need and weaning success in the Guillain-Barre syndrome. *Am Rev Respir Dis.* 1991;144(4):814–818.

Cook D, Meade M, Agency for Healthcare Research and Quality, McMaster University Department of Medicine, Clinical Epidemiology and Biostatistics. *Criteria for Weaning from Mechanical Ventilation.* Rockville, MD: Agency for Healthcare Research and Quality; 2000.

DiNino E, Gartman EJ, Sethi JM, McCool FD. Diaphragm ultrasound as a predictor of successful extubation from mechanical ventilation. *Thorax.* 2014;69(5):423–427.

El-Khatib MF, Jamaleddine GW, Khoury AR, Obeid MY. Effect of continuous positive airway pressure on the rapid shallow breathing index in patients following cardiac surgery. *Chest.* 2002;121(2):475–479.

Esteban A, Frutos F, Tobin MJ, et al. A comparison of four methods of weaning patients from mechanical ventilation. Spanish Lung Failure Collaborative Group. *N Engl J Med.* 1995;332(6):345–350.

Garfield MJ, Lermitte J. Weaning from mechanical ventilation. *Br J Anaesth.* 2005;5(4):113–117.

Jubran A, Mathru M, Dries D, Tobin MJ. Continuous recordings of mixed venous oxygen saturation during weaning from mechanical ventilation and the ramifications thereof. *Am J Respir Crit Care Med.* 1998;158(6):1763–1769.

Jubran A, Tobin MJ. Pathophysiologic basis of acute respiratory distress in patients who fail a trial of weaning from mechanical ventilation. *Am J Respir Crit Care Med.* 1997;155(3):906–915.

Khan N, Brown A, Venkataraman ST. Predictors of extubation success and failure in mechanically ventilated infants and children. *Crit Care Med.* 1996;24(9):1568–1579.

Kim WY, Suh HJ, Hong SB, Koh Y, Lim CM. Diaphragm dysfunction assessed by ultrasonography: influence on weaning from mechanical ventilation. *Crit Care Med.* 2011;39(12):2627–2630. DOI: 10.1097/CCM.0b013e3182266408.

Lemaire F, Teboul JL, Cinotti L, et al. Acute left ventricular dysfunction during unsuccessful weaning from mechanical ventilation. *Anesthesiology.* 1988;69(2):171–179.

MacIntyre NR, Cook DJ, Ely EW Jr, et al. Evidence-based guidelines for weaning and discontinuing ventilatory support: a collective task force facilitated by the American College of Chest Physicians; the American Association for Respiratory Care; and the American College of Critical Care Medicine. *Chest.* 2001;120(6 Suppl):375S–395S.

Mulreany LT, Weiner DJ, McDonough JM, et al. Noninvasive measurement of the tension-time index in children with neuromuscular disease. *J Appl Physiol.* 2003;95(3):931–937.

Patel KN, Ganatra KD, Bates JH, Young MP. Variation in the rapid shallow breathing index associated with common measurement techniques and conditions. *Respir Care.* 2009;54(11):1462–1466.

Pinsky MR. Breathing as exercise: the cardiovascular response to weaning from mechanical ventilation. *Intensive Care Med.* 2000;26(9):1164–1166.

Sahn SA, Lakshminarayan S. Bedside criteria for discontinuation of mechanical ventilation. *Chest.* 1973;63(6):1002–1005.

Sassoon CS, Light RW, Lodia R, et al. Pressure-time product during continuous positive airway pressure, pressure support ventilation, and T-piece during weaning from mechanical ventilation. *Am Rev Respir Dis.* 1991;143(3):469–475.

Shikora SA, Benotti PN, Johannigman JA. The oxygen cost of breathing may predict weaning from mechanical ventilation better than the respiratory rate to tidal volume ratio. *Arch Surg.* 1994;129(3):269–274.

Straus C, Louis B, Isabey D, et al. Contribution of the endotracheal tube and the upper airway to breathing workload. *Am J Respir Crit Care Med.* 1998;157(1):23–30.

Teboul JL, Monnet X, Richard C. Weaning failure of cardiac origin: recent advances. *Crit Care.* 2010;14(2):211.

Tobin MJ, Chadha TS, Jenouri G, et al. Breathing patterns. 1. Normal subjects. *Chest.* 1983;84(2):202–205.

Tobin MJ, Jenouri G, Birch S, et al. Effect of positive end-expiratory pressure on breathing patterns of normal subjects and intubated patients with respiratory failure. *Crit Care Med.* 1983;11(11):859–867.

Tobin MJ, ed. *Principles and Practice of Mechanical Ventilation.* 3rd ed. New York, NY: McGraw-Hill; 2013.

Whitelaw WA, Derenne JP, Milic-Emili J. Occlusion pressure as a measure of respiratory center output in conscious man. *Respir Physiol.* 1975;23(2):181–199.

Yang KL, Tobin MJ. A prospective study of indexes predicting the outcome of trials of weaning from mechanical ventilation. *N Engl J Med.* 1991;324(21):1445–1450.

Zhang B, Qin YZ. Comparison of pressure support ventilation and T-piece in determining rapid shallow breathing index in spontaneous breathing trials. *Am J Med Sci.* 2014;348:300–305.

Pulmonary Measurements

Hess DR. Respiratory mechanics in mechanically ventilated patients. *Respir Care.* 2014;59(11):1773–1794.

Hess D, et al. Mechanical ventilation: initiation, management and weaning. In: Burton GG, Hodgkin JE, Ward JJ, eds. *Respiratory Care: A Guide to Clinical Practice* (3rd ed.). Philadelphia, PA: J.B. Lippincott; 1991.

Marini JJ, Smith TC, Lamb V. 1986. Estimation of inspiratory muscle strength in mechanically ventilated patients: the measurement of maximal inspiratory pressure. *J Crit Care.* 1986;1(1):32–38.

Patel KN, Ganatra KD, Bates JH, Young MP. Variation in the rapid shallow breathing index associated with common measurement techniques and conditions. *Respir Care.* 2009;54(11):1462–1466.

Truwit JD, Marini JJ. Validation of a technique to assess maximal inspiratory pressure in poorly cooperative patients. *Chest.* 1992;102(4):1216–1219.

Traditional Weaning Procedures and Techniques

Figueroa-Casas JB, Connery SM, Montoya R. Changes in breathing variables during a 30-minute spontaneous breathing trial. *Respir Care.* 2015;60(2):155–161.

Girard TD, Alhazzani W, Kress JP, et al. An official American Thoracic Society/American College of Chest Physicians Clinical Practice Guideline: liberation from mechanical ventilation in critically ill adults. Rehabilitation protocols, ventilator liberation protocols, and cuff leak tests. *Am J Respir Crit Care Med.* 2017;195(1):120–133.

Jubran A, Van de Graaff WB, Tobin MJ. Variability of patient-ventilator interaction with pressure support ventilation in patients with chronic obstructive pulmonary disease. *Am J Respir Crit Care Med.* 1995;152(1):129–136.

Mehta S, Nelson DL, Klinger JR, Buczko GB, Levy MM. Prediction of post-extubation work of breathing. *Crit Care Med.* 2000;28(5):1341–1346.

Ouellette DR, Patel S, Girard TD, et al. Liberation from mechanical ventilation in critically ill adults: an official American College of Chest Physicians/American Thoracic Society Clinical Practice Guideline: inspiratory pressure augmentation during spontaneous breathing trials, protocols minimizing sedation, and noninvasive ventilation immediately after extubation. *Chest.* 2017;151(1):166–180.

Perren A, Domenighetti G, Mauri S, et al. Protocol-directed weaning from mechanical ventilation: clinical outcome in patients randomized for a 30-min or 120-min trial with pressure support ventilation. *Intensive Care Med.* 2002;28(8):1058–1063.

Comparison of Weaning Approaches

Brochard L, Rauss A, Benito S, et al. Comparison of three methods of gradual withdrawal from ventilatory support during weaning from mechanical ventilation. *Am J Respir Crit Care Med.* 1994;150(4):896–903.

Esteban A, Alia I, Tobin MJ, et al. Effect of spontaneous breathing trial duration on outcome of attempts to discontinue mechanical ventilation. Spanish Lung Failure Collaborative Group. *Am J Respir Crit Care Med.* 1999;159(2):512–518.

Matić I, Majerić-Kogler V. Comparison of pressure support and T-tube weaning from mechanical ventilation: randomized prospective study. *Croat Med J.* 2004;45(2):162–166.

Technology to Assist Weaning

Guttmann J, Bernhard H, Mols G, et al. Respiratory comfort of automatic tube compensation and inspiratory pressure support in conscious humans. *Intensive Care Med.* 1997;23(11):1119–1124.

Kacmarek RM. Proportional assist ventilation and neurally adjusted ventilatory assist. *Respir Care.* 2011;56(2)140–148.

Otis AB, Fenn WO, Rahn H. Mechanics of breathing in man. *J Appl Physiol.* 1950;2(11):592–607.

Practices to Enhance Weaning Success

Martin AD, Smith BK, Davenport PD, et al. Inspiratory muscle strength training improves weaning outcome in failure to wean patients: a randomized trial. *Crit Care.* 2011;15(2):R84.

Schweickert WD, Pohlman MC, Pohlman AS, et al. Early physical and occupational therapy in mechanically ventilated, critically ill patients: a randomised controlled trial. *Lancet.* 2009;373(9678):1874–1882.

Causes and Correction of Weaning Failure

Heunks LM, van der Hoeven JG. Clinical review: the ABC of weaning failure—a structured approach. *Crit Care.* 2010;14(6):245. doi:10.1186/cc9296. Epub 2010 Dec 8.

Terminal Weaning

Campbell ML, Carlson RW. Terminal weaning from mechanical ventilation: ethical and practical considerations for patient management. *Am J Crit Care.* 1992;1(3):52–56.

Schneiderman LJ, Jecker NS, Jonsen AR. Medical futility: its meaning and ethical implications. *Ann Intern Med.* 1990;112(12):949–954.

12

Neonatal and Pediatric Mechanical Ventilation

Lisa A. Conry, MA, RRT

OUTLINE

OBJECTIVES

1. Compare and contrast anatomical airway differences between neonatal and pediatric patients.
2. Compare and contrast physiologic differences of neonates and adults.
3. Differentiate and appropriately select volume-controlled and pressure-controlled ventilation.
4. Describe the indications and application of CPAP to a neonate.
5. List the initial ventilator settings for neonatal and pediatric patients.
6. Recommend changes in ventilator settings based on arterial blood gas results.
7. Outline the indications and administration of surfactant in neonates.
8. Describe the ventilation methods for pediatric patients.
9. Explain the indications and application of high-frequency oscillatory ventilation and NAVA in the neonate.
10. Describe the indications and application of ECMO in infants and children.

KEY TERMS

barotrauma
epiglottis
eustachian tube
Moro reflex
oscillatory ventilation
oxygenation index
phospholipid
pneumomediastinum
pneumopericardium

pneumoperitoneum
pulmonary interstitial
  emphysema
retractions
tracheostenosis
tracheomalacia
transcutaneous
volutrauma

Introduction

Mechanical ventilation of neonates and children varies from ventilation of adults. Many simplify the differences and assume children are "little adults." This is simply not true. The neonatal population has a different approach to ventilation because the respiratory physiology is very different from that of adults. Although low compliance in either population affects ventilation, the physiologic causes are quite different, so the ventilation approaches must also be different. Children's lungs continue to develop throughout childhood, so their lung physiology also changes. This requires the clinician to fine-tune the ventilator settings for a child. The pediatric/neonatal clinician must be able to quickly assess these patients and make appropriate setting adjustments.

Anatomical Differences

Trachea

The trachea of an adult is much larger than that of an infant. The small tracheal size in newborns means that the airway resistance is much higher in this population. Poiseuille's law indicates the driving pressure must increase by 16 times to maintain flow when the radius decreases by half. In the case of neonates, the tracheal size is about 25% that of an adult, so the work to breathe through these small airways would be immense if they had adult-sized breaths. During childhood, the circumference of the trachea grows as the child grows, but there is no formula to estimate exactly how large a child's trachea may be. It is important to understand that the airway resistance will decrease as the trachea enlarges. The trachea of an infant is also much shorter than that of an adult. The short bronchial length predisposes infants and children to right main stem intubation as shown by Habrat, Shocket, and Braude. Many clinicians use the body weight in kg + 6 to estimate the insertion distance in centimeters (the 7-8-9 rule). This will usually place the tip of the tube between T1 and T2 if the infant is not very low birth weight, <750 g, or >2500 g. Most neonatal endotracheal tubes have a solid black ring on them that should be located just below the vocal cords during intubation.

Head and Spine

In relation to body size, an infant's head is large and the neck provides little support. By age 8, the spine has matured and resembles that of an adult. The anterior fontanelle, which allowed the sutures to override during birth, closes during the first year as well.

Airways

The airways of the child follow the same pattern as those of the adult. As a newborn, the airways are quite small and they grow in circumference throughout childhood as the child grows. As with the trachea, there is no formula to determine the exact size of the airways. However, the younger the child, the higher the airway resistance will be.

Epiglottis

Since the infant respiratory tract is smaller, structures within the airway other than bronchial tree will take up a larger proportion of the airway in an infant or child than these structures do in an adult. One such structure is the **epiglottis**. Not only is it larger in relation to the size of the airway, but it is also shaped a bit differently. In adults it is flat, but in infants it is U-shaped. It is also a bit stiffer in infants and harder to expose the glottis during intubation. For this reason, the straight Miller laryngoscope blade is commonly used as it allows direct lifting of the epiglottis. Fitting the curved MacIntosh blade into the vallecula and raising it upward does not move the epiglottis as well in infants as it does in adults (refer to Chapter 4 for using a MacIntosh blade with an adult).

Tongue

Another structure within the airway that is larger in proportion to the airway in infants versus adults is the tongue, while the oral airway is smaller. This increases the likelihood of airway obstruction by the tongue. As the child grows, the tongue gradually becomes a smaller proportion of the airway. As with other changes throughout childhood, the change in size is gradual and cannot be predicted.

Larynx

Infants have shorter necks than adults and their larynx is more anterior and located opposite C1-C2. As the child grows, the laryngeal position descends. By age 8 it is in the adult position opposite C5-C6. The higher laryngeal position in infants is another reason why the Miller laryngoscope blade is preferred to the MacIntosh blade. It provides better visualization of the glottis during the intubation procedure.

Eustachian Tube

The **eustachian tube** connects the nasopharynx with the middle ear. Normally, air can move freely through these tubes in adults to regulate the pressure within the ear so that it is equal to atmospheric pressure. These passageways are much smaller in infants and children, and more prone to blockage. Secretions and inflammation can easily obstruct the tubes so pressure cannot be equalized and the middle ear can become easily infected. Nasal intubation may physically block the eustachian tube, preventing its function and increasing the risk of middle ear infection.

Lymphatic Tissue

Airway obstruction can occur with inflammation of lymphatic tissues, such as adenoids and tonsils. The adenoids, in the nasopharynx, become inflamed with upper respiratory infections. The tonsils, in the oropharynx, become inflamed with strep throat, epiglottitis, and other infections of the respiratory tract. Physical obstruction of the airway increases the airway resistance during both spontaneous and mechanical ventilation.

Alveoli

The lungs are the only organ that is not completely formed at birth. Alveoli continue to develop up to age 8. This means young children have less surface area for gas exchange.

   Table 12-1 distinguishes between the anatomical differences between adults and infants.

Physiologic Differences
Distribution of Water

Infants and children differ from adults in the amount and the distribution of their body water. Adults are approximately 60% water, with the majority found in the intracellular fluid (within cells). In preterm infants, those born before 38 weeks' gestation, water makes up about 80% of the total weight, with the majority found in the extracellular fluid. A term infant has about equal amounts of intracellular and extracellular fluid. Within a few months

TABLE 12-1
Anatomical Differences Between Adults and Infants

Anatomical Feature	Adults	Infants
Trachea	16 mm	4 mm
Head	Proportionate to body size	Large in relation to body size
Airways	Larger circumference	Smaller circumference
Epiglottis	Paddle-shaped	U-shaped
Tongue	Small in relation to oral cavity	Large in relation to oral cavity
Larynx	Longer neck; less anterior	Shorter neck; more anterior
Eustachian tube	Larger	Smaller
Lymphatic tissue	Small in relation to nasal/oral cavities	Large in relation to nasal/oral cavities
Alveoli	Fully formed	Still developing

Modified from Figaji A. Anatomical and physiological differences between children and adults relevant to traumatic brain injury and the implications for clinical assessment and care. *Front Neurol.* 2017;8:685.

of life, intracellular fluid levels exceed extracellular fluid levels in the same proportion as found in adults. These differences between premature infants, term infants, and children necessitate careful titration of medication doses and intravenous (IV) fluid administration.

Bones and Cartilage

Bones are not completely calcified, and cartilage is softer in infants than in adults. This results in instability of the thorax when the infant work of breathing increases. Infants are prone to exhibiting **retractions** (an inward movement of the chest wall during inspiration) when the work of breathing is high and the compliance is low. Since infants cannot increase their tidal volume, they increase their minute ventilation by increasing the respiratory rate. Tachypnea is a common finding in infants who have respiratory distress.

Liver

Liver development occurs early in gestation, as does most organ development. However, all of the physiologic systems and enzymes needed to metabolize medications and turn blood toxins into metabolites that can be excreted do not develop fully until closer to term, with some enzymes (such as CYP1A, CYP2C, CYP2D, and CYP3A) developing after delivery. Premature infants may not metabolize medications well, requiring dosage adjustments. Because an infant's liver may not be capable of effectively conjugating bilirubin (mainly a byproduct of the breakdown of red blood cells), neonates are also prone to jaundice, recognized by yellowing of the skin and mucous membranes.

Respiratory Rate and Pattern

Periodic breathing is common in infants. It is characterized by short pauses in breathing, less than 20 seconds, that occur periodically. Infants are also obligate nose breathers up to about 5 months of age, so nasal obstructions become quite critical when they occur. By age 8 months, they can breathe through the mouth. The average respiratory rate in infants is also much higher than that of adults. Normal rate in adults is 12 to 20/min; in infants the normal is 40 to 60/min. The exact age at which the respiratory rate has transitioned to the adult normal rate is not known. It is highly variable, but by age 8 or so the child's respiratory rate equals that of the adult.

Cardiac

Heart sounds differ in infants compared to adults. Normal heart rate also varies. Normal adult heart rate is 60 to 100 beats/min. Normal infant heart rate is 120 to 160 beats/min. Because the stroke volume is so much smaller, the rate must be higher to have a cardiac output that perfuses all the tissues in the body. Infants may also exhibit murmurs, or swishing sounds, as blood moves through the heart. These are usually benign and disappear during childhood, unless abnormal cardiac anatomy exists.

Hormones

Growth hormone production is constant and steady throughout childhood, but it surges during puberty. The sex hormones also increase in production during puberty. Children grow throughout childhood because of the presence of growth hormone, but nutrition also has a substantive effect. During puberty, when adult characteristics develop, the presence of both growth hormone and the sex hormones drive the process.

Reflexes

Neonates have several neurological reflexes not found in adults. When the cheek is stroked near the edge of the mouth, the infant will turn the head toward the stroke. This is the rooting reflex. Infants also have an innate suck reflex and will automatically suck on a pacifier placed in the mouth. The **Moro reflex**, or startle reflex, occurs when the infant is allowed to drop an inch from a sitting position toward a lying position. The arms should fly up and out and the legs pull in to the body as the baby startles. The grasp reflex is tested by placing a finger in the baby's palm or just under the toes. The fingers or toes should grasp the finger. If any of these neurological reflexes are absent or abnormal, it signals the presence of a neurological deficit or injury. These reflexes disappear normally by 3 to 6 months of age.

Temperature Regulation

Normally, the hypothalamus regulates body temperature and keeps it steady at 37° C. In cold adults, shivering generates heat to help maintain the body temperature. Conversely, when the temperature rises, sweating helps to cool the body. Infants have difficulty maintaining their body temperature, and the problem is exacerbated in premature infants whose hypothalamus is not completely operational. In infants, a drop in body temperature stimulates release of norepinephrine, which stimulates brown fat metabolism to generate heat. Preterm infants may have few brown fat stores because they develop late in gestation. In addition, an enzyme necessary to regulate the process is not available until close to term. An infant in a cold environment quickly deteriorates and body temperature drops rapidly. Several methods have been used to ensure temperature regulation of infants. They are kept dry to avoid evaporative heat loss. Conductive heat loss is avoided by prewarming anything the baby will contact. This will likewise reduce radiant heat loss to a cool object placed close to the infant. Conductive heat loss to air currents can be reduced by covering and placing the infant in an incubator. Signs of hypothermia include cool skin, acrocyanosis, tachypnea, irritability, poor feeding, and hypotonia. The cold stress and resulting norepinephrine release increase oxygen consumption so hypoxemia and low saturation may also be a sign. Heated humidity is used with all respiratory therapy equipment to reduce cold stress and hypoxemia. On the other hand, heat stress or hyperthermia is equally detrimental to the infant, as the increase in temperature increases oxygen consumption and may quickly deplete the energy stores.

Oxygen Consumption

Oxygen consumption of an infant is greater than that of an adult because infants have higher metabolic requirements. This increases the risk of hypoxemia and desaturation. Since premature infants do not have many energy stores in reserve, they quickly decompensate in the presence of increased oxygen consumption.

Airway Resistance

Because of the smaller tracheal and airway sizes, airway resistance is much higher in infants than adults. Even small amounts of inflammation can have grave consequences because of the increase in work of breathing. Abnormal airway anatomy, such as **tracheostenosis** or **tracheomalacia**, or airway growths, such as granuloma tissue, make an already small airway opening much smaller.

Blood Volume/Blood Pressure

Circulating blood volume is low in infants and young children. This means that even minor blood loss can make a major impact. Blood replacement is a common practice in the neonatal intensive care unit (NICU), based on hemoglobin and hematocrit values. Blood pressure is also lower in infants and children. Pediatric Advanced Life Support (PALS) guidelines for hypotension base their thresholds on the systolic blood pressure. The threshold for neonates is 60 mm Hg, and it is 70 mm Hg for infants younger than 12 months. For children between 1 and 10 years old, $(2 \times$ age in years $+ 70)$ mm Hg determines the hypotension threshold. After the age of 10, the threshold of 90 mm Hg is used.

It is also important to note that prior to using donor blood in the NICU it must be thoroughly tested for compatibility and to make sure it is cytomegalovirus (CMV) negative. CMV in the neonate can have devastating effects, including hepatitis and pneumonia. For this reason, blood that is CMV negative is used preferentially for blood transfusion in the NICU.

Mechanical Ventilation

Volume-Controlled Versus Pressure-Controlled Ventilation

By convention, pressure-controlled ventilation is applied to most neonates. Children may be ventilated with volume-controlled ventilation or pressure-controlled ventilation, depending upon the lung characteristics. If volume-controlled ventilation is used, the same guidelines as for adults are used—the resulting tidal volume is much smaller because the body weight is much smaller. It is only recently that volume ventilation has gained ground in the NICU. Pressure-controlled ventilation was first applied in neonates in the early days of mechanical ventilation. At the time, it was thought that since the premature lungs were so delicate, volume-controlled ventilation would be more harmful than pressure-controlled ventilation. Limiting pressures was thought to have a lung protective effect. With advances in technology and modes, and a better understanding of ventilation, volume ventilation may also be safely applied to this patient population.

Indications for Mechanical Ventilation

Indications for mechanical ventilation in infants and children are the same as those for adults, but the critical values differ. Respiratory failure, defined by a pH <7.25 with a rising $PaCO_2$ or hypoxemia in the face of an FIO_2 >0.50, is an indication for mechanical ventilation. Impending ventilatory failure is another indication. If the trend of a rising $PaCO_2$ and decreasing pH can be seen, it is not necessary to wait until the criteria for respiratory failure are met if the trend cannot be quickly reversed. Additionally, a neonate in distress may be intubated without obtaining an arterial blood gas (ABG) first. Infants can deteriorate quickly and waiting for an ABG may impede a timely response. For this reason, blood gases are not as crucial in clinical decisions with neonates as they are with older children and adults. Apnea is always an indication for mechanical ventilation. It is important, however, to distinguish between apnea and periodic breathing.

Volume-Controlled Ventilation

Volume-controlled ventilation is used to more directly control the minute ventilation and therefore the homeostatic state of the patient. The ABGs can be adjusted by manipulating the volume ventilation settings. In volume-controlled ventilation, the tidal volume and rate are set to achieve a minute ventilation for the patient, and the delivery pressure varies with the patient's lung compliance and airway resistance. The biggest disadvantage to using volume-controlled ventilation is that the pressure can become dangerously high, leading to **barotrauma**. Since volume does not distribute evenly in the lung but will preferentially fill the alveoli with the best lung compliance, **volutrauma** (damage due to overdistended alveoli) can also occur with volume-controlled ventilation. Generally, volume-controlled ventilation is not applied in the neonatal or infant population but may be used with children over the age of 1. The guidelines for setting the tidal volume are to use 4 to 5 mL/kg, outlined by El Hazzani et al. Since

the body weight is much lower, the set tidal volumes are much lower. Volume-controlled ventilation may not work well in the presence of large leaks, although some ventilators can compensate for this. Peng, Zhu, and Liu indicate that volume-controlled ventilation compared to pressure-controlled ventilation may be associated with a lower rate of pneumothoraces, fewer days on the ventilator, less incidence of intraventricular hemorrhage, and lower mortality rate. Because the pressure will increase with decreases in lung compliance or increases in airway resistance, close monitoring of the airway pressure during volume-controlled ventilation is crucial.

Pressure-Controlled Ventilation

Pressure-controlled ventilation is used to reduce lung injury due to excessive inspiratory pressure. It is the most common mode applied when ventilating neonates and infants. With pressure-controlled ventilation, rate and pressure limits are set and volume is variable. Because the tidal volumes are very small, especially in premature infants, very small changes become significant. For example, if an infant has a compliance of 2.5 mL/cm H_2O, and the pressure is increased by 1 cm H_2O, the infant will receive an additional 2.5 mL of tidal volume. If the infant's total tidal volume is 10 mL, 2.5 mL represents a 25% change in the tidal volume! An advantage of pressure-controlled ventilation is that it can accommodate minor leaks around the endotracheal tube and still ventilate the infant. Since the tidal volume is variable with changes in lung compliance and airway resistance, the blood gas parameters are not as well controlled under pressure-controlled ventilation. For instance, respiratory acidosis may occur as the tidal volume drops when the lung compliance decreases or airway resistance increases. Close monitoring of the minute ventilation is essential when utilizing pressure-controlled ventilation.

Properties of Humidification

All patients with an artificial airway require supplemental humidification. There are different ways humidification is applied to the airway, but in neonates and small children, heated humidity is the preferred method. The use of heat moisture exchangers adds too much dead space in the circuit. This can be a problem because the tidal volumes are very small, as in neonates or small children. Consider this example: If the total tidal volume is 10 mL, trapping just 2.5 mL in a heat and moisture exchanger (HME) would trap 25% of the tidal volume, dropping the available tidal volume to just 7.5 mL. This is a huge change when the volumes are that small. In addition, an HME that was only trapping 2.5 mL of volume would not be very efficiently humidifying the inspiratory gas, especially at the respiratory rates encountered in neonates. For these reasons, heated humidity is used. The heated humidifier will usually be a passover or wick type of humidifier used in conjunction with a heated wire circuit. This reduces condensation within the circuit and ensures that the delivered gas will be close to body temperature and with little to no humidity deficit. At 37° C, the gas can hold up to 44 mg/L of water (humidity). If the gas in the circuit cools as it flows through the tubing to the patient, some of that water will condense and rain out within the tubing. Heating the circuit keeps the temperature constant and the humidity in gaseous form. A temperature probe, located close to the patient, works with the humidifier to keep the temperature output constant.

Continuous Positive Airway Pressure

Continuous positive airway pressure (CPAP) is applied to infants to help splint the alveoli open and improve oxygenation while reducing the alveoli opening pressure. Premature infants do not have the same type or quantity of surfactant in their lungs as full-term infants. Very premature infants may have little to no surfactant present at all. This reduced amount or lack of surfactant increases the alveolar surface tension so that the alveoli tend to close with each expiration. This makes the opening pressure of these alveoli very high, and each breath requires a high inspiratory pressure to open the alveoli for gas exchange. Since infants have little energy reserve, they quickly become fatigued and acidotic when the work of breathing is high. CPAP lowers the critical opening pressure for inspiration by splinting and holding the alveoli open during exhalation, reducing the work of breathing for the patient. It is applied when indications of low compliance and high work of breathing are present: grunting, retractions, tachypnea, and nasal flaring.

There are several methods by which CPAP can be applied. Many manufacturers make a CPAP device that is free-standing and can be applied by nasal prongs, mask, or nasopharyngeal tube to the infant. Flow is generated in proportion to the CPAP level selected, and alarms can be set to signal if the pressure increases or decreases past the alarm point. These devices also provide humidification of the gas flow.

The Carden valve is another way to apply CPAP. This is an adapter that has one open end that attaches to the nasal prongs or nasopharyngeal tube. The other end is closed with multiple small openings. There are attachments on the valve for oxygen and a pressure manometer. As gas flows into the Carden valve, the closed end with the multiple openings creates the CPAP pressure. If the pressure manometer used with the Carden valve has alarms that can be set, this system can also alert the clinician if the pressure becomes too high or too low. **Figure 12-1** shows a CPAP setup.

Bubble CPAP is an older method of applying CPAP that is coming back into vogue. With bubble CPAP, gas flow is bubbled through water, which creates the CPAP

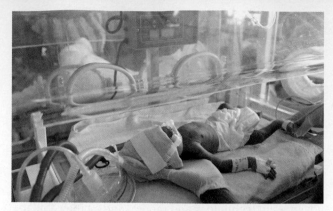

FIGURE 12-1 Neonatal CPAP setup. CPAP, continuous positive airway pressure.
© Jake Lyell/Alamy Stock Photo.

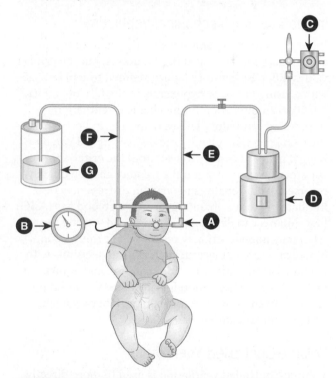

FIGURE 12-2 Bubble CPAP setup **A.** nasal CPAP at nostrils, **B.** manometer, **C.** air/oxygen blender to flow meter, **D.** humidifier, **E.** inhalation, **F.** exhalation, **G.** depth of exhalation tube in water column equals CPAP pressure. CPAP, continuous positive airway pressure.
Modified from Liptsen E, Aghai ZH, Pyon KH, et al. Work of breathing during nasal continuous positive airway pressure in preterm infants: a comparison of bubble vs variable-flow devices. J Perinatol. 2005;25:453–458.

pressure. The depth of the water column determines the CPAP pressure. This device has the advantage of humidifying the gas and it is a simple and easy way to generate CPAP. A bubble CPAP setup is shown in **Figure 12-2**.

Hazards of CPAP are the same as for any pressurized system applied to the thorax. Barotrauma, such as a pneumothorax, may occur as the pressure is applied to delicate alveoli. Other barotraumas, such as **pulmonary interstitial emphysema**, **pneumopericardium**, **pneumoperitoneum**, and **pneumomediastinum**, are also possibilities. Because applied pressure increases the intrathoracic pressure, CPAP can also interfere with venous return and decrease the cardiac output. The increased intrathoracic pressure can also interfere with venous return from the head, increasing the intracranial pressure (ICP) and potentially reducing the cerebral perfusion pressure (CPP), since CPP equals the mean arterial pressure (MAP) minus the ICP (CPP = MAP − ICP or MAP − CVP if central venous pressure [CVP] exceeds the ICP). Autoregulation of cerebral flow is a complex process and not well developed in preterm infants, so increases in ICP have more profound negative effects.

CPAP is contraindicated if the infant has apnea, because there is no set rate with CPAP, and therefore, spontaneous frequency is required. Hemodynamically unstable infants should be intubated rather than placed on CPAP, as decompensation can occur rapidly in this age group. If the infant has an untreated tension pneumothorax, CPAP should not be applied until the pneumothorax has been treated.

Recently, CPAP has been compared to mechanical ventilation with surfactant administration in several studies. These studies suggest that CPAP applied at birth, even to very preterm infants, may reduce the need for mechanical ventilation and surfactant administration and is associated with a lower mortality rate. The American Academy of Pediatrics strongly recommends the use of CPAP at birth, with selective administration of surfactant rather than prophylactic administration for preterm infants as noted by Carlo and Polin. CPAP is usually started at 4 to 6 cm H_2O and titrated based on the clinical response.

Intubation

Because of the shorter neck and more anterior larynx, the straight Miller blade is preferred for neonatal intubation. Determining the size of the endotracheal tube is usually based on age rather than weight. This is because airway growth tends to be constant and unrelated to weight. See **Table 12-2** for neonatal endotracheal tube sizing.

Initial Settings—Neonates

If mechanical ventilation is to be used, the guidelines for initial settings help reduce overventilation and side effects during the placement process. Mode selection is guided by the patient's condition. Advantages of assist-control are a more controlled minute ventilation and a lower work of breathing. Synchronized intermittent mandatory ventilation (SIMV) allows control of the minute ventilation along with preservation of spontaneous breathing. If spontaneous mode is to be used, pressure support is usually added to overcome airflow resistance of the small endotracheal tube. Spontaneous mode with pressure support preserves spontaneous breathing while reducing the work of breathing. If volume-controlled ventilation is being used, El Hazzani et al. recommend the tidal volume be set at 4 to 5 mL/kg. If pressure-controlled ventilation is used, the peak inspiratory pressure (PIP) can be determined by watching for chest rise. If manual ventilation is being done with a resuscitator with a pressure pop-off, the PIP should be set at the ventilating pressure being used—again, chest rise guides the amount of pressure to use. Since tidal volume is variable with pressure-controlled ventilation, and the ventilating volumes are so low for neonates, tidal volume is not a reliable indicator of adequate ventilation. The PIP usually is begun between 12 and 20 cm H_2O.

The rate for infant ventilation is between 30 and 40/min. This should provide an adequate minute ventilation. Rates less than 20/min are discouraged because they fall well below the natural respiratory rate of a neonate.

Positive end-expiratory pressure (PEEP) is usually set between 5 and 6 cm H_2O. Excessive PEEP overdistends the lungs. This can be seen on the chest x-ray by overly hyperlucent lung fields that extend more than nine ribs and flatten the diaphragms. Too little PEEP does not reduce the critical opening pressure of the alveoli enough, requiring a higher PIP to ventilate.

The inspiratory time needs to be short enough to allow at least a 1:2 ratio. When using fast rates, shorter inspiratory times are indicated. The time constant can also be used to guide the inspiratory time setting. If the inspiratory time is set at 3 time constants, inspiration is optimized. Very preterm infants have short time constants because lung compliance is low, so they can tolerate short inspiratory times. Times between 0.35 and 0.5 second are usually sufficient to allow a 1:2 ratio.

The FIO_2 should be kept as low as possible. The target recommended PaO_2 range for a neonate is 50 to 70 mm Hg. Infants can tolerate a much lower PaO_2 because they still have fetal hemoglobin, which has a higher affinity for oxygen. This means even at low PaO_2 levels, the hemoglobin will saturate with oxygen. Keeping the PaO_2 below 100 mm Hg is important to avoid retinopathy of prematurity, which can lead to blindness as the retina detaches. Some facilities titrate the FIO_2 to reach a target saturation range that is based upon the gestational age. There is great controversy as to whether a lower saturation (85% to 89%) or a higher saturation (90% to 95%) should be maintained. Neonates managed with the lower saturation range tend to have more

TABLE 12-2
Endotracheal Tube Sizes

Gestational Age	Tube Size
<30 weeks	2.5 mm
30–35 weeks	3.0 mm
>35 weeks	3.5 mm

BOX 12-1 Ventilator Setting Adjustments for a Desired Paco$_2$ and Pao$_2$

To adjust Paco$_2$:

$$\frac{\text{Known Paco}_2 \times \text{known parameter*}}{\text{Desired Paco}_2}$$

*Parameter can be rate, pressure, or volume.

To adjust Pao$_2$:

$$\frac{\text{Known Fio}_2 \times \text{desired Pao}_2}{\text{Known Pao}_2}$$

---

complications associated with a low Pao$_2$, such as necrotizing enterocolitis and patent ductus arteriosus. However, infants managed with the higher saturation range tend to have higher incidence of retinopathy of prematurity but a lower rate of necrotizing enterocolitis. There is currently no universal standard and a wide range of practice exists.

Higher settings may be needed for some disease processes, such as persistent pulmonary hypertension of the newborn (PPHN). Settings also will need to be increased as the infant gets older.

Once ventilation has been initiated and an ABG drawn, adjustments can be made to normalize the ABG. If the Paco$_2$ is out of range, making the pH out of range, a variety of changes can bring it back into homeostasis. If volume-controlled ventilation is being used, changing the minute ventilation by altering either the rate or tidal volume is appropriate. If pressure-controlled ventilation is being used, changing either the pressure or the rate can bring the Paco$_2$, and therefore the pH, back into balance. If the current Paco$_2$ is known, a calculation can be done to determine the adjustment to make (**Box 12-1**). A calculation can also be performed to adjust the Fio$_2$ to target a Pao$_2$ level (see Box 12-1) as well. These calculations assume there are no significant ventilation-perfusion abnormalities.

If the ABG shows hypoventilation, then the calculation should yield a rate, pressure, or volume that is higher than currently set. If the ABG shows hyperventilation, the calculation will show a reduction of rate, pressure, or volume. If the Pao$_2$ is too high, the calculation should yield a lower Fio$_2$ and vice versa. It is important to double-check the math and make sure the answers make sense with the situation prior to making the change.

When settings are at a minimal level and the ABG values and other clinical signs are favorable, extubation can be considered. The rate is not usually weaned below 15 to 20/min. The airway resistance from the endotracheal tube is so high that it would be difficult for the infant to maintain a normal rate when the set ventilator rate is so low. Spontaneous efforts should be consistent with no apnea spells, indicating intact neurological functioning.

Surfactant Administration

Surfactant is a detergent-like substance that reduces the surface tension in the lung. It helps keep the alveoli from closing with each exhalation, reducing the opening pressure required to ventilate the lungs. Infants start making surfactant at about 24 weeks' gestation. The type that is made first is sphingomyelin. While sphingomyelin is a surfactant, it is not very efficient at reducing surface tension. Phosphatidylcholine, or lecithin, is a more efficient type of surfactant that is made beginning at about 28 weeks' gestation. It is the most prevalent **phospholipid** in surfactant. Closer to term, at about 35 weeks' gestation, phosphatidylglycerol begins to be made. Phosphatidylglycerol plays a role in the reduction of surface tension along with phosphatidylcholine. Other phospholipids in surfactant include phosphatidylinositol, phosphatidylserine, and phosphatidylethanolamine. Their roles are not completely understood, as noted by Chakraborty and Kotecha. Amniotic fluid can be tested for the types of surfactant present and the relative amounts. The lecithin-sphingomyelin ratio, or L/S ratio, is done to determine if any efficient surfactant is present. A 1:2 ratio indicates more sphingomyelin than lecithin. A 2:1 ratio signals that lecithin is present in ratios twice that of sphingomyelin. A 2:1 ratio is associated with low risk for pulmonary disease (e.g., respiratory distress syndrome [RDS]) after birth. An alternate test to the L/S ratio is the lamellar body count assay, which can be performed in most laboratories and is reliable in predicting lung maturity. Lower lamellar body counts are associated with fetal lung immaturity and higher risk of RDS. Tests that require amniocentesis to perform, though, such as the L/S ratio and the lamellar body count assay, are less common currently as the risks associated with the procedure are high. They may, however, be helpful to identify the infant who should receive rescue surfactant immediately upon birth. **Figure 12-3** shows surfactant within an alveolus.

When infants are born prematurely, the fact that surfactant processes develop late in gestation becomes an important factor. Premature infants frequently have increased work of breathing because their alveoli rebound to a smaller circumference during exhalation. The strong inward force within the alveoli must be overcome to open and ventilate them. This imposes a huge work of breathing on the infant, requiring a great deal of energy to breathe. To reduce the surface tension and therefore the opening pressure of the alveoli, surfactant can be given to the infant. When artificial surfactant is given, the infant's immune system treats it as if it were endogenous, or made by the infant. The artificial surfactant is recycled just like endogenous surfactant, so it becomes part of the infant's surfactant pool. This supplies the premature infant with a surfactant pool to use until his or her own type II cells begin to manufacture it.

The composition of surfactant is primarily phosphatidylcholine, phosphatidylglycerol, and four surfactant proteins: A, B, C, and D. As outlined by Chakraborty and Kotecha, protein A is part of the immune system and helps mark bacterial cells so they can be removed by alveolar macrophages. It also seems to play a role in surfactant homeostasis. Protein D also seems to have immune function. Protein B alters the lipid molecules in the cell, reducing surface tension. The manufacture and metabolism of surfactant seem to be the role of protein C. Surfactant preparations that do not contain the surfactant proteins are not as effective as those that do.

There are a variety of sources for exogenous surfactant. It can be made my mincing cow or pig lung and then extracting the surfactant from the minced tissue. It can also be made synthetically in a lab. Since synthetic preparations do not contain the surfactant proteins, they have not been as successful as those extracted from cow or pig lungs. Synthetic analogs for surfactant protein B and C have been tested for improved outcomes. **Table 12-3** summarizes the different surfactant preparations currently on the market.

Surfactant preparations are administered by direct instillation into the endotracheal tube. The preparations are thick solutions. They are administered through a catheter that is inserted through the endotracheal tube into the trachea. Each different brand of surfactant has a specific administration technique. The dosage given is based upon body weight, with each brand having a different dose-to-weight requirement. Once the dose has been calculated, it is divided into portions called aliquots. The number of aliquots depends on the brand of surfactant being used. If the surfactant requires two aliquots, one is given with the infant on the right side and the other given with the infant on the left side. If more aliquots are used, more positions are used in an effort to distribute the surfactant evenly throughout the lung. After an aliquot has been administered, the infant is either manually or mechanically ventilated at a high rate (60 breaths/minute) to distribute the surfactant in the alveoli.

Aerosolized forms of surfactant (Aerosurf [lucinactant] and Survanta) are currently under investigation but have not yet been approved by the Food and Drug Administration (FDA).

The infant's response to the surfactant is immediate. Lung compliance rapidly increases when artificial surfactant is given, so quick ventilator setting changes are required. A reduction in PIP is to be expected because compliance improves quickly after surfactant administration. Because the alveoli are open and more stable, ventilation and perfusion also are better matched, so oxygen exchange improves. Thus, FIO_2 is usually also weaned following surfactant administration. The PIP needs to be reduced to prevent barotrauma and volutrauma. The FIO_2 needs to be reduced to avoid retinopathy of prematurity, since studies in the early 1990s showed that PaO_2 levels greater than 80 mm Hg were

Structure of an Alveolus

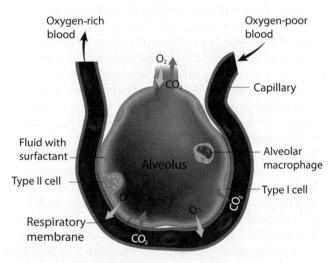

FIGURE 12-3 Surfactant within an alveolus.
© Alila Medical Media/Shutterstock.

TABLE 12-3
Current Surfactant Preparations

Name	Proteins Present	Source	Initial Dose	Number of Aliquots	Subsequent Dose (if indicated)	Dosing Schedule
Survanta (beractant)	B, C	Bovine	4 mL/kg	4	100 mg/kg	Total of four doses given every 6 hours in the first 48 hours of life
Curosurf (poractant)	B, C	Porcine	2.5 mL/kg	2	1.25 mL/kg	Total of three doses given 12 hours apart
Infasurf (calfactant)	B, C	Bovine	3 mL/kg	2	3 mL/kg	Total of four doses given 12 hours apart; can be given in 6 hours if infant requires $FIO_2 > 0.30$

strongly associated with the development of retinopathy of prematurity. Each surfactant preparation has its own administration guidelines, and these guidelines may also vary in the consideration of a second dose. Prior to a second dose of surfactant, the infant must be assessed to determine if clinical signs exist that justify that dose. If clinical signs for more surfactant are not present, the infant is not given a second dose, and no further doses can be given. If clinical signs are present, the infant is given a second dose at a specified time interval determined by the manufacturer.

Ventilating the Pediatric Patient

Intubation of a pediatric patient can be accomplished with either a cuffed or uncuffed endotracheal tube. If the tube leak is too great, reintubation with either a larger tube or a cuffed tube may be required. If a cuffed tube is used, the cuff pressure should be maintained below 20 cm H_2O. The route can be either oral or nasal, with no significant differences in complications between the two as described by Gupta et al. The most common method of determining endotracheal tube size is to use Cole's formula: (age in years/4) + 4 (**Box 12-2**). This formula will determine the appropriate size of an uncuffed tube to use. If using a cuffed tube, the answer should be reduced by 0.5.

The pediatric patient may be ventilated with either volume-controlled or pressure-controlled ventilation. Many use the child's weight to determine the ventilation target: pressure-controlled if less than 20 lb and volume-controlled if over 20 lb. The exact normal respiratory rate for a child is unpredictable: The minute ventilation is guided by the pH and $Paco_2$. If volume-controlled ventilation is used, the recommended tidal volume is 6 mL/kg.

High-Frequency Oscillatory Ventilation

Extremely premature infants may be ventilated with high-frequency **oscillatory ventilation**, rather than conventional ventilation, to lower the risks of ventilator-induced lung injury. The oscillator is the only mechanical ventilator with an active expiratory phase. The oscillations are produced by a piston that moves a diaphragm in and out. As the piston moves toward the diaphragm, it bulges toward the patient. As the piston moves back, the diaphragm moves back. Rapid piston

movement creates rapid diaphragm movement and oscillatory waves that transmit to the patient. In addition, there is a fresh gas flow (termed *bias flow*) that enters the airway to help oxygenate the patient. The oscillations simply shake the air molecules in the lung at tidal volumes smaller than dead space. Some proximal alveoli may be directly ventilated by the oscillation wave, but mostly the oscillations simply enhance diffusion for better gas exchange. Coaxial flow, in which inspiratory gas flows down the center of the airway while expiratory gas flows up the edges of the airway, also helps explain how oscillatory ventilation enhances gas exchange. The physics of oscillatory ventilation are complex and difficult to grasp, but one example that clarifies the principles is to consider filling a glass with water. As water is poured into the middle of the glass, when it hits the bottom it turns and follows the wall of the glass until it spills over the top. There is a continuous stream of water into and out of the glass at the same time. Oscillatory ventilation works in the same fashion: There is a continuous flow of gas into and out of the lung at the same time. **Figure 12-4** outlines the theories of gas exchange with high-frequency oscillatory ventilation.

The oscillator setup is very different from that of conventional ventilation. Following calibration, the oscillator can be set up for use (**Figure 12-5**). There is a specific calibration procedure that must be followed prior to its use. There is no tidal volume or pressure to set. Rather, amplitude (power), which determines the swing of the piston and therefore tidal volume, is set. The amplitude, or power, is set high enough to cause wiggling between the chest and abdomen (as described in the manufacturer's Pocket Guide, CareFusion Inc.). The greater the amplitude, the greater the wiggle. Chest wiggle will also change with altered lung compliance. Wiggle increases as compliance improves and vice versa. Main stem intubation and pneumothoraces also affect wiggle by decreasing it. There is not a true rate set but a frequency in hertz (Hz), which controls how many times per minute the piston moves back and forth, is set instead: 1 Hz is the equivalent of one cycle of the piston per second, so multiplying the hertz setting by 60 will yield the piston stroke rate per minute. The frequency is usually set between 10 and 15 Hz in a neonate and 6 and 10 Hz in children. Once set, it is usually not adjusted further.

Another setting on the oscillator that differs from conventional ventilation is the bias flow setting. A flowmeter on the oscillator determines the bias flow setting. It needs to be high enough to support the mean airway pressure. If it is set too low, it will be difficult to meet the desired mean airway pressure. In premature infants, it may be set between 10 and 15 L/min and as high as 30 L/min in children. Mean airway pressure is set on the oscillator with a dial labeled "Adjust." It is usually set less than 12 cm H_2O in the neonate. Settings higher than this increase the risk of barotrauma. If it is set too low,

---

BOX 12-2 Cole's Formula to Estimate ET Tube Size for Pediatric Patients

(Age in years/4) + 4

Example: A 6-year-old needs intubation. The appropriate size of endotracheal tube would be:

(6/4) + 4
1.5 + 4 = 5.5

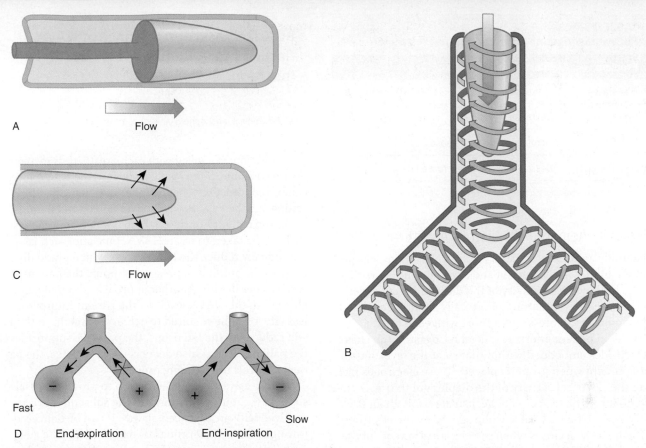

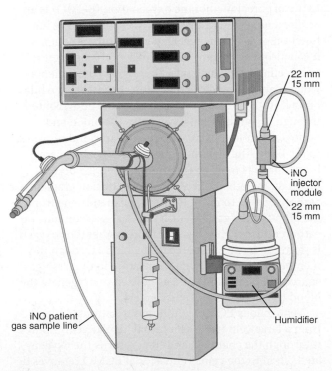

FIGURE 12-4 (A) Spike formation with HFV. **(B)** Helical diffusion with HFV. **(C)** Taylor dispersion with HFV. **(D)** Pendelluft during HFV. HFV, high-frequency ventilation.

B: Modified from Karp TB, Solon JF, Olson DL, et al. High frequency ventilation: a neonatal nursing perspective. *Neonatal Network.* 1986;4(5):43.

FIGURE 12-5 Sensormedics 3100A high-frequency oscillator ventilator. iNO, inhaled nitric oxide.

the risk of atelectasis is increased. The inspiratory time percent is typically set on 33%. It may be increased to 50% to improve recruitment and therefore oxygenation if needed.

When the oscillator is set up and running, breath sounds cannot be determined without stopping the piston and manually ventilating the patient. The infant is evaluated for adequate wiggle, and oxygenation is monitored with pulse oximetry. ABGs can be trended invasively or noninvasively via **transcutaneous** monitoring.

If the $Paco_2$ is too high, and consequently the pH is acidotic, *lowering* the hertz (frequency) setting may allow for an increase in tidal volume and therefore minute ventilation. The amplitude, or power, may also be increased to improve the $Paco_2$ by increasing the piston movement. If the $Paco_2$ is too low, the amplitude/power should be reduced. Oxygenation is adjusted with the mean airway pressure or the Fio_2 setting. Increasing mean airway pressure or Fio_2 should increase the Pao_2 and vice versa. For patients on maximum settings that are not oxygenating well, the inspiratory time percent can be increased from 33% to 50%. **Table 12-4** summarizes patient management strategies with high-frequency oscillatory ventilation.

TABLE 12-4
Patient Management Strategies

Problem	Intervention
High Pa_{CO_2}	Decrease Hz (frequency) or increase amplitude
Low Pa_{CO_2}	Decrease amplitude
Low Pa_{O_2}	Increase mPaw or increase F_{IO_2}
High Pa_{O_2}	Decrease mPaw or decrease F_{IO_2}

mPaw, mean airway pressure.

BOX 12-3 Insertion Distance of NAVA Catheter for Oral (0.8) or Nasal (0.9) Insertion

NEX × 0.8 or 0.9 + catheter factor

NEX, nose, ear, and xiphoid process.

Neurally Adjusted Ventilatory Assist

Neurally adjusted ventilatory assist (NAVA) is a unique mode found on the Servo i and Servo u ventilators that uses the electrical activity of the diaphragm to trigger and cycle the ventilator. It is a totally spontaneous mode that adjusts the pressure support with each breath, based on patient effort. A special nasogastric tube has electrodes embedded within that sit at the level of the diaphragm when properly placed. These electrodes pick up the electrical activity of the diaphragm to trigger the ventilator. The trigger voltage, usually set at about 0.5 mV, opens the flow valve when sensed by the electrodes. The flow valve closes when the electrical activity of the diaphragm (Edi) drops to 70% of the peak electrical level. The peak Edi is multiplied by a NAVA level setting to determine the amount of pressure support applied to the breath. If the ventilator cannot sense the electrodes, or there is a discrepancy in the signal, the ventilator will revert to a backup pressure support level set by the clinician. If the patient becomes apneic, the ventilator reverts to a backup pressure control level. Once spontaneous breaths are detected, the ventilator automatically reverts back to pressure support. NAVA is indicated when mechanical ventilation is required and the infant is spontaneously breathing. It can be applied with invasive ventilation (through an endotracheal tube) or noninvasive ventilation, using a nasal mask or prongs.

Prior to placing the catheter, the distance between the infant's nose, ear, and xiphoid process (NEX) is measured. This measurement is then multiplied by either 0.8 (for an oral tube) or 0.9 (for a nasal tube). The answer is then adjusted by a number based on the size of the catheter used (**Box 12-3**). The size of the NAVA catheter is determined by the weight of the infant.

Once placed, catheter position is verified on the positioning screen of the ventilator. Four electrocardiogram (ECG) patterns appear on this screen. If the middle two are blue, the catheter is in correct position. If only the top ECG is blue, the catheter is too far in and should be pulled back. If only the bottom ECG is blue, the catheter is not in far enough and should be advanced.

If the infant's Pa_{CO_2} is too high, reducing the pH, the NAVA level can be increased to increase the amount of pressure support applied with each breath, thus increasing the tidal volume. If the Pa_{CO_2} is too low, the NAVA level can be reduced. Oxygenation is controlled by the PEEP setting and the F_{IO_2}, as with conventional ventilation.

As the patient improves, there are two approaches that can be taken to wean NAVA. One approach is to gradually reduce the NAVA level, which gradually reduces the amount of pressure support the patient receives per breath. Another approach is to make no changes in the NAVA level. As the patient improves, less effort will be required to achieve a breath, so the Edi will reduce. As the Edi drops, the pressure support level the patient receives also decreases—in essence, the patient controls the weaning process.

Noninvasive NAVA is an option to provide partial support without intubation and the subsequent risks involved with an advanced airway. It can be delivered through either nasal prongs or nasal masks. The advantage to noninvasive NAVA is the reduction of dyssynchrony related to triggering and delays in signaling compared to other noninvasive options.

Extracorporeal Membrane Oxygenation

Extracorporeal membrane oxygenation (ECMO) is an artificial lung system that takes over some of the lung function of gas exchange. Depending on the setup, it can also relieve some of the work of the heart. It is not as efficient as the lungs, however, so the patients will remain on low-level mechanical ventilation while on ECMO. Blood is withdrawn from the body, routed through a chamber that oxygenates the blood and removes carbon dioxide, and then heated and returned to the body. The chamber is a semipermeable membrane that has fresh gas on one side and the body's blood on the other. There is a concentration gradient for carbon dioxide to move through the membrane from the blood to the gas, because the fresh gas contains no carbon dioxide. The concentration gradient for oxygen is from the fresh gas source to the blood through the membrane. The oxygen concentration in the fresh gas source can be manipulated as needed to oxygenate the blood (Rodriguez-Cruz and Berger).

Venovenous ECMO withdraws desaturated blood from a large vein (such as internal jugular vein), routes it through the chamber, and then returns the oxygenated blood to the vein. Venoarterial ECMO removes desaturated blood from a large vein, routes it through the chamber, reheats it, and then returns the oxygenated

BOX 12-4 Calculation of Oxygen Index (OI)

$$OI = \frac{FiO_2 \times mPaw}{PaO_2}$$

mPaw, mean airway pressure; OI, oxygenation index.

blood to an artery. Venoarterial relieves some of the work of the heart because some of the cardiac output bypasses the heart.

ECMO is indicated in neonates with diaphragmatic hernia and those with PPHN. These infants cannot have a low birth weight or significant coagulopathy. They should have a reversible lung disease and should not have been on the ventilator for more than 10 days. Finally, all other types of appropriate medical treatments should be exhausted before ECMO is instituted. If these criteria are not met, Makdisi and Wang recommend that ECMO is contraindicated.

Other criteria to qualify a patient for ECMO include an A-a gradient of 600 mm Hg or more on an FiO_2 of 1.0, an **oxygenation index (OI)** of 40 or more, and acute deterioration, defined as a PaO_2 of 40 mm Hg or less, a pH of 7.25 or less, and intractable hypotension. **Box 12-4** shows the calculation of the oxygenation index.

There is no true normal OI, since one must be on a ventilator to calculate it. However, values <5 are considered good and values >25 are associated with increased mortality risk. An alternative to OI, which seems to correlate well with the OI, is the oxygen saturation index (OSI). It is calculated by substituting SpO_2 for PaO_2 in the OI formula.

In pediatric patients, ECMO may be used in patients with congenital heart defects who have a low cardiac output or severe pulmonary hypertension. It also may be used as a bridge until cardiac surgery can be performed.

Patients on ECMO are still supported on mechanical ventilation, but typically on low settings. Frequent position changes and suctioning are indicated as well. Cardiac output should be maintained, using inotropic medications if needed, so that blood pressure can be maintained. Neurological exams, including head ultrasonography, should be performed routinely. Hypoxia and acidosis should be avoided to reduce serious central nervous system complications. It is not uncommon for urine output to drop and for volume depletion to occur after ECMO has been instituted because ECMO triggers an inflammatory reaction. Fluid retention is common in the first few days. Diuresis signals recovery. If urine output remains low, diuretics may be required. Hemoglobin should be maintained above 12 g/dL, by administering packed red blood cells if necessary. Platelets will need to be given as they are consumed during ECMO and leave the patient vulnerable to bleeding. The circuit is cultured routinely to determine if infection is present. Strict adherence to infection control asepsis is essential.

The most common complication with ECMO is clotting of the circuit. Clots in the circuit can cause emboli in either the pulmonary or systemic circulation. Heparin-coated circuits decrease the tendency of this complication. Another potential complication of ECMO is damage to the vein or artery that the circuit is placed within. This can cause internal bleeding that can be fatal. Air emboli may also occur and can be fatal. Malfunction of the circuit is life threatening to the patient. In these cases, the venous and arterial lines are clamped and the patient is removed from ECMO. The patient may be manually ventilated or the ventilator settings can be increased to ensure ventilation and oxygenation. Electrolyte disorders, gastrointestinal dysfunction, oliguria, arrhythmias, and pneumothorax are other complications associated with ECMO. A final complication is that ECMO alters the concentration of drugs within the bloodstream. Dosage adjustments may be required to titrate medications, and medications with a low therapeutic index should be very closely monitored.

The mortality rates associated with ECMO vary widely, from as low as 18% to as high as 50% for neonates and from 25% to 66% for pediatric patients. The higher the volume of ECMO used at a facility, the lower the mortality rates. Neonates and children who have received ECMO also have a higher rehospitalization rate than those who do not receive ECMO. They also have a higher incidence of asthma. Feeding difficulties are common after ECMO, even if the suck and swallow reflexes are maintained. Seizure activity is not uncommon during ECMO and some patients may continue to have seizure activity for years after. Other central nervous system disabilities, such as developmental delays and hearing loss, may also be seen. Children who have received ECMO have a greater tendency for social problems, academic difficulties, and attention deficit disorders. It is also important to consider the stress of ECMO on the family and provide them with support throughout this process.

The duration of ECMO ranges from 3 to 7 days typically. The longer the patient remains on ECMO, the higher the risk of complications. **Figure 12-6** shows an ECMO circuit.

Assessment of Oxygenation and Ventilation

ABG analysis is commonly used to evaluate oxygenation and ventilation in mechanically ventilated patients. This is true in the neonatal and pediatric population as well. However, in the neonate, the site and the technique are slightly modified. The radial artery, the preferred site for adult ABG sampling, can also be used in neonates and children. It is preferred because the ulnar artery provides collateral circulation to the hand in the event of complications. Rather than using a needle attached to the sampling syringe, however, a butterfly needle is more commonly used (**Figure 12-7**).

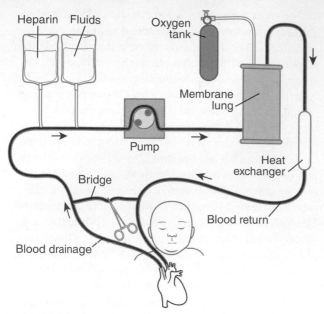

FIGURE 12-6 ECMO circuit. ECMO, extracorporeal membrane oxygenation.
Courtesy of Jessica Hopkins at the University of the District of Columbia, College of Arts and Science, Studio Art.

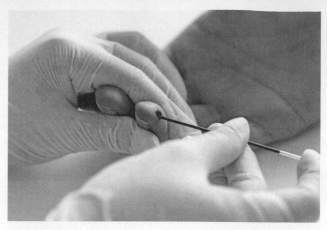

FIGURE 12-8 Capillary blood sampling.
© Pittawut/Shutterstock.

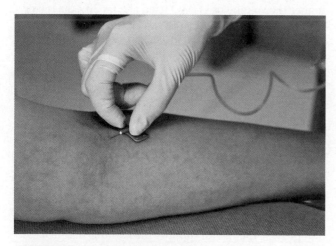

FIGURE 12-7 A butterfly needle.
© Saowanee K/Shutterstock.

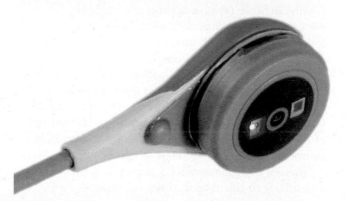

FIGURE 12-9 A sensor for transcutaneous carbon dioxide and oxygen saturation.
Courtesy of SenTec AG.

An alternative site for obtaining an ABG sample in an infant or small child is the dorsalis pedis artery in the foot.

An umbilical artery catheter may also be placed in the neonate, as the umbilical vessels remain patent for a short period of time after birth. The cannula is threaded through the umbilical artery with the tip resting in the thoracic aorta.

Capillary blood draws are common in neonates to avoid the complications of arterial sticks. The site is warmed to draw blood to the area, and a capillary tube is used to collect the sample (**Figure 12-8**). Capillary samples can be obtained from fingers, toes, or the heel of the foot. The puncture site for heel sticks should be on the most medial or lateral portions of the plantar surface of the heel. The posterior curvature of the heel

must not be used to avoid injury to the calcaneus (heel bone). The lancet is a sampling device designed to puncture and enter no deeper than 2 to 3 mm. The same depth caution applies to use of longer scalpel blades.

Transcutaneous blood gas monitoring is a noninvasive method used to monitor oxygenation and ventilation of the neonate, although its popularity has waned since the introduction of pulse oximetry. However, it remains a viable option in the neonatal population to noninvasively monitor the infant. The electrodes used are modified Clark (Pao_2) and Severinghaus ($Paco_2$) electrodes. The skin site is warmed, and oxygen and carbon dioxide diffuse through the skin to the electrode, where they are measured. In the neonatal population, transcutaneous values can correlate closely with arterial, but even if they do not correlate well, they can be used to trend. If the transcutaneous value is changing, the arterial value is also changing. A transcutaneous sensor is shown in **Figure 12-9**.

Summary

Neonatal and pediatric ventilation must be approached with the understanding of the unique physiology of infants and children. They cannot be treated as adults. Their smaller size means even slight variations in ventilation can have a greater impact than the same variation would have on an adult. Although the principles of ventilation are the same, the application

of these principles differs. A thorough understanding of lung development and organ development is crucial to the safe and effective use of mechanical ventilation in this population.

Case Studies

Case Study 12-1 Neonatal Case Study

You are called to assist in the delivery room with a 24-week-old neonate. Following birth, the infant is quickly dried and assessed: The infant is cyanotic and not breathing with a heart rate (HR) of 52 beats/min. She weighs 900 g. Positive pressure ventilation is begun with an increase in the HR to 142 beats/min, and the infant begins to have respiratory effort.

1. **What would you recommend for this infant?**

2. **Upon admission to the neonatal intensive care unit (NICU), the neonatologist orders a dose of Curosurf. What would you administer and how would you give it? If a second dose is given, how long should you wait between doses?**

3. **After surfactant instillation, the neonatologist orders mechanical ventilation. The infant is currently being manually ventilated at a rate of 40/ min with a pressure of 22 cm H_2O required to cause adequate chest rise. What initial settings would you recommend?**

4. **After 12 hours on mechanical ventilation, the infant is not doing well and it is decided to place her on high-frequency oscillatory ventilation. She is started on 12 Hz, amplitude of 20, bias**

flow of 15 L/min, and FIO_2 of 0.55 with a mean airway pressure (mPaw) of 8 cm H_2O. An arterial blood gas (ABG) sample drawn 30 minutes after institution of oscillation shows a $PaCO_2$ of 55 mm Hg with a pH of 7.33 and a PaO_2 of 58 mm Hg. What change would you recommend?

Case Study 12-2 Pediatric Case Study

A 12-year-old, 62-inch 120-lb male is admitted to the pediatric intensive care unit (PICU) following a multiple trauma from a motor vehicle accident. He was thrown from the car and has multiple chest contusions as well as multiple broken bones. Mechanical ventilation is to be initiated.

1. **What size endotracheal tube would you recommend?**

2. **What initial settings would you recommend?**

3. **Thirty minutes after initiation of ventilation, an ABG sample is drawn. The pH is 7.51, the $PaCO_2$ is 30 mm Hg, the PaO_2 is 127 mm Hg, and the HCO_3^- is 23 mEq/L. The patient is on a tidal volume (V_T) of 320 mL, rate 16, positive end-expiratory pressure (PEEP) +4 cm H_2O, and FIO_2 1.0. What changes would you recommend?**

Bibliography
Anatomical Differences

Figaji A. Anatomical and physiological differences between children and adults relevant to traumatic brain injury and the implications for clinical assessment and care. *Front Neurol.* 2017;8:685.

Habra TD, Shocket D, Braude D. Little airways, big challenges: an overview of EMS pediatric airway management. *J Emerg Med Serv.* 2017;42(3):27–37.

Iowa Neonatology Handbook. Available at https://uichildrens.org/health-library/iowa-neonatology-handbook

Saadeh R, Klaunig J. Child's development and respiratory system toxicity. *J Environ Analytic Toxicol.* 2014;4:5. doi:10.4172/2161-0525.100023

Sakhuja P, Finelli M., Hawes J, Whyte H. Is it time to review guidelines for ETT positioning in the NICU? SCEPTIC—Survey of Challenges Encountered in Placement of Endotracheal Tubes in Canadian NICUs. *Int J Pediatr.* 2016;2016:7283179. doi.org/10.1155/2016/7283179

Physiological Differences

Gupta P, Menon P, Ramji S, et al. General pediatrics and neonatology. In: *Textbook of Pediatrics.* New Delhi, India: Jaypee Brothers Medical Publishers; 2015:635–638.

Harless J, Ramajah R, Bhananker S. Symposium: critical airway management. *Int J Crit Illness Inj Sci.* 2014;4:65–70.

Ku L, Smith B. Dosing in neonates: special considerations in physiology and trial design. *Pediatr Res.* 2015;77:2–9.

Lunze K, Hamer DH. Thermal protection of the newborn in resource-limited environments. *J Perinatol.* 2012;32:317–324.

Sohn M, Ahn Y, Lee S. Assessment of primitive reflexes in high-risk newborns. *J Clin Med Res.* 2011;3:285–290.

Mechanical Ventilation

Alapont M, Villanueva A, Fernandez B. Which is the correct tidal volume in neonatal mechanical ventilation? Are we doing it right? *Pediatr Crit Care Med.* 2014;15:687–688.

Arora S, Rana D, Chauhan V, Dhupia JS. Lamellar body count as a predictor of neonatal respiratory distress syndrome in preterm premature rupture of membranes. *Int J Reprod Contracept Obstet Gynecol.* 2017;7:323–328. ISSN 2320-1789. Available at https://www.ijrcog.org/index.php/ijrcog/article/view/3981

Banfi C, Pozzi M, Siegenthaler N, et al. Veno-venous extracorporeal membrane oxygen: cannulation techniques. *J Thoracic Dis.* 2016; 8:3762–3773.

Bockenek A, Osip E, Gohlke A, et al. Aerosolized Survanta in neonatal respiratory distress syndrome: phase I study. *Pediatrics.* 2018;141.

Brew N, Walker D, Wong F. Cerebral vascular regulation and brain injury in preterm infants. *Am J Physiol Regul Integr Comp Physiol.* 2014;306(11):R773–786. Available at www.physiology.org/doi/full/10.1152/ajpregu.00487.2013

Care Fusion. *Pocket Guide.* 2014. Available at www.carefusion.com

Carlo W, Polin R. Policy statement: respiratory support in preterm infants at birth. *Pediatrics.* 2014;133(1):156–163.

Chakraborty M, Kotecha S. Pulmonary surfactant in newborn infants and children. *Breathe.* 2013;9:476–488. doi:10.1183/20734735.006513

Donn S, Sinha, S. *Manual of Neonatal Respiratory Care.* 4th ed. Basel, Switzerland: Springer International Publishing; 2016.

El Hazzani F, Al Hussein K, Al Alaiyan S, et al. Mechanical ventilation in newborn infants: clinical practice guidelines of the Saudi Neonatology Society. *J Clin Neonatol.* 2017;6:57–63.

Figaji A. Anatomical and physiological differences between children and adults relevant to traumatic brain injury and the implications for clinical assessment and care. *Front Neurol.* 2017;8:685.

Gupta P, Menon P, Ramji S, et al. General pediatrics and neonatology. In: *Textbook of Pediatrics.* New Delhi, India: Jaypee Brothers Medical Publishers; 2015:635–638.

Harrison E. *Neonatal Respiratory Care Handbook.* Boston, MA: Jones & Bartlett; 2011.

Hess D, McIntyre N, Galvin W, et al. *Respiratory Care Principles and Practice.* 3rd ed. Boston, MA: Jones & Bartlett; 2016.

Makdisi G, Wang I. Extra corporeal membrane oxygenation (ECMO) review of a lifesaving technology. *J Thorac Dis.* 2015;7: E166–E176.

Murray M, Harrison B, Mueller J, et al. *Faust's Anesthesiology Review.* 4th ed. St. Louis, MO: Elsevier; 2015:chap 192.

Navalesi P, Longhini F. Neurally adjusted ventilatory assist. *Curr Opin Crit Care.* 2015;21:58–64.

Oakes D, Jones S. *Ventilator Management: An Oakes Pocket Guide.* Orono, ME: Health Education Publications; 2018.

Peng W, Zhu H, Shi H, Liu E. Volume-targeted ventilation is more suitable than pressure-limited ventilation for preterm infants: a systematic review and meta-analysis. *Arch Dis Child Fetal Neonatal Ed.* 2014;99(2):F158–165.

Rodriguez-Cruz E, Berger S. Pediatric extracorporeal membrane oxygenation—overview. *Medscape.* 2017. Available at https://emedicine.medscape.com/article/1818617

Tobin M, ed. *Principles and Practices of Mechanical Ventilation.* 3rd ed. New York, NY: McGraw-Hill; 2013.

Assessment of Oxygenation and Ventilation

Askie LM, Darlow BA, Finer N, et al. Association between oxygen saturation targeting and death or disability in extremely preterm infants in the neonatal oxygenation prospective meta-analysis collaboration. *JAMA.* 2018;319:2190–2201.

Harrison E. *Neonatal Respiratory Care Handbook.* Boston, MA: Jones & Bartlett; 2011.

Hess D, McIntyre N, Galvin W, et al. *Respiratory Care Principles and Practice.* 3rd ed. Boston, MA: Jones & Bartlett; 2016.

Kacmarek R, Stoller J, Heuer A. *Egan's Fundamentals of Respiratory Care.* 11th ed. St. Louis, MO: Elsevier; 2017.

Rawat M, Chandrasekharan P, Williams A, et al. Oxygen saturation index and severity of hypoxic respiratory failure. *Neonatology.* 2015;107:161–166.

13

Medical Critical Care Issues

David W. Chang, EdD, RRT

Shannon Harris, DNP, FNP, CCRN

© s_maria/Shutterstock

OUTLINE

OBJECTIVES

1. List the criteria and classification of ARDS.
2. Describe the clinical presentations and treatment algorithm of ARDS.
3. List the criteria and classification of ventilator-associated events (VAEs) and subgroups of VAE (including ventilator-associated pneumonia).
4. Describe the strategies to prevent VAE, including the VAP bundle.
5. Describe the etiology and principles of hypoxic-ischemic encephalopathy.
6. Describe the clinical manifestations and treatment modalities of acute pancreatitis.
7. Differentiate between ischemic and hemorrhagic stroke.
8. Identify evidence-based interventions to treat the sequelae of stroke.
9. List the causes and clinical manifestations of hepatic failure.
10. Describe the clinical manifestations and treatment modalities of sepsis.
11. Describe the causes, assessment findings, and therapy specific to each type of renal failure.
12. Describe the manifestations and management of an acetaminophen and opioid overdose.
13. Describe the clinical manifestations and therapy for an acute pulmonary thrombosis.

KEY TERMS

acute pancreatitis
acute renal failure
acute respiratory
    distress syndrome
amylase
cerebral perfusion
    pressure
hypoxic-ischemic
    encephalopathy
hemorrhagic stroke
hepatic failure
ischemic stroke

jaundice
PADIS
peritonitis
sepsis
septic shock
spontaneous
    awakening trial
spontaneous breathing trial
subglottic secretion
    drainage
ventilator-associated events
vomiting

Introduction

This chapter covers the common ventilator-related and major medical issues for patients in critical care settings. The four main topics in this chapter are acute respiratory distress syndrome (ARDS), ventilator-associated events (including ventilator-associated pneumonia [VAP]), hypoxic-ischemic encephalopathy (hypoxic brain injury), and synopsis of urgent medical conditions. Topics in the urgent medical conditions section are severe conditions and they often cross over to ARDS, VAP, and hypoxic brain injury, depending on the progression and complications of the illness.

Acute Respiratory Distress Syndrome

In 1967, Ashbaugh et al. used the term "adult respiratory distress syndrome" to describe a severe form of respiratory distress caused by critical conditions such as sepsis, severe pancreatitis, and nonthoracic injuries. It is termed a syndrome rather than a disease because although enough is known about the condition to identify it by signs and symptoms, the mechanism and cause of the pathophysiology are not sufficiently understood. The term "*adult* respiratory distress syndrome" was changed in 1994 at the American-European Consensus Conference (AECC) to **acute respiratory distress syndrome** because this syndrome applies to adults and children.

Criteria and Classification of ARDS

The appearance of signs and symptoms of ARDS is acute. They usually appear within 1 week of a known clinical condition or new or worsening respiratory symptoms. Patients typically exhibit progressive hypercapnia and refractory hypoxemia in the early (exudative) phase characterized by high permeability pulmonary edema followed by the formation of hyaline membranes. After 7 to 10 days, a late (proliferative) phase appears with marked interstitial inflammation,

fibrosis, alveolar damage, and disordered healing. Ventilatory and oxygenation failure are the clinical findings in this late phase. On chest radiography, *bilateral* opacities and pulmonary edema are universal findings.

The AECC grades the severity of ARDS by the P/F (Pao_2/Fio_2) ratio. ARDS was defined as P/F <200, and acute lung injury (ALI) P/F <300. This definition of ARDS was further refined in 2011 by a panel of experts (Berlin definition). The ALI designation was replaced by "mild" ARDS. **Table 13-1** summarizes the 2011 criteria and classification of ARDS.

Etiology

There are multiple risk factors for ARDS (things that trigger the destructive immune response) and they include infection (e.g., sepsis), medical conditions (e.g., massive blood transfusion, drug overdose), and traumatic injuries (e.g., chest trauma, burn injury, smoke inhalation, and near drowning). Conditions that increase the risk of ARDS include old age, cigarette and alcohol use, and those critically ill patients with a high Acute Physiology Age Chronic Health Evaluation (APACHE) score (see Appendix G). The APACHE score is an objective evaluation tool to determine the likelihood of death. **Table 13-2** lists the common risk factors for ARDS.

Pathophysiology

ARDS leads to diffuse alveolar damage and pulmonary capillary endothelial injury. These two conditions are the primary causes of the eventual pulmonary edema frequently seen in ARDS. The early phase of ARDS is described as exudative phase characterized by leakage of fluid and cells out of pulmonary capillaries into the lungs. This increase in permeability of the alveolocapillary membrane leads to an influx of protein-rich fluid into the alveolar space and further worsens the osmotic action of fluid movement into the lungs.

Flooding of the lung parenchyma causes damage to the alveolar type I and type II cells. Damage to the type I

TABLE 13-1
Criteria and Classification of ARDS Based on 2011 Berlin Definition

Criteria	Mild ARDS	Moderate ARDS	Severe ARDS
Pao_2/Fio_2 (with PEEP or CPAP ≥5 cm H_2O)	200 to ≤300 mm Hg	100 to ≤200 mm Hg	≤100 mm Hg
Signs and symptoms appear within 1 week of clinical condition *or* new or worsening respiratory symptoms	X	X	X
Radiographic bilateral opacities not fully explained by effusions, consolidation, or atelectasis	X	X	X
Pulmonary edema not fully explained by cardiac failure or fluid overload (i.e., hydrostatic edema not the primary cause of respiratory failure)	X	X	X

ARDS, acute respiratory distress syndrome; CPAP, continuous positive airway pressure; PEEP. positive end-expiratory pressure.

TABLE 13-2
Risk Factors for ARDS

Condition	Examples
Infection	Sepsis Bacteremia Pneumonia Pancreatitis
Medical	Hypotension and shock Transfusion-related acute lung injury (TRALI) Hematopoietic stem cell transplant Fat embolism Postcardiopulmonary bypass Drug overdose or toxicity Aspiration pneumonia
Injury	Chest trauma Pulmonary contusion Fractures (particularly multiple or long bone) Burns Near drowning Smoke inhalation Inhalation of toxins

Table data from Chang DW. *Clinical Application of Mechanical Ventilation.* 4th ed. Clifton Park, NY: Delmar Cengage Learning; 2014; Harman EM. Acute respiratory distress syndrome. *Medscape.* 2018. Available at www.emedicine.medscape.com; Siegel MD. Acute respiratory distress syndrome: clinical features, diagnosis, and complications in adults. *UpToDate.* Available at https://www.uptodate.com/contents/acute-respiratory-distress-syndrome-clinical-features-diagnosis-and-complications-in-adults/print

cells enhances entry of fluid into the alveoli and hinders clearance of fluid from the alveolar space. Damage to the type II cells is more problematic as it decreases the production and recycling of pulmonary surfactant resulting in decreased lung compliance, increased work of breathing, and increased atelectasis. Over time, pulmonary fibrosis may be the outcome as the type II cells cannot adequately carry out the normal functions.

ARDS is a heterogeneous condition that affects how the lungs are ventilated during mechanical ventilation. The percentage of normal or near-normal alveoli often represents a much smaller portion of the lungs, and these functional areas are likened to baby-sized lungs. This normal tissue is relatively compliant and may become overdistended by even a typical tidal volume (whether delivered by volume- or pressure-controlled ventilation). Atelectatic alveoli are difficult to open when conditions are abnormal and may not respond well to mechanical breaths. This uneven ventilation leads to ventilation-perfusion ($\dot{V}/\dot{Q}$) mismatch, intrapulmonary shunting, refractory hypoxemia, and respiratory acidosis.

Barotrauma is a term used to describe lung injury (e.g., pneumothorax) due to pressure, often leading to overdistention of alveoli during mechanical ventilation. *Volutrauma* describes lung injury due to overdistention of alveoli even when inflation pressure may be normal. *Atelectrauma* is lung damage caused by shear forces exerted by the repeated collapse (at end-expiration) and reexpansion (at beginning inspiration) of abnormal

alveoli during mechanical ventilation. These shear forces during positive pressure ventilation enhance production of proinflammatory cytokines. Cytokines are a category of signaling molecules that mediate and regulate immunity, inflammation, and hematopoiesis. These proinflammatory cytokines lead to further worsening of pulmonary inflammation and pulmonary edema. Barotrauma and volutrauma are terms often used interchangeably. Their occurrence may be prevented or minimized by using appropriate mechanical ventilation strategies.

ARDS is a progressive critical condition and afflicted patients typically require prolonged intensive care unit (ICU) and hospital stay. They are also prone to develop nosocomial infection, especially ventilator- or hospital-associated pneumonia. Physically, these patients lose body mass and may have muscle weakness and functional impairment. If managed promptly, the acute phase of ARDS can resolve promptly and without serious complications. In prolonged cases, nonreversible residual pulmonary fibrosis may occur. Progression to pulmonary fibrosis may be identified by an increased level of procollagen peptide III (PCP-III) in the bronchoalveolar lavage (BAL) sample.

Clinical Presentations

ARDS is characterized by signs that may include acute dyspnea, tachypnea, tachycardia, hypotension, peripheral vasoconstriction, hypoxemia, and cyanosis. The onset of ARDS can be within hours to days of the onset of a clinical condition (e.g., sepsis, trauma). In this early stage (up to 7 days), the patients may respond to oxygen/continuous positive airway pressure (CPAP) therapy, high-flow nasal cannula, or noninvasive ventilation. If the initial clinical condition is not corrected, the oxygenation status progressively worsens primarily due to low $\dot{V}/\dot{Q}$ mismatch and intrapulmonary shunting. The Pao_2/Fio_2 ratio continues to decrease as the condition worsens. Refractory hypoxemia becomes evident with development of atelectasis, hypercapnia, decreased lung compliance, and increased myocardial work and work of breathing. When the patient develops respiratory muscle fatigue due to increased work of breathing and oxygen demand, the $Paco_2$ begins to increase and progresses to severe respiratory acidosis. In this late stage, most patients develop diffuse alveolar infiltrates and eventual respiratory failure within 48 hours of the onset of severe signs and symptoms such as refractory hypoxemia. The immune response that produces ARDS affects all organs of the body, but the lungs are typically one of the first systems to show signs of abnormal function. An adverse outcome is more likely in patients who experience greater impairment of multiple organ systems.

During the exudative phase of ARDS, fluid is leaked from the cells of the capillaries into the interstitial or alveolar space as a result of inflammation. Chest radiographs show a progression from diffuse interstitial infiltrates to diffuse, fluffy, alveolar opacities. **Figure 13-1** shows the typical chest radiograph of a patient with severe ARDS. The radiographic presentation of infiltrates and opacities is typically bilateral. Reticular opacities (crisscrossing lines that form a mesh pattern) on the chest radiograph suggest the development of interstitial fibrosis in late phase ARDS.

Pulmonary Edema

Although the radiographic signs of cardiogenic (e.g., congestive heart failure) and noncardiogenic pulmonary edema (e.g., ARDS) are similar, patients with ARDS often lack cardiogenic signs such as cardiomegaly, intravascular volume overload, jugular vein and pulmonary artery distention, cardiac murmurs and gallops, hepatomegaly, and pedal edema. In addition, the pulmonary artery occlusion pressure (PAOP) measurement should be near normal in noncardiogenic pulmonary edema (i.e., ARDS).

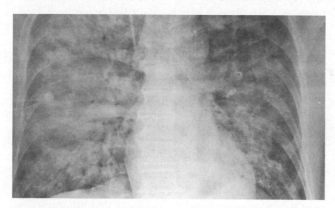

FIGURE 13-1 Chest radiograph of a patient with severe acute respiratory distress syndrome.
© Casa nayafana/Shutterstock.

Workup

The primary goals of a detailed workup are to confirm a diagnosis of ARDS and to classify its severity for a treatment plan. Since ARDS is a clinical diagnosis, there are no absolute laboratory abnormalities beyond the commonly used P/F ratio and chest radiographic findings. Computed tomography, echocardiography, and invasive hemodynamic monitoring are accurate and useful but do not provide significant information in the ARDS workup. For this reason, their use should be based on whether the benefit-to-risk yield is worthwhile for each patient. **Table 13-3** provides an overview of the laboratory tests and other diagnostic evaluations that could be used in the workup. Some of these laboratory and diagnostic findings are especially useful when the patient has significant multisystem organ failure.

Treatment Algorithm

The treatment algorithm for patients with ARDS begins with a confirmation of ARDS and classification of its severity. For mild ARDS, the patient may be managed initially with high-flow nasal cannula or noninvasive ventilation. If the patient is clinically stable and the P/F is >200 mm Hg, noninvasive ventilation is continued until weaned to spontaneous breathing. If the patient is clinically unstable or cannot tolerate noninvasive ventilation, controlled mechanical ventilation is initiated.

For moderate and severe ARDS, volume- or pressure-controlled ventilation is started with an initial tidal volume (V_T) of 8 mL/kg predicted body weight. The V_T is titrated to 6 mL/kg while keeping plateau pressure (Pplat) ≤30 cm H_2O. A higher positive end-expiratory pressure (PEEP) may be used to keep Pa_{O_2}

TABLE 13-3
Laboratory Tests and Diagnostic Evaluations for Acute Respiratory Distress Syndrome (ARDS)

Evaluation	Threshold for ARDS
Pa_{O_2}/F_{IO_2}	<300 mm Hg with evidence of ARDS
Arterial blood gases	Refractory hypoxemia, hypercapnia, and acidosis (partially or fully compensated)
Chest radiograph	Bilateral infiltrates/opacities Infiltrates may be interstitial or alveolar
Plasma B-type natriuretic peptide (BNP)	<100 pg/mL with bilateral infiltrates and hypoxemia points to ARDS because of unlikely cardiac impairment
Echocardiogram	Normal left ventricular ejection fraction (rule out cardiogenic pulmonary edema)
Bronchoalveolar lavage (BAL)	Differential diagnosis of pneumonia types (e.g., >20% eosinophils in BAL fluid indicates acute eosinophilic pneumonia)

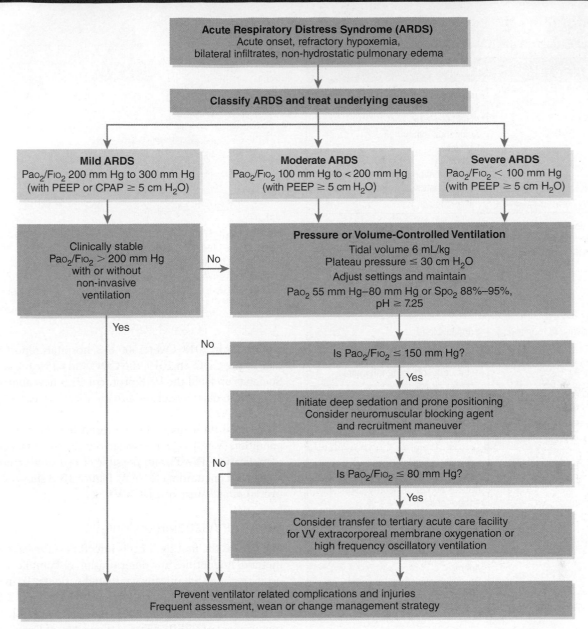

FIGURE 13-2 Treatment algorithm for ARDS. ARDS, acute respiratory distress syndrome; CPAP, continuous positive airway pressure; ECMO, extracorporeal membrane oxygenation; HFOV, high-frequency oscillatory ventilation; PEEP, positive end-expiratory pressure; VV, venovenous.

Fan E, Brodie D, Slutsky AS. Acute respiratory distress syndrome: advances in diagnosis and treatment. JAMA. 2018;319:698–710. doi: 10.1001/jama.2017.21907

from 55 to 80 mm Hg or Spo_2 88% to 95%. Respiratory frequency may be adjusted to maintain appropriate $Paco_2$ and pH ≥7.25. **Figure 13-2** shows a sample treatment algorithm for ARDS.

Complications

Essentially all patients with severe ARDS are intubated and mechanically ventilated. Complications related to these two invasive procedures are numerous. Complications related to intubation and use of endotracheal (ET) tube include traumatic intubation, esophageal

intubation, main stem intubation, accidental extubation, cuff leaks, aspiration, postextubation laryngeal edema, and subglottic stenosis. For patients requiring a tracheostomy tube and hemodynamic monitoring, the primary complications are surgical bleeds, infection, and line sepsis. Intubated patients are also at risk for VAP. Complications related to mechanical ventilation include barotrauma, hypotension, muscle wasting, functional impairment, and infection.

Patients with ARDS are also at risk for other complications frequently seen in the ICU population (**Table 13-4**).

TABLE 13-4
Complications in the ICU and ARDS Population

Type	Examples
Airway	Traumatic intubation
	Esophageal intubation
	Main stem intubation
	Accidental extubation
	Cuff leaks
	Aspiration
	Postextubation laryngeal edema
	Postextubation subglottic stenosis
	Infection
Intubation	Ventilator-associated pneumonia
Mechanical ventilation	Barotrauma and volutrauma
	Hypotension
	Muscle wasting
	Functional impairment
	Infection
Hemodynamic monitoring	Surgical bleed
	Infection
	Line sepsis (red streaks or lines indicate spreading infection)
Enteral tube feeding	Sinusitis (nasal)
	Aspiration
Urinary catheter	Urinary tract infection
Multiple antibiotic use	Drug-resistant pathogens (e.g., methicillin-resistant *Staphylococcus aureus*, vancomycin-resistant enterococcus)
Others	Renal failure
	Ileus (intestinal obstruction)
	Stress gastritis
	Anemia
	Posttraumatic stress disorder

ARDS, acute respiratory distress syndrome; ICU, intensive care unit.

Ventilator-Associated Events

VAP is a severe complication of intubation and mechanical ventilation. Prevention of VAP is challenging because many diagnostic criteria are *not* based on objective clinical or laboratory data. For example, infiltrates on chest radiograph are often considered a sign of VAP. However, infiltrates may be due to different causes other than consolidation of lung parenchyma. Presence of pneumonia may sometimes be evident only by computed tomography but not on regular chest radiograph.

The traditional metric for VAP detection and prevention has been criticized because it is subjective, labor intensive, and prone to bias, and accounts for a small population of ICU deaths. In response to these concerns, the National Healthcare Safety Network of the Centers for Disease Control and Prevention (CDC) replaced the VAP definitions with VAE (**ventilator-associated event**)

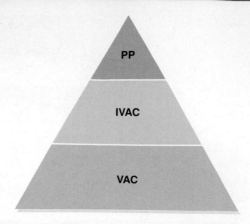

FIGURE 13-3 The CDC's ventilator-associated events have 3 tiers based on the predetermined criteria for each tier (see text): ventilator-associated conditions (VAC), infection-related ventilator-associated complications (IVAC), and possible or probable pneumonia (PP).

Modified from Klompas M, Anderson D, Trick W, et al. The preventability of ventilator-associated events. The CDC Prevention Epicenters Wake Up and Breathe Collaborative. *Am J Respir Crit Care Med.* 2015;191(3):292–301. doi: 10.1164/rccm.201407-1394OC.

definitions in 2013. Over 1500 U.S. hospitals report VAE data to the CDC. In 2019, the CDC and Critical Care Societies updated the VAE protocol. This new approach is based on objective criteria to identify different VAEs, including VAP.

VAE has three distinct tiers: ventilator-associated condition (VAC), infection-related ventilator-associated complication (IVAC), and possible or probable ventilator-associated pneumonia (PVAP). **Figure 13-3** shows the overlapping feature of CDC's VAEs.

Ventilator-Associated Conditions

The VAC is the first tier of this infection surveillance method. It identifies any deterioration or complication occurring in mechanically ventilated patients. To meet the VAC definition, the patient must have at least 2 days of clinical stability or improvement based on a reduced requirement of PEEP or F_{IO_2}, followed by at least 2 days of worsening oxygenation (i.e., increase PEEP [≥ 3 cm H_2O] or increase F_{IO_2} [$\geq 20\%$]).

Infection-Related Ventilator-Associated Complications

The IVAC is the second tier and it identifies the subgroup of VACs that may be related to presence of infection. The objective data include an abnormal white blood cell count ($\leq 4,000$ or $\geq 12,000$ cells/mm^3) or an abnormal temperature ($< 36°$ C or $> 38°$ C) and the use of a new antimicrobial agent for infection treatment continued for at least 4 days.

Possible or Probable Ventilator-Associated Pneumonia

PVAP (or PP) is the third tier. The evidence for *possible* VAP includes the evidence of IVAC plus presence of purulent secretions and/or positive microbiological tests on respiratory tract specimens. The *possible* VAP becomes *probable* VAP when the lower respiratory tract culture meets certain quantitative or semiquantitative thresholds of pathogen growth.

Ventilator-associated tracheobronchitis (VAT) is a distinct category separated from the three tiers described previously. VAT is defined as a condition related to VAC, IVAC, or PVAP during the course of mechanical ventilation (at least 48 hours) plus presence of positive respiratory culture obtained by bronchoalveolar lavage. The patient does not have *new* radiographic infiltrates and may or may not have clinical or biological signs of sepsis. See **Table 13-5** for a summary of the criteria for the identification of different VAEs.

Prevention of Ventilator-Associated Events

Patient management bundles have been developed to prevent VAP. However, the ideal bundle or combination of bundle components remains unknown. In the review of literature, many bundle components are used to reduce the duration of mechanical ventilation.

Studies have shown that early liberation from mechanical ventilation reduces the incidence of VAEs. Since duration of intubation/mechanical ventilation and occurrence of VAEs are codependent, the ideal VAE bundle should include strategies to reduce the duration of intubation and mechanical ventilation. The following sections provide current information on the prevention of VAEs.

Paired Spontaneous Awakening Trials and Spontaneous Breathing Trials

Increasing the frequency of paired **spontaneous awakening trials** (SATs) and **spontaneous breathing trials** (SBTs) has been shown to significantly lower the incidence of VAEs. This strategy also leads to shorter duration of mechanical ventilation, as well as shorter ICU and hospital stays.

For the SAT, sedatives are discontinued to allow "awakening" and return of spontaneous breathing efforts. The SBT is done to evaluate the patient's ability to breathe spontaneously without ventilatory support.

SAT and SBT can be performed separately but when they are paired together, the combined trials reduce the

TABLE 13-5
Criteria for the Identification of Different Ventilator-Associated Events

Type*	Oxygenation	Temperature/WBC Count	Antibiotic	Sputum Culture
Ventilator-associated condition (VAC)	≥2 days of stability (↓Fio$_2$ or ↓PEEP) followed by ≥2 days of worsening oxygenation (↑PEEP ≥3 cm H$_2$O or ↑Fio$_2$ ≥20%)			
Infection-related ventilator-associated complications (IVAC)	VAC plus →	Temp (<36°C or >38°C) or WBC count (≤4000 or ≥12,000 cells/mm^3)	Use of one or more new antibiotics continued for ≥4 days within 2 days of VAC onset	
Possible or probable ventilator-associated pneumonia (PVAP or PP)			IVAC plus →	Sputum/BAL with ≥25 neutrophils and ≤10 epithelial cells per field (low power field, ×100) *and/or* positive sputum culture**
Ventilator-associated tracheobronchitis (VAT)			VAE, VAC, *or* VAP plus →	Purulent sputum/BAL with positive respiratory culture, no *new* radiographic infiltrates, with or without clinical or biological signs of sepsis

BAL, bronchoalveolar lavage; PEEP, positive end-expiratory pressure; VAE, ventilator-associated event; WBC, white blood cell.
*All evaluations done during mechanical ventilation.
**For additional recommended laboratory criteria, see Figure 1 at https://www.cdc.gov/nhsn/pdfs/pscmanual/10-vae_final.pdf
Data from Centers for Disease Control and Prevention. Ventilator-associated events (VAE) protocol. Centers for Disease Control and Prevention: Atlanta, GA; 2019. Available at https://www.cdc.gov/nhsn/pdfs/pscmanual/10-vae_final.pdf; Neuville M, Mourvillier B, Bouadma L, et al. Bundle of care decreased ventilator-associated events—implications for ventilator-associated pneumonia prevention. *J Thorac Dis.* 2017;9(3):430–433. doi: 10.21037/jtd.2017.02.72; Torres A, Niederman MS, Chastre J, et al. International ERS/ESICM/ESCMID/ALAT guidelines for the management of hospital-acquired pneumonia and ventilator-associated pneumonia. *Eur Respir J.* 2017;50(3):1700582. doi:10.1183/13993003.00582-2017

number of mechanical ventilation days and length of hospital stay when compared to SBT alone. This combined technique is also called "wake up and breathe."

Spontaneous Awakening Trial

Unless contraindicated, SAT should be done at least once daily because it is a simple, noninvasive procedure that can be done readily at the bedside. Frequent SATs also allow an ongoing evaluation of the patient's clinical progress. SAT should be deferred if the patient requires sedation to (1) control seizures, (2) control agitation, (3) accompany use of neuromuscular blockers, (4) mitigate recent myocardial ischemia, and (5) control elevated intracranial pressure.

If no contraindications are present, the awakening trial is initiated by discontinuing all sedatives and analgesics unless analgesics are needed for pain. The SAT is considered successful when the patient is able to perform three of four simple tasks on command: (1) open eyes, (2) look at the clinician, (3) squeeze the hand of clinician, and (4) stick out the tongue. For a detailed discussion on SAT, refer to Element B of the ABCDEF Bundle in Chapter 15.

Spontaneous Breathing Trial

SBT should be considered if the patient has met the following conditions: (1) cause leading to mechanical ventilation has been reversed, (2) patient is able to breathe spontaneously for a sustained time period, (3) patient has an adequate cough mechanism and does not have excessive secretions, and (4) neuromuscular blocker has been stopped and use of sedative is at the lowest appropriate dose.

Along with normal vital signs, P/F ratio ≥ 200 mm Hg and rapid shallow breathing index (RSBI) <105 cycles/L indicate adequate ventilation and oxygenation to support sustained spontaneous breathing during the trial. Contraindications for SBT include refractory hypoxemia, apnea, agitation, elevated intracranial pressure, and use of high-dose vasopressors or inotropes to maintain blood pressure and circulation. For a detailed discussion on SBT, refer to Element B of the ABCDEF Bundle in Chapter 15.

Pain Analgesic and Delirium Guidelines

In 2018, the Society of Critical Care Medicine (SCCM) revised the original Pain, Agitation/sedation, Delirium guidelines by adding two categories: Immobilization and Sleep (new guideline acronym **PADIS**). In the agitation/sedation category, the guideline recommends reduction or elimination of sedatives and analgesics to facilitate return of spontaneous breathing. A study by Klompas et al. finds that the PADIS guidelines reduce the duration of mechanical ventilation, length of stay, and incidence of VAE. This finding coincides with the spontaneous

awakening trial in which the use of sedatives/analgesics is discontinued. For a detailed discussion on this topic, refer to PADIS guidelines in Chapter 15.

Intensive Care Society VAP Bundle

The VAP bundle recommended by the Intensive Care Society has four components: (1) elevation of head of bed (30 to 45 degrees), (2) daily sedation interruption and assessment of readiness to extubate, (3) use of **subglottic secretion drainage**, and (4) avoidance of scheduled ventilator circuit changes.

Elevation of Head of Bed (30 to 45 Degrees)

Aspiration of oropharyngeal or gastric contents is the primary cause of VAP in critical care settings. In a study using technetium (Tc)-99m-labeled sulfur colloid as a marker in the stomach, aspiration of gastric content is more likely when feeding is done in a supine position. Risk of aspiration is also increased with the use of ET tube. Microaspiration can occur when the ET tube is moved deliberately (e.g., during routine oral care) or inadvertently (e.g., during patient movement). Events such as insufficient cuff inflation and faulty cuff add to the risk of aspiration. Elevating the head of bed to 45 degrees has been shown to reduce incidence of aspiration and VAP. In clinical practice, this elevation may not be achievable, especially in the mechanically ventilated patient. The exact degree of elevation to prevent VAP is unclear but the general consensus is to avoid supine position and keep the head of bed elevated to at least 30 degrees (up to 45 degrees).

Daily Sedation Interruption and Assessment of Readiness to Extubate

Prolonged or continuous sedation can lead to systemic accumulation of sedatives (oversedation). This outcome is associated with increased duration of intubation and mechanical ventilation. Two strategies that have been used to reduce the duration of mechanical ventilation are daily sedation interruption (DSI) and daily spontaneous breathing trial (SBT). The bundled DSI and SBT is essentially same as the SAT and SBT bundle.

Paired SAT and SBT are associated with a significant reduction in duration of mechanical ventilation, VAE risk, and infection-related ventilator associated complications. It should be emphasized that reducing time on mechanical ventilation limits the at-risk ventilator duration that could lead to associated complications such as aspiration, lung injuries, and VAE. Research studies have produced evidence to support a strategy of DSI to prevent oversedation and use of paired SAT and SBT to enhance liberation from mechanical ventilation.

Use of Subglottic Secretion Drainage

Traditional ET tubes tend to have secretions pooled above the cuff because this area is not accessible by conventional suction methods. Subglottic secretion drainage (SSD) is a special feature of some ET tubes in which a suction port with vacuum channel is present posteriorly above the cuff. SSD reduces the incidence of microbiologically confirmed VAP and the percentage of ICU days on antibiotic therapy. It is a recommended procedure in the VAP bundle.

Avoidance of Scheduled Ventilator Circuit Changes

As the expired gases cool during expiration, the heated and humidified gases condense into water in the ventilator circuit. Frequent manipulation of the circuit (e.g., circuit changes) is a risk factor for the aspiration of contaminated condensate into the bronchial tree and lung parenchyma. This condition increases the incidence of VAP.

Research has shown that changing the ventilator circuit only when clinically indicated (soiled or faulty) does not increase the incidence of VAP. This practice also results in significant cost savings compared to routine daily circuit changes.

Additional Strategies to Prevent VAE

Additional strategies to prevent VAE include procedures to reduce pulmonary secretions, prevent aspiration, implement fluid balance and transfusion thresholds, use a weaning algorithm, and decontaminate oral and gastric microbial colonization. **Table 13-6** summarizes these strategies to prevent or reduce the incidence of VAE

Hypoxic-Ischemic Encephalopathy

Hypoxic-ischemic encephalopathy (HIE) is a type of acute brain injury caused by conditions leading to a severe or prolonged lack of oxygen. In neonates, HIE often occurs during the birthing process (prolonged or traumatic birth). In adults, HIE may be caused by a variety of conditions, including sepsis, cardiac arrest, and drowning.

TABLE 13-6
Strategies to Prevent or Reduce Incidence of VAEs

Strategy	Notes
Sedation protocol	Conduct early and frequent spontaneous awakening trial (SAT) and spontaneous breathing trial (SBT)
Paired SAT and SBT	Facilitate early liberation from mechanical ventilation and extubation
Handwashing	Reduce cross-contamination and nosocomial infection
Closed suctioning	Reduce cross-contamination and nosocomial infection
Same ventilator circuit	Change only when clinically indicated (soiled or faulty) to reduce cross-contamination and nosocomial infection
Head of bed elevation (30 to 45 degrees)	Reduce incidence of aspiration
ET tube with subglottic secretion drainage	Reduce incidence of aspiration
Conservative fluid management	Reduce work of heart and incidence of pulmonary edema
Conservative transfusion thresholds	Reduce incidence of transfusion-related acute lung injury (TRALI)
Automatic weaning algorithm	Facilitate early extubation and spontaneous breathing
Oral decontamination with chlorhexidine	Reduce lower respiratory tract infections including VAP (inconclusive)
Oropharyngeal decontamination	Reduce incidence of VAP (inconclusive) Reduce incidence of mortality (inconclusive) Antimicrobial resistance caution
Digestive decontamination	Reduce episodes of ICU bacteremia or candidemia Reduce incidence of mortality (inconclusive) Antimicrobial resistance caution

ET, endotracheal; ICU, intensive care unit; VAE, ventilator-associated event; VAP, ventilator-associated pneumonia.
Table data from Benson AB. Pulmonary complications of transfused blood components. *Crit Care Nurs Clin North Am.* 2012;24(3):403–418. doi: 10.1016/j.ccell.2012.06.005; Hellyer TP, Ewan V, Wilson P, et al. The Intensive Care Society recommended bundle of interventions for the prevention of ventilator-associated pneumonia. *J Intensive Care Soc.* 2016;17(3):238–243. doi:10.1177/1751143716644461; Torres A, Niederman MS, Chastre J, et al. International ERS/ESICM/ESCMID/ALAT guidelines for the management of hospital-acquired pneumonia and ventilator-associated pneumonia. *Eur Respir J.* 2017;50(3):1700582. doi:10.1183/13993003.00582-2017

HIE is also called cerebral anoxia or cerebral hypoxia. A complete stoppage of oxygen supply to the brain is called cerebral anoxia. If there is partial oxygen supply but at a level inadequate to maintain normal brain function, it is called cerebral hypoxia. These two terms are used interchangeably.

Signs and symptoms of mild HIE range from poor concentrating to lethargy. In severe HIE, seizures and coma may be the outcome. Most patients with lung diseases and hypoxia may show signs of mild HIE, but this condition can be treated readily with supplemental oxygen. In conditions refractory to oxygen therapy (e.g., respiratory arrest, ARDS, brain injury, and sepsis), severe oxygen deficient and HIE can occur. The next section, "Synopsis of Urgent Medical Conditions," describes those critical conditions that could lead to HIE.

Etiology

There are two main causes of cerebral hypoxia: (1) inadequate ventilation or oxygenation (e.g., respiratory arrest, carbon monoxide poisoning, drowning) and (2) inadequate perfusion (e.g., cardiac arrest, sepsis, blocked or ruptured blood vessels), indicated by a decrease in **cerebral perfusion pressure** (CPP).

Principles of HIE

The brain is a small organ with extremely high metabolic rate and oxygen demand. It has about 2% of the total body weight but requires 15% of the energy generated by the body. Unlike the muscle cells in the body, the brain does not hold or store any energy source (e.g., glucose) except for a small amount of glycogen in the astrocytes. Furthermore, the brain cells cannot utilize fatty acids because they cannot cross and enter the brain capillaries. For this reason, normal cerebral metabolism solely depends on a constant supply of oxygen and glucose in the blood. Lack of cerebral blood flow (e.g., ischemic stroke), red blood cells (e.g., severe anemia), glucose (e.g., hypoglycemia, starvation), and many other similar conditions can hinder the normal cerebral functions and lead to HIE.

In cardiac arrest, a lack of cerebral circulation depletes the neuronal oxygen stores within 20 seconds. This can render the patient unconscious. Within 5 minutes of complete cerebral anoxia, brain glucose and adenosine triphosphate (ATP) stores are lost. Energy depletion, irreversible brain cell injury, and brain death are the outcomes.

The first event following energy depletion is failure of the Na^+ and K^+ pumps, leading to depolarization of the neuronal membrane. Depolarization causes neurons to release excessive glutamate into the synaptic cleft. Since some glutamate receptors are nonselective cation-permeable ion channels, influx of excessive cations (Ca^{2+} ions) into neurons leads to activation of catabolic or destructive enzymes, as well as activation of

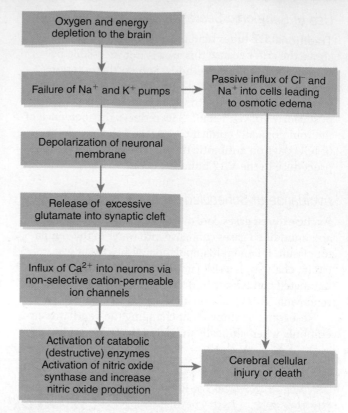

FIGURE 13-4 Mechanism of cerebral cellular injury as a result of energy depletion to the brain.

Modified from Chang DW. *Clinical Application of Mechanical Ventilation.* 4th ed. Clifton Park, NY: Delmar Cengage Learning; 2014.

nitric oxide (NO) synthase and increase of nitric oxide production. Furthermore, passive influx of Ca^{2+} and Na^+ into the brain cells can cause osmotic edema and rapid death of the brain cells. **Figure 13-4** outlines the mechanism of cerebral cellular injury as a result of energy depletion to the brain.

The most common cause of energy depletion to the brain cells is a lack of cerebral perfusion (global ischemia). Cerebral perfusion is mainly determined by the CPP, the pressure gradient between the mean arterial pressure (MAP) and intracranial pressure (ICP) or central venous pressure (CVP), if it is greater. Either a drop in MAP or an increase in ICP effectively reduces the CPP and the cerebral perfusion.

In critical care settings, perfusion-related conditions (e.g., cardiac arrest) can lead to a decrease in MAP and a direct reduction in CPP ($\downarrow$CPP = $\downarrow$MAP − ICP). Nonperfusion-related conditions (e.g., closed head injury) can cause an increase in ICP and an indirect reduction in CPP ($\downarrow$CPP = MAP − $\uparrow$ICP).

Cerebral Perfusion Pressure

CPP is the pressure required to provide blood flow, oxygen, and metabolites to the brain. Under normal conditions, the brain is able to maintain adequate blood flow within a range of systemic blood pressure and cerebral vascular resistance. However, the brain becomes vulnerable in conditions of severe hypotension (e.g., cardiac arrest, massive blood loss). The autoregulation ability of the brain may also be lost following head trauma in which the cerebral vascular resistance is often greatly elevated. Depending on the severity of reduction in cerebral perfusion, neurological effects on the brain may range from cerebral ischemia to brain death.

The clinical safety threshold for CPP ranges from 70 to 80 mm Hg. The mortality rate increases about 20% for each 10 mm Hg *decrease* in CPP. In studies involving severe head injuries, a 35% reduction in mortality rate was achieved when the CPP was maintained above 70 mm Hg.

Decrease in CPP Due to Severe Hypotension

Cardiac arrest and shock are two common causes of severe hypotension. Based on the American Heart Association statistical update, the 2016 out-of-hospital cardiac arrest had an incidence of >350,000 and an overall survival rate of 12%. For in-hospital cases, the incidence count is >209,000 with a survival rate of 24.8%.

Another study described a vast majority of cardiac arrest survivors who remained in a coma for different durations, in which about 40% remained in a persistent vegetative state and 80% were dead at 1 year. The comatose state is caused by the lack of CPP and cerebral oxygenation during and following resuscitation. Therapeutic hypothermia (32° to 34° C) has been used to lower the oxygen utilization and to improve the neurological outcomes in cardiac arrest victims.

Decrease in CPP Due to Shock

Hypotension or lack of circulating volume in critical care settings is primarily due to severe blood loss (absolute hypovolemia) or vasodilation (relative hypovolemia, as in **septic shock**). As in cardiac arrest, hypotension causes abnormally low systolic, diastolic, and mean arterial pressures.

Based on CPP = MAP − ICP, a higher CPP is achievable by increasing the MAP or by decreasing the ICP. In hypotension, the MAP can be improved by giving fluid or using vasopressors. In the absence of severe blood loss, the MAP should be managed initially by providing intravenous fluids, followed by a vasopressor such as norepinephrine or dopamine. Systemic hypotension (systolic blood pressure <90 mm Hg) should be avoided because it is associated with increased morbidity and mortality rates following severe brain injury.

Decrease in CPP Due to Brain Injury

In clinical practice, ICP control is typically not necessary because it tends to stay below its clinical threshold (20 mm Hg), unless the ICP increase is due to closed head trauma. Traumatic brain injury raises the ICP due to swelling of the brain within a confined fixed space (skull). The increase in ICP reduces the CPP and blood supply to the brain ($\downarrow$CPP = MAP − $\uparrow$ICP). The end result is energy depletion and development of HIE.

Evaluation and Treatment of HIE

The severity of anatomic and physiologic changes in the brain and spinal cord may be evaluated by examining the results of computed tomography (CT) or magnetic resonance imaging (MRI) scan, electroencephalography (EEG), ultrasonography, and evoked potential test (analysis of brain waves). These tests may also be used to evaluate the effectiveness of treatments for HIE. Treatments for HIE must be immediate. The treatment plan should include supportive care (e.g., oxygen therapy) and reversal of the underlying causes of cerebral hypoxia (e.g., cerebral perfusion). See the following sections for critical conditions that could lead to hypotension and HIE.

Synopsis of Urgent Medical Conditions

This section covers a collection of urgent medical conditions that are often seen in critical care settings. A brief summary of the important principles and concepts is presented for each condition.

Sepsis

Severe sepsis affects more than 1 million patients in the United States annually and of those 15% to 30% die (2019 CDC data). **Sepsis** is a systemic response triggered by a current infection and is considered a life-threatening emergency (Surviving Sepsis Campaign data). Timing of the initiation of therapy is crucial as the quick spread of the systemic inflammatory response could lead to tissue damage and organ failure (Surviving Sepsis).

Adequate tissue perfusion and oxygenation are essential for metabolic processes in cells and the influencing element regarding tissue repair and resistance to infectious organisms. The concept of tissue oxygen perfusion is related to blood flow, oxygen delivery, and oxygen consumption. Tissue perfusion is dependent on blood flow affected by the circulating volume, cardiac pump function, and peripheral vascular resistance. These three factors formulate cardiac output (CO), which determines blood flow to tissues (CO = stroke volume × heart rate). Stroke volume is affected by preload or the amount of blood returning from the body and to the heart, the cardiac contractility, and the afterload or arterial blood pressure the heart must overcome to push blood through the aortic and pulmonic valves.

Clinical Findings

Patients who are diagnosed with severe sepsis and septic shock will have insufficient arterial circulation due to the vasodilatation of blood vessels associated with infection or impaired cardiac output (Story). Inadequate tissue perfusion can result in tissue hypoxia, which can be associated with an elevated serum lactate. A serum lactate value of >4 mmol/L is concomitant with increased severity of illness and mortality rates even if treatment is initiated before hypotension and compensation begin

TABLE 13-7
Sepsis Diagnosis Based on Surviving Sepsis Guidelines Criteria

A Sepsis Diagnosis Must Meet Two of the Following Criteria	Definitions
• Temperature >38° C or <36° C • HR >90 beats/minute • Tachypnea with RR >20/min or P_{CO_2} <33 mm Hg • WBC count >12,000 or <4000 cells/mm^3 or >10% bands	• Sepsis: SIRS with an infection • Severe sepsis: sepsis with at least one organ dysfunction with hypotension • Multiple organ dysfunction syndrome: two or more organ dysfunctions with the need for interventions to assist with hemodynamic support

HR, heart rate; RR, respiratory rate; SIRS, systemic inflammatory response syndrome; WBC, white blood cell.

(Story). Patients who are hypotensive or have a lactate >4 mmol/L will require intravenous fluid resuscitation to expand the circulating volume and effectively establish tissue perfusion (Story). Sepsis is an extreme inflammatory response that is life threatening and caused by the body's response to a bacterial infection that gets into the bloodstream. Proinflammatory cytokines are released, causing an increase of total white blood cell count and neutrophils. Another proinflammatory enzyme, myocardial depressant factor, is released causing a decrease in ejection fraction and vasodilator effect. Hypotension occurs in severe sepsis and may be refractory to intravenous fluid resuscitation and vasopressors (Story). See **Table 13-7** for sepsis criteria.

Management

Sepsis bundles permitted an early goal-directed therapy, and implementation resulted in an improved outcome of patients in septic shock. The application is timely and consistent using evidence-based care and reduced healthcare team practice inconsistencies (Jozwiak et al.). Severe Sepsis 3-Hour Resuscitation Bundle is used by most emergency departments and ICUs (**Box 13-1**). This bundle instructs the clinician to administer a crystalloid (normal saline or Ringer's lactate solution) fluid challenge of 30 mL/kg if hypovolemia is suspected or serum lactate is greater than 4 mmol/L (Story). Ringer's lactate solution is preferred when giving boluses because of normal saline being more acidic. Intravenous fluid resuscitation should be initiated as early as possible for the treatment of septic shock. Quantitative resuscitation targets a CVP of 8 mm Hg, S_{vO_2} of 70%, and normalization of lactate (Story).

Acute Hepatic Failure

Acute hepatic or liver failure (ALF) is an emergent condition with a poor prognosis if untreated, so early recognition and management of patients with ALF are critical and patients should be monitored in an ICU. An estimated 1600 patients die annually of acute liver failure with acetaminophen overdose being the top cause (Saraswat et al.). There are two types of acute liver failure: fulminant and subfulminant. Fulminant liver failure is classified as the development of severe liver injury and acute hepatic encephalopathy in a person with a normal

BOX 13-1 Three-Hour Bundle Based on Surviving Sepsis Guidelines Criteria for Sepsis

Measure lactate

Draw blood cultures

Administer broad-spectrum antibiotics

Administer 30 mL/kg crystalloid intravenous bolus

BOX 13-2 Causes of Hepatic Failure

Viral hepatitis

Hepatotoxic drugs
- Acetaminophen
- Chemotherapy
- Antibiotics (penicillin, sulfa drug, and tetracycline)
- Nonsteroidal anti-inflammatory drugs

Toxins
- Industrial solvents
- Yellow phosphorus
- Mushroom species

Metabolic
- Wilson's disease

or compensated liver. Subfulminant liver failure is classified as a person who develops hepatic encephalopathy 8 to 26 weeks after the onset of illness (Murali and Menon). ALF can be associated with acute liver injury, hepatic encephalopathy, and an elevated international normalized ratio (INR) of >1.5. Fulminant **hepatic failure** occurs within 8 weeks of acute liver injury and subfulminant hepatic failure occurs up to 26 weeks after an acute liver injury (Papadakis and McPhee).

The etiology of ALF can be discovered in about 60% to 80% of patients (Saraswat et al.). Identifying the cause of the patient's liver failure is essential to determine the course of treatment (**Box 13-2**). A diagnosis is usually

BOX 13-3 Hepatic Encephalopathy Grading Scale

- Grade I: Changes in behavior, mild confusion, slurred speech, disordered sleep
- Grade II: Lethargy, moderate confusion
- Grade III: Marked confusion (stupor), incoherent speech, sleeping but wakes with stimulation
- Grade IV: Coma, unresponsive to pain

made with a combination of obtaining a history of present illness, laboratory results, and radiological studies. A liver biopsy may be necessary if the initial workup does not reveal the cause.

Clinical Findings

Clinical manifestations may include **jaundice**, hepatomegaly, and right upper quadrant tenderness. Markedly elevated aminotransferase levels, elevated bilirubin level, and a low platelet count of $\leq 150,000/mm$ (Singh et al.). Increased plasma ammonia level (PAL) appears to have a significant correlation with the severity of encephalopathy. Patients being treated for ALF with associated renal insufficiency or failure encounter a higher ammonia level due to decreased renal function. Cerebral edema may develop in patients with ALF with hepatic encephalopathy grades III and IV (Papadakis and McPhee). The criteria for grading hepatic encephalopathy are given in **Box 13-3**.

The MELD Score (Model for End-Stage Liver Disease) is used by clinicians to calculate the severity of liver disease. The calculation is determined by the patient's creatinine, sodium, bilirubin, and INR, and if he or she has had hemodialysis at least twice in the past 2 weeks (Singh et al.). If the score is >10, then there is a need for a referral to hepatologist or liver transplant center. It assesses mortality risk in acute alcoholic hepatitis, acute variceal hemorrhage, and after a transjugular intrahepatic portosystemic shunt.

Management

Determining the cause of ALF is essential so that a specific treatment can be initiated. Perform plasma toxicology screen, acetaminophen level, and serologic testing for hepatitis A, hepatitis B, hepatitis C, herpes simplex virus, autoimmune hepatitis, and serum copper (Singh et al.). Start a broad-spectrum antibiotic and a proton pump inhibitor. Hepatic encephalopathy grade II to III warrants a CT scan of the brain to rule out additional causes of encephalopathy. If a patient has a hepatic encephalopathy grade III or IV, intubation should be performed to protect the airway and mannitol administered to prevent or decrease cerebral edema (Papadakis and McPhee).

Acute Renal Failure

Kidneys remove waste and extra fluid from the body. Cells in the body produce acid, which is filtered and removed by the kidneys, which maintain a healthy balance of water, sodium, calcium, phosphorus, and potassium. The lungs partially compensate for acidosis or alkalosis in a few minutes by adjusting the excretion of carbon dioxide. The kidneys are ultimately responsible for maintaining body pH over a few hours to days by adjusting the excretion of hydrogen ions within narrow limits (Nagami and Hamm).

Acute renal failure (ARF) is a rapid decline in renal function, and often accompanies shock, hyperkalemia, hyperphosphatemia, hypocalcemia, and decreased volume status. Renal cell death begins to occur when the systolic blood pressure is less than 75 mm Hg (Story). The risk of ARF is related to the severity of hypotension. For each hour the mean arterial pressure is less than 70 mm Hg, the risk for ARF increases by 2%; if MAP is less than 60 mm Hg, the risk for ARF increases by 5%; if MAP is less than 50 mm Hg, the risk of ARF increases by 22% (Lehman et al.). Treatment will depend on the cause and degree of ARF when discovered; however, it is reversible if aggressive management is timely (Fry and Farrington).

The renin-angiotensin system (RAS) is a hormone system that has powerful effects in the control of blood pressure and sodium homeostasis (**Figure 13-5**). If renal blood flow is reduced, juxtaglomerular cells in the kidneys convert the precursor prorenin into renin and secrete it directly into circulation. The major biologically active hormone generated by this system is angiotensin II, which is produced by sequential cleavage of peptides derived from the substrate molecule angiotensinogen. Angiotensin II binds to specific receptors, triggering a broad range of biological actions impacting virtually every system of the body, including the brain, heart, kidney, vasculature, and immune systems. The primary functions of the RAS are circulatory homeostasis and protecting body fluid volumes. An abnormal activation of the RAS can contribute to the development of hypertension, cardiac hypertrophy, and heart failure. Pharmacological inhibitors of the synthesis or activity of angiotensin II have proved immensely useful in cardiovascular therapeutics (Sparks et al.).

Nephrotoxic drugs such as angiotensin-converting enzyme inhibitors and angiotensin receptor blockers can play a role in acute kidney insufficiency and postoperative renal dysfunction. Following an ischemic injury to the kidney, intrinsic vasodilators are released, which contributes to loss of glomerular filtration rate and poor blood flow. Insufficient tissue perfusion and hypoxic injury causes tubular necrosis and acute renal failure (Kaplow and Hardin).

Clinical Findings

There are three types of ARF: prerenal, intrarenal, and postrenal (**Table 13-8**). Causes of prerenal ARF include

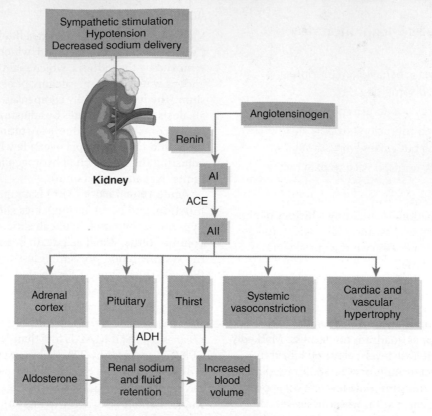

FIGURE 13-5 The renin-angiotensin system. AI, angiotensin I; AII, angiotensin II; ACE, angiotensin-converting enzyme; ADH, antidiuretic hormone.

TABLE 13-8
The Three Types of Acute Renal Failure

Types of Acute Renal Failure	Causes	Laboratory Results
Prerenal	Decreased blood volume Vasodilation Poor cardiac output Renal artery stenosis Renal impairment	Urine output <400 cm³/24 hours Increased BUN Decreased sodium and urinary urea Serum creatinine normal or high
Intrarenal	Exposure to nephro-toxic agents Hemolysis Trauma Intrarenal obstruction Prolonged prerenal ARF	Oliguria Increased BUN Elevated serum creatinine Isosthenuria (urinary osmolality approximates plasma osmolality)
Postrenal	Postrenal blockage • Urethral or bladder neck obstruction • Enlarged prostate • Pelvic tumors Exposure to drugs • Antihistamines Pregnancy	BUN increased Creatinine increased Anuria, oliguria, or polyuria Increase in urinary sodium and urea

ARF, acute renal failure; BUN, blood urea nitrogen.
Data from Kaplow R, Hardin S. *Critical Care Nursing: Synergy for Optimal Outcomes.* Sudbury, MA: Jones and Bartlett Publishers, Inc; 2007.

a change in blood volume status, vasodilation, poor cardiac output, renal artery stenosis, and renal impairment. Intrarenal ARF involves acute renal failure or acute tubular necrosis, which is usually caused by sepsis. Postrenal ARF occurs when there is an obstruction in the urinary tract below the kidney, preventing urine from leaving the kidney. Examples of obstructions leading to postrenal ARF include benign prostatic hyperplasia, ureteral stones, obstructed urinary catheter, and bladder stones (Kaplow and Hardin).

Management

An assessment of hemodynamics, physical examination, and volume status is essential to determine initial therapy. Critically ill patients may require an arterial line, central venous pressure assessment, or cardiac output monitoring to determine tissue perfusion. Urine sodium and urea levels are helpful in diagnosing decreased kidney perfusion in a patient who has oliguria. Urinary microscopy for renal tubular epithelial cells and granular casts may be helpful to make the concomitant diagnosis of acute tubular necrosis, which is the primary cause of ARF in hospitalized patients. A nephrology consult is crucial to assist with the timely management of the patient with ARF. Therapy may include blood pressure control, intravenous fluid resuscitation, and/or emergency hemodialysis (Moore et al.). Hemodialysis serves as an artificial kidney, which is used to filter wastes and water from blood. Peritoneal dialysis is another type of artificial kidney (more limited in function) but is not used in emergency situations. This type of dialysis can be done at home or while at work. A cleaning solution called dialysate is instilled through a surgically placed catheter, passing over the vasculature of the peritoneum, and absorbs waste along with fluid from the blood.

Acute Pancreatitis

The pancreas is an organ located in the upper left abdomen. It plays an essential role in converting ingested food into fuel for the cells. The pancreas has two main functions: (1) an exocrine function that assists in digestion and (2) an endocrine function that regulates blood sugar. Ninety-five percent of the pancreas consists of exocrine tissue, which produces pancreatic enzymes for digestion. The remaining pancreatic tissue consists of endocrine cells called islets of Langerhans, which produce hormones that regulate blood sugar and pancreatic secretions, (Columbia University Irving Medical Center).

Acute pancreatitis is an acute inflammatory process associated with severe abdominal pain (Papadakis and McPhee). Cholelithiasis is the most common cause of acute pancreatitis, and it occurs when gallstones pass through the ampulla of Vater causing an obstruction of the pancreatic duct. This obstruction allows bile to back up in the pancreas, causing an enzymatic response. Stimulation of pancreatic enzymes (lipase to break down fat, protease to assist with digestion of protein, and **amylase** for carbohydrates) inside the pancreatic ducts will cause autodigestion of pancreatic tissue, causing severe inflammation and tissue necrosis (Papadakis and McPhee). Pancreatic enzymes that leak into the circulatory system may cause shock, acute respiratory distress syndrome, and/or disseminated intravascular coagulation due to the activation of immunity mediators. Some of other causes of pancreatitis include hepatotoxic drugs, metabolic disorders, hypertriglyceridemia, trauma, and hyperglycemia, which can all cause damage and/or autodigestion of the pancreas. Acute pancreatitis is a medical emergency with a 15% mortality rate, which can increase with comorbidities (Papadakis and McPhee). Severe pain, hemorrhage, **peritonitis**, and shock can occur with active enzymes leaking into the peritoneum and causing breakdown of tissues.

Clinical Findings

Clinical findings will start quickly and be severe, warranting an ICU admission. Upper abdominal pain is described as radiating to the back and becomes worse after meals but improves with knee to chest position. Nausea, **vomiting**, low-grade fever, and jaundice are other associated symptoms. Serum amylase, a level three times normal (0 to 137 units/L), is the most significant laboratory finding in the diagnosis of acute pancreatitis (Papadakis and McPhee). Leukocytosis, hyperglycemia, hypercalcemia, and high levels of

TABLE 13-9
Ranson's Criteria for Acute Pancreatitis

Leukocyte count >16,000 mm^3	BUN level increase >5 mg/dL
Serum glucose >200 mg/dL	Serum calcium <8 mg/dL
Serum amylase >390 U/L	Base deficit >4 mEq/L
LDH >350 IU/L	Estimated fluid deficit >6 L
AST >250 IU/L	Arterial Pao$_2$ <60 mm Hg
Age >55 years	Decrease in hematocrit >10%

AST, aspartate aminotransferase; BUN, blood urea nitrogen; LDH, lactate dehydrogenase.
Data from Kaplow R, Hardin S. *Critical Care Nursing: Synergy for Optimal Outcomes.* Sudbury, MA: Jones and Bartlett Publishers, Inc; 2007.

C-reactive protein are also present in acute pancreatitis (**Table 13-9**). Hypercalcemia and hyperlipidemia are related to fat necrosis related to pancreatic tissue necrosis. Transabdominal ultrasonography will determine the condition of the pancreas and if gallstones are the culprit (Papadakis and McPhee).

Pancreatitis is a disease process with parenchymal inflammation of the pancreas, and acute pancreatitis can be associated with lung injury and hypoxia. The exact etiology is unknown; however, it is believed that acute lung injury is due to singular or multiple system organ failure. Acute lung injury and acute respiratory distress syndrome are seen in one-third of patients with severe pancreatitis and have a 60% mortality rate (Manohar et al.).

Management

Treatment begins with resting the pancreas by nothing by mouth status and initiating aggressive intravenous fluids resuscitation initially and intravenous nutrition such as total parenteral nutrition (Papadakis and McPhee). Monitor strict intravenous intake and urinary output. Monitor laboratory data closely and correct any metabolic abnormalities. Use antiemetics as needed; insert a nasogastric tube and place to intermittent suction for persistent nausea and vomiting. Perform pain assessments every 2 hours (ask patient for numerical rating on a pain scale) and as needed, as acute pancreatitis causes severe, stabbing abdominal pain. The drug of choice for pain management is meperidine (Demerol). If a stone is lodged in the duct, the drug of choice is morphine (Story).

The clinician should monitor the continuous pulse oximetry and check the arterial blood gas results as needed for signs of hypoxia. Supplemental O_2 can be used as needed. Turn, cough, and deep breathing every 2 hours will prevent atelectasis. Intubation along with mechanical ventilation is necessary if there is severe hypoventilation. If infection is a concern, then antibiotic therapy is appropriate. Temporary or permanent insulin replacement may be needed depending on the extent of the pancreatic damage. Once an oral diet is resumed, pancreatic enzyme supplements will need to be initiated. Early identification and treatment of anemia, renal failure, acute respiratory distress syndrome, draining of an abscess, and/or repair of biliary obstruction are crucial to prevent death (Papadakis and McPhee).

Acetaminophen Overdose

Acetaminophen is used to treat mild to moderate pain and reduce fever. Acetaminophen is the drug of choice for overdose and triggers more than 100,000 calls to poison control annually. Acute liver failure is a variable syndrome characterized by coagulopathy and encephalopathy. Acetaminophen overdose is the leading cause of liver failure in the United States with a 70% survival rate with emergency liver transplant (Fontana). More ICU admissions occur related to acetaminophen exposure than for any other medication (Papadakis and McPhee).

Clinical Findings

The recommended dose of acetaminophen is 650 to 1,000 mg every 4 to 6 hours, not to exceed 4 g/day (4000 mg/day). Toxicity develops with ingestion of 7.5 to 10 g/day (7,500 to 10,000 mg/day) or 140 mg/kg with an acetaminophen level of greater than 20 mcg/mL (Agrawal and Khazaeni). Acetaminophen toxicity signs and symptoms are divided into three phases. Phase I starts as early as a half an hour to 24 hours with nausea, vomiting, anorexia, and diaphoresis. Phase II begins at 24 to 72 hours, after ingestion of toxic levels, with renal insufficiency, elevated liver enzymes, and right upper quadrant pain. Phase III occurs at 72 to 96 hours, following toxic ingestion, with coagulation deficits, hepatic encephalopathy, jaundice, and renal failure. Multisystem organ failure can be caused by hemorrhage, shock, and/or sepsis; however, hepatic failure is the main cause of death (Papadakis and McPhee).

Management

ICU admission is necessary for the patient who ingested a toxic amount of acetaminophen to closely monitor vital signs, laboratory data, and neurological status. Nearly half of persons admitted with acetaminophen overdose require mechanical ventilation for airway protection. The majority of acetaminophen absorption occurs within the first 2 hours and levels peak within 4 hours (Story). The antidote for acetaminophen overdose is oral N-acetylcysteine (NAC), also known as Mucomyst. NAC halts liver damage by preventing toxic metabolites from attaching to protein molecules within the liver. If NAC is administered within 8 hours of a toxic ingestion of acetaminophen, the incidence of hepatotoxicity is significantly reduced. NAC comes in concentrations of 10% (100 mg/mL) and 20% (200 mg/mL). The loading dose of NAC is 140 mg/kg followed by 17 doses of 70 mg/kg every 4 hours. The dose can be diluted to a 1:4 concentration using juice or water to allow the NAC to be more pleasant tasting. If the patient experiences emesis following a dose of NAC, then the dose is repeated within 1 hour. An antiemetic may be given as needed or a nasogastric tube may be inserted if emesis persists. Intravenous NAC may also be used if not tolerated by mouth (Papadakis and McPhee).

Opioid Overdose

In 2014, a total of 47,055 drug overdose deaths occurred in the United States. In 2016, 63,632 people died of an opioid overdose (Rudd et al.). The steady increase in synthetic opioid deaths is being blamed on the increased availability of manufactured unlawful fentanyl. However, the death certificate cannot differentiate between unlawfully manufactured fentanyl and prescription fentanyl. There is an intense need for opioid abuse prevention, improvement in treatment of dependence, and reducing the supply of unlawful opioids and overdose deaths (Seth et al.).

Unlawful and prescription opioids are popular drugs for abuse and the cause for overdose requiring an ICU admission. Some examples of these opioids are fentanyl, heroin, codeine, and morphine. Fentanyl is 2,000 times more potent than its cousin morphine (Rudd et al.). These drugs attach to opioid receptors in the brain and then decrease central nervous system activity, block pain, slow respirations, and promote an antidepressant effect.

Clinical Findings

Mild opioid ingestion effect is euphoria and drowsiness; however, a more severe effect is bradycardia, hypotension, and respiratory depression. Death from an opioid overdose is usually the result of apnea or aspiration of emesis into the airway and lungs. The half-life of heroin is 2 to 30 minutes, with the duration of the effect from 3 to 5 hours. Methadone has a duration from 48 to 72 hours. Morphine half-life is 1.5 to 7 hours (Papadakis and McPhee).

Management

If the patient is obtunded or comatose, intubation and mechanical ventilation are warranted to protect the airway. Place a nasogastric tube and give 60 to 100 g activated charcoal (Papadakis and McPhee). Activated charcoal is given to absorb any toxins or drugs in the stomach or colon. Naloxone (Narcan) is an opioid antagonist, as it blocks the opioid receptor and reverses the effects of the opioid overdose. The dose of naloxone is 0.2 to 2 mg given intravenously, and the dose may be repeated to restore adequate respirations (Papadakis and McPhee). Fentanyl and codeine will require multiple doses to achieve results. The duration of activated charcoal is 2 to 3 hours, so if the patient has taken a long-acting opioid, then a repeated dose will be necessary to continue the opioid receptor blockade.

Stroke

Every year, about 795,000 people are affected by a stroke and over 140,000 people die each year from a stroke in the United States (Strokecenter.org). Stroke is the leading cause of serious, long-term disability in the United States. Cerebral circulation involves anterior circulation by the two internal carotid arteries and posterior circulation by the two vertebral arteries. The cause of a stroke can be ischemic or hemorrhagic. An **ischemic stroke** is a severe reduction in blood flow to the brain. A **hemorrhagic stroke** is a ruptured blood vessel preventing blood flow to the brain.

Ischemic Stroke

Ischemic strokes account for 80% to 85% of all strokes (Strokecenter.org). An ischemic stroke is a disturbance of blood flow to an area of the brain due to a clot obstruction. The goal of therapy is to increase cerebral blood flow to the brain and prevent further damage by decreasing the vulnerability of the brain tissue.

Hemorrhagic Stoke

Cerebral blood flow (CBF) fluctuates with the mean arterial pressure and is critical to intracerebral function. Cerebral perfusion pressure propels oxygen transport to brain tissue. If the MAP decreases, there is cerebral vasodilation to enhance CBF (Mount and Das). If the MAP increases, there is cerebral vasoconstriction and it tends to reduce CBF. The normal CPP is 60 to 80 mm Hg and it depends on the intracranial pressure (ICP) and the MAP. To calculate the CPP, subtract the ICP from the MAP.

Subdural hematoma (SDH) and an intracranial hemorrhage (ICH) are the two types of hemorrhagic stroke. An SDH is usually caused by a ruptured cerebral aneurysm with bleeding into the subarachnoid space beneath the arachnoid mater. The patient will present complaining of the worst headache of his or her life. SDH is classified using a scale of stage I asymptomatic to stage V comatose (**Table 13-10**). An ICH is usually due to traumatic brain injury, and brain tissue is compressed. ICH is often associated with poor patient outcomes and increased mortality rate. Patients with concurrent ICH and SDH, 10% will die suddenly before receiving treatment and 20% to 30% will present for treatment comatose and die within 3 months (Papadakis and McPhee).

Management of Ischemic Stroke

The goal of therapy for an acute ischemic stroke is to preserve tissue where cerebral perfusion is poor and to optimize collateral circulation. Administration of a tissue-type plasminogen activator, also known as tPA, along with a cerebral arterial thrombectomy can restore CBF to affected areas. The quicker CBF is restored, the less long-term harmful effects of ischemia (Jauch). The goal of therapy is to keep the central venous pressure 10 to 12 mm Hg and the hematocrit between 33% and 38% (Papadakis and McPhee). Hypervolemia with the use of volume expanders, hemodilution, and induction of hypertension are used to prevent vasospasms and increase CBF. Blood pressure control, a dark and quiet room, pain management, and keeping the head of the bed elevated 30 degrees are also important. Glycemic control following stoke is essential because hyperglycemia worsens clinical outcomes and increases mortality risk (Kim et al.).

Management of a Hemorrhagic Stroke

Emergency treatment of a hemorrhagic stroke involves controlling the bleeding and decreasing ICP. Pharmaceutical interventions or blood products to reverse anticoagulation or antiplatelet medication may be given (Mayo Clinic). Maintaining a lower MAP will lower ICP and prevent vasospasm. A neurosurgeon may place a clip to the neck of the aneurysm or perform an endovascular coiling if necessary (Papadakis and McPhee). A summary of ischemic stroke management is provided in **Box 13-4**.

Pulmonary Thromboembolism

Pulmonary thromboembolism (PTE) is a condition that may become life threatening if not promptly diagnosed so that initiation of appropriate therapy can be done. A PTE is the development of a thrombus in the pulmonary artery and is the third leading cause of death among patients admitted to the hospital (Papadakis and McPhee). A saddle embolism straddles the main pulmonary arterial trunk at its bifurcation and is one of the few types of emboli that may merit surgical removal. Virchow's triad lists the risk factors for PTE as venous stasis, injury to a blood vessel lumen, and hypercoagulopathy (Papadakis and McPhee). Protein C, protein S, and antithrombin deficiencies can cause hypercoagulopathy. Other risk factors are obesity, stroke, increased CVP, and immobility. High-resolution CT images of two types of PTE findings are shown in **Figure 13-6**. A reduced end-tidal CO_2 correlates with an increase of dead space ventilation, a unique V/Q mismatch feature of PTE.

TABLE 13-10
Hunt and Hess Subdural Hematoma (SDH) Scale

Stage I	Asymptomatic with mild headache
Stage II	Moderate to severe headache, meningism (stiff neck, photophobia, and headache), and no weakness
Stage III	Mild alteration in mental status
Stage IV	Depressed level of conciousness and/or hemiparesis
Stage V	Posturing or comatose

Modifed from The Joint Commission. Manual for joint commission national quality measures. Available at https://www.jointcommission.org/specifications _manual_joint_commission_national_quality_core_measures.aspx

BOX 13-4 Ischemic Stroke Management

Thrombolytic Therapy

- Thrombolytic therapy (clot lysis and reopen blood vessel)
- Low molecular weight heparin (prevent clot from becoming larger)
- Increased intracranial pressure (control with Mannitol and/or hyperventilation)
- Blood Pressure control (keep MAP 80–100 mm Hg)
- Strict glycemic control (improve patient outcomes)
- Induced hypothermia (reduce metabolic rate)

Data from Kaplow R, Hardin S. *Critical Care Nursing: Synergy for Optimal Outcomes*. Sudbury, MA: Jones and Bartlett Publishers, Inc: 2007; Strokecenter.org. Stroke statistics. Available at http://www.strokecenter.org/patients/about-stroke/stroke-statistics. Published 2019.

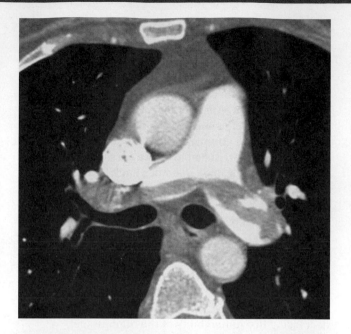

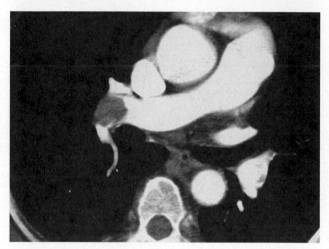

FIGURE 13-6 Computed tomography scans of pulmonary thromboembolism: **(Top)** saddle embolism with filling defects on left and right; **(Bottom)** right-sided embolism with filling defect on left, patient's right.

Clinical Findings

Clinical findings are related to the size of the PTE and the patient's cardiopulmonary health. Tachypnea is a symptom in half of the patients with PTE. Dyspnea and pleuritic pain are noted in 65 to 70% of the patients diagnosed with a PTE. The electrocardiogram will show sinus tachycardia in 70% of patients. Because of tachypnea, acute respiratory alkalosis with profound hypoxia will most likely be revealed by the arterial blood gas analysis. Capnography is an effective method to emergently rule out a PTE by checking if the alveoloarterial P_{CO_2} gradient is widened (sudden decrease in end-tidal CO_2 value without similar change in Pa_{CO_2}). The degradation product of cross-linked fibrin (D-dimer) is elevated >500 mcg/L. A chest radiograph will appear normal unless other lung disease is present (Papadakis and McPhee).

Diagnostic Testing

A computed tomography pulmonary angiography (CTPA) with intravenous radiocontrast dye is the gold standard in diagnosing or excluding a PTE (Doğan et al.). A ventilation-perfusion ($\dot{V}/\dot{Q}$) scan can be performed instead of CT in the case of a creatinine value >2.0 mg/dL and/or allergy to intravenous radiocontrast dye. A perfusion scan involves radiolabeled microaggregated albumin intravenously, and these particles of albumin embolize to the pulmonary capillaries. The ventilation portion of the scan involves the patient inhaling a radioactive gas and the distribution in the pulmonary system is recorded. Defects in the pulmonary system will be highlighted on the scan and be graded as low, medium, or high probability of a PTE (Papadakis and McPhee).

Management

A patient with a PTE needs an ICU admission in order to be observed closely. Echocardiography should be performed to determine if there is right-sided heart strain present. Heparin and Lovenox can be used for immediate protection to keep the embolus from becoming larger (Papadakis and McPhee). Heparin accelerates the function of antithrombin, which blocks thrombin and halts thrombus formation. Lovenox blocks the clotting factor Xa, and the patient's body will break down the clot faster than thrombin can be activated by coagulation factors and bind with fibrinogen, which makes fibrin. Fibrin forms strands that attach to platelets and increase the clot size and burden. Heparin has a short half-life of about 30 minutes, so it is the drug of choice if an intervention is pending (Papadakis and McPhee).

If large clot burden is present, there are several options for therapy. Streptokinase can be given intravenously to lyse the intravascular clot if the patient does not have any indications for major hemorrhagic complications. The EKOS® is an ultrasound-assisted catheter-directed thrombolysis procedure that reduces treatment risks for pulmonary emboli. A cardiovascular surgeon can perform a surgical thrombectomy to remove a clot from the pulmonary artery (Papadakis and McPhee).

Summary

This chapter includes many medical care events and conditions that frequently occur in critical care settings. These medical conditions (e.g., sepsis, opioid overdose, pulmonary thromboembolism) often lead to pulmonary complications such as ARDS, VAP, and HIE or hypoxic brain injury. The authors hope that our readers may integrate this information into other aspects of patient care, especially during patient assessment and management of mechanical ventilation.

Case Studies

You are doing the morning rounds in the intensive care unit (ICU). The first patient, Mary, has a PaO_2 of 60 mm Hg while breathing spontaneously on an air entrainment device with FIO_2 of 0.4.

1. **What is the P/F ratio?**

2. **Does Mary have acute respiratory distress syndrome (ARDS)?**

The second patient, Cat, received a massive transfusion 12 hours ago because of an unrecognized large internal bleed. She is being mechanically ventilated with a tidal volume setting of 6 mL/kg of predicted body weight. Her chest radiograph shows severe bilateral infiltrates with no evidence of cardiomegaly. Her recent arterial blood gas (ABG) shows PaO_2 of 100 mm Hg on an FIO_2 of 0.4.

3. **Does Cat have ARDS? If yes, classify her severity of ARDS.**

4. **Are Cat's conditions likely caused by large internal bleed, massive transfusion, or excessive tidal volume setting?**

A third patient, Rock, is being mechanically ventilated and he has been improving the last 3 days. His FIO_2 and PEEP have been weaned down to 0.4 and 5 cm H_2O, respectively. The night shift clinician reports that Rock suddenly developed "lung problems" around 3 a.m. The FIO_2 and PEEP are up to 0.6 and 8 cm H_2O for acceptable ABGs.

5. **Which of the following terms best describe Rock's condition: ventilator-associated condition (VAC), infection-related ventilator-associated complications (IVAC), or possible or probable ventilator-associated pneumonia (PVAP)?**

On your way leaving the ICU, the infection control coordinator asks you about the strategies to prevent or reduce the incidence of ventilator-associated events (VAEs).

6. **List the methods to reduce the incidence of VAE.**

Bibliography
Acute Respiratory Distress Syndrome

Ashbaugh DG, Bigelow DB, Petty TL, Levine BE. Acute respiratory distress in adults. *Lancet*. 1967; 12;2(7511):319–323.

Chang DW. *Clinical Application of Mechanical Ventilation*. 4th ed. Clifton Park, NY: Delmar Cengage Learning; 2014.

Fan E, Brodie D, Slutsky AS. Acute respiratory distress syndrome: advances in diagnosis and treatment. *JAMA*. 2018;319:698–710. doi:10.1001/jama.2017.21907

Harman EM. Acute respiratory distress syndrome. *Medscape*. 2018. Available at www.emedicine.medscape.com

Ranieri VM, Rubenfeld GD, Thompson BT, et al. Acute respiratory distress syndrome: the Berlin definition. ARDS Definition Task Force. *JAMA*. 2012;307:2526–2533.

Siegel MD. Acute respiratory distress syndrome: clinical features, diagnosis, and complications in adults. *UpToDate*. Available at https://www.uptodate.com/contents/acute-respiratory-distress-syndrome-clinical-features-diagnosis-and-complications-in-adults/print

Ventilator-Associated Events

Benson AB. Pulmonary complications of transfused blood components. *Crit Care Nurs Clin North Am*. 2012;24:403–418. doi:10.1016/j.ccell.2012.06.005

Centers for Disease Control and Prevention. Ventilator-associated events (VAE) protocol. Centers for Disease Control and Prevention: Atlanta, GA; 2019. Available at https://www.cdc.gov/nhsn/pdfs/pscmanual/10-vae_final.pdf

Hamilton VA, Grap MJ. The role of the endotracheal tube cuff in microaspiration. *Heart Lung*. 2012;41:10.

Hellyer TP, Ewan V, Wilson P, et al. The Intensive Care Society recommended bundle of interventions for the prevention of ventilator-associated pneumonia. *J Intensive Care Soc*. 2016;17:238–243. doi:10.1177/1751143716644461

Klompas M, Anderson D, Trick W, et al. The preventability of ventilator-associated events. The CDC Prevention Epicenters Wake Up and Breathe Collaborative. *Am J Respir Crit Care Med*. 2015;191(3):292–301. doi:10.1164/rccm.201407-1394OC

Neuville M, Mourvillier B, Bouadma L, et al. Bundle of care decreased ventilator-associated events—implications for ventilator-associated pneumonia prevention. *J Thorac Dis.* 2017;9:430–433. doi:10.21037/jtd.2017.02.72

Torres A, Niederman MS, Chastre J, et al. International ERS/ESICM/ESCMID/ALAT guidelines for the management of hospital-acquired pneumonia and ventilator-associated pneumonia. *Eur Respir J.* 2017;50(3):1700582. doi:10.1183/13993003.00582-2017

Hypoxic-Ischemic Encephalopathy

American Heart Association. CPR & first aid emergency cardiovascular care. Available at https://cpr.heart.org/AHAECC/CPRAndECC/ResuscitationScience/UCM_477263_AHA-Cardiac-Arrest-Statistics. jsp%5BR=301,L,NC%5D

Bouma GJ, Muizelaar JP. Relationship between cardiac output and cerebral blood flow in patients with intact and with impaired autoregulation. *J Neurosurg.* 1990;73:368–374.

Chang DW. *Clinical Application of Mechanical Ventilation.* 4th ed. Clifton Park, NY: Delmar Cengage Learning; 2014.

Changaris DG, McGraw CP, Richardson JD, et al. Correlation of cerebral perfusion pressure and Glasgow Coma Scale to outcome. *J Trauma.* 1987;27:1007–1013.

Chesnut RM, Marshall SB, Piek J, et al. Early and late systemic hypotension as a frequent and fundamental source of cerebral ischemia following severe brain injury in the Traumatic Coma Data Bank. *Acta Neurochir Suppl (Wien).* 1993;59:121–125.

Kanyal N. The science of ischemic stroke: pathophysiology & pharmacological treatment. *Int J Pharm Res Rev.* 2015;4:65–84.

Madl C, Holzer M. Brain function after resuscitation from cardiac arrest. *Curr Opin Crit Care.* 2004;10:213–217. doi:10.1097/01.ccx.0000127542.32890.fa

Marion DW, Darby J, Yonas H. Acute regional cerebral blood flow changes caused by severe head injuries. *J Neurosurg.* 1991;74:407–414.

Marmarou A, Anderson RL, Ward JD, et al. Impact of ICP instability and hypotension on outcome in patients with severe head trauma. *J Neurosurg.* 1991;75:S59–S66.

Rosner MJ, Daughton S. Cerebral perfusion pressure management in head injury. *J Trauma.* 1990;30:933–940.

Synopsis of Urgent Medical Conditions

Agrawal S, Khazaeni B. Acetaminophen toxicity. *StatPearls.* 2018. Available at www.nlm.nih.gov/books/NBK441917

Centers for Disease Control and Prevention. What is sepsis? Available at https://www.cdc.gov/sepsis/what-is-sepsis.html

Columbia University Irving Medical Center. The pancreas center. Available at http://columbiasurgery.org/pancreas/pancreas-and-its-functions

Doğan H, de Roos A, Geleijns J, et al. The role of computed tomography in the diagnosis of acute and chronic pulmonary embolism. *Diagn Intervent Radiol.* 2015;21:307–316. doi:10.5152/dir.2015.14403

Fontana R. Acute liver failure including acetaminophen overdose. *Med Clin North Am.* 2008;92(4):961–794. doi:10.1016/j.mcna.2008.03.005

Fry A, Farrington K. Management of acute renal failure. *Postgrad Med J.* 2006;82:106–116. doi:10.1136/pgmj.2005.038588

Jauch E. Ischemic stroke treatment & management. *Medscape.* 2019. Available at https://www.emedicine.medscape.com/article/1916852-treatment

Jozwiak M, Monnet X, Teboul J. Implementing sepsis bundles. *Ann Transl Med.* 2016;4(17):332. doi:10.21037/atm.2016.08.60

Kaplow R, Hardin S. *Critical Care Nursing: Synergy for Optimal Outcomes.* Sudbury, MA: Jones and Bartlett; 2007.

Kim N, Jhang Y, Park JM, et al. Aggressive glucose control for acute ischemic stroke patients by insulin infusion. *J Clin Neurol.* 2009;5(4):167–172. doi:10.3988/jcn.2009.5.4.167

Lehman L, Saeed M, Moody G, et al. Hypotension as a risk factor for acute kidney injury in ICU patients. *Comput Cardiol.* 2010;37:1095–1098.

Manohar M, Verma AK, Venkateshaiah SU, et al. Chronic pancreatitis associated acute respiratory failure. *MOJ Immunol.* 2017;5(2):00149. doi:10.15406/moji.2017.05.00149

Mayo Clinic. Stroke. Available at https://www.mayoclinic.org/diseases-conditions/ stroke/...treatment/drc-20350119

Moore P, Hsu R, Liu K. Management of acute kidney injury: core curriculum 2018. *Am J Kidney Dis.* 2018;72:136–148. doi:10.1053/j.ajkd.2017.11.021

Mount C, Das J. Cerebral perfusion pressure. *StatPearls.* 2019. Available at http:// www.ncbi.nlm.nih.gov/books/NBK537271

Murali A, Menon K. Acute liver failure. Cleveland Clinic Center for Continuing Education. Available at https://www.clevelandclinicmeded.com/medicalpubs/diseasemanagement/hepatololgy/acute-liver-failure. Published 2017.

Nagami G, Hamm L. Regulation of acid-base balance in chronic kidney disease. *Adv Chronic Kidney Dis.* 2017;24(5):274–279. doi:10.1053/j.ackd.2017.07.004

Papadakis M, McPhee S, Rabow M. *Current: Medical Diagnosis & Treatment.* 58th ed. New York, NY: McGraw Hill Education; 2019.

Rudd R, Aleshire N, Zibbell J, et al. Increases in drug and opioid overdose deaths—United States, 2000–2014. *Am J Transplant.* 2016;64:1378–1382. doi:10.1111/ajt.13776

Saraswat VA, Saksena S, Nath K, et al. Evaluation of mannitol effect in patients with acute hepatic failure and acute-on-chronic liver failure using conventional MRI, diffusion tensor imaging and in vivo proton MR spectroscopy. *World J Gastroenterol.* 2008;14(26):4168–4178. doi:10.3748/wjg.14.4168

Seth P, Rudd R, Noonan R, et al. Quantifying the epidemic of prescription opioid overdose deaths. *Am J Pub Health.* 2018;108:500–502. doi:10.2105/AJPH.2017.30426

Singh T, Gupta N, Alkhouri N, et al. A guide to management of acute liver failure. *Cleveland Clin J Med.* 2016;83(6):453–462. doi:10.3949/ccjm.83a.15101

Sparks MA, Crowley SD, Gurley SB, et al. Classical renin-angiotensin system in kidney physiology. *Comp Physiol.* 2014;4:1201–1228. doi:10.1002/cphy.c130040

Story L. *Pathophysiology: A Practical Approach.* Burlington, MA: Jones & Bartlett; 2018.

Stroke Center. Stroke statistics. Strokecenter.org. Available at http://www.strokecenter.org/patients/about-stroke/stroke-statistics. Published 2019.

Surviving Sepsis Campaign. 3 hour bundle. Available at http://www.survivingsepsis.org/SiteCollectionDocuments/Bundle-3-Hour-Step4-Fluids.pdf

14

Traumatic Critical Care Issues

Ruben D. Restrepo, MD, RRT

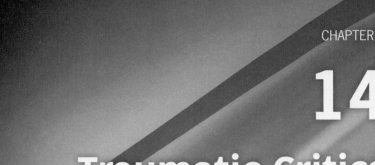

OUTLINE

Chest Trauma
  Classification of Chest Trauma
  Diagnosis of Chest Trauma
  Monitoring of Patients with Chest Trauma
  Treatment
Burn and Inhalation Injury
  Smoke Inhalation
  Pathophysiology of Inhalation Injury
  Diagnosis
  Monitoring
  Treatment
  Complications and Prognosis
Traumatic Brain Injury
  Classification of TBI
  Pathophysiology
  Management of TBI
Summary
Case Study
Bibliography

OBJECTIVES

1. Describe the components of a primary survey on a chest trauma patient.
2. Describe the radiographic findings associated with a pneumothorax and a hemothorax.
3. Define flail chest and describe its management.
4. Summarize the physical exam findings in the most common types of chest trauma.
5. List the classic signs of tension pneumothorax in the physical exam.
6. Explain when chest drainage systems can be removed.
7. Review the pathophysiology of inhalation injury.

8. Describe the symptoms associated with different COHb levels.
9. Explain the role of nebulized heparin in the management of inhalation injury.
10. List and explain the clinical parameters used to calculate the Glasgow Coma Scale.
11. Review the management of traumatic brain injury.
12. Explain the mechanical ventilation strategy recommended for patients with traumatic brain injury.

KEY TERMS

acute respiratory
  distress syndrome
barbiturate coma
blunt chest injury
bronchoscopy
carbon monoxide
cardiac tamponade
cerebral blood flow
cerebral herniation
cerebral perfusion pressure
computed tomography
CO-oximeter
craniectomy
Cushing triad
dry suction systems
external ventricular drain
flail chest
focused abdominal
  sonography for trauma
Glasgow Coma Scale
Heimlich valve
hemothorax
high-frequency percussive
  ventilation

hydrogen cyanide
intracranial pressure
N-acetylcysteine
nebulized heparin
non-tension pneumothorax
penetrating chest injury
pneumothorax
primary survey
pulmonary contusion
secondary survey
smoke inhalation
subcutaneous emphysema
sulcus sign
tension pneumothorax
thermal injury
thoracostomy
thoracotomy
traumatic brain injury
underwater seal
video-assisted
  thoracoscopic surgery

Chest Trauma

The World Health Organization estimates that by 2020 vehicular injury will be the second most common cause of mortality and morbidity worldwide. In the United States, trauma is the leading cause of death, morbidity, and hospitalization among people younger than 50 years of age. Estimates of thoracic trauma frequency indicate that injuries occur in 12 per 1 million individuals per day. Approximately a third of these injuries require hospitalization. Blunt chest injuries (BCIs) are the second leading cause of death among trauma patients. Overall, BCIs are directly responsible for 20% to 25% of all deaths, and chest trauma is a major contributor in another 50% of deaths. High-velocity trauma in motor vehicle accidents (MVAs) accounts for 70% to 80% of all BCIs. A recent analysis of flail chest injury conducted by the National Trauma Data Bank revealed that lung contusion was present in 59% of the patients whereas 15% of the patients had significant head trauma. Chest trauma can affect any one or all components of the chest wall and thoracic cavity (**Box 14-1**).

The most significant disruption to the normal physiology encountered in BCI involves abnormalities in the flow of air, blood, or both in combination. The pain associated with chest trauma can cause dyspnea, altered respiratory pattern, and ultimately abnormalities in gas exchange. Shunting and dead space ventilation produced by these injuries can also impair oxygenation. Therefore, hypoxia and hypoventilation are considered the primary killers in acute trauma patients. Assessment of breathing should therefore be given high priority in the initial evaluation or primary survey.

The presence of air and/or fluid in the pleural space interferes with lung expansion and may compress the healthy lung. If pressure builds up, such as in the case of a tension pneumothorax, the structures in the mediastinum can shift and lead to decreased venous return to the heart, circulatory compromise, and shock. Release of inflammatory mediators during chest trauma is also believed to cause lung injury and lead to cases of multiple organ failure.

Direct injury to the heart and blood vessels can cause rapid and catastrophic exsanguination and frequently results in death before any resuscitation effort is initiated.

Classification of Chest Trauma

The **primary survey** is designed to evaluate any chest trauma that could be potentially life threatening and to determine the best therapeutic approach to stabilize the patient (**Box 14-2**). In severe trauma, assessment and resuscitation should be performed simultaneously. Life-threatening chest traumas include tension pneumothorax, open pneumothorax, massive hemothorax, cardiac tamponade, and flail chest.

A **secondary survey** is a more detailed and complete (head-to-toe) examination, aimed at identifying all other injuries that could have been missed or appear not life threatening and planning further investigation and treatment. It is performed only after the primary survey of airway, breathing, and circulation has been completed and/or the initial resuscitation is in progress. Chest injuries identified during a secondary survey are listed in **Box 14-3**.

Although several types of chest trauma will be discussed individually in this section of the chapter, each clinician should be prepared to ask specific questions during the physical exam of patients with chest trauma (**Table 14-1**).

Depending on the mechanism of injury, chest trauma can be classified in two categories: blunt and penetrating. They have different pathophysiology and clinical courses. **Blunt chest injury** (BCI) results from kinetic energy forces and is caused by three very distinct mechanisms: blast, compression, and deceleration. The majority of **penetrating chest injuries** result from stab wounds (low-energy trauma) or gunshot wounds (high-energy trauma).

Although the diagnosis of blunt injuries may be more difficult and require additional investigations such as

---

BOX 14-2 Components of the Primary Survey

- Airway maintenance with cervical spine protection
- Breathing and ventilation
- Circulation and hemorrhage control
- Disability/neurologic status
- Exposure/environmental control

BOX 14-1 Distribution of Organ Injury in Chest Trauma

- Chest wall (70%)
- Lung (21%)
- Heart (7%)
- Diaphragm (7%)
- Esophagus (7%)
- Aorta (4.8%)
- Tracheobronchial tree (0.8%)

BOX 14-3 Chest Injuries Typically Identified on the Secondary Survey

- Rib fractures and flail chest
- Pulmonary contusion
- Simple pneumothorax
- Simple hemothorax
- Blunt aortic injury
- Blunt myocardial injury

TABLE 14-1
Questions to Ask During the Chest Physical Exam of Patients with Chest Trauma

Component of Physical Exam	Questions
Inspection	What is the respiratory rate and depth? Is the chest wall symmetric? (see Figure 14-14) Is the patient displaying paradoxical chest wall motion? Does the patient have bruising, seat belt or steering wheel marks, or penetrating wounds? Is the trachea midline?
Palpation	Is the trachea midline upon palpation of the suprasternal notch? Is there adequate and equal chest wall movement? Does the patient complain of chest wall tenderness? Does it feel like rib "crunching" indicating rib fractures? Is there subcutaneous emphysema?
Percussion	Is the percussion note increased (pneumothorax) or decreased (hemothorax)?
Auscultation	Are breath sounds diminished or absent? Are these changes in breath sounds unilateral or bilateral?

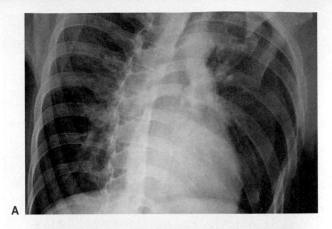
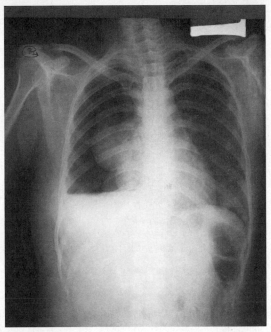

FIGURE 14-1 Anterioposterior radiograph of the chest showing a non-tension pneumothorax on the left hemithorax (**A**). The other radiograph (**B**) shows a pneumothorax on the right hemithorax where the pleural line of the collapsed lung is clearly visible.
A: © Casa Nayafana/Shutterstock; B: © Santibhavank P/Shutterstock.

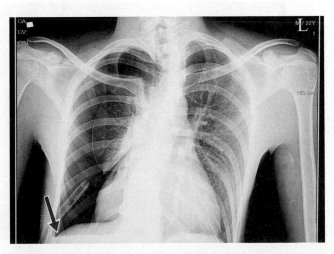

FIGURE 14-2 Posteroanterior chest radiograph showing the sulcus sign (black arrow) in a patient with a right-sided pneumothorax.
© Sopone Nawoot/iStock/Getty Images Plus/Getty Images.

computed tomography (CT) scanning, they are typically managed nonoperatively. However, the recovery time may be lengthy. On the other hand, penetrating injuries are more likely to require operation, and complex investigations are required infrequently. Patients with penetrating trauma may also deteriorate rapidly but recover much faster than patients with blunt injury.

Pneumothorax

Pneumothorax is the collection of air in the pleural space. Air may come from an injury to the lung tissue, a bronchial tear, or a chest wall injury allowing air to be sucked in from the outside. Traumatic pneumothoraces are often classified as non-tension and tension pneumothorax.

Non-tension Pneumothorax

A **non-tension pneumothorax** is defined as a nonexpanding collection of air in the pleural space where the lung is collapsed, to a variable extent. The classic signs of decreased chest expansion upon inspection, increased resonance to percussion, and diminished breath sounds are often difficult or impossible to appreciate. Although the chest radiograph is the standard diagnostic tool, it may not show small pneumothoraces, particularly if the film is taken with the patient in supine position (**Figure 14-1**).

A deep **sulcus sign**, abnormal deepening of the costophrenic angle when the pleural air collects laterally, is indicative of an anterior pneumothorax (**Figure 14-2**).

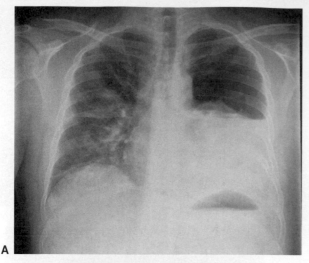

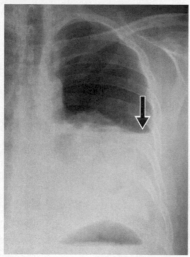

FIGURE 14-3 Anteroposterior radiograph of the chest showing a hemopneumothorax in the left hemithorax (**A**). A closeup view of the left lower section of the chest (**B**) shows the flat meniscus of the hemothorax (black arrow).

de Wolf SP, Deunk J, Cornet AD, Elbers PW. Case report: bilateral reexpansion pulmonary edema following treatment of a unilateral hemothorax. *F1000Res.* 2014;3:318. doi:10.12688/f1000research.6000.1

When a pneumothorax is visible on the erect chest radiograph, the presence of a flat meniscus indicates the presence of an associated hemothorax (**Figure 14-3**).

Chest CT scanning is more sensitive for detecting the presence of small or occult pneumothoraces than a plain chest radiograph (**Figure 14-4**).

Tension Pneumothorax

A lung laceration allows air to move into the pleural space, which will build up pressure without immediate intervention. In the presence of a **tension pneumothorax**, the one-way valve effect keeps air from moving out during exhalation. Every subsequent breath can further increase the intrapleural pressure. As the pressure inside the pleural space increases, the mediastinum shifts to the opposite side of the chest and venous return to the heart is compromised. One of the most important features of the tension pneumothorax is the hemodynamic compromise, which is proportional to the size of the collection of air in the hemithorax. Patients are often tachycardic, tachypneic, and hypoxic. When the collection of air (and pressure) in the pleural space is large enough, the patient may become hypotensive due to circulatory collapse, leading to pulseless electrical activity (PEA) and possible cardiac arrest. Some of the classic signs of tension pneumothorax are listed in **Box 14-4**.

Tension pneumothorax develops abruptly when trauma is the cause. However, when it results as a consequence of using positive pressure ventilation, its presentation may be more insidious. An unexplained tachycardia, hypotension, and rise in airway pressure are strongly suggestive of a developing tension pneumothorax.

The typical radiographic features of a tension pneumothorax are the contralateral deviation of both trachea and mediastinum, and depression of the diaphragm (**Figure 14-5**).

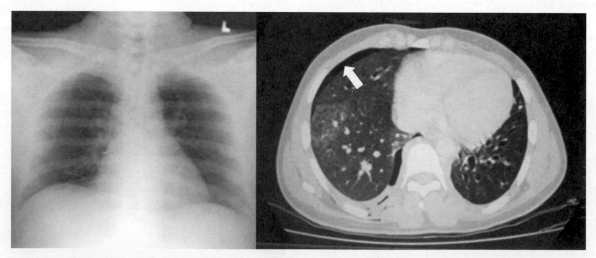

FIGURE 14-4 An anteroposterior chest radiograph interpreted as normal. The computed tomography scan (right) shows the presence of a pneumothorax on the right hemithorax (white arrow).

Khan HS, Wadood A, Ayyaz M. Occult pneumothorax: what do we need to do? *J Coll Physicians Surg Pak.* 2018;28(3):S31–S32.

BOX 14-4 Classic Signs of Tension Pneumothorax in the Physical Exam of the Chest

Inspection

- Tracheal deviation
- Hyperexpanded chest
- Decreased chest expansion

Palpation

- Decreased tactile/vocal fremitus

Percussion

- Increased percussion note

Auscultation

- Diminished to absent breath sounds

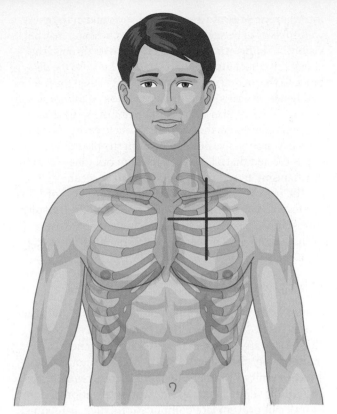

FIGURE 14-6 Schematic depiction of the anatomical landmark used for insertion of a cannula during decompression thoracostomy. The needle should be inserted in the second intercostal space with midclavicular line.

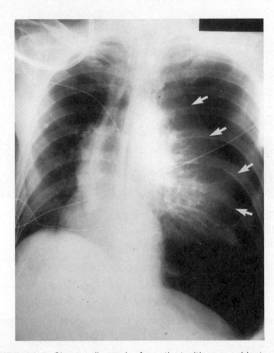

FIGURE 14-5 Chest radiograph of a patient with severe blunt trauma to the chest demonstrating the classic features of a left tension pneumothorax: deviation of both trachea and mediastinum to the right, and depression of the left hemidiaphragm.

Courtesy of Leonard V. Crowley, MD, Century College.

The diagnosis of bilateral tension pneumothoraces can be challenging since in most cases the trachea is midline and the percussion and auscultatory findings are similar on both sides of the chest. Tension pneumothoraces should therefore be presumed and bilateral decompression undertaken in all cases of traumatic arrest. Any unexplained acute deterioration of the respiratory and hemodynamic status in a patient undergoing mechanical ventilation should alert the clinician of the possibility of a tension pneumothorax. Unilateral or bilateral tension pneumothoraces require emergent chest decompression to prevent traumatic arrest.

The classic management of a tension pneumothorax is chest decompression with needle thoracostomy. A 14- to16-gauge intravenous cannula should be inserted into the upper border of the third rib in the second intercostal space with midclavicular line. The needle is advanced until air can be aspirated into a syringe connected to the needle (**Figure 14-6**).

Once the needle is withdrawn and the cannula is left open to air, a rush of air should leave the chest indicating the presence of a tension pneumothorax. However, absence of air rush does not rule out the presence of a tension pneumothorax, as the needle may have not reached the pleural cavity. Regardless of the hemodynamic status of the patient, if a tension pneumothorax is suspected, a form of decompression is indicated even before chest radiograph. Clinicians responsible for this procedure in the emergency setting need to remember needle decompression can be associated with complications. The presence of distended neck veins, reduced or absent breath sounds, and deviated trachea are typically excellent indicators for needle decompression until a definitive treatment (chest tube placement) is performed.

Open Pneumothorax

Open pneumothorax is rare in blunt chest trauma, but it can occur when injury results in a substantial loss of the chest wall. During inspiration, since a negative intrathoracic pressure is generated, a wound in the chest wall appears to be sucking air into the chest and may be visibly bubbling. Air enters the chest cavity through the chest wall defect instead of the trachea because the distance to the pleural space is much shorter than the trachea, and hence provides less resistance to flow. If the chest wall opening is more than 75% the diameter of the trachea, air preferentially enters through the thoracic cavity. This results in a progressive buildup of air in the pleural space. If a flap is created that allows air in but not out (one-way valve mechanism), tension pneumothorax may occur.

The use of oxygen at inspired fraction (F_{IO_2}) of 1.0 is recommended unless clear deterioration of the respiratory status is present. Chest tube placement, closure of the wound, and placement of an occlusive dressing should not be delayed.

Massive Hemothorax

Hemothorax is a collection of blood in the pleural space. It may result from direct blunt trauma (BT) to the chest or by any object that penetrates the chest cavity (**penetrating chest injury** [PCI]). Most hemothoraces are the result of rib fractures, lung parenchymal injury, and minor venous injuries. Early identification of hemothorax can prevent late complications such as retained hemothorax and empyema (collection of pus in the pleural space). The classic signs of hemothorax during physical exam of the chest are summarized in **Box 14-5**.

A chest radiograph, a CT scan, or a focused assessment with sonography for trauma (FAST) can confirm the diagnosis and size of the blood collection in the pleural space.

The upright chest radiograph remains the primary diagnostic study in the acute evaluation of hemothorax. It takes approximately 400 to 500 mL of blood to obliterate the costophrenic angle on the upright chest radiograph. The presence and size of a hemothorax are much more difficult to evaluate on supine films. As much as 1000 mL of blood may be missed when viewing a portable supine chest x-ray film. In the normal unscarred pleural space, a hemothorax is noted as a meniscus of fluid blunting the costophrenic angle or diaphragmatic surface and tracking up the pleural margins of the chest wall (**Figure 14-7**).

In the supine position (most BT patients) no fluid level is visible as the blood lies posteriorly along the posterior chest. The chest x-ray shows a diffuse opacification of the hemithorax, through which lung markings can be seen. It may be difficult to differentiate a unilateral hemothorax from a pneumothorax on the opposite side (**Figure 14-8**).

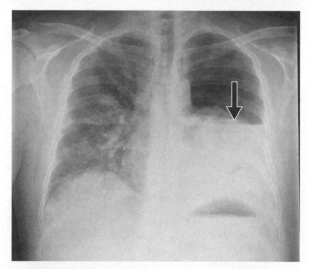

FIGURE 14-7 Anteroposterior radiograph of a patient in an erect position showing the presence of the classic meniscus of a hemothorax in the left hemithorax (arrow).

de Wolf SP, Deunk J, Cornet AD, Elbers PW. Case report: bilateral reexpansion pulmonary edema following treatment of a unilateral hemothorax. *F1000Res*. 2014;3:318. doi:10.12688/f1000research.6000.1

BOX 14-5 Classic Signs of Hemothorax During Physical Exam of the Chest

Inspection

- External bruising, lacerations
- Evidence of penetrating chest injury
- Decreased chest expansion
- Mediastinal shift on massive hemothorax

Palpation

- Crepitus, indicating rib fracture

Percussion

- Dull percussion note

Auscultation

- Diminished to absent breath sounds

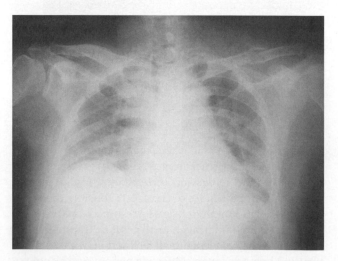

FIGURE 14-8 Anteroposterior radiograph of a patient in a supine position showing the presence of diffuse opacification of the right hemothorax consistent with a hemothorax.

© Santibhavank P/Shutterstock.

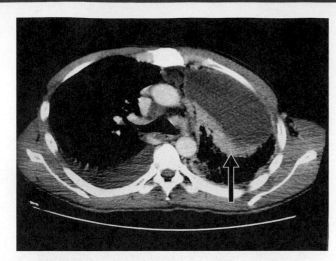

FIGURE 14-9 Computed chest tomography of a patient showing the presence of diffuse opacification of the left hemithorax (arrow) consistent with a hemothorax.
© Karan Bunjean/Shutterstock.

FAST has the advantage of detecting amounts of blood as little as 200 mL. However, in the presence of a pneumothorax or subcutaneous air, it may be difficult to detect or be inaccurate. Although computed chest tomography is more sensitive than the plain chest radiograph in diagnosing hemothoraces, most cases of thoracic trauma do not require it (**Figure 14-9**).

Cardiac Tamponade

Cardiac tamponade is defined as an increased pressure around the heart that occurs when blood or fluid builds up in the space between the heart muscle (myocardium) and the outer covering sac of the heart (pericardium). In traumatic cardiac tamponade, the presence of blood in the pericardial space impairs ventricular filling and venous return. The worst outcome is ventricular collapse causing a precipitous drop in cardiac output, hypotension, and possible cardiac arrest. The majority of patients who arrive at the emergency room with cardiac tamponade due to a penetrating chest injury have no vital signs. Therefore, traumatic pericardial tamponade is considered a serious and rapidly fatal injury. Every penetrating injury to the chest (especially in hypotensive patients) is a cardiac injury until proved otherwise.

The classic signs of cardiac tamponade, known as Beck's triad, include hypotension, distended neck veins, and muffled heart sounds. However, these signs are not present in many patients or are attenuated. The diagnosis is challenging since patients can be relatively stable in early stages, and other associated injuries may distract attention from the chest and mask the clinical features.

A chest radiograph in erect and straight position should be ordered whenever possible. Radiological signs suggestive of cardiac injury are enlarged cardiac shadow, pneumopericardium (air in the pericardium), and widened upper mediastinum.

If a central catheter is in place, central venous pressure (CVP) can be measured. If the CVP is higher than 12 cm H_2O tamponade should be suspected. However, conditions such as hemopneumothorax, restlessness, fluid overload, mechanical ventilation, and a misplaced catheter may give a raised CVP. On the other hand, severe hypovolemia may not show a raised CVP.

There is growing evidence that acute tamponade may also be precipitated by rapid administration of large volumes of fluid. Thus it is recommended that hypotensive but stable patients should have delayed and controlled fluid replacement.

Pericardiocentesis, also called a pericardial tap, is an invasive procedure in which a needle and catheter remove fluid from the pericardium. Although sometimes lifesaving, it is a dangerous procedure and considered of limited value. Needle pericardiocentesis may also fail as a diagnostic measure due to blood in the pericardial sac being clotted. Ventricular puncture and damage to the coronary arteries may result from pericardiocentesis.

A high degree of clinical suspicion for cardiac tamponade in patients with chest trauma, together with close monitoring and reevaluation, particularly during volume replacement, is essential.

According to a 2012 practice management guideline from the Eastern Association for the Surgery of Trauma (Clancy et al.), electrocardiogram (ECG) alone should not be considered sufficient for ruling out blunt cardiac injury. The guideline recommends obtaining an admission ECG and troponin I (muscle protein released from damaged cells, especially cardiac) from all patients in whom blunt cardiac injury is suspected and states that such injury can be ruled out only if both the ECG and the troponin I level are normal.

Pulmonary Contusion

Pulmonary contusion is an injury to lung parenchyma, leading to inflammation of the alveolar spaces and collection of blood in alveolar spaces. It occurs in approximately 20% of severe blunt traumas, and it is the most common chest injury in children. This type of lung injury develops over the course of 24 hours, leading to poor gas exchange, increased pulmonary vascular resistance, and decreased lung compliance. More than 50% to 60% of patients with significant pulmonary contusions develop **acute respiratory distress syndrome** (ARDS), and the mortality rate could be as high as 60% in patients who require mechanical ventilation.

The physical exam does not routinely provide any specific clues to pulmonary contusion. However, the presence of bruising, seat belt sign, rib fractures, or flail chest makes pulmonary contusion a strong possibility. Crackles may be heard on lung auscultation due to accumulation of fluid in the alveoli.

The plain chest radiograph is the standard method of diagnosing pulmonary contusions. However, it tends to lag behind the clinical picture, and the signs of pulmonary contusion may not be apparent until 24 to 48 hours following the chest trauma.

Rib Fractures and Flail Chest

Blunt trauma is associated with a wide spectrum of injuries to the chest wall. It can go from an isolated rib fracture to severe crush injuries of both hemithoraces, leading to respiratory compromise. Rib fractures are the most common blunt trauma injury. Pulmonary contusion may not be apparent on the initial chest radiograph, but it should be suspected in the presence of multiple rib fractures. The presence of pain aggravated by breathing or coughing or compression of the chest are common signs of rib fractures. Crepitus over the site of the fracture is a very common finding. Ribs 4 to 10 are the ones most frequently involved. Fractures of ribs 8 to 12 may be associated with diaphragmatic tears and spleen or liver injuries but are less commonly associated with injuries to adjacent great vessels. Since significant force is required to fracture the first or second ribs, their fractures should prompt a careful evaluation of more severe trauma and associated vascular injuries (**Figure 14-10**).

Flail chest is a condition in which there are at least two fractures per rib (producing a free segment) in at least two ribs. This area of the chest wall is flail, meaning it will move inward during inspiration while the rest of the chest wall moves outward. It is unable to contribute to lung expansion and produces a paradoxical movement of that segment of the chest wall. Although the management of flail chest consists of standard management of the rib fractures, in severe cases of chest wall disruption that lead to alteration of pulmonary mechanics, patients may require mechanical ventilation.

The presence of bruising, grazes, or seat belt signs upon inspection as well as crepitus from the broken ribs are the most significant changes in the physical exam of the chest (**Figure 14-11**).

Anteroposterior chest radiographs identify the majority of rib fractures (**Figure 14-12**).

The management of rib fractures and flail chest is directed toward protecting the lungs and sustaining adequate gas exchange. Adequate pulmonary hygiene is important to prevent the development of pneumonia,

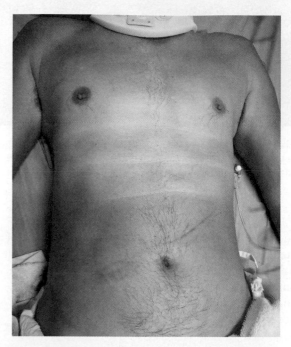

FIGURE 14-11 Presence of seat belt sign in the abdomen on a patient admitted for severe chest trauma as a result of a car crash.
© Happysuttinee/Shutterstock.

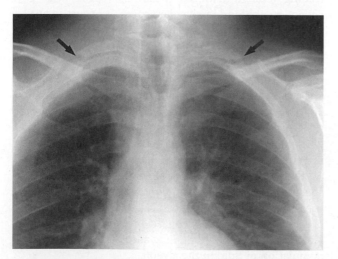

FIGURE 14-10 Anteroposterior chest radiograph showing a bilateral fracture of the first rib (arrows).
Reproduced with permission from Hacking D, Werring DJ. Bilateral first rib fractures due to tardive dystonia. *J Neurol Neurosurg Psychiatry*. 2005;76(7):983.

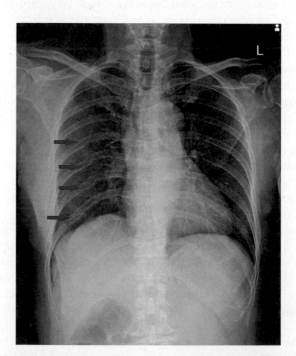

FIGURE 14-12 Anteroposterior chest radiograph showing four lower rib fractures.
© Richman Photo/Shutterstock.

which is the most common complication of chest wall injury. Adequate analgesia is the cornerstone of the management of rib fractures. Strapping the chest to splint rib fractures may impede chest wall movement and prevents adequate inspiration and clearance of secretions. Although patient-controlled analgesia (PCA) of an opioid infusion is the best method for cooperative patients, patients with severe chest wall injury benefit more from epidural infusion of local anesthetic. Respiratory depression and impairment of cough associated with the use of opioids needs to be considered.

Diaphragmatic Injuries

Any penetrating chest injury (PCI) in the left lower chest (between nipple and costal margin) has the potential to cause diaphragmatic injury. Injuries to the right diaphragm rarely have any clinical significance, except for anterior injuries. In left diaphragmatic injuries, the positive intra-abdominal pressure might cause migration of abdominal viscera into the chest and formation of diaphragmatic hernia. This herniation into the left hemithorax significantly decreases lung expansion and leads to severe respiratory distress. In blunt trauma (BT) the diaphragmatic rupture is usually due to severe abdominal trauma, which results in a sudden, major increase of the intra-abdominal pressure. The tear is usually 7 to 10 cm long. Broken ribs can also cause a diaphragmatic tear. Deceleration injuries may result in avulsion of the diaphragm from its peripheral attachments. Most (80%) of the injuries involve the left diaphragm. Rupture of the right diaphragm requires a much more intense force and is almost always associated with other intra-abdominal injuries.

A high degree of suspicion is the most important factor for early diagnosis. About 30% of all asymptomatic penetrating left thoracoabdominal injuries are associated with diaphragmatic perforation. Signs of hypovolemic shock are present in large diaphragmatic tears, and severe respiratory distress with audible bowel sounds in the chest may indicate massive left diaphragmatic herniation.

The chest radiograph may reveal an elevated hemidiaphragm and the presence of air-fluid levels in the chest. However, in about half the cases of diaphragmatic injuries the chest x-ray usually shows a nonspecific hemopneumothorax, in about 40% the chest x-ray is normal, and in only about 10% is there cause for suspicion of diaphragmatic injury. Laparoscopic evaluation should be considered in all PCI below the nipple line and above the costal margin on the left side. In cases when left diaphragmatic herniation is suspected, a chest radiograph after insertion of a gastric tube showing its tip in the chest may confirm the diagnosis of diaphragmatic perforation (due to upward migration of the stomach).

Surgical repair via open laparotomy or laparoscopically is the recommended treatment. If a diaphragmatic hernia is suspected, a thoracostomy tube should not be placed preoperatively.

Diagnosis of Chest Trauma

Although the physical exam of the chest is a critical element in the recognition of life-threatening chest traumas, imaging studies are considered the guiding test to confirm specific chest injuries, determine the extent of the trauma, determine the problems that require intervention, and anticipate potential complications. All patients with stab wounds between the neck and the umbilicus as well as gunshot wounds between the neck and the pelvis should have a chest film or other imaging study. Additional laboratory studies may be included as well.

Physical Exam

The physical evaluation should precede other diagnostic approaches. The primary survey or initial evaluation should follow a systematic approach that includes inspection, palpation, percussion, and auscultation. The clinician responsible for the evaluation of the patient with chest trauma should answer specific questions (see Table 14-1) when approaching the physical exam (**Table 14-2**). Palpation of the chest wall and apices may

TABLE 14-2
Physical Exam Findings in Chest Trauma

Chest Injury	Trachea	Chest Expansion	Percussion	Auscultation
Tension pneumothorax	Away	Decreased; chest may be fixed in hyperexpansion	Hyperresonant	Diminished or absent
Simple pneumothorax	Midline	Decreased	May be hyperresonant; usually normal	May be diminished
Hemothorax	Midline (if small) Away (if large)	Decreased	Dull, especially posteriorly	Diminished if large; normal if small
Pulmonary contusion	Midline	Normal	Normal	Normal; may have crackles
Lung collapse	Toward	Decreased	Normal	May be reduced

reveal **subcutaneous emphysema** (presence of air in the subcutaneous tissues) and rib fractures as the only sign of an underlying pneumothorax. Its presence is an important sign, but it has no clinical significance per se.

Examples of asymmetrical chest expansion observed in a tension pneumothorax and palpation technique used to confirm the presence of subcutaneous emphysema are observed in **Figure 14-13**.

A special situation needs to be considered when conducting the physical exam to confirm the presence of a pneumothorax. When an endotracheal tube is mistakenly placed in the right main bronchus, two different case scenarios may present. In the first scenario, obstruction of the right upper lobe bronchus can lead to collapse of the right upper lobe and shift of the trachea to the right. Upon percussion, the left side of the chest may appear to be hyperresonant compared to the right and give the impression of a left-sided pneumothorax. In the second scenario, preferential gas flow

of the right lung may lead to collapse of the left lung and hyperexpansion of the right. Although an obvious decrease in breath sounds on the left should indicate possible lung collapse, auscultation may be challenging in an emergent situation when noise is unavoidable. On the other hand, the hyperexpansion of the right side of the chest, increased percussion noted, and possible deviation of the trachea to the left caused by the left lung collapse may be misinterpreted as a potential pneumothorax on the right. In both scenarios, the unnecessary placement of a chest drain should be avoided by performing a very thorough physical exam of the chest and monitoring the hemodynamic status. (**Figure 14-14**).

Chest Radiograph

A chest radiograph (CXR) should be obtained on every patient with chest trauma. It helps in determining diagnosis of injuries, progression, complications, and placement of tubes and lines, according to Aukema et al. The plain anteroposterior CXR provides a rapid screening examination and thus it is considered the standard initial evaluation for all patients with chest trauma.

The indications and techniques are slightly different for blunt and penetrating trauma. It is recommended that CXR be routinely taken in the supine position until spinal injuries are ruled out. In addition, they should be slightly overpenetrated (additional x-ray exposure) to allow better visualization of the thoracic spine, and to facilitate the recognition of air in the pleural space. If the spine appears stable, the CXR in penetrating trauma

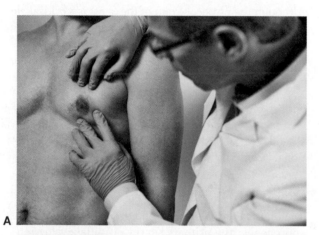

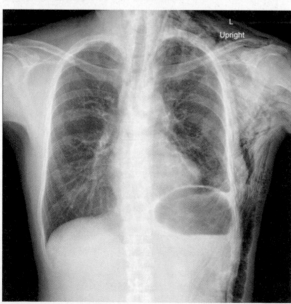

FIGURE 14-13 Palpation of the anterior part of the left hemithorax (**A**) performed to confirm the presence of subcutaneous emphysema observed on the chest radiograph (**B**).

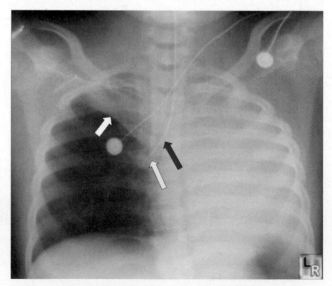

FIGURE 14-14 This portable chest radiograph shows an endotracheal tube in the right main bronchus (yellow arrow), far from the carina (red arrow). The right upper lobe is collapsed causing the lung fissure to be displaced upward (white arrow). In addition, there is hyperexpansion of the remaining areas of the right lung and important lung volume loss on the left.

should be taken with the patient sitting upright. This position improves the detection of small hemothorax, pneumothorax, or diaphragmatic injury.

Methods to estimate the correct size of pneumothorax are controversial. If the lateral edge of the lung is >2 cm from the thoracic cage, it implies the pneumothorax is at least 50% and should be considered a large pneumothorax for treatment purposes.

Routine CXR following placement of a chest tube is a standard practice in most trauma centers worldwide. However, the yield is relatively low. In about 15% of the cases, the results of a postinsertion chest tube CXR influence clinical management of the cases. Therefore, good clinical examination after tube insertion should provide enough information for the clinician to recognize whether problems are likely to result. However, in the more rural setting, and in resource-challenged environments, there is a relatively high yield from the CXR, which alters management.

Computed Chest Tomography

Advancements in CT imaging have changed the management of blunt lung trauma and permitted the detection of blood in bronchi and interstitial air or blood with greater accuracy. Contrast-enhanced CT helps in the screening of patients with suspected aortic injuries. CT scans also help in the demonstration of serious thoracic injuries that may have been overlooked on initial CXRs. These include tracheobronchial tears, diaphragmatic rupture, esophageal tears, thoracic spine injuries, chest wall and seat belt injuries, lung contusion, cardiac injuries, pneumothorax, hemothorax, and chest tube complications.

Focused Abdominal Sonography for Trauma

Focused abdominal sonography for trauma (FAST) is a rapid ultrasound examination performed in patients who are hemodynamically unstable to identify potentially life-threatening hemorrhages in the peritoneal, pericardic, or thoracic spaces. In many trauma centers, FAST has become an extension of the physical exam. It is very sensitive to detecting hemothoraces, but its application for the detection of pneumothoraces has yet to be established (**Figure 14-15**). FAST is particularly important since several reports have shown that during the primary survey, clinical examination and supine chest radiography may have low accuracy in the assessment of pneumothorax in unstable patients with major chest trauma. In the presence of a pneumothorax, FAST demonstrates loss of both lung sliding and comet-tail artifacts.

Arterial Blood Gas

Arterial blood gas (ABG) analyses should be drawn on all intubated and ventilated trauma patients and any patient with significant chest trauma or evidence of hemodynamic

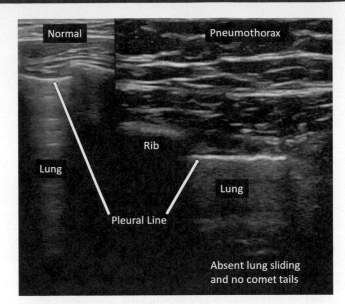

FIGURE 14-15 Chest ultrasound image of a victim of blunt trauma with left-sided pleuritic chest pain and dyspnea but no evidence of pneumothorax on the plain chest x-ray suggesting the presence of a left-sided pneumothorax.

Used with permission from Cirilli, A, REBEL EM. Ultrasound for detection of pneumothorax. Available at https://rebelem.com/ultrasound-detection-pneumothorax

instability. However, ABG testing should not replace physical diagnosis, nor should treatment be delayed while awaiting results if the patient with chest trauma is symptomatic. However, ABG analysis may be useful in evaluating hypoxia, hypercapnia, and respiratory acidosis.

Complete Blood Count

A complete blood count is a routine laboratory test for most trauma patients. Although it can help gauge blood loss, it is not entirely reliable when determining acute blood loss. A baseline platelet count and white blood cell count should be obtained upon admission since complications such as coagulopathy and infection may occur during the hospital course and affect these values.

Other Laboratory Studies

Additional laboratory tests can provide valuable information at the time of admission and throughout the time required for management all injuries associated with chest trauma (**Table 14-3**).

Monitoring of Patients with Chest Trauma

Pulse oximetry (SpO_2) should be used during the resuscitation of all trauma patients. End-tidal carbon dioxide ($EtCO_2$) monitoring should be used when placement of an endotracheal tube needs to be confirmed, and it also should be considered as an important tool to determine effectiveness of cardiopulmonary resuscitation in any trauma setting. In addition, it could assist in monitoring CO_2 levels for those patients who in addition to the chest trauma suffered traumatic brain injuries.

TABLE 14-3
Additional Laboratory Tests for Patients with Chest Trauma

Test	Rationale
Electrolytes	Fluid resuscitation may affect concentration of sodium and chloride
Coagulation profile	Massive transfusions; presence of unexplained hemorrhage
Troponin I and creatine kinase-MB	Elevated in blunt cardiac injuries
Lactate	Measure of tissue perfusion

Treatment

The treatment of chest trauma greatly depends on the clinical status of the patient. Life-threatening injuries require more prompt attention and often more invasive procedures. Oxygen administration, placement of a chest drainage, thoracotomy, surgical fixation of ribs, mechanical ventilation, fluid management, and analgesia are some of the therapeutic alternatives considered in the treatment of patients with chest trauma.

Oxygen Therapy

Oxygen at 100% should be administered immediately, particularly if pneumothorax is suspected. Administration of supplemental oxygen accelerates the rate of pleural air absorption. By breathing 100% oxygen instead of air, alveolar pressure of nitrogen falls, and nitrogen is gradually washed out of tissues and oxygen is taken up by the vascular system. This causes substantial gradient between the tissue capillary and the pneumothorax space, and it results in a substantial increase in absorption from the pleural space. Normally, 1.25% of the volume is absorbed in 24 hours; hence, 10% of the volume is absorbed in 8 days, 20% would be absorbed in 16 days, and so on. This must be balanced with the knowledge that high concentrations of inhaled oxygen over an extended period (>2 days) can cause lung injury (oxygen toxicity). The majority of patients with small pneumothoraces often are managed with oxygen administration and no treatment other than repeat observation via CXRs may be required.

Chest Tube

Thoracostomy is the placement of a pleural chest tube. It is the most common intervention in chest trauma since it offers a definitive treatment to the majority of issues that arise from the injuries.

The presence of air (pneumothorax) and/or blood (hemothorax) is the main indication for chest tube placement in chest trauma. If the pneumothorax is stable and less than 20%, it can be managed without a chest drain. In cases in which the patient undergoes a surgical opening of the chest (**thoracotomy**), a chest tube can prevent pleural collection of fluid. Chest tube placement may be diagnostic as well as prophylactic and therapeutic. Although radiographic confirmation of a pneumothorax or hemothorax is ideal prior to insertion of a chest tube, patients with traumatic arrest with no cardiac output may require chest decompression to confirm or exclude tension pneumothorax. Other relative indications include presence of rib fractures in a patient undergoing positive pressure ventilation to prevent pneumothorax. Patients with profound hypoxia and hypotension and either penetrating chest injury or unilateral abnormal exam of the chest may also be considered for chest tube placement.

Clinicians should pay close attention to the characteristics of the material drained from the chest. Frank, red, bright blood may indicate vascular damage and could require thoracotomy to repair the injury. Intestinal contents are associated with diaphragmatic injuries or esophageal tears. Persistent air leaks often occur when there is lung laceration, and, when large, they may indicate bronchial disruption.

Chest tube placement is a procedure routinely performed in a variety of clinical settings where either air and/or fluid needs to be drained from the pleural space. However, its technique requires special attention to obtain the best results and minimize complications.

The chest tube should be placed in the mid- or anterior axillary line of the hemithorax affected. Since the diaphragm rises to the fifth rib at the level of the nipple on expiration, chest tubes should be placed above this level. Rib spaces are counted down from the second rib at the sternomanubrial joint. Practically, the highest rib space that can be easily felt in the axilla (usually the fourth or fifth) is the most appropriate.

Chest tube insertion is a painful procedure, and thus, a combination of intravenous analgesia (opioid such as morphine) and local anesthesia (lidocaine) is recommended. The local anesthetic should be infiltrated under the skin along the line of the incision. The needle is then directed perpendicular to the skin and local anesthetic infiltrated through the layers of the chest wall down onto the rib below the actual intercostal space. The needle is then angled above the rib and advanced slowly until air is aspirated. The last 5 mL or so of local anesthetic should then be injected into the pleural space.

The steps in insertion of a chest drain are as follows:

1. The area is prepped and draped appropriately.
2. An incision is made along the upper border of the rib below the intercostal space to be used. The drain track will be directed over the top of the lower rib to avoid the intercostal vessels lying below each rib. The incision should easily accommodate the operator's finger (**Figure 14-16**).

3. Using a curved clamp, the track is developed by blunt dissection only. The clamp is inserted into muscle tissue and spread to split the fibers. The track is developed with the operator's finger. Once the track comes onto the rib, the clamp is angled just over the rib and dissection continued until the pleural space is entered (**Figure 14-17**).

4. Once the track comes onto the rib, the clamp is angled just over the rib and dissection continued until the pleural space is entered. A finger is inserted into the pleural cavity and the area explored for pleural adhesions.

5. A large-bore (32F or 36F) chest tube is mounted on the clamp and passed along the track into the pleural cavity.

6. The tube is connected to an underwater seal and sutured/secured in place (**Figure 14-18**).

7. The chest is reexamined and a CXR is taken to confirm placement and position.

8. Chest tubes should be inserted so that the last hole of the drain is inside the thoracic cavity. If passed too far into the chest, drains can cause severe pain due to direct trauma to the mediastinum.

The chest tube should be placed anteriorly in the chest if the patient has to lie supine to prevent the development of a tension pneumothorax if the chest tube is blocked by dependent lung tissue. This is often the case with blunt trauma. When patients are not restricted to the supine position, such as in penetrating chest trauma, hemothoraces may be more efficiently drained with a posterior, basally directed drain.

An **underwater seal** is used to allow air to escape through the drain but not to reenter the thoracic cavity. The drainage bottle should always be kept below the level of the patient; otherwise its contents will siphon back into the chest cavity. Persistent bubbling of air through the water indicates an air leak from the lung. To avoid the development of a tension pneumothorax, chest tubes should never be clamped. The air outlet of the underwater seal may be connected to moderate suction (-20 cm H_2O) to assist in lung reexpansion. This is more important in the presence of an air leak.

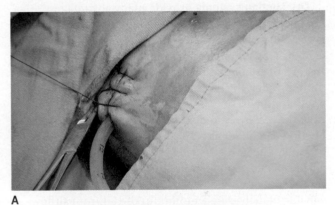

A

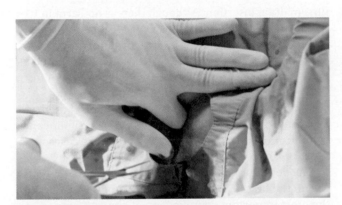

FIGURE 14-16 Insertion of a finger in the intercostal space confirming palpation of the upper border of the rib.
© Casa nayafana/Shutterstock.

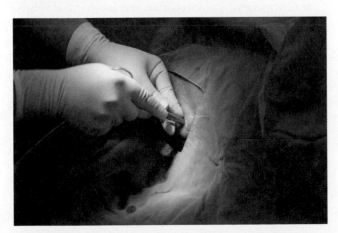

FIGURE 14-17 Use of curved clamp to direct the chest tube through the tissues until the pleura is entered.
© Samrith Na Lumpoon/Shutterstock.

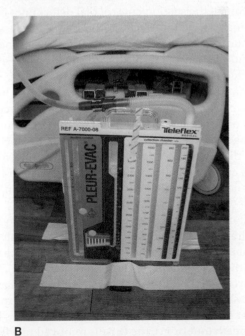

B

FIGURE 14-18 Chest tube secured in place (**A**) and connected to underwater seal (**B**).
A: © Casa Nayafana/Shutterstock; **B:** © Barry Slaven/Medical Images.

The **Heimlich valve** is a rubber flutter one-way valve within a rigid plastic tube that connects to a standard chest drain. It does not need to be kept upright like the underwater sealed drain and therefore is suitable for outpatient use. However, the efferent portal of the Heimlich valve must be kept open to the atmosphere making control of the fluid effluent difficult. The device is bulky under clothing and staining is a constant problem. To avoid this problem, the valve should be attached to a perforated plastic bag, or a specifically designed one-way valve including a small reservoir can be used. Other units for outpatient management incorporating a system for checking air leaks are available but are more expensive than a classic Heimlich or a plastic bag. The use of this one way valve has been proposed in the outpatient management of first episodes of primary spontaneous pneumothorax, in the early postoperative discharge after lobectomy or segmentectomy for lung cancer in fast-tracking protocols, and in complicated postoperative air leaks.

Dry suction systems provide many advantages: higher suction pressure levels can be achieved, set-up is easy, and there is no fluid to evaporate which would decrease the amount of suction applied to the patient. Instead of regulating the level of suction with a column of water, the dry suction units are controlled by a self-compensating regulator. To set the suction setting, the dial is rotated at the prescribed suction level. Suction can be set at -10, -15, -20, -30, or -40 cm of water. The unit is usually preset at -20 cm of water when opened. Connect the short suction tubing or suction port to the suction source. Source suction must be capable of delivering a minimum of 16 L/min airflow. The setting of the suction control dial determines the approximate amount of suction imposed regardless of the amount of source suction. Patient situations that may require higher suction pressures of -30 or -40 cm H_2O include a large air leak from the lung surface, empyema or viscous pleural effusion, a reduction in pulmonary compliance, or anticipated difficulty in expansion of the pulmonary tissue to fill the hemithorax. A drawback to the dry suction system is that it does not provide the same level of patient assessment information as a conventional water seal; for example, the clinician cannot see changes in the water level reflecting pressure changes in the chest.

Chest drains may be removed when they are no longer draining any fluid and any air leak has resolved. Removal is ideally performed with two people, one to remove the tube and one to occlude the drain site. To avoid further air being entrained into the pleural cavity, the tube should be removed either at the end of expiration or at peak inspiration. While the patient holds his or her breath (out or in), the tube is removed rapidly and the occlusive dressing applied.

Some surgeons prefer to use a purse-string or U-suture to close the wound. This may be placed at the

> **BOX 14-6 Acute and Late Complications of Chest Tube Placement**
>
> **Technique Complications**
> - Hemothorax, usually from laceration of the intercostal vessel
> - Lung laceration
> - Diaphragm/abdominal cavity penetration
> - Stomach/liver/colon injury
> - Tube placed subcutaneously, too far, or not deep enough
>
> **Acute Complications**
> - Early-onset pneumonia
>
> **Late Complications**
> - Blockage by clot or lung tissue
> - Retained hemothorax
> - Empyema
> - Pneumothorax after removal (poor technique)

time of drain insertion. Although there is no harm in using a closing suture, they probably serve little purpose and the purse-string especially may produce an ugly scar.

Although a relatively simple procedure, chest tube insertion is invasive and considered by many an almost barbaric procedure that requires brutal force. The piercing of organs in the chest and abdomen caused by a chest drain has been well documented. Significant complications may occur in 2% to 10% of the cases (**Box 14-6**).

The development of an early-onset pneumonia, within the first 72 hours after admission, is considered the most important complication of chest trauma. Some independent predictors of early-onset pneumonia include the following:

- The necessity of intubation and mechanical ventilation in the field
- A history of aspiration
- The presence of pulmonary contusion
- The occurrence of a hemothorax

Thoracotomy

Thoracotomy is defined as the surgical opening of the chest. Indications and contraindications are listed in **Box 14-7**. The majority of emergent thoracotomies (ETs) are performed in penetrating chest injuries (PCIs) and are associated with a better survival rate than when performed in patients with blunt trauma.

In cases of hemothorax, thoracotomy is also indicated in cases of persistent bleeding from the chest, defined as 150 to 200 mL/hour for 2 to 4 hours if persistent blood transfusion is required to maintain hemodynamic stability.

BOX 14-7 Indications and Contraindications for Emergent Thoracotomy

Indications

Penetrating lung injury

- Traumatic arrest with previously witnessed cardiac activity (prehospital or in-hospital)
- Unresponsive hypotension (BP <70 mm Hg)

Blunt chest trauma

- Unresponsive hypotension (BP <70 mm Hg)
- More than 1500 mL of blood evacuated by the chest tube

Contraindications

Blunt injuries

- Blunt thoracic injuries with no witnessed cardiac activity
- Multiple blunt traumas
- Severe head injury

BP, blood pressure.

BOX 14-8 Benefits of VATS Over Open Thoracotomy in Patients with Chest Trauma

- Reduction in the incidence of postoperative complications
- Lower chest tube drainage volume
- Shorter duration of tube drainage
- Shorter duration of hospitalization
- Shorter operation time
- Smaller amount of bleeding
- Smaller transfusion volume

VATS, video-assisted thorascopic surgery.

Video-Assisted Thoracoscopy

Video-assisted thoracoscopic surgery (VATS) is a type of thoracic surgery performed using a small video camera that is introduced into the patient's chest via a scope. It is considered a minimally invasive technique, and the surgeon is able to view both the instruments being used and the anatomy on which the surgeon is operating. The camera and instruments are inserted through separate holes in the chest wall also known as ports. These small ports have the advantage of fewer observed infections and a faster recovery. VATS minimally invasive technique has replaced in many cases thoracotomy or sternotomy. Systematic reviews comparing perioperative outcomes of VATS with open thoracotomy for chest trauma patients have shown significant benefits (**Box 14-8**).

Mechanical Ventilation

The need for ventilatory support in patients with chest trauma greatly depends on the severity of their ventilatory dysfunction, degree of deterioration in gaseous exchange, and any associated injuries.

Noninvasive ventilation (NIV) may reduce the need to intubate patients with trauma-related hypoxemia, which may or may not be associated with hypercapnia. It could be considered in patients who remain hypoxic despite regional anesthesia. NIV significantly reduces complications related to endotracheal intubation, mainly ventilator-associated pneumonia. According to the British Thoracic Society guidelines, the indications and efficacy of NIV in respiratory distress induced by trauma have been inconsistent and have merely received a low-grade recommendation. Similarly, the Canadian Critical Care Trials Group/Canadian Critical Care Society Noninvasive Ventilation Guidelines Group did not propose recommendations for its use for chest trauma patients. Selection of appropriate patients is crucial for optimizing NIV success rates and resource utilization. Otherwise, application of NIV in trauma-associated ARDS may be challenging. Implementing NIV for some of these patients may prove inadequate and may simply prolong the time to an inevitable endotracheal intubation. Delaying the time to endotracheal intubation is known to lead to further respiratory instability and increased risk of mortality.

Endotracheal intubation and mechanical ventilation are rarely indicated for chest wall injury alone. Rapid sequence intubation and mechanical ventilation should be immediately performed in the presence of hypoxic arrest or when the Glasgow Coma Scale score is <8. If endotracheal intubation is not possible due to extensive facial trauma, a cricothyroidotomy may be necessary. In many instances, ventilation with 100% oxygen could rapidly reverse hypoxic traumatic arrest without the need for further interventions.

Positive pressure ventilation may be required for severe chest wall instability that causes inadequate spontaneous ventilation and gas exchange. It essentially provides an internal stabilization to the thoracic cage as well as improving oxygenation and ventilation for the management of pulmonary contusion. Early intubation and mechanical ventilation should be considered particularly in elderly or severely traumatized patients.

The clinical impact of pulmonary contusion tends to develop over 24 to 48 hours following chest trauma. Therefore, close monitoring and supplemental oxygen may be the only necessary measures during that period. If the lung contusion leads to severe hypoxemia, mechanical ventilation may be necessary until gas exchange is restored. Healing and stabilization of rib fractures are rarely the limiting step in weaning from mechanical ventilation, except in the most severe chest injuries. A general optimal ventilatory strategy that is applicable to all patients after chest trauma does not exist but should be directed to using a lung protective strategy and preventing ventilator-induced lung injury (VILI).

Burn and Inhalation Injury

Inhalation injury is defined as the toxic and deleterious effects of heat and the chemical products of combustion on the airways and lungs. Inhalation injury is particularly important because it has traditionally been recognized as the third most important factor, after age and extent of burn, in determining mortality following thermal injury. With federal organizations such as the Occupational Safety and Health Administration (OSHA) providing explicit guidelines for the handling and storage of potential workplace dangers such as chemicals, and various regulatory bodies enforcing those guidelines, employers are increasingly compliant to avoid the sanctions and penalties that OSHA can impose for failing noncompliance. Despite these fairly comprehensive safety guidelines, accidents can and do happen and can lead to injuries including inhalation and thermal injury.

Patients with burns and inhalation injuries often have significant fluid resuscitation requirements and present with a higher incidence of pulmonary complications of thermal injury. Although the classic paper describing the effects of inhalation injury was published over two decades ago, its findings are still relevant to this day. Total body surface area (TBSA) cutaneous injury has a strong correlation with a corresponding rise in the incidence of inhalation injury. The diagnosis of pneumonia is typically made at approximately 10 days for patients experiencing inhalation injury. There is an incremental increase when inhalation injury is complicated by pneumonia. Expected mortality rate can increase by a maximum of 20% in the presence of inhalation injury alone and 60% when both inhalation injury and pneumonia are present. The contributions of inhalation injury and pneumonia to mortality rate are independent and additive. Percent TBSA cutaneous injury, age, and Pao_2/Fio_2 ratio have been found to be strong mortality predictors.

Smoke Inhalation

Smoke inhalation injuries occur when a patient's respiratory system is exposed to direct heat from fire as well as toxic chemicals that formed during combustion. It affects one-third of all burn injury victims. The composition of smoke varies with each fire depending on the materials being burned, the amount of oxygen available to the fire, and the nature of the fire. High-oxygen and high-temperature fires often do not produce large amounts of smoke. Low-oxygen fires are often lower temperature fires, and these lower temperatures often give rise to more toxic chemicals, such as **carbon**

monoxide. Other common toxic compounds created in smoke are ammonia, carbon dioxide, **hydrogen cyanide**, aldehydes, sulfur dioxides, and nitrogen dioxide. These different elements give rise to a combination of gases, airborne solids, and liquid vapors that mix with the ambient air to create smoke. Inhalation of these components, when exposed to smoke, causes both upper and lower airway injury. The great majority of lower respiratory tract injury is from smoke particles and the chemicals that they carry.

Pathophysiology of Inhalation Injury

Thermal injury to the upper airway, chemical irritation of the lower (subglottic) airway by smoke, and systemic chemical or metabolic injury caused by specific noxious chemicals such as hydrogen cyanide are the most significant pathophysiologic changes that occur in inhalation injury. Progressive inflammation leads to pulmonary shunting and hypoxemic respiratory failure. While direct thermal injury is rare past the vocal cords, chemical toxins may cause damage to just the airways or the alveoli, or both. The less soluble fumes and aerosols may cause more significant injury to the lung parenchyma. Injury of the airways causes increased mucus production, edema, denudation of epithelium, and mucosal ulceration and hemorrhage. These insults are responsible for the airway obstruction routinely observed with these patients. Alveolar damage extends to both epithelial and endothelial layers resulting in pulmonary edema and possibly ARDS.

Diagnosis

Since few diagnosis-specific therapeutic options have been identified for patients with inhalation injury, the clinical assessment continues to be paramount in determining the extent of the lung injury. Tachypnea, wheezing, stridor, and desaturation can be early signs of inhalation injury.

History and Physical Exam

Before completing a physical exam, it is important to determine the type of exposure (smoke, flames, chemicals), duration of exposure, and the location of exposure (enclosed vs. opened space), and if there is loss of consciousness. If the patient is unconscious, interviewing first responders will be necessary to obtain the information. It is important to remember that a significant number of patients with smoke inhalation show no outward signs of burns. Some of the most frequent symptoms and signs from smoke inhalation include a burning sensation in nose or throat, cough with increased sputum production, stridor, and dyspnea with rhonchi or wheezing (**Box 14-9**). If patients complain of painful swallowing (odynophagia) after smoke exposure, inhalation injury possibly occurred. Altered mental status (delirium, hallucinations, coma) could indicate the presence

BOX 14-9 Clinical Manifestations of Aspiration and Inhalation Injury

Chemical

Shortness of breath, dry to progressive cough, tachypnea, cyanosis

Progressive worsening radiograph

Accessory muscle use

Altered level of consciousness

Progressive fever

Prolonged ventilator time

If smoke, soot around the nares or in the upper airway and sputum; concomitant increases in carboxyhemoglobin

Physical

Partial or complete obstruction of the affected side

Extreme respiratory distress

Wheezing unaffected by aerosol treatments

Possible absent breath sounds

Atelectasis

Potential ipsilateral shift of mediastinal structures

Progressive fever

Potential respiratory arrest

Paradoxical cough or inability to cough

BOX 14-10 Workup of Inhalation Injury

- Chest imaging: Serial chest radiographs (often negative early in smoke inhalation injury), computed tomography of the chest
- Complete blood count (CBC), complete metabolic panel (CMP), lactate
- Pulse oximetry (may be falsely elevated with carbon monoxide exposure)
- Arterial blood gas (ABG) assessment
- Carboxyhemoglobin level
- Cyanide level (often not readily available, therefore limited use in the acute setting)
- Pulmonary function testing: flow-volume loop is a very sensitive noninvasive test
- Bronchoscopy and direct laryngoscopy

TABLE 14-4
The Abbreviated Injury Score System for Bronchoscopic Appearances in Inhalation Injury

Grade	Class	Description
0	No injury	Absence of carbonaceous deposits, erythema, edema, bronchorrhea, or obstruction
1	Mild injury	Minor or patchy areas of erythema, carbonaceous deposits in proximal or distal bronchi
2	Moderate injury	Moderate degree of erythema, carbonaceous deposits, bronchorrhea, or bronchial obstruction
3	Severe injury	Severe inflammation with friability, copious carbonaceous deposits, bronchorrhea, or obstruction
4	Massive injury	Evidence of mucosal sloughing, necrosis, endoluminal obliteration

of hypoxia, hypercapnia, carbon monoxide poisoning, or hydrogen dioxide poisoning (see Box 14-9).

Inspection is designed to initially determine the presence of facial burns, singed nasal hair, loss of facial and intranasal hair, and carbonaceous material or soot in the mouth or sputum. The presence of accessory muscle usage, tachypnea, cyanosis, and rhonchi/rales/wheezing indicate a more significant inhalation injury. Stridor is often an ominous sign of impending airway compromise, and prompt intubation should be considered. Delayed symptoms are not uncommon, particularly related to compromise of the lower airway. Damage due to chemical toxin exposure such as nitric oxide may take up to 72 hours to manifest clinically. **Box 14-10** suggests the workup for inhalation injury.

Bronchoscopy

Bronchoscopy helps in determining severity of airway injury, can be used to provide a functional washout of the bronchial tree, and could be used for bronchoalveolar lavage.

The Abbreviated Injury Score (AIS) system has been used to correlate bronchoscopic findings with risk of mortality (**Table 14-4**).

Laboratory

The presence of leukopenia, thrombocytopenia, and high urea and creatinine levels on admission have been

associated with increased risk of death in patients with inhalation injury. An elevated urokinase plasminogen activator receptor (uPAR), a new biological marker of disease, in bronchial lavage fluid of inhalation injury patients has been associated with a significantly longer period of mechanical ventilation and intensive care unit (ICU) stay.

Monitoring

It is important to note that noninvasive monitoring of oxygenation status of patients demonstrating signs or suspected of having carbon monoxide poisoning is very challenging. **Carbon monoxide** (CO) has 200 times the affinity for hemoglobin (Hb) that oxygen has, so as

TABLE 14-5
Levels of Carboxyhemoglobin (CoHb) and Associated Symptoms

Level of CoHb	Symptom
10%	No symptoms; heavy smokers can have as much as 10% to 15% COHb
15%	Mild headache
25%	Nausea and a serious headache, fairly quick recovery after treatment with oxygen and/or fresh air
30%	Symptoms intensify; potential for long-term effects especially in the case of infants, children, the elderly, victims of heart disease, and pregnant women
40–60%	Mental confusion, weakness, loss of coordination, and unconsciousness
>60%	Death

a result it binds to the hemoglobin, leaving little to no ability for oxygen transport. Normal levels of carboxyhemoglobin (COHb) in nonsmokers are <2.3% and in adult smokers 2.1% to 4.2% but could reach 8% to 9% in heavy smokers (**Table 14-5**). Most pulse oximeters are unable to distinguish between O_2Hb and COHb, and as a result will read falsely high. The pulse oximeter may read that hemoglobin is 100% saturated with oxygen when in fact the patient's actual PaO_2 is <40 mm Hg. To avoid this error, it is necessary to obtain an arterial sample and run it through a **CO-oximeter**, which will quantify the levels of dysfunctional Hb, giving a true picture of the patient's oxygenation status. (A pulse oximeter capable of monitoring COHb% noninvasively is available, but it is not as accurate as oximetry that utilizes a blood sample.) Patients with elevated levels of COHb should be treated with 100% oxygen to flush the CO out of their system. There is some evidence that suggests hyperbaric therapy will expedite this process, but recent studies have called this practice into question.

Treatment

Management of patients with inhalation injury is also complex as injured pulmonary tissue cannot be simply excised as the burned skin and is constantly needing to be protected against secondary injury from the effects of mechanical ventilation (ventilator-induced lung injury [VILI]), resuscitation, and infection. In addition, these patients represent a challenge as they have a significantly increased fluid demand.

Heat exposure and inhaled toxins explain in great extent the morbidity associated with inhalation injury. Management of toxin exposure in smoke inhalation is particularly focused on carbon monoxide and cyanide.

TABLE 14-6
Management Concerns and Strategies for Inhalation Injuries

Management Concern	Approach
Increasing hypoxia (ambient PO_2 may be as little as 10%)	Patient extraction from hypoxic environment and administration of supplemental oxygen
Progressive edema	Establish venous access for fluid administration if necessary
CO poisoning; possible cardiac arrest	Administration of 100% high-flow oxygen
Early intubation	Observe patient for progressive airway inflammation and edema, the development of stridor or an increasingly hoarse voice; respiratory rate is also a sensitive marker of increasing distress
Mechanical ventilation	Settings should be dialed in to improve oxygenation, with low tidal volume lung protective strategies and high PEEP; permissive hypercapnia and high-frequency ventilation are also used often
Possible need for fluids	Fluid management typically only needed for burns and thermal injury; monitor urine output and hemodynamic parameters to assess for need as some chemicals can be caustic
Inhaled anticoagulants	Typically reserved for thermal injury
Infection	Prophylactic antibiotics have been shown to reduce mortality risk, but routine use remains controversial
Underlying conditions such as asthma or COPD	Manage as per usual

CO, carbon monoxide; COPD, chronic obstructive pulmonary disease; PEEP, positive end-expiratory pressure.

Hyperbaric oxygen treatment, cyanide antidote strategies, and other medical strategies such as β-agonists, pulmonary blood flow modifiers, anticoagulants, and anti-inflammatory agents remain as the most important therapeutic strategies for these events. A summary of management considerations is outlined in **Table 14-6**.

Airway Management

Removing the patient from the exposure area and maintaining a secure airway are paramount. Clinicians need to be prepared for early and preemptive intubation for patients with inhalation injury as often as may be required. Airway obstruction, when occurs, could develop suddenly as airway edema worsens. Airway management strategies are summarized in **Box 14-11**.

BOX 14-11 Airway Management Strategies Used During Inhalation Injury

- Have a high degree of suspicion as to the need for an artificial airway: *Better too early than too late.*

- Ensure there are endotracheal tube alternatives such as laryngeal mask airways (LMAs) available in the event the patient is unable to be traditionally intubated: *This includes smaller tubes and even cricothyroidotomy kits.*

- Consider a nasal intubation, particularly if there are burns present on the patient's face: *Utilize the McGill forceps to aid in airway placement if necessary.*

- If possible, have a bronchoscope or video laryngoscope on hand: *An edematous inflamed airway lumen can get quite small rather quickly.*

- Do not fear using a smaller tube than what would normally be indicated: *Having an airway is better than not having one at all.*

- Be prepared to suction the airway and to obtain moderate to large amounts of carbonaceous sputum with or without sloughing airway epithelium: *Mucus plugging is a real problem due to the damaged mucociliary escalator; suctioning and humidification is key; mucosal sloughing typically takes a few days to occur.*

- Maintain secure airway: Intubation, tracheostomy if necessary.

- Nebulized N-acetylcysteine (NAC) used as a mucolytic. Since NAC may irritate airways causing bronchoconstriction, pretreatment with a bronchodilator should always be considered.

- β_2-Adrenergic agonists improve pulmonary functioning.

- Nebulized heparin reduces the inflammatory response and fibrin cast formation, which helps to reduce airway obstruction.

Carbon Monoxide and Hydrogen Cyanide Poisoning

CO treatment includes high oxygen therapy. Although most clinicians could administer 100% oxygen, hyperbaric oxygen (HBO) treatment is preferred as it increases clearance of CO from blood. However, its limited availability to specific centers restricts its usage. Since testing for hydrogen cyanide poisoning is not readily available, it is often challenging to detect. When suspected, hydroxycobalamin may be given.

Nebulized Therapy

Nebulized anticoagulants are thought to have beneficial effects as they could attenuate pulmonary coagulopathy and maybe even affect pulmonary inflammation. Heparin breaks down the fibrin binding of airway casts formed during inhalation injury and is often alternated with **N-acetylcysteine** (NAC) every 2 hours. **Nebulized heparin** has been associated with a reduction of lung injury scores and duration of mechanical ventilation with no adverse effects.

Although the use of short-acting bronchodilators is widespread, the evidence supporting or disputing it is not substantial. Inhaled corticosteroids appear to provide no benefit in patients with inhalation injury.

Mechanical Ventilation

When required, mechanical ventilation should follow similar guidelines to those used for patients with ARDS. A lung protective strategy that includes low tidal volumes ($\leq$6 mg/kg) and low pressures should be used. There is emerging evidence that higher tidal volumes can decrease the incidence of ARDS and ventilator days in pediatric patients with inhalation injury. Permissive hypercapnia is not only frequent but also a safe strategy in patients with inhalation injury.

NIV can be considered in selected cases where mild edema is present or as part of a de-escalation strategy to implement early extubation. When in doubt, endotracheal intubation and mechanical ventilation continue to be the best ventilatory strategies for these patients.

High-frequency percussive ventilation (HFPV) mechanically enhances the clearance of carbon and other debris from the bronchial tree and improves oxygenation (frequency ranging from 60 to 300 cycles/min). It can be used as a rescue strategy and as a planned ventilation strategy.

Complications and Prognosis

Long-term complications from smoke inhalation injury are much less common. They include subglottic stenosis, bronchiectasis, and bronchiolitis obliterans. Patients who have been exposed to carbon monoxide are also known to have long-term neurologic complications. Severe brain damage may occur with carbon monoxide poisoning but is uncommon. More commonly patients will describe persistent or delayed neurologic symptoms after carbon monoxide poisoning. These symptoms are often subjective but will include depressed mood, poor concentration, and issues with short-term memory. Neurologic sequelae after carbon monoxide exposure seem to be more common in patients who had a loss of consciousness. Symptoms often develop 1 to 3 weeks after poisoning.

In burned patients, inhalation injury is, along with percent of total body surface area (%TBSA) and age, one of the strongest predictors of mortality risk. Victims of inhalation injury are at high risk for complications. The majority of fatal burn cases are caused by respiratory failure, either from direct injury or complications such as pneumonia. Severe injuries often will lead to long-term complications such as bronchiectasis, bronchiolitis obliterans, and need for artificial airways; however, many patients will have no long-term sequelae from a single episode of smoke inhalation injury.

Traumatic Brain Injury

Traumatic brain injury (TBI) contributes to 30% of all injury-related deaths in the United States. It is also one of the leading causes of disability, having a tremendous financial impact in health care. According to data from the Centers for Disease Control and Prevention in the United States during 2013, the highest rates of TBI were observed in older adults ($\geq$75 years), very young (0 to 4 years), and young adults (15 to 24 years). Males had higher rates of TBI than females. The most common mechanisms of TBI, adjusted for age, were falls, followed by being struck by an object and motor vehicle crashes. The primary cause of TBI-related death also changed, from motor vehicle crashes in 2007 to intentional self-harm in 2013. Lower socioeconomic status, alcohol and drug use, and underlying psychiatric and cognitive disorders are also risk factors for head injury. The proportion of TBI secondary to violence has risen over the past decade and now accounts for 7% to 10% of cases.

Classification of TBI

TBI is classified according to clinical severity, mechanism of injury, and pathophysiology. Clinical severity scores as well as neuroimaging have been extensively used to classify TBI.

Clinical Severity Scores

The most commonly used injury severity score is the **Glasgow Coma Scale** (GCS) (**Table 14-7**). The GCS is routinely assessed following the initial resuscitation and within 48 hours of injury. It is scored between 3 and 15. It is composed of three parameters: best eye response (E), best verbal response (V), and best motor response (M). The components of the GCS should be recorded individually; for example, E3V3M4 results in a GCS score of 10. A score of 13 or higher correlates with mild brain injury, a score of 9 to 12 correlates with moderate injury, and a score of 8 or less represents severe brain injury.

Although the GCS is simple, reproducible, and predictable, sedation and paralysis, endotracheal intubation, and intoxication should be considered as confounding factors. An alternative scoring system, the Full

TABLE 14-7
Glasgow Coma Scale

Parameter	Score
Eye Opening	
Spontaneous	4
Response to verbal command	3
Response to pain	2
No eye opening	1
Best Verbal Response	
Oriented	5
Confused	4
Inappropriate words	3
Incomprehensive sounds	2
No verbal response	1
Best Motor Response	
Obeys commands	6
Localizing response to pain	5
Withdrawal response to pain	4
Flexion to pain	3
Extension to pain	2
No motor response	1
Total	

Outline of UnResponsiveness (FOUR) Score, includes a brain stem examination to minimize the effects of the confounding factors mentioned earlier.

Neuroimaging Classification

Computed tomography is the preferred imaging modality in the acute phase of head trauma and should be performed as quickly as possible. CT can reveal the most common pathologic injuries, including skull fractures, epidural hematoma (EDH), subdural hematoma (SDH), subarachnoid hemorrhage (SAH), intraparenchymal hemorrhage, cerebral contusion, intraventricular hemorrhage, and focal and diffuse patterns of axonal injury with cerebral edema. A noncontrast CT scan routinely detects skull fractures, intracranial hematomas, and cerebral edema (**Figures 14-19** to **14-21**).

Two currently used CT-based grading scales are the Marshall scale and the Rotterdam scale. Routine follow-up CT scans should be performed in the presence

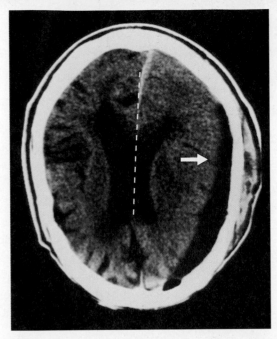

FIGURE 14-19 Computed tomography scan showing a left traumatic subdural hematoma (arrow) with the typical crescent shape causing significant mass effect (shift of midline structures to the right).
© Callista Images/Image Source/Getty Images.

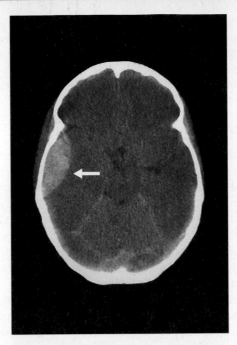

FIGURE 14-21 Computed tomography scan demonstrating a right epidural hematoma (arrow) with the typical lenticular shape.
© ISM/Sovereign/Medical Images.

Pathophysiology

There are two separate but related categories: primary brain injury and secondary brain injury.

Primary Brain Injury

The different mechanisms of primary brain injury include direct impact, rapid acceleration/deceleration, penetrating injury, and blast waves. A combination of focal contusions and hematomas, as well as shearing of white matter tracts (diffuse axonal injury [DAI]) along with cerebral edema and swelling is largely responsible for the damage associated with TBI. Patients with severe DAI typically present with profound coma without elevated **intracranial pressure** and often have poor outcome.

Focal cerebral contusions are by far the most frequently encountered lesions in TBI. Extra-axial (outside the brain) lesions include epidural, subdural, and subarachnoid hemorrhage. In adults, epidural hematomas (EDHs) are almost always associated with a skull fracture and rupture of the middle meningeal artery but tend not to be associated with underlying brain damage, and these patients may have a better prognosis than individuals with other traumatic hemorrhage types. Subdural hematomas (SDHs) result from damage to bridging veins and are often associated with underlying cerebral injury. Subarachnoid hemorrhage (SAH) can occur with disruption of small pial vessels, and intraventricular hemorrhages are believed to result from

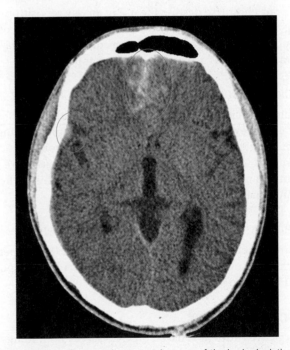

FIGURE 14-20 Computed tomography scan of the brain depicting frontal cerebral contusions.
© O_Akira/Shutterstock.

of clinical deterioration or changes in physiologic parameters such as intracranial pressure (ICP). Repeat CT scan has been considered reasonable in patients with a hematoma present on the initial scan, particularly in patients with a GCS score <9.

tearing of subependymal veins, or by extension from adjacent intraparenchymal or subarachnoid hemorrhage.

Approximately one-third of patients with severe TBI develop a coagulopathy, which is associated with an increased risk of hemorrhage enlargement, poor neurologic outcomes, and death.

Secondary Brain Injury

Secondary brain injury in TBI initiates at the time of initial trauma but continues for hours or days. It is believed to be a combination of free-radical injury to cell membranes, electrolyte imbalances, mitochondrial dysfunction, inflammatory responses, and secondary ischemia from vasospasm, focal microvascular occlusion, and vascular injury. These mechanisms turn into cerebral edema and increased ICP with a potential for neuronal cell death.

To reduce the effects of secondary brain injury, emphasis is placed on the avoidance of secondary brain insults as a result of hypotension and hypoxia, fever and seizures, and hyperglycemia. The incidence of hypotension and hypoxia in TBI could be as high as 50% and 30%, respectively.

Management of TBI

The Brain Trauma Foundation (BTF) has designed a series of guidelines for the management of severe TBI. It is important to remember that patients with severe head injury may frequently have other traumatic injuries to internal organs, lungs, limbs, or the spinal cord.

Prehospital Management

The primary goal of prehospital management for severe TBI in the first 24 hours is the prevention of hypotension (blood pressure [BP] <90 mm Hg) and hypoxia (Pao_2 <60 mm Hg). Although hypotension increases risk of death, a low to normal BP may be associated with poor outcomes. Changes in prehospital management that aim to normalize oxygenation and BP may be associated with improved outcomes.

Airway Management

Endotracheal intubation is recommended in patients with TBI and a GCS score <9, an inability to protect their airway, or an Spo_2< 90% despite the administration of supplemental oxygen. Patients who are not intubated should receive supplemental oxygen as necessary to maintain an Spo_2 >90% to 93%. Bag-mask ventilation should be performed in conjunction with basic airway-opening maneuvers or use of a supraglottic airway device in cases in which intubation cannot be performed. The benefit of prehospital intubation on functional outcomes of patients with TBI is uncertain.

Box 14-12 lists factors that should be considered by emergency medical service (EMS) systems when

---

> ## BOX 14-12 Factors to Consider Before Prehospital Intubation by EMS Personnel
>
> - Appropriate hands-on training in rapid-sequence intubation.
> - Both hypoventilation and hyperventilation should be avoided following intubation.
> - Quantitative capnography should be used to assess ventilation.
> - Hemodynamic instability may occur following rapid-sequence intubation, and immediate measures should be taken to manage hypotension prior to emergency department (ED) arrival.
> - The Glasgow Coma Scale score should not be the sole factor in making decisions on prehospital intubation. Patients with a poor initial neurologic exam will often improve prior to ED arrival.

addressing the use of prehospital intubation in patients with severe TBI.

Trained clinicians may make the decision to intubate in the following circumstances: GCS score <9, presence of poor chest rise despite the use of airway repositioning and adjuncts, Spo_2 <90% to 93% despite the use of supplemental oxygen, clinical signs of cerebral herniation, evidence of aspiration, and long transport time.

Fluid Resuscitation and Neurologic Assessment

Fluid resuscitation using isotonic crystalloids adequately prevents hypotension in the prehospital setting. Neurologic assessment: Patients with TBI should be assumed to have a spinal fracture and appropriate precautions must be taken to stabilize and immobilize the spine during transport.

Management in the Emergency Department

Management in the emergency department (ED) is performed according to the Advanced Trauma Life Support (ATLS) protocol (**Box 14-13**).

Surgical Treatment

Surgical treatment is based on GCS score and findings on the CT scan (**Box 14-14**).

Intensive Care Management

In cases of TBI, ICU care should focus on the prevention or control of the secondary brain injury by managing ICP, maintaining adequate cerebral perfusion, optimizing oxygenation and BP, and managing temperature, glucose, seizures, and other potential secondary brain insults. This section of the chapter will focus on cerebral perfusion pressure.

BOX 14-13 ATLS Guidelines Specific to TBI

- Vital signs including heart rate, BP, respiratory status (pulse oximetry, capnography), and temperature require ongoing monitoring.
- The patient should be assessed for other systemic trauma, per the ATLS algorithm.
- A neurologic examination, including the GCS, should be completed as soon as possible to determine the clinical severity of the TBI. The pupillary examination is crucial in the patient with TBI.
- Neurologic status should be frequently assessed as deterioration typically occurs in the initial hours after the TBI.
- Evaluation and management of increased ICP should begin in the ED, particularly in patients demonstrating clinical signs of impending or ongoing **cerebral herniation** (significant pupillary asymmetry, unilateral or bilateral fixed and dilated pupils, decorticate or decerebrate posturing, respiratory depression, and the **Cushing triad** of hypertension, bradycardia, and irregular respiration).
- A complete blood count, electrolytes, glucose, coagulation parameters, blood alcohol level, and urine toxicology should be checked. Efforts to reverse a coagulopathy should begin immediately.

ATLS, Advanced Trauma Life Support; BP, blood pressure; ED, emergency department; GCS, Glasgow Coma Scale; ICP, intracranial pressure; TBI, traumatic brain injury.

BOX 14-14 Indications for Surgical Evacuation in TBI

- EDH larger than 30 mL in volume regardless of a patient's GCS score.
- Acute EDH and coma (GCS score ≤8) in patients who have pupillary abnormalities (anisocoria).
- Acute SDH >10 mm in thickness or associated with midline shift >5 mm
- GCS score is ≤8 in acute SDH or if the GCS score has decreased by ≥2 points from the time of injury to hospital admission.
- Asymmetric or fixed and dilated pupils, and/or ICP measurements are consistently >20 mm Hg.
- Traumatic ICH in the posterior fossa when there is evidence of significant mass effect.
- Decompressive craniectomy may be lifesaving in patients with refractory elevations of ICP.

EDH, epidural hematoma; GCS, Glasgow Coma Scale; ICH, intracranial hematoma; ICP, intracranial pressure; SDH, subdural hematoma.

Mechanical Ventilation

Mechanical ventilation is required in most patients with TBI. Close monitoring of ventilation with the use of end-tidal carbon dioxide is important as acute hypercapnia may result in elevations in ICP, and hypocapnia ($Paco_2$ <30 mm Hg) may precipitate cerebral ischemia. Hyperventilation-induced cerebral vasoconstriction decreases $Paco_2$ and ICP, but significantly reduces CBF, leading to cerebral hypoperfusion. It should be avoided in the first 24 to 48 hours following TBI and should be reserved for emergencies such as impending cerebral herniation (**Box 14-15**).

A target Pao_2 of at least 60 mm Hg should be achieved in all patients with TBI. In some patients this goal may require the use of higher than usual positive end-expiratory pressure (PEEP) levels (15 to 20 cm H_2O) or even modes of ventilation associated with high mean airway pressures such as airway pressure release ventilation (APRV). While elevated intrathoracic pressure decreases venous return and increases ICP, high PEEP and APRV have no significant effect on ICP.

Antiseizure Drugs

Early posttraumatic seizures could be present in approximately 30% of the patients with TBI. Antiseizure drugs are generally recommended to prevent and treat posttraumatic seizures in patients with severe TBI. Levetiracetam every 12 hours for 7 days is often recommended.

Cerebral Perfusion Pressure

The normal cerebral vasculature maintains an adequate **cerebral blood flow** (CBF) across a wide range (50 to 150 mm Hg) of mean arterial pressure (MAP). In patients with TBI, a rise in MAP can lead to elevated CBF, while drops in MAP may be associated with hypoperfusion and ischemia. Since bedside measurement of CBF is not easily obtained, **cerebral perfusion pressure** (CPP = MAP − ICP) has been used as a surrogate. Although there is not a strong consensus on the desired CPP, a minimum between 60 and 80 mm Hg is usually recommended to improve survival and favorable outcomes. Efforts to optimize CPP should first focus on treatment of ICP elevations. Continuous monitoring of cerebral oximetry or the pressure reactivity index (PRx) may help determine the adequacy of autoregulation and identify the optimal CPP in individual patients.

BOX 14-15 Techniques to Reduce ICP in Patients with TBI

- Head of bed (HOB) elevation to 30 degrees, to permit adequate venous drainage from the brain while not compromising cerebral perfusion
- Optimization of venous drainage: keeping the neck in neutral position, loosening neck braces if too tight

If impending cerebral herniation is suspected:

- Endotracheal intubation
- Brief hyperventilation to a P_{CO_2} of approximately 30 mm Hg ($ETCO_2$ 25 to 30 mm Hg)
- Bolus dose of an osmotic agent (mannitol and hypertonic saline)
- Maintenance of a higher MAP (80 to 100 mm Hg)

ICP, intracranial pressure; MAP, mean arterial pressure; TBI, traumatic brain injury.

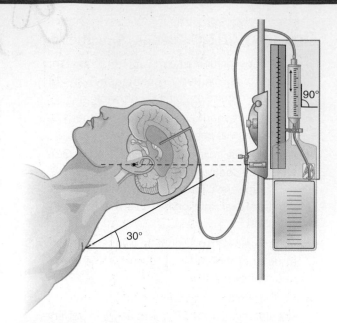

FIGURE 14-22 An **external ventricular drain** (EVD) is a small catheter inserted through the skull, usually into the lateral ventricle, which is typically connected to a closed collecting device to allow for drainage of cerebrospinal fluid and can record intracranial pressure.

Temperature Management

Fever appears to worsen outcome after severe TBI by increasing ICP and aggravating secondary brain injury. Although hypothermia has been suggested in a few studies, current approaches emphasize maintaining normothermia through the use of antipyretic medications, surface-cooling devices, or endovascular temperature management catheters.

ICP Management

Since elevated ICP is associated with increased mortality risk in patients with TBI, specific strategies need to be instituted as soon as possible (see Box 14-15).

ICP Monitoring

Although the presence of a GCS score ≤8 and an abnormal CT scan showing evidence of mass effect are indications for ICP monitoring, patients with a normal CT scan may also require ICP monitoring when age is >40 years, motor posturing is present, and systolic BP is <90 mm Hg.

A ventricular catheter connected to a strain gauge transducer is the most accurate and cost-effective method of ICP monitoring and has the therapeutic advantage of allowing for cerebrospinal fluid (CSF) drainage to treat high ICP levels (**Figure 14-22**).

An ICP <22 mm Hg and a CPP of 50 to 80 mm Hg are recommended as thresholds that predict survival and favorable outcome following TBI.

Other Management Strategies

Light sedation can lower ICP and also reduce the risk of patient-ventilator asynchrony. Deeper levels of sedation are only required when ICP elevation is refractory to conventional treatment. Propofol is one of the most common and effective sedatives used in TBI as it appears to be neuroprotective. Analgesics are essential in the management of patients with TBI. Fentanyl is commonly used in this setting as it minimizes the hemodynamic instability associated with administration of morphine.

Decompressive **craniectomy** (removal of a portion of the skull) should be considered in patients with TBI who have failed medical therapy.

The induction of a **barbiturate coma** with either pentobarbital or thiopental (barbiturates) profoundly decreases cerebral metabolic demand, CBF, and cerebral blood volume. However, this strategy has not been shown to improve outcomes following TBI.

Summary

Traumatic critical care includes many medical care events and conditions that frequently occur in the clinical setting. Chest trauma, inhalation injury, and traumatic brain injury are among the most frequent medical emergencies critical care events. They could be encountered and managed in the emergency setting or critical care areas.

In the vast majority of these traumatic critical care events, a multidisciplinary approach is required as clinicians are often challenged with the wide range of conditions imposed by patient conditions as many body systems can be adversely affected.

Case Study

Gerry is a 21-year-old male, admitted to the surgical emergency department after crashing his car frontally against another car at approximately 40 miles per hour. He was driving while not wearing a seat belt. At admission, he was complaining of jabbing pain in the right hemithorax and in the sternal region, thoracic constriction, and considerable dyspnea. During review of his symptoms, he only complained of having a cough for the last 2 days and suffering from an acute rhinitis. The patient was an occasional smoker but did not have any history of pulmonary or other diseases.

Gerry was oriented and had no neurologic deficit with stable vital signs. Some small superficial wounds and hematoma in the lower part of the sternum and the right hemithorax were found. A discrete cyanosis of the lips was seen. Upon physical exam of the chest, Gerry was found to have hyperresonant percussion on the right side as well as diminished breath sounds, while the exam of the left hemithorax was within normal limits. He complained of excruciating pain on the right side of the chest when trying to take a deep breath. The same area was tender to palpation and some crepitus was present.

1. **Which of the following symptoms and signs are most suggestive of a pneumothorax?**
   a. Tenderness to palpation
   b. Presence of a crepitus
   c. Hyperresonant percussion
   d. Diminished breath sounds

A chest radiograph (CXR) after insertion of the chest tube showed lungs expanded correctly; however, increased and diffuse radio-opacity on the right side near the point where chest tube was inserted was noticed.

2. **What does this change on the CXR suggest?**
   a. Pneumonia
   b. Hemothorax
   c. Pulmonary contusion
   d. Atelectasis

Bibliography

Chest Trauma

Aukema TS, Beenen LF, Hietbrink F, et al. Initial assessment of chest x-ray in thoracic trauma patients: awareness of specific injuries. *World J Radiol.* 2012;4:48–52.

Centers for Disease Control and Prevention. *Web-Based Injury Statistics Query and Reporting System (WISQARS) Online.* Atlanta, GA: National Center for Injury Prevention and Control; 2015. Available at http://www.cdc.gov/injury/wisqars

Clancy K, Velopulos C, Bilaniuk JW, et al. Screening for blunt cardiac injury: an Eastern Association for the Surgery of Trauma practice management guideline. *J Trauma Acute Care Surg.* 2012;73(5 Suppl 4):S301–S306.

Farooq U, Raza W, Zia N, et al. Classification and management of chest trauma. *J Coll Physicians Surg Pak.* 2006;16:101–103.

Waydhas C, Nast-Kolb D, Jochum M, et al. Inflammatory mediators, infection, sepsis, and multiple organ failure after severe trauma. *Arch Surg.* 1992;127:460–467.

Diagnosis of Chest Trauma

Ianniello S, Di Giacomo V, Sessa B, et al. First-line sonographic diagnosis of pneumothorax in major trauma: accuracy of e-FAST and comparison with multidetector computed tomography. *Radiol Med.* 2014;119:674–680.

Roberts DJ, Leigh-Smith S, Faris PD, et al. Clinical presentation of patients with tension pneumothorax: a systematic review. *Ann Surg.* 2015;261:1068–1078.

Sabbar S, Nilles EJ. Images in clinical medicine. Deep sulcus sign. *N Engl J Med.* 2012;366:552.

Treatment of Chest Trauma

Chadha TS, Cohn MA. Noninvasive treatment of pneumothorax with oxygen inhalation. *Respiration.* 1983;44:147–152.

Cotte J, Cungi PJ, Lacroix G, et al. Needle thoracostomy for tension pneumothorax. *J Trauma Acute Care Surg.* 2013;74:949.

Cubuk S, Yucel O. Importance of tube position after tube thoracostomy. *Am J Emerg Med.* 2015;33:592.

de Jong MB, Kokke MC, Hietbrink F, Leenen LP. Surgical management of rib fractures: strategies and literature review. *Scand J Surg.* 2014;103:120–125.

Dehghan N, de Mestral C, McKee MD, et al. Flail chest injuries: a review of outcomes and treatment practices from the National Trauma Data Bank. *J Trauma Acute Care Surg.* 2014;76:462–468.

Doben AR, Eriksson EA, Denlinger CE, et al. Surgical rib fixation for flail chest deformity improves liberation from mechanical ventilation. *J Crit Care.* 2014;29:139–143.

Heydary MB, Hessami MA, Setayeshi K, et al. Use of prophylactic antibiotics following tube thoracostomy for blunt chest trauma in the prevention of empyema and pneumonia. *J Inj Violence Res.* 2014;6:91–92.

Jafarpour S, Nassiri SJ, Bidari A, et al. Principles of primary survey and resuscitation in cases of pediatric trauma. *Acta Med Iran.* 2014;52:943–946.

Jayle CP, Allain G, Ingrand P, et al. Flail chest in polytraumatized patients: surgical fixation using stracos reduces ventilator time and hospital stay. *Biomed Res Int.* 2015;2015:624723.

Jin H, Tang LQ, Pan ZG, et al. Ten-year retrospective analysis of multiple trauma complicated by pulmonary contusion. *Mil Med Res.* 2014;1:7.

Karcz MK, Papadakos PJ. Noninvasive ventilation in trauma. *World J Crit Care Med.* 2015;4:47–54.

Keenan SP, Sinuff T, Burns KE, et al. Clinical practice guidelines for the use of noninvasive positive-pressure ventilation and noninvasive continuous positive airway pressure in the acute care setting. *Can Med Assoc J.* 2011;183:E195–E214.

Kong VY, Oosthuizen GV, Clarke DL. What is the yield of routine chest radiography following tube thoracostomy for trauma? *Injury.* 2015;46:45–48.

Marasco SF, Davies AR, Cooper J, et al. Prospective randomized controlled trial of operative rib fixation in traumatic flail chest. *J Am Coll Surg.* 2013;216:924–932.

McClintick CM. Open pneumothorax resulting from blunt thoracic trauma: a case report. *J Trauma Nurs.* 2008;15:72–76.

Michelet P, Couret D, Bregeon F, et al. Early onset pneumonia in severe chest trauma: a risk factor analysis. *J Trauma.* 2010;68:395–400.

Mowery NT, Gunter OL, Collier BR, et al. Practice management guidelines for management of hemothorax and occult pneumothorax. *J Trauma.* 2011;70:510–518.

Paliouras D, Barbetakis N, Lazaridis G, et al. Video-assisted thoracic surgery and pneumothorax. *J Thorac Dis.* 2015;7:S56–S61.

Partrick DA, Moore EE, Moore FA, et al. Release of anti-inflammatory mediators after major torso trauma correlates with the development of postinjury multiple organ failure. *Am J Surg.* 1999;178:564–569.

Protti A, Andreis DT, Monti M, et al. Lung stress and strain during mechanical ventilation: any difference between statics and dynamics? *Crit Care Med.* 2013;41:1046–1055.

Roumen RM, Redl H, Schlag G, et al. Inflammatory mediators in relation to the development of multiple organ failure in patients after severe blunt trauma. *Crit Care Med.* 1995;23:474–480.

Subhani SS, Muzaffar MS, Khan MI. Comparison of outcome between low and high thoracic trauma severity score in blunt trauma chest patients. *J Ayub Med Coll Abbottabad.* 2014;26(4):474–477.

Tan BK, Pothiawala S, Ong ME. Emergency thoracotomy: a review of its role in severe chest trauma. *Minerva Chir.* 2013;68(3):241–250.

Weilemann Y, Thali MJ, Kneubuehl BP, et al. Correlation between skeletal trauma and energy in falls from great height detected by postmortem multislice computed tomography (MSCT). *Forensic Sci Int.* 2008;180:81–85.

Wu N, Wu L, Qiu C, et al. A comparison of video-assisted thoracoscopic surgery with open thoracotomy for the management of chest trauma: a systematic review and meta-analysis. *World J Surg.* 2015;39(4):940–952.

Inhalation Injury

Antonio ACP, Castro PS, Freire LO. Smoke inhalation injury during enclosed-space fires: an update. *J Bras Pneumol.* 2013;39(3):373–381.

Cui P, Xin HM, Zhan Q, et al. Mechanism of lung injury of rats induced by inhalation of white smoke from burning smoke pot. *Zhonghua Shao Shang Za Zhi.* 2018;20:476–480.

Dries D, Endorf FW. Inhalation injury: epidemiology, pathology, treatment strategies. *Scand J Trama Resusc Emerg Med.* 2013;21(1):31.

Gupta K, Mehrotra M, Kumar P, et al. Smoke inhalation injury: etiopathogenesis, diagnosis, and management. *Indian J Crit Care Med.* 2018;22:180–188.

Palmieri TL. Inhalation injury: research progress and needs. *J Burn Care Res.* 2007;28:549–554.

Park GY, Park JW, Jeong DH, et al. Prolonged airway and systemic inflammatory reactions after smoke inhalation. *Chest.* 2003;123:475–480.

Rehberg S, Maybauer MO, Enkhbaatar P, et al. Pathophysiology, management and treatment of smoke inhalation injury. *Expert Rev Respir Med.* 2009;3:283–297.

Sen S, Greenhalgh D, Palmieri T. Review of burn research for the year 2010. *J Burn Care Res.* 2012;33:577–586.

Sheridan RL. *Burns: A Practical Approach to Immediate Treatment and Long-Term Care.* London, UK: Manson Publishing; 2012:48–54.

Shirani KZ, Pruitt BA Jr, Mason AD Jr. The influence of inhalation injury and pneumonia on burn mortality. *Ann Surg.* 1987;205:82–87.

Diagnosis

Backes Y, van der Sluijs KF, Tuip de Boer AM, et al. Soluble urokinase-type plasminogen activator receptor levels in patients with burn injuries and inhalation trauma requiring mechanical ventilation: an observational cohort study. *Crit Care.* 2011;15:R270.

Badulak JH, Schurr M, Sauaia A, et al. Defining the criteria for intubation of the patient with thermal burns. *Burns.* 2018;44:531–538.

Burn and Trauma Branch of Chinese Geriatrics Society, Guo F, Zhu YS, et al. National experts consensus on clinical diagnosis and treatment of inhalation injury. *Zhonghua Shao Shang Za Zhi.* 2018;34(11):E004.

Carr J, Phillips BD, Bowling WM. The utility of bronchoscopy after inhalational injury complicated by pneumonia in burn patients: results from the National Burn Repository. *J Burn Care Res.* 2009;30:967–974.

Ching JA, Shah JL, Doran CJ, et al. The evaluation of physical exam findings in patients assessed for suspected burn inhalation injury. *J Burn Care Res.* 2015;36:197–202.

Clark WR. Smoke inhalation: diagnosis and treatment. *World J Surg.* 1992;16:24–29.

Liffner G, Bak Z, Reske A, et al. Inhalation injury assessed by score does not contribute to the development of acute respiratory distress syndrome in burn victims. *Burns.* 2005;31:263–268.

Liodaki E, Kalousis K, Schopp BE, et al. Prophylactic antibiotic therapy after inhalation injury. *Burns.* 2014;11:S305–S417. doi:10.1016/j.burns.2014.01.022

Marek K, Piotr W, Stanisław S, et al. Fibreoptic bronchoscopy in routine clinical practice in confirming the diagnosis and treatment of inhalation burns. *Burns.* 2007;33:554–560.

Masanes MJ, Legendre C, Lioret N, et al. Fiberoptic bronchoscopy for the early diagnosis of subglottal inhalation injury: comparative value in the assessment of prognosis. *J Trauma.* 1994;36:59–67.

Mosier MJ, Pham TN, Park DR, et al. Predictive value of bronchoscopy in assessing the severity of inhalation injury. *J Burn Care Res.* 2012;33:65–73.

Murtaza B, Sharif MA, Tamimy MS, et al. Clinico-pathological profile and outcome of inhalational burns. *J Coll Physicians Surg Pak.* 2009;60:613.

Wittnebel LD. Diagnosis and management of burn injury and associated complications in the geriatric population. *AARC Times.* 2005;26.

Monitoring

Megahed MA, Ghareeb F, Kishk T, et al. Blood gases as an indicator of inhalation injury and prognosis in burn patients. *Ann Burns Fire Disasters.* 2008;21:192–198.

Treatment

Bourdeaux C, Manara A. Burns and smoke inhalation. *Anaesth Intensive Care Med.* 2008;9:404–408.

Cha SI, Kim CH, Lee JH, et al. Isolated smoke inhalation injuries: acute respiratory dysfunction, clinical outcomes, and short-term evolution of pulmonary functions with the effects of steroids. *Burns.* 2007;33:200–208.

Colohan SM. Predicting prognosis in thermal burns with associated inhalational injury: a systematic review of prognostic factors in adult burn victims. *J Burn Care Res.* 2010;31:529–539.

Cui P, Xin HM, Zhan Q, et al. Mechanism of lung injury of rats induced by inhalation of white smoke from burning smoke pot. *Zhonghua Shao Shang Za Zhi.* 2018;20:476–480.

Deutsch CJ, Tan A, Smailes S, et al. The diagnosis and management of inhalation injury: an evidence based approach. *Burns.* 2018;44:1040–1051.

Fujioka M, Yakabe A. Does inhalation injury increase the mortality rate in burn patients? Investigation of relationship between inhalation injury and severity of burn surface. *Signa Vitae.* 2009;4(2):20–22.

Gigengack RK, van Baar ME, Cleffken BI, et al. Burn intensive care treatment over the last 30 years: improved survival and shift in case-mix. *Burns.* 2019;45(5):1057–1065. doi:10.1016/j.burns.2019.02.005

Goh CT, Jacobe S. Ventilation strategies in paediatric inhalation injury. *Paediatr Respir Rev.* 2016;20:3–9.

Gupta K, Mehrotra M, Kumar P, et al. Smoke inhalation injury: etiopathogenesis, diagnosis, and management. *Indian J Crit Care Med.* 2018;22:180–188.

Hall JJ, Hunt JL, Arnoldo BD, et al. Use of high-frequency percussive ventilation in inhalation injuries. *J Burn Care Res.* 2007;28:396–400.

Holt J, Saffle JR, Morris SE, et al. Use of inhaled heparin/N-acetylcystine in inhalation injury: does it help? *J Burn Care Res.* 2008;29:192–195.

Juschten J, Tuinman PR, Juffermans NP, et al. Nebulized anticoagulants in lung injury in critically ill patients: an updated systematic review of preclinical and clinical studies. *Ann Transl Med.* 2017;5:444.

Maybauer MO, Greenwood JE, Maybauer DM, et al. Management of acute smoke inhalation injury. *Crit Care Resusc.* 2010;12:53–61.

McCall JE, Cahill TJ. Respiratory care of the burn patient. *J Burn Care Rehabil.* 2005;26:200–206.

McIntire AM, Harris SA, Whitten JA, et al. Outcomes following the use of nebulized heparin for inhalation injury (HIHI Study). *J Burn Care Res.* 2017;38:45–52.

Newberry JA, Bills CB, Pirrotta EA, et al. Timely access to care for patients with critical burns in India: a prehospital prospective observational study. *Emerg Med J.* 2019;36:176–182.

Palmieri TL. Use of beta-agonists in inhalation injury. *J Burn Care Res.* 2009;30:156–159.

Sheridan RL, Kacmarek RM, McEttrick MM, et al. Permissive hypercapnia as a ventilatory strategy in burned children: effect on barotrauma, pneumonia, and mortality. *J Trauma.* 1995;39:854–859.

Sousse LE, Herndon DN, Andersen CR, et al. High tidal volume decreases adult respiratory distress syndrome, atelectasis, and ventilator days compared with low tidal volume in pediatric burned patients with inhalation injury. *J Am Coll Surg.* 2015;220:570–578.

Traumatic Brain Injury

Butcher I, McHugh GS, Lu J, et al. Prognostic value of cause of injury in traumatic brain injury: results from the IMPACT study. *J Neurotrauma.* 2007;24(2):281–286.

Coronado V, McGuire L, Faul M, et al. Epidemiology and public health issues. In: Zasler ND, Katz DI, Zafonte RD, et al., eds. *Brain Injury Medicine: Principles and Practice.* 2nd ed. New York, NY: Demos Medical Publishing; 2012.

Defense and Veterans Brain Injury Center. *DoD Numbers for Traumatic Brain Injury.* Washington, DC: Department of Defense; 2017.

Finkelstein E, Corso P, Miller T. *The Incidence and Economic Burden of Injuries in the United States.* New York, NY: Oxford University Press; 2006.

Li M, Zhao Z, Yu G, et al. Epidemiology of traumatic brain injury over the world: a systematic review. *Austin Neurol Neurosci.* 2016;1:1007.

Liao CC, Chiu WT, Yeh CC, et al. Risk and outcomes for traumatic brain injury in patients with mental disorders. *J Neurol Neurosurg Psych.* 2012;83:1186.

Schiller JS, Lucas JW, Ward BW, et al. Summary health statistics for U.S. adults: National Health Interview Survey, 2010. *Vital Health Stat.* 2012;10:1.

Taylor CA, Bell JM, Breiding MJ, Xu L. Traumatic brain injury–related emergency department visits, hospitalizations, and deaths—United States, 2007 and 2013. *MMWR Surveill Summ.* 2017;66(9):1–16.

Classification of TBI

Eken C, Kartal M, Bacanli A, et al. Comparison of the full outline of unresponsiveness score coma scale and the Glasgow coma scale in an emergency setting population. *Eur J Emerg Med.* 2009;16:29.

Maas AI, Hukkelhoven CW, Marshall LF, et al. Prediction of outcome in traumatic brain injury with computed tomographic characteristics: a comparison between the computed tomographic classification and combinations of computed tomographic predictors. *Neurosurgery.* 2005;57:1173.

Saatman KE, Duhaime AC, Bullock R, et al. Classification of traumatic brain injury for targeted therapies. *J Neurotrauma.* 2008;25:719.

Teasdale G, Jennett B. Assessment of coma and impaired consciousness. A practical scale. *Lancet.* 1974;2:81.

Pathophysiology

Wafaisade A, Lefering R, Tjardes T, et al. Acute coagulopathy in isolated blunt traumatic brain injury. *Neurocrit Care.* 2010;12:211.

Management of TBI

Badjatia N, Carney N, Crocco TJ, et al. Guidelines for prehospital management of traumatic brain injury. *Prehosp Emerg Care.* 2008;12:S1.

Badri S, Chen J, Barber J, et al. Mortality and long-term functional outcome associated with intracranial pressure after traumatic brain injury. *Intensive Care Med.* 2012;38:1800.

Bernard SA, Nguyen V, Cameron P, et al. Prehospital rapid sequence intubation improves functional outcome for patients with severe traumatic brain injury: a randomized controlled trial. *Ann Surg.* 2010;252:959.

Boone MD, Jinadasa SP, Mueller A, et al. The effect of positive end-expiratory pressure on intracranial pressure and cerebral hemodynamics. *Neurocrit Care.* 2017;26(2):174–181.

Brain Trauma Foundation, American Association of Neurological Surgeons, Congress of Neurological Surgeons, et al. Guidelines for the management of severe traumatic brain injury. I. Blood pressure and oxygenation. *J Neurotrauma.* 2007;24:S7.

Bullock MR, Chesnut R, Ghajar J, et al. Surgical management of acute epidural hematomas. *Neurosurgery.* 2006;58(Suppl 1):S7.

Cadena R, Shoykhet M, Ratcliff JJ. Emergency neurological life support: intracranial hypertension and herniation. *Neurocrit Care.* 2017;27:82.

Carney N, Totten AM, O'Reilly C, et al. Guidelines for the management of severe traumatic brain injury. *Neurosurgery.* 2017;80(1):6–18.

Davis DP, Peay J, Sise MJ, et al. Prehospital airway and ventilation management: a trauma score and injury severity score-based analysis. *J Trauma.* 2010;69:294.

Diringer MN, Yundt K, Videen TO, et al. No reduction in cerebral metabolism as a result of early moderate hyperventilation following severe traumatic brain injury. *J Neurosurg.* 2000;92:7.

Fletcher JJ, Wilson TJ, Rajajee V, et al. Changes in therapeutic intensity level following airway pressure release ventilation in severe traumatic brain injury. *J Intensive Care Med.* 2018;33:196.

Fuller G, Hasler RM, Mealing N, et al. The association between admission systolic blood pressure and mortality in significant traumatic brain injury: a multi-centre cohort study. *Injury.* 2014;45:612.

Koenig MA, Bryan M, Lewin JL III, et al. Reversal of transtentorial herniation with hypertonic saline. *Neurology.* 2008;70:1023.

McHugh GS, Engel DC, Butcher I, et al. Prognostic value of secondary insults in traumatic brain injury: results from the IMPACT study. *J Neurotrauma.* 2007;24:287.

Qureshi AI, Geocadin RG, Suarez JI, et al. Long-term outcome after medical reversal of transtentorial herniation in patients with supratentorial mass lesions. *Crit Care Med.* 2000;28:1556.

Roberts I, Sydenham E. Barbiturates for acute traumatic brain injury. *Cochrane Database Syst Rev.* 2012;12:CD000033.

Rosner MJ, Daughton S. Cerebral perfusion pressure management in head injury. *J Trauma.* 1990;30:933.

Sadaka F, Veremakis C. Therapeutic hypothermia for the management of intracranial hypertension in severe traumatic brain injury: a systematic review. *Brain Inj.* 2012;26:899.

Stocchetti N, Maas AI, Chieregato A, et al. Hyperventilation in head injury: a review. *Chest.* 2005;127:1812.

Vandromme MJ, Melton SM, Griffin R, et al. Intubation patterns and outcomes in patients with computed tomography-verified traumatic brain injury. *J Trauma.* 2011;71:1615.

von Elm E, Schoettker P, Henzi I, et al. Pre-hospital tracheal intubation in patients with traumatic brain injury: systematic review of current evidence. *Br J Anaesth.* 2009;103:371.

15

Critical Care Guidelines and Bundles

David W. Chang, EdD, RRT

OUTLINE

OBJECTIVES

1. Outline the algorithm of ACLS.
2. Discuss three procedures or drugs with limited or no benefits based on the AHA guidelines for adult cardiovascular life support.
3. Discuss three key recommendations of the 2015 AHA guidelines.
4. List three common crash cart usage errors in an acute care setting.
5. Name and discuss the PADIS categories.
6. Name and discuss the ABCDEF categories.
7. Discuss the advantages and disadvantages of enteral and parenteral feeding.
8. Explain the significance of gastric residual volume.

KEY TERMS

ABCDEF Bundle
Behavioral Pain Scale (BPS)
Confusion Assessment
  Method (CAM)
Critical Care Pain
  Observation Tool (CPOT)
early mobility
enteral nutrition
extracorporeal CPR
gastric residual volume
intraosseous (IO) access
numerical rating
  scale (NRS)
nutritional bundle

nutritional risk screening
  (NRS 2002)
PADIS guidelines
parenteral nutrition
Richards-Campbell Sleep
  Questionnaire (RCSQ)
Richmond Agitation and
  Sedation Scale (RASS)
Riker Sedation-Agitation
  Scale (SAS)
spontaneous awakening
  trial
spontaneous breathing trial
visual analog scale

Introduction

This chapter covers several key critical care practice guidelines and bundles. Among them are the 2010 and 2015 American Heart Association (AHA) Guidelines for adult Advanced Cardiovascular Life Support (ACLS). The 2010 guidelines cover items no longer recommended by the AHA but are still occasionally used in clinical practice. The 2015 guidelines cover the updated key recommendations for ACLS. Also included in this chapter are the use of crash cart, two critical care practice bundles (PADIS Bundle and ABCDEF Bundle), and nutritional support therapy for critically ill patients.

Adult Advanced Cardiovascular Life Support

In adult critical care, cardiac arrest is the most serious event that calls for immediate intervention. The actions for full and prolonged cardiac arrest typically include interpretation of the electrocardiogram (ECG) rhythm, cardiopulmonary resuscitation (CPR), shock energy for defibrillation, drug therapy, advanced airway, and procedures following return of spontaneous circulation (ROSC). In 2018, the American Heart Association updated the cardiac arrest algorithm (**Figure 15-1**).

This topic is divided into two subsections. The first subsection provides an overview of the key recommendations based on the 2010 AHA guidelines for CPR and ECC (emergency cardiovascular care). The second subsection provides the updated recommendation published in 2015.

Key Recommendations Based on 2010 AHA Guidelines

A quick review of the key recommendations in the 2010 AHA guidelines is provided here because they are the most common procedures or devices used during adult CPR. For a complete discussion of the 2010 AHA guidelines, refer to 2010 AHA Guidelines for CPR and ECC, "Part 8: Adult Advanced Cardiovascular Life Support."

- For airway care, oropharyngeal airways can be used in unconscious or unresponsive patients with no cough or gag reflex. The oral airway is preferred for patients with known or suspected basal skull fracture or severe coagulopathy. Following successful intubation, the endotracheal should be secured with tape or a similar device.
- For mechanical ventilation, automatic transport ventilators (pneumatically powered and time- or pressure-cycled) can be used in adult patients with a correctly placed functional advanced airway.
- CPR should be continued while a defibrillator is being readied for use.

- **Intraosseous (IO) access** should be established if an intravenous (IV) access is not readily available or cannot be established because of collapsed veins or severe hypotension. If IO and IV access is not available, epinephrine, vasopressin, and lidocaine may be administered via a correctly placed endotracheal tube.
- For symptomatic bradycardia, atropine is the first-line drug. If the patient is unresponsive to atropine, IV β-agonists with rate accelerating effects (dopamine, epinephrine) or transcutaneous pacing should be considered and used.
- For symptomatic tachycardia (heart rate <150/min), immediate cardioversion with proper sedation should be performed. A trial of adenosine may be considered for selected narrow complex tachycardia before cardioversion.

Procedures or Drugs with Limited or No Benefits

The ACLS procedures are updated when new scientific evidence becomes available. However, some procedures have been taken off the recommended list. It is important for clinicians to keep up with the changes in each update. **Table 15-1** summarizes the procedures or drugs that are deemed as having uncertain or no benefits or are not recommended.

Key Recommendations Based on 2015 AHA Guidelines

The following information highlights the key recommendations in the *2015 American Heart Association Guidelines Update for Cardiopulmonary Resuscitation and Emergency Cardiovascular Care*. These recommendations are based on an extensive review completed by the ILCOR (International Liaison Committee on Resuscitation) in 2015. They are grouped into three categories: (1) adjuncts to CPR, (2) adjuncts for airway control and ventilation, and (3) management of cardiac arrest (**Tables 15-2** to **15-4**).

Adjuncts to CPR

Tables 15-2 to 15-4 provide a summary of the 2015 key recommendations and guidelines update for cardiopulmonary resuscitation and emergency cardiovascular care.

Adjuncts for Airway Control and Ventilation

For airway control and ventilation, the key recommendations are summarized in Table 15-3.

Management of Cardiac Arrest

Table 15-4 summarizes the key recommendations for use of equipment, medications, and defibrillator energy dose during CPR.

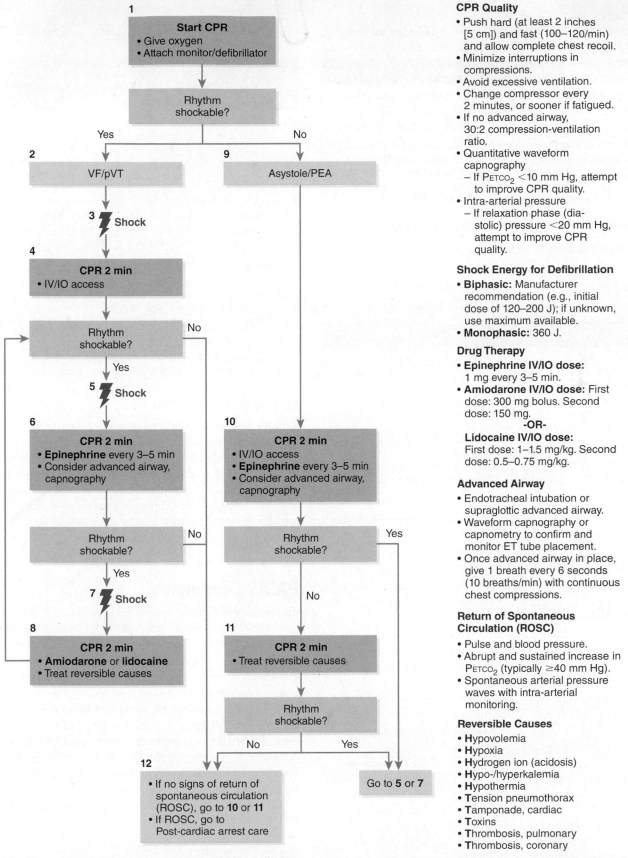

FIGURE 15-1 AHA cardiac arrest algorithm. AHA, American Heart Association; CPR, cardiopulmonary resuscitation; ET, endotracheal; IO, intraosseous; IV, intravenous; PEA, pulseless electrical activity; pVT, pulseless ventricular tachycardia; VF, ventricular fibrillation.

TABLE 15-1
Routine ACLS Procedures or Drug Therapy with Limited or No Benefits

Procedure or Drug Therapy	Notes
ABG measurements during CPR	Uncertain value
Cricoid pressure during endotracheal intubation	Not recommended
Atropine during pulseless electrical activity (PEA) or asystole	Unlikely to have a therapeutic benefit
Sodium bicarbonate in cardiac arrest	Not recommended
Calcium for cardiac arrest	Not recommended

ABG, arterial blood gas; ACLS, advanced cardiovascular life support; CPR, cardiopulmonary resuscitation.

TABLE 15-2
2015 Key Recommendations for Adjuncts to CPR

Adjuncts to CPR	Recommendation
Supplemental oxygen	Use highest FIO_2 during CPR.
Physiologic monitoring parameters	Resuscitation efforts may be guided by: Capnography waveforms (ventilation and perfusion) Arterial relaxation diastolic pressure (perfusion) Arterial pressure monitoring (perfusion) Central venous oxygen saturation (oxygen extraction)
Cardiac and non-cardiac ultrasound	Ultrasound may be performed when it does not interfere with standard cardiac arrest protocol.

CPR, cardiopulmonary resuscitation.

Crash Cart

Crash cart (emergency cart) is a portable storage of essential equipment and supplies for cardiovascular life support. It typically includes a defibrillator, cardiovascular drugs, and devices for establishing an airway, providing ventilation and oxygenation, and initiating intravenous access. Since the crash cart is not used frequently by clinicians, mishaps can happen. In one report by the Pennsylvania Patient Safety Authority (PPSA), 56 incidences occurred over a 12-month period in which equipment or supplies in a crash cart were either missing or malfunctioning. It should be noted that these data cover only *reported* incidences in one state. The magnitude of this problem in the United States as a whole could be much higher had the *unreported* incidences been included.

There are many contributing factors affecting patient safety due to crash cart errors. **Table 15-5** outlines three types of common errors relating to crash cart use.

TABLE 15-3
2015 Key Recommendations for Adjuncts for Airway Control and Ventilation

Adjuncts for Airway Control and Ventilation	Recommendation
Basic airway	Bag-mask device may be used as an *initial* basic airway for ventilation and oxygenation.
Advanced airway	Supraglottic airway or endotracheal tube may be used as an *initial* advanced airway during CPR.
Capnography	Continuous CO_2 waveform device should be used to confirm placement of ETT or monitor changes in perfusion status.
Colorimetric CO_2 detector (no waveform)	Color-change CO_2 detecting device, esophageal detector, or ultrasound may be used when continuous capnography is not available.
Ventilation frequency	Following placement of an advanced airway, manual ventilation should be delivered at a frequency of 10/min (1 breath every 6 sec).

CPR, cardiopulmonary resuscitation; ETT endotracheal tube.

Airway and Ventilation

Common airways and supplies in a crash cart may include oropharyngeal airway, King airway, laryngoscope and blades, Magill forceps (for nasotracheal intubation), flexible stylet (for orotracheal intubation), bag-mask device for manual ventilation, nasal cannula, and oxygen masks. Different sizes of airways and laryngoscopy blades are also provided for individual patient needs. Blood gases kits, syringes, needles, and color-change CO_2 detectors are some additional supplies found in a crash cart.

PADIS Guidelines

The Society of Critical Care Medicine (SCCM) published the Pain, Agitation/sedation, Delirium, Immobility (rehabilitation/mobilization), and Sleep (disruption) (PADIS) guidelines in 2018. It is an update to the 2013 guidelines to which two clinical topics (immobility and sleep) were added.

The **PADIS guidelines** are very similar to the topics in the ABCDEF Bundle (to be discussed in a later section). **Table 15-6** compares the coverage of PADIS and ABCDEF. Since sleep disruption in the PADIS guidelines is not fully discussed in the ABCDEF Bundle, this topic will be discussed in this section.

Refer to the ABCDEF Bundle for similar topics in PADIS guidelines.

Sleep Disruption

According to the PADIS guidelines on sleep disruption, the quality of sleep and other sleep attributes may be based on the patient's self-reporting (e.g.,

TABLE 15-4
2015 Key Recommendations for Management of Cardiac Arrest

Management of Cardiac Arrest	Recommendation
Defibrillators	Biphasic (biphasic truncated exponential [BTE] or rectilinear biphasic [RLB]) defibrillators are preferred for atrial and ventricular arrhythmias.
Defibrillator energy dose for first shock	Use manufacturer's recommended energy dose for first shock (or maximum dose if no recommendation).
Defibrillator energy dose for subsequent shocks	Use manufacturer's recommended energy dose (fixed or escalating) for second and subsequent shocks.
Single shock or stacked shock	Single shock is preferred with chest compressions between shocks.
Drug for VF/pVT unresponsive to CPR, defibrillation, and vasopressor therapy	Amiodarone (or lidocaine as an option)
Magnesium for VF/pVT	Routine use of magnesium is *not* recommended.
Lidocaine for VF/pVT	Routine use of lidocaine after cardiac arrest is *not* recommended. Lidocaine may be considered immediately after ROSC (return of spontaneous circulation) from cardiac arrest due to VF/pVT.
Beta-blocker for VF/pVT	Routine use of beta-blocker after cardiac arrest is *not* recommended. Beta-blocker may be considered early after hospitalization from cardiac arrest due to VF/pVT.
Epinephrine for cardiac arrest	Standard dose (1 mg) of epinephrine is recommended. Epinephrine should be administered as soon as feasible after onset of cardiac arrest due to an initial nonshockable rhythm. *High* single-dose epinephrine is *not* recommended. Vasopressin offers *no* advantage over epinephrine.
Steroids during CPR	Use of steroids during CPR is of *uncertain* benefit to patients with out-of-hospital cardiac arrests (OHCAs).
Intra-arrest vasopressin, epinephrine, and methylprednisolone combination and postarrest hydrocortisone	Routine use is *not* recommended for intra-arrest vasopressin, epinephrine, and methylprednisolone combination and postarrest hydrocortisone.
$ETCO_2$ to end resuscitation	In intubated patient, failure to achieve $ETCO_2$ of >10 mm Hg after 20 min of CPR may be considered as *one* component of ending resuscitation. In nonintubated patients, a specific $ETCO_2$ cutoff value should *not* be used as an indication to end resuscitation.
Extracorporeal CPR (ECPR)	Routine use of ECPR is *not* recommended.

CPR, cardiopulmonary resuscitation; pVT, pulseless ventricular tachycardia; VF, ventricular fibrillation.

Modified from Link MS, Berkow LC, Kudenchuk PJ, et al. Part 7: adult advanced cardiovascular life support: 2015 American Heart Association guidelines update for cardiopulmonary resuscitation and emergency cardiovascular care. *Circulation*. 2015;132(18 Suppl 2):S444–S464.

TABLE 15-5
Common Crash Cart Errors

Type of Error	Example
Procedural error	Medication dosage Medication identification
Readiness error	Missing or expired equipment or medications Missing or empty oxygen cylinder Dead or insufficiently charged batteries Locked crash cart with misplaced key Incorrect size of equipment or supplies
Staff error	Unable to locate crash cart Unfamiliar with location of crash cart contents Unfamiliar with procedures for using, stocking, restocking crash cart

Modified from Pennsylvania Patient Safety Authority. Clinical emergency: are you ready in any setting? *Pennsylvania Patient Safety Advisory*. 2010;7(2):52–60.

TABLE 15-6
Comparison of PADIS and ABCDEF Bundles

PADIS	ABCDEF
Pain	**A**ssess, prevent and manage pain
Agitation/sedation	**C**hoice of analgesia and sedation
Delirium	**D**elirium assess and manage
Immobility	**E**arly mobility and exercise
Sleep disruption	
	Both SATs and SBTs
	Family engagement/empowerment

Modified from Devlin JW, Skrobik Y, Gélinas CR, et al. Executive summary: clinical practice guidelines for the prevention and management of pain, agitation/sedation, delirium, immobility, and sleep disruption in adult patients in the ICU. *Crit Care Med*. 2018;46:1532–1548. doi:10.1097/CCM.0000000000003259

"I slept soundly last night"). Alternatively, sleep quality and disruption may be assessed by the **Richards-Campbell Sleep Questionnaire (RCSQ)**. The RCSQ approximates the patient's perception with a continuum of values (e.g., **visual analog scale** of 0 to 100 mm, in intervals of 1 mm). For example, the sleep depth can be described by the patient as between 0 (light sleep) and 100 (deep sleep). Since there are 100 mm intervals on the visual scale, the perception scale appears to be continuous to the patient. **Figure 15-2** shows a 100 mm visual analog scale for sleep depth.

The RCSQ with its five categories of sleep attributes is shown in **Figure 15-3**.

Monitoring of Sleep

The PADIS guidelines do not recommend using physiologic sleep monitoring of critically ill patients in a clinic setting. These monitoring techniques (e.g., actigraphy, bispectral analysis, polysomnography) should not be used to determine if a patient is asleep or awake. Instead, bedside assessment by patient self-reporting or

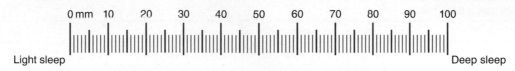

FIGURE 15-2 A visual analog scale for describing sleep depth.

Sleep attribute last night	Interval rating		
1. Sleep depth	Light sleep (0) Deep sleep (100)		
2. Sleep latency	Never could fall asleep (0) Fell asleep almost immediately (100)		
3. Awakenings	Awake all night long (0) Awake very little (100)		
4. Returning to sleep	Couldn't get back to sleep (0) Got back to sleep immediately (100)		
5. Sleep quality	Bad night's sleep (0) Good night's sleep (100)		

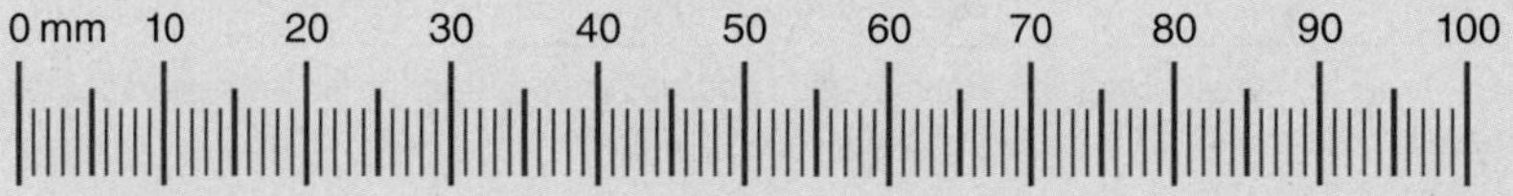

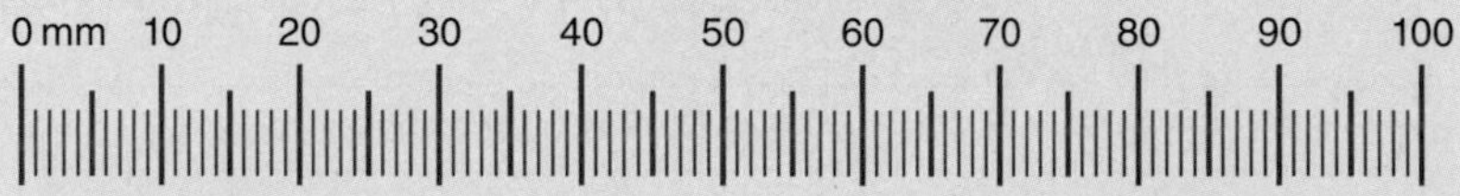

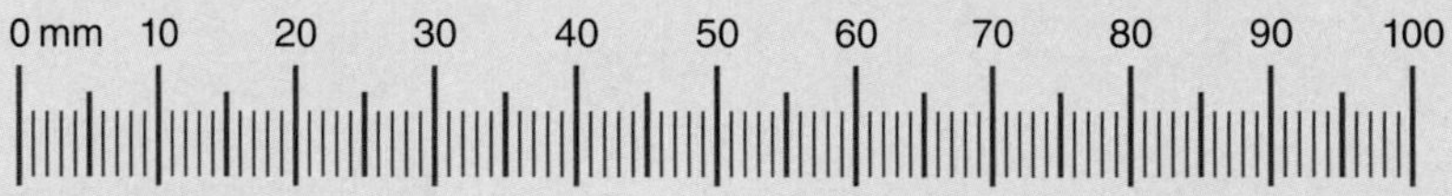

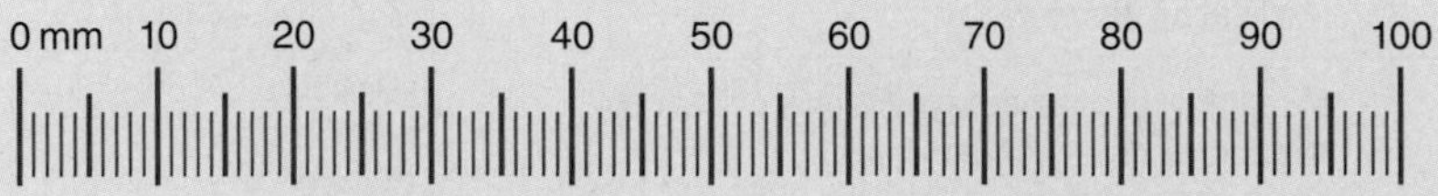

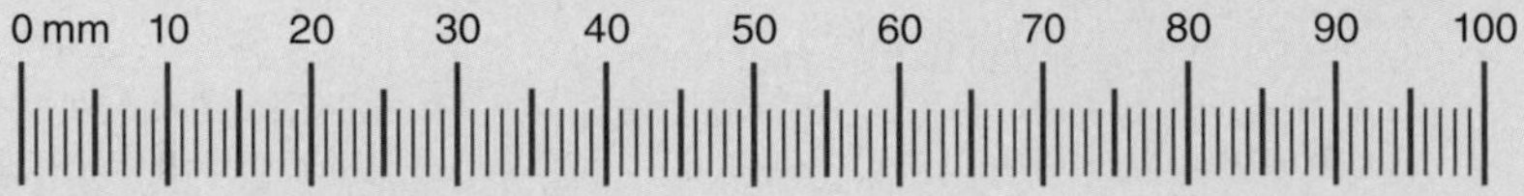

FIGURE 15-3 Richards-Campbell Sleep Questionnaire (RCSQ).

a validated assessment tool (e.g., RCSQ) should be used to assess sleep.

Ventilation During Sleep

For mechanically ventilated patients, the assist/control mode (vs. pressure support ventilation) is recommended for improving sleep. For patients using noninvasive ventilation (NIV) during sleep, the type of ventilator may be the traditional intensive care unit (ICU) ventilator or a NIV-dedicated ventilator. There is no recommendation in regard to the use of an adaptive mode of ventilation (vs. pressure support ventilation) for improving sleep.

Adjunctive Therapies for Sleep

Aromatherapy, acupressure, or music therapy should not be used to improve sleep in critically ill patients. An appropriate level of sedatives may be used if the patient is sleep deprived due to anxiety or pain.

ABCDEF Bundle

The **ABCDEF Bundle** is an integrated, interprofessional strategy intended to facilitate and improve management of critically ill patients in the hospital. There are six elements in the ABCDEF Bundle. From A to F, these six elements are listed in **Table 15-7**, and a discussion of each element follows.

According to a study published in 2018 by Pun, benefits of using the six elements in the ABCDEF Bundle (completely or proportionally) provide significant and dose-related improvements in patient outcomes. The improvements include positive impact on survival, duration of mechanical ventilation, brain organ dysfunction such as delirium and coma, agitation, ICU readmission, and ICU survival. The results of the bundle also point to potential opportunities for future research in patient-centered care and interprofessional collaboration in a critical care setting.

Element A (Assess, Prevent, and Manage Pain)

Many critically ill patients are unable to express presence of pain due to different clinical conditions (e.g., head trauma, endotracheal tube). The clinicians must rely on other tools to evaluate the presence of pain and the degree of pain. The ICU Liberation program and its implementation tools suggest a stepwise pain assessment approach, and it includes (1) patient self-report of pain when capable, (2) evaluating behavioral changes of the patient, and (3) asking family member to identify unique pain behaviors. The assessment of pain should be ongoing so that the pain may be managed appropriately without using excessive or insufficient analgesics.

Numerical Rating Scale for Pain

Patient self-report of pain can be done easily using a **numerical rating scale (NRS)**. This is an interval scale

TABLE 15-7
The ABCDEF Bundle

Element	Notes
Assess, prevent, and manage pain	Techniques to assess pain may include: 1. Numerical Rating Scale (NRS) 2. Behavioral Pain Scale (BPS) 3. Critical Care Pain Observation Tool (CPOT)
Both SATs and SBTs	SAT (spontaneous awakening trial) is related to reduction in use of sedatives SBT (spontaneous breathing trial) is related to the patient's ability to sustain spontaneous breathing for at least 30 min while intubated and with only minimal pressure support ventilation
Choice of analgesia and sedation	Titrate analgesic/sedative to achieve RASS scale of −2 (light sedation) to 0 (calm and alert) *or* SAS scale of 3 (sedated) or 4 (calm and cooperative)
Delirium assess and manage	Using CAM, delirium is present when patient presents acute change of mental status and inattention plus *one* of the following: altered level of consciousness or disorganized thinking
Early mobility and exercise	Complications during mobility exercise may include hypoxia, respiratory and circulatory adverse outcomes, falling, disconnection of access lines and ET tube
Family engagement/ empowerment	Team approach to patient care Positive psychological and social support

CAM, confusion assessment method; ET, endotracheal; RASS, Richmond Agitation and Sedation Scale; SAS, Riker Sedation-Agitation Scale.

Modified from Devlin JW, Skrobik Y, Gélinas C, et al. Clinical practice guidelines for the prevention and management of pain, agitation/sedation, delirium, immobility, and sleep disruption in adult patients in the ICU. *Crit Care Med.* 2018;46: 825–873; Pun BT. ABCDEF Bundle. Society of Critical Care Medicine. Available at http:// www.sccm.org/ICULiberation/ABCDEF-Bundles. Published 2018.

ranging from 0 (no pain) to 10 (extreme pain). Use of this scale requires that the patient is alert and able to communicate the numerical choice by verbalizing or signaling the intended number. For patients who are unable to self-report presence of pain, the Behavioral Pain Scale (BPS) and Critical Care Pain Observation Tool (CPOT) may be used. These two methods are discussed next.

Behavioral Pain Scale

The **Behavioral Pain Scale (BPS)** assesses a patient's facial expression, upper limb movement, and compliance with ventilation (intubated patients) or vocalization (nonintubated patients). **Table 15-8** describes the scoring of the BPS. The total score ranges from 3 (no pain) to 12 (extreme pain). It should be noted that evaluation of upper limb movement must take into account of any preexisting neuromuscular conditions.

TABLE 15-8
Behavioral Pain Scale

Item	Description	Score
Facial expression	Relaxed	1
	Partially tightened (e.g., brow lowering)	2
	Fully tightened (e.g., eyelid closing)	3
	Grimacing	4
Upper limbs	No movement	1
	Partially bent	2
	Fully bent with finger flexion	3
	Permanently retracted	4
Compliance with ventilation	Tolerating movement	1
	Coughing but tolerating ventilation for most of the time	2
	Fighting ventilator	3
	Unable to control ventilation	4

Reproduced from Wolters Kluwer Health. Payen J, Bru O, Bosson J, et al. Assessing pain in critically ill sedated patients by using a behavioral pain scale. *Crit Care Med.* 2001;29:2258–2263.

Critical Care Pain Observation Tool

The **Critical Care Pain Observation Tool (CPOT)** is another tool for assessing pain by observation. It uses four categories to evaluate the patient: facial expression, body movements, muscle tension, and compliance with mechanical ventilation (or verbalization of pain for nonintubated patients). **Table 15-9** describes the scoring method. The total score ranges from 0 (no pain) to 8 (extreme pain). As in the BPS assessment, evaluation of body movements and muscle tension must take into account any preexisting neuromuscular conditions.

Element B (Both SATs and SBTs)

The **spontaneous awakening trial** (SAT) evaluates the patient's comfort level after the sedatives are discontinued. The **spontaneous breathing trial** (SBT) evaluates the patient's ability to breathe for up to 30 minutes spontaneously or with minimal pressure support ventilation (e.g., 5 cm H_2O of PSV).

SAT and SBT are traditionally performed separately. In a study by Girard et al., the combined SAT and SBT reduced the number of mechanical ventilation days and length of hospital stay when compared to SBT alone. This combined technique is also known as "wake up and breathe."

Spontaneous Awakening Trial

The SAT consists of a safety screen prior to the awakening trial. The patient safety screen checks for

TABLE 15-9
Scoring Method for Critical Care Pain Observation Tool (CPOT)

Indicator	Description		Score
Facial expression	No muscle tension observed	Relaxed, neutral	0
	Presence of frowning, brow lowering, orbit tightening, and levator contraction	Tense	1
	All of the above facial movements plus eyelids tightly closed	Grimacing	2
Body movements	Does not move at all (does not necessarily mean absence of pain)	Absence of movements	0
	Slow, cautious movements, touching or rubbing the pain site, seeking attention through movements	Protection	1
	Pulling tube, attempting to sit up, moving limbs/thrashing, not following commands, striking at staff, trying to climb out of bed	Restlessness	2
Muscle tension Evaluation by passive flexion and extension of upper extremities	No resistance to passive movements	Relaxed	0
	Resistance to passive movements	Tense, rigid	1
	Strong resistance to passive movements, inability to complete them	Very tense or rigid	2
Compliance with the ventilator (intubated patients) OR Vocalization (extubated patients)	Alarms not activated, easy ventilation	Tolerating ventilator or movement	0
	Alarms stop spontaneously	Coughing but tolerating	1
	Asynchrony: blocking ventilation, alarms frequently activated	Fighting ventilator	2
	Talking in a normal tone or no sound	Talking in normal tone or no sound	0
	Sighing, moaning	Sighing, moaning	1
	Crying out, sobbing	Crying out, sobbing	2
Total score range			0-8

Reproduced from Gélinas C, Fillion L, Puntillo KA, et al. Validation of the critical-care pain observation tool in adult patients. Am *J Crit Care.* 2006;15(4):420–427. Available at http://ajcc.aacnjournals.org/content/15/4/420.full.pdf+html

contraindications, including (1) use of continuous sedative infusion for different clinical conditions (e.g., seizures), (2) use of increasing doses of sedative (e.g., agitation), (3) use of neuromuscular blockers, (4) recent myocardial ischemia within 24 hours, and (5) elevated intracranial pressure.

If no contraindications are present, the awakening trial is initiated by discontinuing all sedatives and analgesics unless analgesics are needed for pain. The SAT is considered successful when the patient is able to perform three of four simple tasks on command: (1) open eyes, (2) look at the clinician, (3) squeeze the hand of the clinician, and (4) stick out the tongue.

When the patient is unable to follow a command, signs and symptoms may be used to evaluate the outcome of SAT. The SAT is deemed *unsuccessful* when the patient shows signs and symptoms in any *one* of five categories in **Table 15-10** within 4 hours following sedation discontinuance. If a patient fails the SAT, sedation is started at half the last dosage and titrated for an appropriate level of sedation.

Spontaneous Breathing Trial

The SBT is indicated under 4 conditions: (1) The cause leading to mechanical ventilation has been reversed, (2) patient is able to breathe spontaneously for a sustained time period (may use vital capacity or maximal inspiratory pressure for assessment of ventilatory reserve), (3) patient has an adequate cough mechanism and does not have excessive secretions, and (4) neuromuscular blocker has been stopped and use of sedative is at the lowest appropriate dose.

TABLE 15-10
Untoward Signs and Symptoms of Spontaneous Awakening Trial

Category*	Notes
1. Prolonged anxiety, agitation, or pain	By observation
2. Tachypnea for at least 5 min	Spontaneous frequency $\geq$35/min
3. Desaturation for at least 5 min	SpO_2 <88%
4. Acute dysrhythmia	Tachycardia Bradycardia Atrial or ventricular dysrhythmias
5. Respiratory distress (two or more)	Use of accessory respiratory muscles Abdominal paradox Diaphoresis Marked dyspnea (subjective reporting)

*Presence of any one category indicates *unsuccessful* spontaneous awakening trial.

The vital signs, indicators for adequate ventilation and oxygenation, must be within patient's normal range to support sustained spontaneous breathing during the trial. Positive objective indicators include $PaO_2/FIO_2 \geq 200$ mm Hg and rapid shallow breathing index (RSBI) <105 cycles/L.

Some contraindications for SBT include refractory hypoxemia, apnea, agitation, elevated intracranial pressure, and use of high-dose vasopressors or inotropes to maintain blood pressure and circulation. SBT may begin once the patient is deemed to be ready. During the trial, the patient must be monitored closely, especially the first few minutes. **Table 15-11** summarizes the key points for a well-planned SBT.

During SBT, the patient should be monitored for respiratory distress, which is defined as having two or more of the following: heart rate >20% of baseline, marked use of accessory muscle, abdominal paradox, diaphoresis, marked cyanosis, or dyspnea. Most patients fail the SBT within the first 30 minutes of the trial. If a patient fails the SBT, mechanical ventilation is resumed with the latest ventilator settings. The SBT may be repeated in 24 hours.

Element C (Choice of Analgesia and Sedation)

Analgesia and sedatives are often used to manage patients with pain, agitation, and delirium. The primary goal of pharmacotherapy for these conditions is to use

TABLE 15-11
Key Points for a Spontaneous Breathing Trial

Key Point	Note
Mechanical breaths	Assist/control or SIMV must be off
Pressure support ventilation	May use 5 to 8 cm H_2O of PSV if ventilator is used to conduct SBT
Device (off ventilator)	T-piece connected to an endotracheal or tracheostomy tube
Oxygen	Titrate oxygen to maintain SpO_2 (e.g., $\geq$88%)
CPAP	Level same as PEEP while on ventilator
Duration	At least 30 min
Breathing pattern	Regular in frequency and tidal volume Without use of accessory muscles
Criteria of success SBT	Spontaneous frequency <35/min Heart rate <140 beats/min or <20% change from baseline $SpO_2 \geq$88% or $PaO_2 \geq$60 mm Hg on $FIO_2 \leq$40% for $\geq$5 min Systolic BP 80 to 180 mm Hg or <20% change from baseline No arrhythmia

CPAP, continuous positive airway pressure; BP, blood pressure; PEEP, positive end-expiratory pressure; PSV, pressure support ventilation; SBT, spontaneous breathing trial; SIMV, synchronized intermittent mandatory ventilation.

Modified from Zein H, Baratloo A, Negidal A, et al. Ventilator weaning and spontaneous breathing trials; an educational review. *Emergency*. 2016;4:65–71.

the least amount of drugs and for the shortest duration possible. For this reason, a consistent plan for patient assessment is a necessity.

Element D (Delirium Assess and Manage)

All patients in the critical care unit should be evaluated for presence of pain, agitation (anxiety), and delirium. Refer to Element A for a detailed discussion on assessment of pain. For agitation, two common assessment tools are often used. The **Richmond Agitation and Sedation Scale (RASS)** ranges from −5 (unarousable) to +4 (combative) (**Table 15-12**). Titration of sedatives should target a RASS scale from −2 (light sedation) to 0 (alert and calm).

As shown in **Table 15-13**, the **Riker Sedation-Agitation Scale (SAS)** ranges from 1 (unarousable) to 7 (dangerous). The titration target is an SAS score of 3 (sedated) or 4 (calm and cooperative) for optimal sedation.

TABLE 15-12
Richmond Agitation and Sedation Scale (RASS)

Scale	Degree of Agitation
+4	Combative
+3	Very agitated
+2	Agitated
+1	Restless
0	Alert and calm
−1	Drowsy
−2	Light sedation
−3	Moderate sedation
−4	Deep sedation
−5	Unarousable

TABLE 15-13
Riker Sedation-Agitation Scale (SAS)

Scale	Degree of Agitation
7	Dangerous
6	Very agitated
5	Agitated
4	Calm and cooperative
3	Sedated
2	Very sedated
1	Unarousable

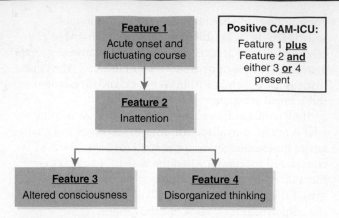

FIGURE 15-4 Assessment of CAM-ICU. CAM, confusion assessment method; ICU, intensive care unit.

For delirium, the **Confusion Assessment Method (CAM)** is a common assessment tool done at bedside (**Figure 15-4**). This assessment tool assesses four features. The patient is deemed to have delirium if the patient presents clinical features 1 (acute change of mental status) and 2 (inattention) plus one of features 3 or 4 (altered level of consciousness or disorganized thinking).

Before pharmacotherapy or treatments are initiated, the patient must be thoroughly evaluated for other clinical conditions that may also cause delirium. Some examples include alcohol or drug toxicity, stroke, heart attack, lung or liver disease, head injury, hyponatremia, hypocalcemia, acute infection, carbon monoxide or other toxins, malnutrition or dehydration, sleep deprivation or severe emotional distress, pain, and effects of anesthesia.

Element E (Early Mobility and Exercise)

Early mobility may be defined as a clinical procedure that is done as soon as feasible to provide a range of physical activities to the patient. Typically, it involves a set of prescribed physical activities that occurs within 48 to 72 hours from admission to the ICU.

The range of early mobility activities may be as simple as sitting up on the edge of bed or as involved as walking in the hallway with life-supporting equipment, monitoring devices, and related supplies. The feasibility of early mobility depends on several factors: stable and improving clinical condition, patient willingness and readiness, absence of contraindications, and availability of an adequate number of support staff (e.g., respiratory therapist, nurse, physical or occupational therapist).

Adverse Outcomes of Early Mobilization

Early mobility can be a safe procedure when performed with a protocol and a team of support staff. Because of the critical nature of the patient and use of numerous medical and monitoring devices during mobility, adverse outcomes may occur (**Table 15-14**). The most common adverse outcome of early mobilization is oxygen desaturation (SpO_2 <88%). This condition can often

TABLE 15-14
Adverse Outcomes of Early Mobilization

Adverse Outcome	Notes
Oxygen desaturation	Pulse oximetry
Cardiorespiratory instability	Vital signs
Falling	Falling to ground if walking Falling to bed if sitting on edge of bed
Mechanical ventilation asynchrony	Changes in tidal volume, frequency, I:E ratio, and triggering of high pressure or other alarms
Extubation	Patient and ventilator circuit are not moved at the same time or in the same direction
Device/line disconnection	Intravenous, arterial, and central line

Data from Pun BT. ABCDEF Bundle. Society of Critical Care Medicine. Available at http:// www.sccm.org/ICULiberation/ABCDEF-Bundles. Published 2018.

be resolved by increasing the F_{IO_2} or by slowing down or discontinuing the mobility (e.g., walking) or activity (e.g., limb exercise while sitting). Cardiorespiratory instability is another common occurrence, and signs may include changing heart rate, blood pressure, spontaneous respiratory frequency, and tidal volume. Baseline value of these parameters should be obtained prior to mobility. In general, significant changes from the baseline of each parameter (e.g., heart rate >15% or >20/min change from baseline) indicate patient intolerance, and the mobility should be slowed or stopped. Patient subjective expressions (e.g., "I am feeling weak") must be used as an important sign of intolerance.

Element F (Family Engagement/ Empowerment)

Family engagement and empowerment means providing patient-centered care. Patients and family members are better educated or informed about the illness, and they share and take an active role in the self-management and decision-making process. At the same time, the patients and family members are offered ongoing physical and emotional supports.

Patients benefit from family engagement and empowerment in many ways. They may experience less anxiety, confusion, and agitation; have fewer cardiovascular complications; and feel more secure about their illness and surroundings. They also have a higher level of satisfaction. In some patients, the ICU stay is shortened.

Nutritional Support Therapy

Nutritional support is defined as adjunctive nutritional care to preserve or maintain lean body mass. Nutritional therapy goes one step further. Its goals are to reduce metabolic response to stress. Nutritional therapy also helps to prevent oxidative cellular injury and enhance immune responses.

The Society of Critical Care Medicine (SCCM) and American Society of Parenteral and Enteral Nutrition (ASPN) reviewed available literature through the end of 2013 and published the guidelines for the provision and assessment of nutritional support therapy in critically ill adult patients. The target population of these guidelines is for critically ill adults who stayed in the medical ICU or surgical ICU for at least 2 days. Since the nutritional guidelines are based on scientific evidence derived from a wide spectrum of study designs and sampling populations, the clinical decision on nutritional therapy must be based on individual patient needs and clinical conditions.

Nutritional Therapy

Nutritional therapy in the hospital is provided by feeding via the gastrointestinal route (**enteral nutrition**) or the intravenous route (**parenteral nutrition**).

Enteral nutrition therapy is administered by a feeding tube. It is the preferred route for delivery of nutritional support because it promotes gut functions. The tip of the feeding tube may be placed in the stomach, different segments of the duodenum, or the jejunum. Patient tolerance to enteral feeding is better (less regurgitation, vomiting, or aspiration) when the tip is at a lower gastrointestinal position. If the patient cannot use enteral nutrition due to diminished gut function, or poor tolerance to enteral feeding, the parenteral route should be used to avoid malnutrition and depletion of macronutrients (proteins, carbohydrates, and fats) and micronutrients (e.g., minerals, electrolytes, vitamins).

Parenteral nutrition therapy is administered by an intravenous line. Since all prescribed macronutrients and micronutrients are included in the intravenous fluid, this route of administration is also called total parenteral nutrition (TPN) therapy. The TPN solutions are more concentrated than a traditional intravenous solution with saline or 5% dextrose in water (D5W). Clotting and injury to a smaller peripheral vein are common complications from using fluid with high solute concentrations and a higher fluid osmotic gradient. To avoid these complications, central lines are required for TPN. A central line is often inserted via the right internal jugular vein or left subclavian vein as they are closest to the right atrium than other routes, especially the femoral vein.

Nutritional Bundle Statements

There are six major recommendations in the **nutritional bundle**. They include (1) assessment of need, (2) initiation of enteral nutrition as soon as feasible, (3) reduction of risk of aspiration during enteral feeding, (4) implementation of enteral feeding protocol to maximize delivery of enteral nutrients, (5) discontinuation of residual volume assessment, and (6) initiation of parenteral nutrient when enteral therapy is not sufficient or tolerated. Refer to McClave et al. for a complete discussion on these and additional recommendations.

Assessment of Need

Following admission to the ICU, all patients should be evaluated for nutritional needs and risk of inadequate nutrition. There are many screening tools and methods for this assessment, but most do not account for the patient's nutritional risk due to the disease state. Two methods of nutritional risk assessment (**nutritional risk screening [NRS 2002]** and nutrition risk in the critically ill [NUTRIC]) are most useful as they account for the patient's nutrition status and disease severity.

The NRS 2002 is recommended by the American College of Gastroenterology (ACG) clinical guideline on nutrition therapy. There are four yes/no assessment questions (ICU patient, BMI <20.5 kg/m^2, weight loss within 3 months, decrease dietary intake in last week). If the answer is yes to any one question, three additional final screening questions are done: nutritional impairment (0 to +3 points), severity of disease (0 to +3 points), and age of 70 (0 or 1 point) for a total maximum score of 7. A score of 4 or 5 on the NRS 2002 is considered nutrition risk and a score of 6 or 7 is considered high risk.

The NUTRIC assessment consists of the patient's age, APACHE II (Acute Physiology and Chronic Health Evaluation), SOFA (Sequential Organ Failure Assessment) Score, number of comorbidities, days in hospital to ICU admission, and IL-6 (interleukin 6). With the NUTRIC assessment method, a score of 0 to 4 indicates low malnutrition risk and 5 to 9 high malnutrition risk. (Note: The latter score becomes 6 to 10 if IL-6 is used and ≥ 400 μ/ml.)

For energy (caloric) need in critically ill patients, indirect calorimetry (metabolic study) should provide an accurate determination providing that there is no major testing and analytical errors. If indirect calorimetry is not available, the daily energy requirement for maintenance in the medical ICU may be estimated by using 25 to 30 kcal/kg/day. Trauma, burns, and related critical conditions may call for a higher energy requirement (e.g., 30 to 35 kcal/kg/day).

Initiation of Enteral Nutrition

For critically ill patients who are unable to maintain volitional intake by mouth (e.g., unconscious or intubated patients), enteral nutrition should be provided as early as feasible, preferably within 24 to 48 hours following admission to the ICU. Early enteral feeding helps to maintain gut function and integrity. It also reduces the likelihood of infection and multiorgan dysfunction syndrome. In addition, early enteral nutrition enhances the stress and system immune response and minimizes disease severity.

Reduction of Aspiration

One of the major risks of oral or enteral feeding is aspiration. Aspiration is defined as unwanted movement of foreign substances into the airway and lungs. For spontaneously breathing patients who are not intubated, enteral feeding can be a risk factor for aspiration if the patient cannot tolerate the volume or speed of feeding. To minimize the risk of aspiration during enteral feeding, the tip of the feeding tube should be placed at a lower gastrointestinal position (e.g., section D4 of duodenum or jejunum). For intubated patients, the cuff of the endotracheal tube does not guarantee aspiration-free enteral feeding. However, tubes with subglottic suctioning port can be useful in removing feeding solution that has already been aspirated. Under-inflated cuff and microchannels along the cuff can lead to low-volume aspiration. Clinicians must ensure proper placement of feeding tube, proper endotracheal tube cuff volume, and pressure. Any signs of aspiration (e.g., presence of enteral feeding formula in suction catheter) must be investigated promptly.

Enteral Feeding Protocol

For patients who are deemed to have low nutrition risk (i.e., NRS 2002 of 0 to 3 or NUTRIC score of 0 to 4), nutrition therapy may not be necessary during the first week of hospitalization. For patients with acute respiratory distress syndrome who are on mechanical ventilation for ≥ 72 hours, enteric feeding with trophic or full nutrition is recommended.

Residual Volume Assessment

Gastric residual volume (GRV) is an assessment tool commonly used to determine the patient's tolerance of enteral feeding. Accuracy of GRV is affected by several factors (e.g., composition of enteral nutrient, sampling technique, bolus or continuous feeding, use of motility agent). A high GRV implies that the digestive tract cannot process and eliminate the enteric feeding in a timely manner. Excessive GRV may lead to abdominal distention, fullness, discomfort, vomiting, and aspiration. According to one surgical guideline, a GRV of 200 mL to 500 mL suggests patient tolerance, and additional feeding volume may be increased by 10 mL every 4 hours to reach feeding target. If GRV is >500 mL and signs of intolerance are present, use of gastric motility agent, a lower feeding position, or total parenteral nutrition should be considered.

According to the recommendations by McClave et al., gastric residual volumes should not be used routinely to monitor patient tolerance. Enteral therapy may continue unless the patient shows other signs of intolerance (e.g., vomiting) or the residual volume exceeds 500 mL. For patient safety, risks of aspiration should be assessed on a regular basis. A lower enteral access should be used in patients at high risk for aspiration. In addition, a continuous infusion of enteric nutrient provides better tolerance to patients who are intolerant of bolus infusion. Elevating the head of the bed by 30 to 45 degrees is a strategy to reduce aspiration and ventilator-assisted pneumonia in intubated patients receiving enteral feeding.

Initiation of Parenteral Nutrient

Parenteral nutrient should be initiated in patients who are at high nutrition risk (i.e., NRS 2002 of 6 or 7 or NUTRIC score ≥6 with IL-6), or severely malnourished, or in whom enteral feeding is not feasible. This strategy improves patient outcome and reduces

mortality risk. The American Society for Parenteral and Enteral Nutrition (ASPEN) offers a vast amount of resources on parenteral nutrition.

Summary

This chapter provides a useful discussion on several critical care guidelines and critical care bundles. They include the key elements of the AHA ACLS guidelines, precautions of crash cart use, PADIS Bundle, and ABCDEF Bundle, as well as nutritional support therapy in critical care settings. It is our hope that the critical care team can enhance patient care by integrating the knowledge and clinical practice from each health profession.

Case Studies

The clinician is called to the intensive care unit (ICU) for an urgent assessment of a mechanically ventilated patient. The patient's radial pulse is 160 beats/min, which matches the sinus rhythm on the cardiac monitor. The SpO_2 is 88%, vital signs are stable, and basic ventilator parameters are within normal limits. As the clinician is further assessing the patient and ventilator, the cardiac rhythm changes to ventricular tachycardia at a rate of 150 beats/min.

1. **What should the clinician do immediately?**
   a. Check for pulse
   b. Perform defibrillation
   c. Perform cardioversion
   d. Perform cardiopulmonary resuscitation

Ms. Greene was admitted to the ICU 3 days ago secondary to a drug overdose. She was comatose, unresponsive, calm, and without spontaneous movements for 2 days. She was intubated upon arrival, but she was

not given sedation to allow for reevaluations of her neurological status.

Today, the patient is agitated and is biting her endotracheal tube. She is restrained because she has tried to extubate herself several times. She does not make eye contact or respond to orders. The ventilator's alarm is constantly ringing.

1. **Is this patient in pain? Please provide justification to support your answer that may include the use of a bedside assessment scale/tool discussed in this chapter.**

2. **What is her level of sedation? Please provide justification to support your answer that may include the use of a bedside assessment scale or tool.**

3. **Is she delirious? Please provide justification to support your answer that may include the use of a bedside assessment scale or tool.**

Bibliography
Adult Advanced Cardiovascular Life Support

American Heart Association. Adult cardiac arrest algorithm. Available at https:// eccguidelines.heart.org/wp-content/uploads/2018/10/ACLS-Cardiac-Arrest-Algorithm-2018.png

Link MS, Berkow LC, Kudenchuk PJ, et al. Part 7: adult advanced cardiovascular life support: 2015 American Heart Association guidelines update for cardiopulmonary resuscitation and emergency cardiovascular care. *Circulation.* 2015;132:S444–464.

Crash Cart

Pennsylvania Patient Safety Authority. Clinical emergency: are you ready in any setting? *Pennsylvania Patient Safety Advisory.* 2010;7(2):52–60.

PADIS Guidelines

Devlin JW, Skrobik Y, Gélinas CR, et al: Executive summary: clinical practice guidelines for the prevention and management of pain, agitation/sedation, delirium, immobility, and sleep disruption in adult patients in the ICU. *Crit Care Med* 46:1532–1548, 2018. doi:10.1097/CCM.0000000000003259.

ABCDEF Bundle

Agency for Healthcare Research and Quality. *Coordinated Spontaneous Awakening and Breathing Trials Protocol.* Rockville, MD: Agency for Healthcare Research and Quality; 2017. Available at http://www.ahrq.gov/professionals/quality-patient-safety/hais/tools/mvp/modules/technical/sat-sbt-protocol.html

Devlin JW, Skrobik Y, Gélinas C, et al. Clinical practice guidelines for the prevention and management of pain, agitation/sedation, delirium, immobility, and sleep disruption in adult patients in the ICU. *Crit Care Med.* 2018;46:825–873.

Girard TD, Kress JP, Fuchs BD, et al. Efficacy and safety of a paired sedation and ventilator weaning protocol for mechanically ventilated patients in intensive care (awakening and breathing controlled trial): a randomised controlled trial. *Lancet.* 2008;371:126–134.

Inouye SK, van Dyck CH, Alessi CA, et al. Clarifying confusion: the confusion assessment method. *Ann Intern Med.* 1990;113:941–948.

Mayo Clinics. Delirium. Available at https://www.mayoclinic.org/diseases-conditions/delirium/symptoms-causes/syc-20371386

Payen J, Bru O, Bosson J, et al. Assessing pain in critically ill sedated patients by using a behavioral pain scale. *Crit Care Med.* 2001;29:2258–2263.

Pun BT. ABCDEF Bundle. Society of Critical Care Medicine. Available at http:// www.sccm.org/ICULiberation/ABCDEF-Bundles. Published 2018.

Zein H, Baratloo A, Negidal A, et al. Ventilator weaning and spontaneous breathing trials; an educational review. *Emergency.* 2016;4:65–71.

Nutritional Support Therapy

McClave SA, Taylor BE, Martindale RG, et al. Guidelines for the provision and assessment of nutrition support therapy in the adult critically ill patient: Society of Critical Care Medicine (SCCM) and American Society for Parenteral and Enteral Nutrition (A.S.P.E.N.). *J Parenteral Enteral Nutr.* 2016;40:159–211.

Surgical Critical Care. ICU enteral feeding guidelines (revised 2017). Available at http://www.surgicalcriticalcare.net/Guidelines/ICU%20nutrition%202017.pdf

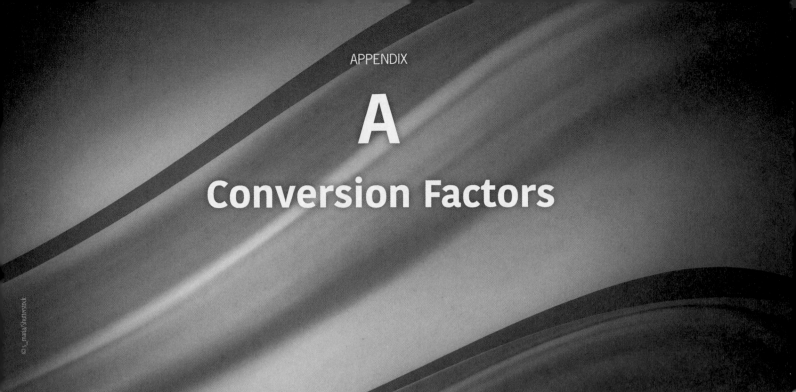

A

Conversion Factors

Parameter	Conversion Factor
Temperature	Centigrade to Fahrenheit: °C = (°F − 32) × 5/9 Fahrenheit to Centigrade: °F = (°C × 9/5) + 32
Pressure	1 mm Hg = 1.36 cm H_2O 1 cm H_2O = 0.74 mm Hg 1 atmosphere at sea level = 760 mm Hg, 1033 cm H_2O, 14.7 psig, or 101.325 kPa
Length	inch to centimeter: 1 in = 2.54 cm centimeter to inch: 1 cm = 0.394 in millimeter to French: 1 mm = 3 Fr French to millimeter: 1 Fr = 0.33 mm
Weight	kilogram to pound: 1 kg = 2.2 lb pound to kilogram: 1 lb = 0.454 kg
Energy	1 joule = 1 watt · sec 1 joule = 0.1 kilogram-force · meter

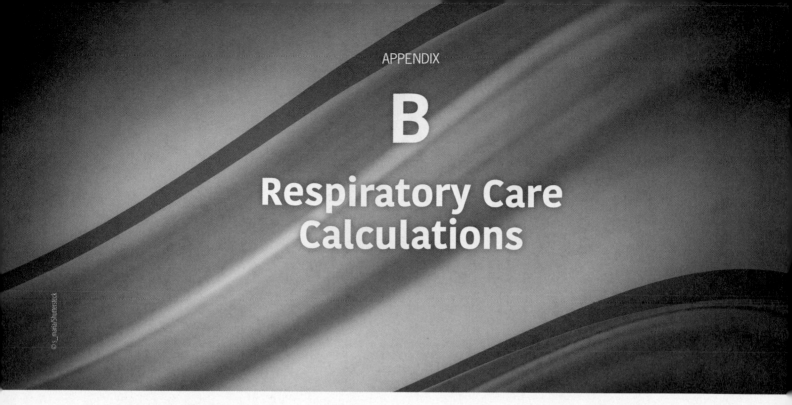

B
Respiratory Care Calculations

Airway Resistance: Estimated (Raw)

Equation

$$Raw = \frac{(PIP - Pplat)}{Flow}$$

Raw   : Airway resistance in cm H_2O/L/sec
PIP   : Peak inspiratory pressure in cm H_2O
Pplat   : Plateau pressure in cm H_2O (static pressure)
Flow   : Flow rate in L/sec

Normal Value

0.6 to 2.4 cm H_2O/L/sec at flow rate of 0.5 L/sec (30 L/min). If the patient is intubated, use serial measurements to establish trend.

Alveolar-Arterial O_2 Tension Gradient: $P(A–a)O_2$

Equation $P(A–a)O_2 = PAO_2 - PaO_2$

$P(A–a)O_2$: Alveolar-arterial oxygen tension gradient in mm Hg
PAO_2 : Alveolar oxygen tension in mm Hg
PaO_2 : Arterial oxygen tension in mm Hg

Normal Value

(1) On *room air*, the $P(A–a)O_2$ should be less than 4 mm Hg for every 10 years in age. For example, the $P(A–a)O_2$ should be less than 24 mm Hg for a 60-year-old patient.

(2) On *100% oxygen*, every 50 mm Hg difference in $P(A–a)O_2$ approximates 2% shunt.

Anion Gap

Equation   Anion gap = $Na^+ - (Cl^- + HCO_3^-)$

Na^+ : Serum sodium concentration in mEq/L
Cl^- : Serum chloride concentration in mEq/L
HCO_3^- : Serum bicarbonate concentration in mEq/L

Normal Values

10 to 14 mEq/L

15 to 20 mEq/L if potassium (K^+) is included in the equation

Arterial/Alveolar Oxygen Tension (a/A) Ratio

Equation $a/A\ ratio = \dfrac{PaO_2}{PAO_2}$

a/A ratio   : Arterial/alveolar oxygen tension ratio in percent
PaO_2 : Arterial oxygen tension in mm Hg
PAO_2 : Alveolar oxygen tension in mm Hg

Normal Value

>60%

Arterial-Mixed Venous Oxygen Content Difference [$C(a - \bar{v})O_2$]

Equation $\quad C(a - \bar{v})O_2 = CaO_2 - C\bar{v}O_2$

$C(a - \bar{v})O_2$: Arterial–mixed venous oxygen content difference in vol%

CaO_2 : Arterial oxygen content in vol%

$C\bar{v}O_2$: Mixed venous oxygen content in vol%

Normal Values

5 vol% for spontaneously breathing patients
3 to 5 vol% for patients on mechanical ventilation

Cardiac Index (CI)

Equation $\quad CI = \dfrac{CO}{BSA}$

CI : Cardiac index in L/min/m^2
CO : Cardiac output in L/min ($\dot{Q}T$)
BSA : Body surface area in m^2

Normal Value

2.5 to 3.5 L/min/m^2

Cardiac Output (CO): Fick's Estimated Method

Equation 1 $\quad CO = \dfrac{O_2 \text{ consumption}}{CaO_2 - C\bar{v}O_2}$

Equation 2 $\quad CO = \dfrac{130 \times BSA}{CaO_2 - C\bar{v}O_2}$

CO : Cardiac output in L/min; same as total perfusion ($\dot{Q}T$)

O_2 consumption : Estimated to be $130 \times BSA$, in mL/min ($\dot{V}O_2$)

CaO_2 : Arterial oxygen content in vol%

$C\bar{v}O_2$: Mixed venous oxygen content in vol%

130 : Estimated O_2 consumption rate of an adult, in mL/min/m^2

BSA : Body surface area in m^2

Normal Value

4 to 8 L/min

Cerebral Perfusion Pressure

Equation $\quad CPP = MAP - ICP$

CPP : Cerebral perfusion pressure
MAP : Mean arterial pressure
ICP : Intracranial pressure

Normal Value

70 to 80 mm Hg

Compliance: Dynamic (Cdyn)

Equation $\quad Cdyn = \dfrac{\Delta V}{\Delta P}$

Cdyn : Dynamic compliance in mL/cm H$_2$O
ΔV : Corrected tidal volume in mL
ΔP : Pressure change (PIP – PEEP) in cm H$_2$O

Normal Value

30 to 40 mL/cm H$_2$O

If the patient is intubated, use serial measurements to establish trend.

Compliance: Static (Cst)

Equation $\quad Cst = \dfrac{\Delta V}{\Delta P}$

Cst : Static compliance in mL/cm H$_2$O
ΔV : Corrected tidal volume in mL
ΔP : Pressure change (Pplat – PEEP) in cm H$_2$O

Normal Value

40 to 60 mL/cm H$_2$O

If the patient is intubated, use serial measurements to establish trend.

Compliance: Total (CT)

Equation $\quad \dfrac{1}{C_T} = \dfrac{1}{C_L} + \dfrac{1}{Ccw}$

$\dfrac{1}{C_T}$: Reciprocal of total compliance (lung and chest wall)

$\dfrac{1}{C_L}$: Reciprocal of lung compliance

$\dfrac{1}{Ccw}$: Reciprocal of chest wall compliance

Dead Space to Tidal Volume Ratio (V_D/V_T)

Equation $\quad \dfrac{V_D}{V_T} = \dfrac{(Pa_{CO_2} - P\bar{E}_{CO_2})}{Pa_{CO_2}}$

$\dfrac{V_D}{V_T}$: Dead space to tidal volume ratio in %

Pa_{CO_2} : Arterial carbon dioxide tension in mm Hg

$P\bar{E}_{CO_2}$: Mixed expired carbon dioxide tension in mm Hg*

Normal Values

20 to 40% in patients breathing spontaneously
40 to 60% in intubated patients receiving mechanical ventilation

I:E Ratio

Equation $\quad I:E = \left(\dfrac{I\ time}{I\ time} \right) : \left(\dfrac{E\ time}{I\ time} \right)$

Normal Values

1:2 to 1:4

Mean Airway Pressure ($\bar{P}aw$)

Equation $\bar{P}aw = \left[\dfrac{f \times I\ time}{60} \right] \times (PIP - PEEP) + PEEP$

(Pressure-controlled or constant pressure ventilation)

$\bar{P}aw = 0.5 \left[\dfrac{f \times I\ time}{60} \right] \times (PIP - PEEP) + PEEP$

(Constant flow ventilation)

$\bar{P}aw$: Mean airway pressure in cm H_2O
f : Frequency/min
I time : Inspiratory time in sec
PIP : Peak inspiratory pressure in cm H_2O
PEEP : Positive end-expiratory pressure in cm H_2O

Normal Value

<30 cm H_2O during mechanical ventilation

Mean Arterial Pressure (MAP)

Equation $\quad MAP = \dfrac{BP_{systolic} + 2\ BP_{diastolic}}{3}$

MAP : Mean arterial pressure in mm Hg
$BP_{systolic}$: Systolic blood pressure in mm Hg
$BP_{diastolic}$: Diastolic blood pressure in mm Hg

Normal Value

>60 mm Hg

Minute Ventilation

Equation 1

Expired Minute Ventilation

$$\dot{V}_E = V_T \times f$$

Equation 2

Alveolar Minute Ventilation

$$\dot{V}_A = (V_T - V_D) \times f$$

Equation 3

Minute Ventilation in Intermittent Mandatory Ventilation

$$\dot{V}_E = (V_T\ mech \times f\ mech) + (V_T \times f)$$

$\dot{V}_E$: Expired minute ventilation in L/min
$\dot{V}_A$: Alveolar minute ventilation in L/min
V_T : Spontaneous tidal volume in mL
$V_T\ mech$: Ventilator tidal volume in mL
f : Spontaneous frequency/min
f mech : Ventilator frequency/min
V_D : Dead space volume in mL

Oxygen:Air (O_2:Air) Entrainment Ratio and Total Flow

Equation 1

O_2:Air Entrainment Ratio

$$O_2:air = 1 : \dfrac{100 - F_{IO_2}}{F_{IO_2} - 21}$$

O_2:air : Oxygen:air entrainment ratio
F_{IO_2} : Fraction (concentration) of inspired oxygen in %

---

* $P\bar{E}_{CO_2}$ is measured by analyzing the P_{CO_2} of a sample of expired gas collected on the exhalation port of the ventilator circuit or via a one-way valve for spontaneously breathing patients. A 5-L bag can be used for sample collection. To prevent contamination of the gas sample, sigh breaths should not be included in this sample, and exhaled gas should be completely isolated from the patient circuit. The Pa_{CO_2} is measured by analyzing an arterial blood gas sample obtained while collecting the exhaled gas sample.

Equation 2
Total Flow of O_2:Air Entrainment Device

$$\text{Total Flow} = \text{Sum of } O_2\text{:Air Ratio} \times \text{Oxygen Flow}$$

Total flow : Oxygen flow + Air entrained
Sum of O_2:Air ratio : O_2 + Air
Oxygen flow : Oxygen flow on the O_2:air entrainment device

Oxygen Consumption ($\dot{V}_{O_2}$) and Index ($\dot{V}_{O_2}$ index)

Equation 1 $\quad \dot{V}_{O_2} = \dot{Q}_T \times C(a - \bar{v})_{O_2}$

Equation 2 $\quad \dot{V}_{O_2} \text{ index} = \dfrac{\dot{V}_{O_2}}{BSA}$

$\dot{V}_{O_2}$: Oxygen consumption in mL/min; same as oxygen uptake
$\dot{V}_{O_2}$ index : Oxygen consumption index in L/min/m^2
$\dot{Q}_T$: Total perfusion; same as cardiac output (CO) in L/min
$C(a - \bar{v})_{O_2}$: Arterial–mixed venous oxygen content difference in vol%
BSA : Body surface area in m^2

Normal Values

$\dot{V}_{O_2}$ = 200 to 350 mL/min
$\dot{V}_{O_2}$ index = 125 to 165 mL/min/m^2

Oxygen Content: Arterial (Ca_{O_2})

Equation $\quad Ca_{O_2} = (Hb \times 1.34 \times Sa_{O_2}) + (Pa_{O_2} \times 0.003)$

Ca_{O_2} : Arterial oxygen content in vol%
Hb : Hemoglobin content in g%
1.34 : Amount of oxygen in 1 g of fully saturated hemoglobin
Sa_{O_2} : Arterial oxygen saturation in %
Pa_{O_2} : Arterial oxygen tension in mm Hg
0.003 : Amount of dissolved oxygen for 1 mm Hg of Pa_{O_2} in vol%

Normal Value

16 to 20 vol%

Oxygen Content: End-Capillary (Cc_{O_2})

Equation $\quad Cc_{O_2} = (Hb \times 1.34 \times Sa_{O_2}) + (Pa_{O_2} \times 0.003)$

Cc_{O_2} : End-capillary oxygen content in vol%
Hb : Hemoglobin content in g%

1.34 : Amount of oxygen in 1 g of fully saturated hemoglobin
Sa_{O_2} : Arterial oxygen saturation in % (100%)
Pa_{O_2} : Alveolar oxygen tension in mm Hg, used in place of end-capillary P_{O_2} (Pc_{O_2})
0.003 : Amount of dissolved oxygen for 1 mm Hg of Pa_{O_2}

Normal Value

Varies according to the hemoglobin level and the $F_{I_{O_2}}$.

Oxygen Content: Mixed Venous ($C\bar{v}_{O_2}$)

Equation $\quad C\bar{v}_{O_2} = (Hb \times 1.34 \times S\bar{v}_{O_2}) + (P\bar{v}_{O_2} \times 0.003)$

$C\bar{v}_{O_2}$: Mixed venous oxygen content in vol%
Hb : Hemoglobin content in g%
1.34 : Amount of oxygen in 1 g of fully saturated hemoglobin
$S\bar{v}_{O_2}$: Mixed venous oxygen saturation in %
$P\bar{v}_{O_2}$: Mixed venous oxygen tension in mm Hg
0.003 : Amount of dissolved oxygen for 1 mm Hg of $P\bar{v}_{O_2}$

Normal Value

12 to 15 vol%

Oxygen Extraction Ratio (O_2ER)

Equation $\quad O_2ER = \dfrac{Ca_{O_2} - C\bar{v}_{O_2}}{Ca_{O_2}}$

O_2ER : Oxygen extraction ratio in %
Ca_{O_2} : Arterial oxygen content in vol%
$C\bar{v}_{O_2}$: Mixed venous oxygen content in vol%

Normal Value

20% to 28%

P/F Ratio

Equation $\quad P/F = Pa_{O_2}/F_{I_{O_2}}$

P/F : $Pa_{O_2}/F_{I_{O_2}}$ ratio (index) in mm Hg
Pa_{O_2} : Partial pressure of oxygen in arterial blood, in mm Hg
$F_{I_{O_2}}$: Inspired oxygen concentration in %

Normal Value

>300 mm Hg

pH (Henderson-Hasselbalch)

Equation 1 $$pH = 6.1 + \log\left[\frac{HCO_3^-}{H_2CO_3}\right]$$

Equation 2 $$pH = 6.1 + \log\left[\frac{HCO_3^-}{P_{CO_2} \times 0.03}\right]$$

pH   : Puissance hydrogen, negative logarithm of H^+ ion concentration
HCO_3^- : Serum bicarbonate concentration in mEq/L
H_2CO_3 : Carbonic acid in mEq/L
P_{CO_2} : Carbon dioxide tension in mm Hg

Normal Values

Arterial pH   = 7.40 (7.35 to 7.45)
Mixed venous pH = 7.36

Shunt Equation ($Q_{SP}/\dot{Q}_T$): Classic Physiologic

Equation $$\frac{Q_{SP}}{\dot{Q}_T} = \frac{C_{CO_2} - C_{aO_2}}{C_{CO_2} - C\overline{v}_{O_2}}$$

$Q_{SP}/\dot{Q}_T$: Physiologic shunt to total perfusion ratio in %
C_{CO_2} : End-capillary oxygen content in vol%
C_{aO_2} : Arterial oxygen content in vol%
$C\overline{v}_{O_2}$: Mixed venous oxygen content in vol%

Normal Value

Less than 10%

Shunt Equation ($Q_{SP}/\dot{Q}_T$): Estimated

Equation 1

For individuals who are breathing spontaneously with or without CPAP:

$$\frac{Q_{SP}}{\dot{Q}_T} = \frac{C_{CO_2} - C_{aO_2}}{5 + (C_{CO_2} - C_{aO_2})}$$

Equation 2

For critically ill patients who are receiving mechanical ventilation with or without PEEP:

$$\frac{Q_{SP}}{\dot{Q}_T} = \frac{C_{CO_2} - C_{aO_2}}{3.5 + (C_{CO_2} - C_{aO_2})}$$

$Q_{SP}/\dot{Q}_T$: Physiologic shunt to total perfusion ratio in %
C_{CO_2} : End-capillary oxygen content in vol%
C_{aO_2} : Arterial oxygen content in vol%

Normal Value

Less than 10%

Stroke Work: Left Ventricular (LVSW) and Index (LVSWI)

Equation 1 (LVSW)

$$LVSW = (MAP - PAOP) \times SV \times 0.0136$$

Equation 2 (LVSWI)

$$LVSWI = \frac{LVSW}{BSA}$$

LVSW   : Left ventricular stroke work in $g \cdot m/beat$
LVSWI : Left ventricular stroke work index in $g \cdot m/beat/m^2$
MAP   : Mean arterial pressure in mm Hg
PAOP   : Pulmonary artery occlusion pressure in mm Hg
SV   : Stroke volume in mL
BSA   : Body surface area in m^2

Normal Values

LVSW = 60 to 80 $g \cdot m/beat$
LVSWI = 40 to 60 $g \cdot m/beat/m^2$

Stroke Work: Right Ventricular (RVSW) and Index (RVSWI)

Equation 1 (RVSW)

$$RVSW = (\overline{PA} - \overline{RA}) \times SV \times 0.0136$$

Equation 2 (RVSWI)

$$RVSWI = \frac{RVSW}{BSA}$$

RVSW   : Right ventricular stroke work in $g \cdot m/beat$
RVSWI : Right ventricular stroke work index in $g \cdot m/beat/m^2$)
$\overline{PA}$: Mean pulmonary artery pressure in mm Hg
$\overline{RA}$: Mean right atrial pressure (central venous pressure) in mm Hg
SV   : Stroke volume in mL
BSA   : Body surface area in m^2

Normal Values

RVSW = 10 to 15 $g \cdot m/beat$
RVSWI = 7 to 12 $g \cdot m/beat/m^2$

Vascular Resistance: Pulmonary

Equation $\qquad PVR = (\overline{PA} - PCWP) \times \dfrac{80}{CO}$

PVR : Pulmonary vascular resistance in dyne · sec/cm^5
$\overline{PA}$: Mean pulmonary artery pressure in mm Hg
PCWP : Pulmonary capillary wedge pressure in mm Hg
80 : Conversion factor from mm Hg/L/min to dyne · sec/cm^5
CO : Cardiac output in L/min ($\dot{Q}_T$)

Normal Value

50 to 150 dyne · sec/cm^5

Vascular Resistance: Systemic

Equation $\qquad SVR = \left(MAP - \overline{RA}\right) \times \dfrac{80}{CO}$

SVR : Systemic vascular resistance in dyne · sec/cm^5
$\underline{MAP}$: Mean arterial pressure in mm Hg
$\overline{RA}$: Mean right atrial pressure in mm Hg, same as central venous pressure (CVP)
80 : Conversion factor from mm Hg/L/min to dyne · sec/cm^5
CO : Cardiac output in L/min ($\dot{Q}_T$)

Normal Value

800 to 1500 dyne · sec/cm^5

Weaning Index: Rapid Shallow Breathing (RSBI)

Equation $\qquad RSBI = f/V_T$

RSBI : Rapid shallow breathing index, in breaths/ min/L or cycles/L
f : Spontaneous frequency in breaths/min (cycles)
V_T : Spontaneous tidal volume, in L

Normal Value

≤100 breaths/min/L or cycles/L
(rounded from <103 breaths/min/L)

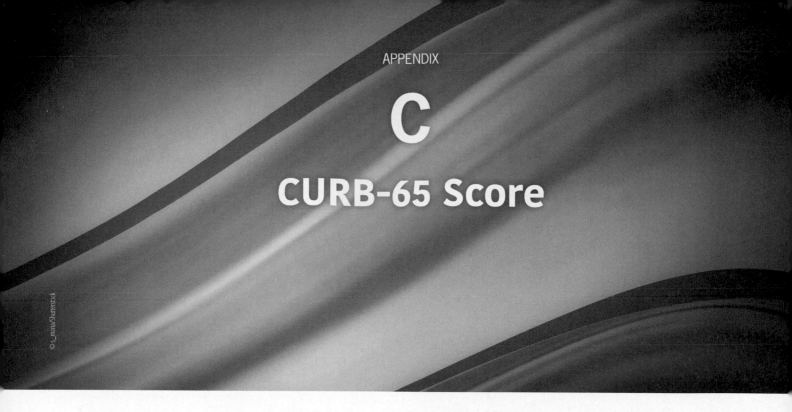

C

CURB-65 Score

CURB-65 is a scoring method for evaluation of severity of community-acquired pneumonia. The score may be used to estimate risk of death and suggested treatment plan.

CURB-65 Criterion	Yes	No
Confusion (mental test score ≤8; disorientation of person, place or time)	1	0
Urea (BUN) >20 mg/dL or >7 mmol/L	1	0
Spontaneous respiratory frequency ≥30/min	1	0
Blood pressure (SBP <90 mm Hg or DBP ≤60 mm Hg)	1	0
Age ≥65 years	1	0

BUN, blood urea nitrogen; DBP, diastolic blood pressure; SBP, systolic blood pressure.

Modified from CURB-65 Score for Pneumonia Severity. Available at https://www.mdcalc.com/curb-65-score-pneumonia-severity; https://reference.medscape.com/calculator/curb-65-pneumonia-severity-score

Interpretation

Point	Risk of Death	Treatment
0–1	Low	Home treatment
2	Moderate	Hospital supervised or outpatient
3–4	High	Inpatient treatment
5	High	Inpatient treatment with possible ICU admission

ICU, intensive care unit.

Modified from CURB-65 Score for Pneumonia Severity. Available at https://www.mdcalc.com/curb-65-score-pneumonia-severity; https://reference.medscape.com/calculator/curb-65-pneumonia-severity-score

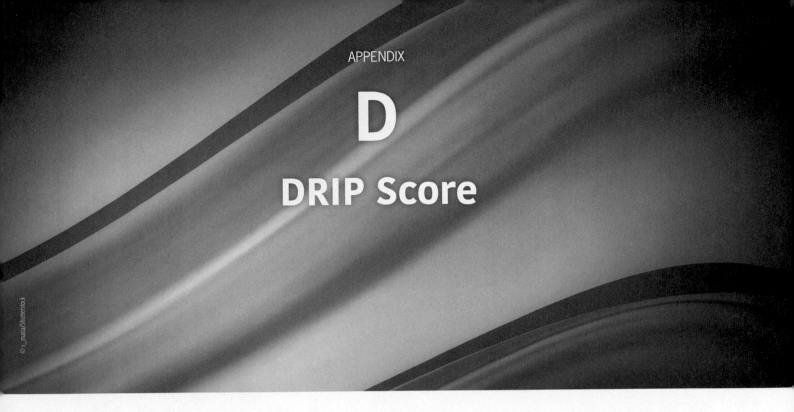

D
DRIP Score

Drug resistance in pneumonia (DRIP) score evaluates risk for community-acquired pneumonia due to drug-resistant pathogens.

Major Risk Factor	Points
Antibiotic use within 60 days	2
Long-term care resident (not including assisted living or group home)	2
Tube feeding (nasogastric, nasojejunal, or percutaneous endoscopic gastrostomy)	2
Drug-resistant pneumonia within last year	2
Hospitalization within 60 days	1
Chronic pulmonary disease	1
Poor function status, Karnofsky score* of <70 or non-ambulatory	1
H2 blocker or proton pump inhibitor (PPI) use within 14 days	1
Active wound care	1
Methicillin-resistant *Staphylococcus aureus* (MRSA) colonization within 1 year	1
Total points**	

*Karnofsky score of 70 = Basic care for self but unable to carry on normal activity or to do active work.
**Total points of ≥4 suggests high risk of drug-resistant pneumonia and extended-spectrum antibiotic coverage is recommended.

Reproduced from Webb BJ, Dascomb K, Stenehjem E, et al. Derivation and multicenter validation of the drug resistance in pneumonia clinical prediction score. *Antimicrob Agents Chemother.* 2016;60(5):2652–2663. doi: 10.1128/AAC.03071-15

E

Multiple Organ Dysfunction Score (MODS)

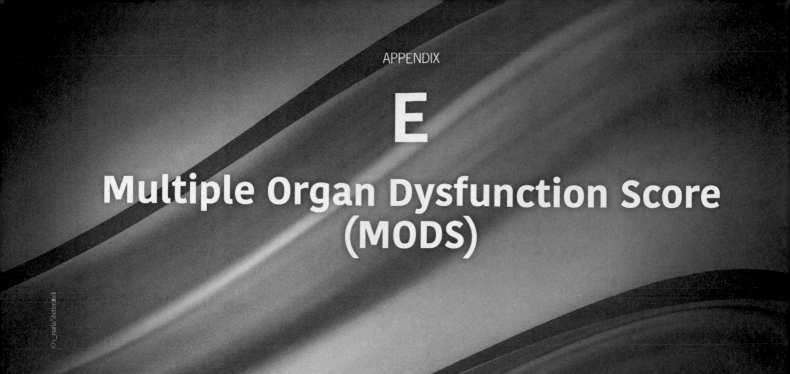

The MODS is used to estimate the ICU and hospital mortality rates in critically ill patients.

Organ System/Points	0	1	2	3	4
Respiratory (P/F), mm Hg	>300	226–300	151–225	76–150	<75
Renal (serum creatinine), mmol/L	≤100	101–200	201–350	351–500	>500
Hepatic (serum bilirubin), mmol/L	≤20	21–60	61–120	121–240	>240
Cardiovascular (R/P ratio)*	≤10	10.1–15	15.1–20	20.1–30	30
Hematologic (platelet count)	>120	81–120	51–80	21–50	≤20
Neurologic (Glasgow Coma Scale score)	15	13–14	10–12	7–9	≤6

*R/P ratio = (Heart rate × Central venous pressure) / Mean blood pressure
Reproduced from Marshall JC, Cook DJ, Christou, NV, et al. Multiple Organ Dysfunction Score: A reliable descriptor of a complex clinical outcome. *Crit Care Med.* 1995;23(10):1638–1652.

Interpretation of MODS:

Points	ICU Mortality	Hospital Mortality
0	0%	0%
1–4	1–2%	7%
5–8	3–5%	16%
9–12	25%	50%
13–16	50%	70%
17–20	75%	82%
≥21	100%	100%

Data from Marshall JC, Cook DJ, Christou, NV, et al. Multiple Organ Dysfunction Score: A reliable descriptor of a complex clinical outcome. *Crit Care Med.* 1995;23(10):1638–1652.

F

Systemic Inflammatory Response Syndrome (SIRS), Sepsis, Septic Shock, and Multiple Organ Dysfunction Syndrome (MODS)

The sepsis definitions have been evolving over the years and there is no single gold standard. The criteria for identification of sepsis are difficult to finalize because differences exist among many sepsis definitions. This table should be used as a supplemental tool for the identification of sepsis and related conditions.

Criteria	SIRS (any 2 items below)	Sepsis	Severe Sepsis	Septic Shock	MODS
Temp >38°C or <36° C	Y/N	SIRS + source of infection	Sepsis + lactic acidosis or SBP changes	Severe sepsis + hypotension	Septic shock + ≥2 organs failing
Heart rate >90/min	Y/N				
Respiratory rate >20/min	Y/N				
WBC >12,000/mm³ or <4,000/mm³ or >10% bands	Y/N				
Suspected or present source of infection		Y/N	Y/N	Y/N	Y/N
Lactic acidosis, SBP <90 or SBP decrease by ≥ 40 mm Hg of normal			Y/N	Y/N	Y/N
Hypotension despite fluid resuscitation				Y/N	Y/N
≥2 organs failing					Y/N

SBP, systolic blood pressure; WBC, white blood cell.

Data from Balk RA. SIRS, Sepsis, and Septic Shock Criteria. Available at https://www.mdcalc.com/sirs-sepsis-septic-shock-criteria; Comstedt P, Storgaard M, Lassen AT. The Systemic Inflammatory Response Syndrome (SIRS) in acutely hospitalised medical patients: a cohort study. *Scand J Trauma Resusc Emerg Med.* 2009;27;17:67. doi: 10.1186/1757-7241-17-67

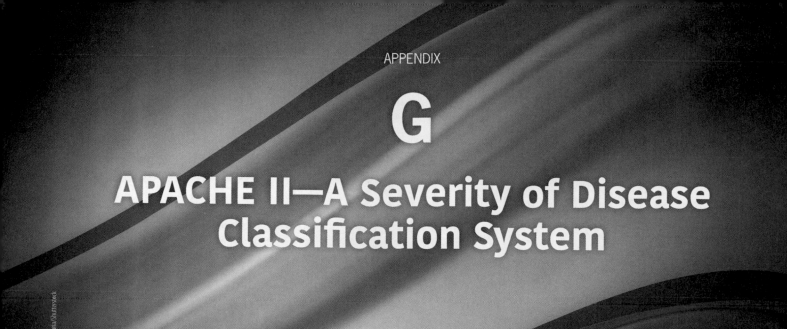

APPENDIX

G

APACHE II—A Severity of Disease Classification System

Patient Data	Significance of Data
Temperature (°C)	Hyperthermia or hypothermia
Mean arterial pressure (mm Hg)	Perfusion
Heart rate (beats/min)	Cardiac output
Respiratory frequency (breaths/min)	Ventilation
Oxygenation Use A-aDo$_2$ if Fio$_2$ ≥0.5 Use Pao$_2$ if Fio$_2$ <0.5	Oxygenation
Arterial pH (preferred) or serum HCO$_3^-$	Acid-base status
Serum sodium (mEq/L)	Electrolyte
Serum potassium (mEq/L)	Electrolyte
Serum creatinine (mg/dL) Double point score for acute renal failure)	Renal function
Hematocrit	Low: anemia, blood loss High: dehydration, polycythemia
White blood cell count (×1000/mm^3)	Infection
Glasgow coma score (GCS)	Brain injury
Age points	
Chronic health points	Comorbidity

Modified from Knaus WA, Draper EA, Wagner DP, Zimmerman JE. APACHE II: a severity of disease classification system. *Crit Care Med.* 1985;13(10): 818–829.

The APACHE II (Acute Physiology, Age, Chronic Health Evaluation II) is a disease severity classification system. This score can be calculated on all patients admitted to the intensive care unit (ICU) and it is a useful tool for mortality risk assessment. To calculate the APACHE II score, the patient data in the table are needed. Input data with this online calculator at https://www.mdcalc.com/apache-ii-score.

Interpretation of APACHE II score:

Total Point Score	Likely Mortality Risk*
0–4	4%
5–9	8%
10–14	15%
15–19	25%
20–24	40%
25–29	55%
30–34	75%
≥35	85%

*The mortality risk should also account for the patient's indication for ICU (intensive care unit) admission.
Modified from Knaus WA, Draper EA, Wagner DP, Zimmerman JE. APACHE II: a severity of disease classification system. *Crit Care Med.* 1985;13(10):818–829.

Glossary

A

ABCDEF Bundle A management strategy for critically ill patients that includes: Assess, Prevent, and Manage Pain, Both Spontaneous Awakening Trials (SAT) and Spontaneous Breathing Trials (SBT), Choice of analgesia and sedation, Delirium: Assess, Prevent, and Manage, Early mobility and Exercise, and Family engagement and empowerment.

absolute shunt A pulmonary condition in which capillary blood flow is not matched by alveolar ventilation (i.e., complete or near complete absence of ventilation), also called true shunt or capillary shunt.

absorption Movement of a drug from the site of administration to the bloodstream.

acute exacerbation of COPD A severe form of COPD characterized by acute airflow obstruction, severe dyspnea and hypoxemia, and increased sputum production.

acute pancreatitis An acute inflammatory of the pancreas associated with severe abdominal pain.

acute renal failure A rapid decline in renal function associated with decreased urine output, hyperkalemia, hyperphosphatemia, hypocalcemia.

acute respiratory distress syndrome A rapid onset of ventilatory failure characterized by refractory hypoxemia, bilateral infiltrates or non-cardiogenic pulmonary edema.

acute ventilatory failure An inability of the respiratory system to adequately eliminate carbon dioxide from the body that develops over a short period of time.

agonists Drugs that stimulate the receptor site, mimicking the body's function.

air leak A clinical phenomenon that is associated with loss of tidal volume.

air trapping An abnormal retention of air in the lungs where it is difficult to exhale completely.

airflow resistance The opposition to flow caused by frictional forces and expressed as the ratio of driving pressure to the rate of gas flow.

airway pressure Pressure applied to the airway during administration of positive pressure ventilation.

airway resistance The resistance of the respiratory tract to airflow during inhalation and expiration.

alveolar-arterial oxygen pressure gradient The difference between the alveolar (calculated) and arterial (measured) oxygen pressures.

amylase A protein mainly produced by the pancreas for breakdown of carbohydrates and starches into sugar.

analgesia Medication that provides pain relief

anion gap A difference between the cations and anions in the blood.

antagonists Drugs that lessen or block a biological response by binding to and blocking a receptor.

antimicrobials Agents that kill microbes or stop their growth.

apnea test Used to monitor a patient to determine if brain death is present.

ARDSNet A research network formed to study the pathophysiology and management strategies of acute respiratory distress syndrome.

arterial catheter A catheter placed into an artery (e.g., radial or brachial artery) for collection of blood gas samples or measurement of arterial blood pressure.

asystole The absence of cardiac electrical conduction.

auto-PEEP An abnormal positive end-expiratory pressure due to incomplete exhalation or persistent air trapping.

B

barbiturate coma Temporary coma (a deep state of unconsciousness) induced by a controlled dose of a barbiturate drug.

barotrauma Damage to lung tissue as a result of rapid or excessive pressure changes. These may occur in patients receiving mechanical ventilation who are subjected to high airway pressures.

baseline variable Describes what occurs between the end of one ventilator breath and the start of the next ventilator breath, or the expiratory phase of ventilation.

Behavioral Pain Scale (BPS) A pain assessment scale ranging from 3 (no pain) to 12 (extreme pain). It is based on the patient's facial expression, upper limbs movement, and compliance with ventilation.

benzodiazepines A commonly used, fairly safe group of drugs that treat anxiety and insomnia.

bilevel positive airway pressure The application of positive airway pressure during inspiration (inspiratory positive airway pressure) and exhalation (expiratory positive airway pressure or baseline pressure) during spontaneous ventilation.

biopsy Collection and analysis of a sample of tissues for determination of the presence or extent of a disease.

Biot's respirations An abnormal breathing pattern associated with CNS disorders that is characterized by clusters of rapid breaths interspersed with periods of apnea.

biovariable targeting This allows the ventilator to adapt its output (tidal volume, for example) to mimic normal physiologic spontaneous ventilation.

blunt chest injury Results from kinetic energy forces and is caused by three very distinct mechanisms: blast, compression, and deceleration.

bradypnea Occurs when the ventilator rate is less than 12/min, such as when weaning in the SIMV mode.

bronchial alveolar lavage A diagnostic procedure by which cells and other components from bronchial and alveolar spaces are washed out and aspirated for various laboratory studies.

bronchoscopy Diagnostic procedure useful in determining severity of airway injury. It can be used to provide a functional washout of the bronchial tree, and could be used for bronchoalveolar lavage.

brushing Collection of samples using a brush at sites where biopsy samples cannot be obtained.

bubble study A technique in which blood flow through the heart can be monitored using echocardiography.

C

caloric test Used to assess the level of trauma to the brain stem using different temperatures to diagnose damage to the acoustic nerve.

capnogram A direct monitor of the exhaled concentration or partial pressure of CO_2, and an indirect monitor of the CO_2 partial pressure in the arterial blood.

carbon monoxide A colorless, odorless, and tasteless flammable gas that is slightly less dense than air.

cardiac tamponade An increased pressure around the heart that occurs when blood or fluid builds up in the space between the myocardium and the pericardium.

carina The point of division of the two main bronchi in the trachea.

central venous catheter A catheter that is placed into the vena cave or right atrium for measurement of right atrial pressure or collection of venous blood sample.

cerebral blood flow The blood supply to the brain in a given period of time.

cerebral herniation Refers to shift of cerebral tissue from its normal location, into an adjacent space as a result of mass effect. It is a life-threatening condition that requires prompt diagnosis.

cerebral perfusion pressure The net pressure gradient between the mean arterial pressure and intracranial pressure.

Cheyne-Stokes respirations An abnormal breathing pattern characterized by periods of progressively increasing then decreasing tidal volume interspersed with periods of apnea, associated with CNS disorders.

chronic ventilator dependence Patients who require mechanical ventilation permanently (i.e., patients with high spinal cord injuries) or for a very long time (i.e., patients who are difficult to wean).

colony-forming units A count of viable bacterial cells in a given volume of sample, expressed in U/L.

computed tomography An imaging procedure that uses special x-ray equipment to create detailed pictures, or scans, of areas inside the body.

Confusion Assessment Method (CAM) A delirium assessment tool. The patient is deemed to have delirium if three clinical features are met: acute change of mental status *and* inattention *plus* altered level of consciousness *or* disorganized thinking.

continuous positive airway pressure (CPAP) The application of positive baseline pressure (pressure is elevated above ambient pressure), during continuous spontaneous ventilation.

control circuit The mechanism the ventilator uses to control its drive mechanism.

control variable A variable that is measured and used as feedback to control the ventilator's output.

Cook catheter A hollow, semirigid type of tube with blunt tips that can be used to exchange an ET tube with a leaking cuff.

CO-oximeter A device that quantifies the levels of dysfunctional Hb, giving a true picture of the patient's oxygenation status.

CO-oximetry Provides the means for automated spectrophotometric measurement of the concentration of total hemoglobin (ctHb) in blood and the percentages of the hemoglobin derivatives that total hemoglobin commonly comprises: oxyhemoglobin, deoxyhemoglobin, carboxyhemoglobin, and methemoglobin.

craniectomy Removal of a portion of the skull.

Critical Care Pain Observation Tool (CPOT) A pain assessment scoring tool ranging from 0 (no pain) to 8 (severe pain). It is based on the patient's facial expression, body movements, muscle tension, and compliance with mechanical ventilation (or verbalization of pain for nonintubated patients).

cuff leak test This test monitors for the presence or absence of airway swelling in a patient with an ET tube

Cushing triad A clinical triad variably defined as having irregular, decreased respirations (caused by impaired brainstem function), and bradycardia.

cycle variable Describes how the ventilator changes from inspiration to exhalation. Cycle variables may include pressure, volume, and time.

cytology A study of cells.

D

dead space ventilation The portion of tidal volume that does not take part in gas exchange. It is also called *wasted ventilation* or *ventilation in excess of perfusion*. Dead space ventilation has three distinct types: anatomic, alveolar, and physiologic.

decompensated heart failure A sudden worsening of the signs and symptoms of heart failure characterized by hypoxemia, pedal edema or pulmonary edema.

decremental recruitment maneuver A method of titration for optimal PEEP by setting a high CPAP (and PEEP) and gradually decreasing the pressure and F_{IO_2}.

deep vein thrombosis (DVT) A blood clot in the veins, most commonly in the leg or pelvis.

distribution Movement of a drug from the bloodstream to the tissues/cells.

diuretics Medications that block reabsorption of sodium and water in the nephron, which increases urine output (UO) and depletes blood volume (reducing cardiac output (CO) and lowering blood pressure).

Doll's eyes test A test to monitor the extent of injury in patients with head trauma is the test of the vestibulo-ocular reflex, commonly called the doll's eyes test. Normally, when the head is moved from side to side, the eyes deviate to the opposite side of the head and then gradually move midline. When the head is move upward, the eyes deviate down and vice versa.

drive mechanism Describes the method used by the ventilator to convert the input power into ventilatory work.

dry suction systems A type of chest tube drainage system (without a water seal chamber) where fluids drain from the patient directly into a large collection chamber via a 6-foot patient tube.

dynamic compliance The change in volume for a given unit of applied pressure when gas is moving in the respiratory system (usually measured just before the end of inspiration).

E

early mobility A procedure that provides a range of physical activities to the critically ill patient.

elimination Removal of drugs and their metabolites from the body, primarily by the kidneys.

endotracheal intubation Placement of an artificial airway into the trachea to maintain a patent airway.

endotracheal tube A flexible plastic tube that is placed through the airway opening into the trachea to connect to a mechanical ventilator and help a patient breathe.

enteral nutrition Feeding via the oral or gastrointestinal route.

epiglottis A leaf-shaped structure in the throat that prevents food from entering the trachea when swallowing, protecting the lungs from aspiration.

esophageal pressure An indirect measurement of pleural pressure obtained from a catheter inserted into the esophagus.

eustachian tube A canal that connects the nasopharynx with the middle ear.

external ventricular drain A small catheter inserted through the skull, usually into the lateral ventricle, which is typically connected to a closed collecting device to allow for drainage of cerebrospinal fluid and can record intracranial pressure.

extracorporeal CPR A method of cardiopulmonary life support outside the body using a machine that provides perfusion and oxygenation.

extubation The process of removing an endotracheal tube from an intubated patient.

F

fentanyl (Duragesic) An opioid used as a pain medication.

flail chest A condition in which there are at least two fractures per rib (producing a free segment) in at least two ribs.

flexible bronchoscopy A procedure that provides visual images of the airways and it allows collection of a clinician to examine the breathing passages (airways) of the lungs.

flow controller If during inspiration the volume delivery remains unchanged when patient resistance and compliance change, and if volume is not measured and used to control the ventilator's output, it is classified as a flow controller.

flow triggering Breath triggering when a patient's inspiratory flow meets a flow threshold.

focused abdominal sonography for trauma A rapid ultrasound examination performed in patients who are hemodynamically unstable to identify potentially life-threatening hemorrhages in the peritoneal, pericardial, or thoracic space.

forceps An instrument used for grasping and holding objects.

G

gastric residual volume A procedure to measure the gastric volume at different time intervals to determine the patient's tolerance to enteral feeding.

Glasgow Coma Scale The most common scoring system used to describe the level of consciousness in a person following a traumatic brain injury.

H

Heimlich valve A rubber flutter one-way valve within a rigid plastic tube that connects to a standard chest drainage system.

hemorrhagic stroke Brain injury caused by rupture of cerebral blood vessels.

hemothorax A collection of blood in the pleural space. It may result from direct blunt trauma to the chest or by any object that penetrates the chest cavity (penetrating chest injury).

hepatic failure The inability of the liver to perform its normal metabolic functions.

high-frequency percussive ventilation Combines diffusive (high-frequency mini-bursts) and convective ventilation patterns. Benefits include enhanced oxygenation and hemodynamics, and alveolar recruitment, while providing lung-protective ventilation.

hydrogen cyanide A chemical compound with the chemical formula HCN. It is a colorless, extremely poisonous, and flammable liquid that boils slightly above room temperature, at 25.6°C.

hypoxemia A lower than normal level of oxygen in blood (typically arterial blood).

hypoxia A lack of sufficient oxygen in the tissues or organs.

hypoxic-ischemic encephalopathy brain injury caused by lack of circulation or oxygen to the cerebral circulation.

hysteresis Surface tension and frictional forces contribute to differences in the shape of the PVL during expansion and deflation. This difference results from one measured variable changing at a faster rate than another plotted against it, referred to as hysteresis.

I

I:E ratio The ratio of time spent in inspiration to the time spent in expiration.

impending ventilatory failure A situation in which a patient may still be within normal ranges for blood gas values (usually marginal) but is progressing to ventilatory failure because of significant effort required to overcome increased WOB with blood gas values trending toward $Paco_2$ >50 mm Hg and a pH <7.25.

inotropic Modifying the myocardial strength of contraction (myocardial contractility).

intelligent targeting Automatically adjusts ventilator set points using rule-based systems.

intracranial pressure The pressure inside the skull and thus reflects the pressure in the brain tissue and cerebrospinal fluid.

intraosseous (IO) access A route similar to intravenous access that can be used to provide fluids, medications or blood draw through the bone marrow.

intraosseous infusion The process of providing fluid directly into the marrow of a bone.

intrapulmonary shunting A condition in which blood flowing through a lung area is exposed to under-ventilated or unventilated alveoli, resulting in significant hypoxemia (an extreme ventilation-perfusion mismatch).

ischemic stroke Brain injury caused by reduction of blood flow to the brain due to constriction of cerebral blood vessels.

J

jaundice A yellow discoloration of the skin, mucous membranes, and the whites of the eyes caused by increased amounts of bilirubin in the blood.

K

ketamine A medication typically used for starting and maintaining anesthesia.

L

laryngoscope An instrument that is used to obtain a view of the vocal cords and the glottis to facilitate endotracheal intubation.

likelihood ratio An expression of the odds that a given test result will be present in a patient with a given condition, compared to a patient without the condition (for ventilator weaning, greater likelihood of success above one and greater likelihood of failure below one).

limit variable A variable that increases and then plateaus or stops increasing during inspiration.

loops Formed by plotting inspiratory and expiratory curves of two of these three variables: pressure, flow, volume. There are two loops routinely available for interpretation: pressure-volume (i.e., compliance) loop and flow-volume loop.

M

Macintosh blade A **laryngoscope blade** that is curved with a tip that is inserted into the vallecula (the space between the base of the tongue and the pharyngeal surface of the epiglottis).

Mallampati classification An assessment used to predict the ease of endotracheal intubation. It involves a visual assessment of the distance from the tongue base to the roof of the mouth, to estimate the difficulty of endotracheal intubation.

mandatory breath A breath for which the machine triggers and/or cycles the breath.

mass casualty An unexpected situation in which the large number of severely injured or deaths exceeds the capacity of acute care centers to respond in a timely manner.

maximal expiratory pressure (MEP) The positive pressure measured during a maximal expiratory effort by a patient against an occluded airway. It serves as an indicator of the strength of respiratory muscles used to clear the airway.

maximal inspiratory pressure (MIP) The negative pressure measured during a maximal inspiratory effort by a patient against an occluded airway. It serves as an indicator of inspiratory muscle strength.

mechanical insufflation-exsufflation A non-invasive ventilation technique that uses adjustable positive and negative pressures during a respiratory cycle.

medical futility Medical procedures/interventions that are unlikely to produce any meaningful benefit to a given patient.

metabolism The Chemical processes that occur in living organisms in order to maintain life.

methemoglobinemia A form of dysfunctional hemoglobin caused by an elevated level of methemoglobin in the blood.

midazolam (Versed) A benzodiazepine used for anesthesia, procedural sedation, and relief of anxiety.

Miller blade A laryngoscope blade that is straight. The tip is passed over the epiglottis so that it can be lifted to expose the vocal cords.

mini-bronchoalveolar lavage A blind, non-bronchoscopic procedure to obtain a wash-out sample from the lungs.

Moro reflex An infantile reflex that develops between 28 and 32 weeks of gestation and disappears between 3 and 6 months of age. It is a startle reflex that is also seen when infants are overstimulated or stressed. The arms fly out to the side and then return to the side when the infant relaxes.

MRI conditional This term is applied to devices that pose no known hazards in a specific *MRI* environment under certain device and *MRI* scanner conditions.

MRI safe A term to describe the equipment or device that poses no hazards in an MRI environment.

N

N-acetylcysteine A medication well-known as a mucolytic that is used to treat paracetamol (acetaminophen) overdose.

nebulized heparin Therapeutic use of heparin to the airways when smoke inhalation occurs that exerts a local anticoagulant effect in the lungs and without significant systemic effects.

neurally adjusted ventilatory assist (NAVA®) A proportional ventilatory mode that uses the electrical activity of the diaphragm to offer ventilatory assistance in proportion to patient effort.

neuromuscular blocking agents Drugs that interrupt transmission of nerve impulses at the skeletal neuromuscular junction, causing paralysis. They can be nondepolarizing or depolarizing.

non-invasive ventilation A technique of ventilation without using an artificial airway.

non-tension pneumothorax A nonexpanding collection of air in the pleural space where the lung is collapsed, to a variable extent.

numerical rating scale (NRS) An interval scale for the patient to report perception of pain, ranging from 0 (no pain) to 10 (extreme pain).

nutritional bundle A strategy to provide appropriate nutrition to critically ill patients. It includes six categories ranging from assessment of need to initiation of parenteral nutrient.

nutritional risk screening (NRS 2002) A tool to determine levels of malnutrition, ≤ 3 (no nutritional risk), 4 or 5 (nutritional risk), 6 or 7 (high nutritional risk).

O

operative tube thoracostomy A technique of placing a chest tube by dissection into the pleura, digitally inspecting the pleural space, and insertion guided with the finger and hemostat.

opioids Class of drugs used to treat moderate to severe pain. Medically they are primarily used for pain relief, including anesthesia.

optimal targeting Allows a ventilator set-point to be adjusted to optimize another ventilator set-point.

oscillatory ventilation A type of mechanical ventilation that uses a constant mean airway pressure with pressure variations oscillating around the MAP at high rates. It is the only type of ventilation with an active expiratory phase.

overdistention Excessive stretching, insufflation, or inflation of the lung.

oxygenation failure Severe hypoxemia due to any condition (i.e., high altitude, smoke inhalation, cardiopulmonary diseases) that leads to persistent tissue hypoxia.

oxygenation index A calculation used in intensive care medicine to measure severity of hypoxic respiratory failure using mean airway pressure, $F_{I}O_2$, and P_aO_2. It indicates the degree of ventilatory support required to maintain oxygenation.

P

P/F ratio An abbreviation for the ratio of P_aO_2 to $F_{I}O_2$ that is used to assess the degree of hypoxemia in patients.

PADIS Clinical Practice Guidelines for the Prevention and Management of Pain, Agitation/Sedation, Delirium, Immobility, and Sleep Disruption in Adult Patients in the ICU.

PADIS guidelines A set of Clinical Practice Guidelines for the prevention and management of pain, agitation/sedation, delirium, immobility, and sleep disruption in critically ill patients

parenteral nutrition Nutritional feeding via the intravenous route.

patient–ventilator asynchrony A condition in which a mismatching between neural (patient) and mechanically (ventilator) assisted breaths occurs.

patient–ventilator interaction Condition that allows observation of the clinical reaction of a patient to a preset number of ventilator parameters.

peak inspiratory pressure The largest pressure attained during inspiration (usually at end inspiration).

penetrating chest injury Type of injury where a penetrating object enters the chest with the potential to cause lung or other organ damage.

peptic ulcers Ulcers (sores) that affect the stomach or duodenum.

peripherally inserted central catheter A catheter placed into a peripheral vein for central venous access to administer medication or fluid.

peritonitis Inflammation of the peritoneum, typically caused by bacterial infection either via the blood or after rupture of an abdominal organ.

permissive hypercapnia A lung protection strategy that allows a high P_aCO_2 by reducing the volume or pressure during mechanical ventilation.

phospholipid A class of lipids that contain a phosphate group in the molecule. An example is lecithin, which is found in surfactant.

pilot balloon a small inflatable pouch that is connected to the cuff at the end of an endotracheal tube by a thin tube. It remains outside of the body to serve as an indicator of the degree to which the endotracheal tube cuff is inflated.

plateau pressure A stable pressure measured at the end of an inspiratory breath hold.

pneumomediastinum The abnormal presence of air in the mediastinum. It can occur as a result of trauma to the lungs or trachea.

pneumopericardium The abnormal presence of air in the pericardial cavity. It can occur as a result of severe lung disease or mechanical ventilation.

pneumoperitoneum The abnormal presence of air in the peritoneal cavity, a potential space within the abdominal cavity.

pneumothorax The collection of air in the pleural space.

pressure control Ventilator modes where the control variable is pressure, and this variable is used as a feedback signal to control inspiration (pressure, volume, or flow).

pressure controller A ventilator that measures pressure and uses it as a feedback signal to control inspiration.

pressure support or pressure support ventilation (PSV), uses a preset inspiratory pressure to augment the patient's spontaneous tidal volume (and indirectly the spontaneous frequency).

pressure support ventilation (PSV) An assisted spontaneous mode of ventilation. The patient initiates every breath and the ventilator delivers support with a preset pressure value to boost tidal volume.

pressure target Pressure becomes the set point for breath cycling. Once the set pressure is met, inspiration is terminated and exhalation begins.

pressure targeted Airway pressure is held constant while alveolar pressure rises during inspiration. Tidal volume delivered to the airways is variable and depends on airway resistance and alveolar compliance.

pressure triggering Pressure is set as a threshold to initiate inspiration (trigger a breath). Once the patient meets the set trigger threshold (pressure), inspiration begins.

pressure-time index A calculated value that expresses the respiratory load on the diaphragm and its capacity to handle it (the amount of pressure generated over the time required for an inspiratory volume) obtained from noninvasive ventilator measurements.

pressure-time product Another measure of the efficiency of respiratory muscles at performing the work of breathing. It involves calculating the integral of the pressure curve developed by the contraction of respiratory muscles over the duration of inspiration.

pressure-volume slope The rate of change observed in a pressure-volume plot of a breath (indicates a patient's respiratory system compliance characteristics during mandatory breaths delivered by a ventilator).

primary survey Designed to evaluate any chest trauma that could be potentially life-threatening and to determine the best therapeutic approach to stabilize the patient.

prolonged ventilator dependence The need for mechanical ventilation for more than 6 hours per day for more than 21 days.

prone positioning A method to improve V/Q matching by placing the patient in a prone position.

prophylactic support The use of a medical modality (i.e., mechanical ventilation) indicated for patients with clinical conditions that have a high risk of ventilatory failure, before failure occurs.

propofol (Diprivan) A short-acting, lipophilic intravenous general anesthetic that provides sedation for mechanically ventilated patients, and procedural sedation during unpleasant or painful procedures.

pulmonary artery catheter A balloon-tipped catheter that is inserted via a large vein and floated into the pulmonary artery.

pulmonary compliance The measure of the lungs' ability to stretch or to distend. Pulmonary compliance is calculated by dividing the lungs change in volume by the change in pressure required to distend them.

pulmonary contusion An injury to lung parenchyma, leading to inflammation of the alveolar spaces and collection of blood in alveolar spaces.

pulmonary interstitial emphysema A condition in which air enters the interstitial space around the lungs as a result of injury from mechanical ventilation.

pulse pressure The difference between the systolic and diastolic blood pressure—the diastolic is subtracted from the systolic to obtain the pulse pressure.

R

rapid sequence intubation A procedure that uses a medication to produce immediate unresponsiveness or muscular relaxation to allow the fastest and most effective means of endotracheal intubation, especially when a patient resists in an emergency situation.

rapid shallow breathing index (RSBI) A weaning predictor calculated by dividing the respiratory frequency by the average tidal volume (in Liters).

respiratory muscle training A technique that aims to improve pulmonary function, exercise capacity, sensation of dyspnea and quality of life by strengthening the *respiratory muscles* through specific exercises.

retractions An inward movement of the chest wall during inspiration.

reversal agent Drugs used to reverse the effects of anesthetics, narcotics, or potentially toxic agents.

Richards-Campbell Sleep Questionnaire (RCSQ) A survey instrument for assessment of sleep quality and disruption.

Richmond Agitation and Sedation Scale (RASS) An evaluation method to assess the patient's level of agitation and sedation, ranging from -5 (unarousable) to +4 (combative). The optimum RASS scale is -2 (light sedation) to 0 (alert and calm).

Riker Sedation-Agitation Scale (SAS) An evaluation method to assess the patient's level of agitation and sedation, ranging from 1 (unarousable) to 7 (dangerous). The optimum SAS scale is 3 (sedated) to 0 (calm and cooperative).

rise time Also called slope control on a ventilator that allows the practitioner to fine-tune how quickly the flow valve opens during inspiration, and peak flow and PIP are achieved when pressure ventilation modes are used.

S

scalar Any single variable displayed against time.

secondary survey A more detailed and complete (head-to-toe) examination, aimed at identifying all other injuries that could have been missed or appear not life-threatening and planning further investigation and treatment.

septic shock A severe hypovolemic condition associated with infection, low blood pressure and decreased cardiac output.

servo targeting Allows the output of the ventilator (pressure, volume, or flow) to automatically follow a varying input.

set-point targets Targets that are established by the clinician.

shunt fraction The percentage of venous blood that bypasses oxygenation in the lung capillaries or that anatomically bypasses the lung.

smoke inhalation Occurs when a patient's respiratory system is exposed to direct heat from fire as well as toxic chemicals that formed during combustion.

sniffing position Extending a patient's neck forward without tilting the head to provide an optimal view of the vocal cords for placement of an endotracheal tube. It mimics the position when a person leans forward to sniff something.

SOFA Sequential Organ Failure Assessment score is a mortality prediction tool for critically ill patients and it is based on the degree of dysfunction of six organ systems (respiration, cardiovascular, renal, coagulation, liver, and central nervous system).

spontaneous awakening trial A method to evaluate the patient's comfort level after the sedatives and most analgesics are discontinued.

spontaneous breath A breath in which the patient initiates the breath, determines the aspiratory flow and tidal volume, and determines when the breath ends.

spontaneous breathing trial (SBT) An assessment of a patient's ability to *breathe* while receiving minimal (PSV of 5 cm H_2O and/or CPAP of 5 cm H_2O) or no ventilator support for a period of 30–120 minutes.

START Simple triage and rapid treatment is a sorting method used by first responders to quickly classify victims during a mass casualty incident (MCI) based on the severity of their condition.

static compliance The change in volume in the respiratory system for a given unit of applied pressure at the end of inspiration but before exhalation (when no gas movement occurs).

stylet A bendable metal wire/tube (coated or uncoated) that is placed within an endotracheal tube to shape it to facilitate tracheal intubation.

subcutaneous emphysema Presence of air in the subcutaneous tissues.

subglottic secretion drainage A special design in the endotracheal tube that is capable of removing secretions above the cuff by low level suction.

suction control chamber This chamber regulates the amount of vacuum (suction) to the pleural cavity.

sulcus sign Deep, lucent, ipsilateral costophrenic angle indicator of a pneumothorax within the nondependent portions of the pleural space as opposed to the apex (of the lung) on the supine chest radiograph.

synchronized intermittent mandatory ventilation (SIMV) A weaning mode of ventilation that guarantees a set number of mandatory ventilator breaths in synchrony with a patient's breathing. Additional spontaneous breaths are permitted between the mandatory breaths.

T

tension pneumothorax Accumulation of air in the pleural space under pressure, compressing the lungs and decreasing venous return to the heart.

therapeutic hyperventilation Intentional excess ventilation via mechanical ventilation to lower abnormally high intracranial pressure. The over-ventilation lowers arterial CO_2, which reduces cerebral blood flow, decreases cerebral swelling, and ultimately lowers intracranial pressure (temporarily).

thermal injury A frequent cause owing to electrocautery and occurs often during normal dissection or as an attempt at coagulation of adjacent tissue bleeding.

thoracostomy The placement of a pleural chest tube.

thoracotomy A surgical opening of the chest.

time controller When the volume and pressure waveforms change during inspiration when subjected to changes in the patient's resistance and compliance, the ventilator is termed a time controller.

time triggering Inspiration begins at pre-set time intervals. Triggering (the start of inspiration) occurs in the absence of any spontaneous patient efforts to breathe.

tolerance The reaction to a specific drug where its concentration is progressively reduced, requiring increased concentration or amounts of the drug to achieve the desired effect (you have to take more and more of the drug to produce the same effect).

tracheal gas insufflation An adjunctive ventilatory technique that delivers fresh gas into the trachea either continuously or as a phasic flow.

tracheomalacia A process in which the tracheal walls weaken and collapses during breathing. It is associated with tracheostomy tubes.

tracheostenosis Abnormal narrowing of the lumen of the trachea that can occur with prolonged intubation.

tracheostomy tube A curved tube that is inserted into a tracheostomy stoma (an opening made in the neck and trachea) through which ventilation occurs.

transbronchial lung biopsy A procedure in which a flexible, multi-channel bronchoscope is used to collect lung tissue samples.

transbronchial needle aspiration A sheathed needle is used to collect lung tissue samples for the diagnosis of primary and metastatic peripheral lung cancers as well as submucosal, peribronchial, and mediastinal tumors.

transcutaneous Through the skin, such as transcutaneous oxygen monitoring.

transesophageal echocardiography A test that produces images of your heart. It uses high-frequency sound waves (ultrasound) to make detailed images of your heart and the arteries that lead to and from it. It differs from transthoracic echocardiography in the placement of the transducer. It is on the chest wall with transthoracic echocardiography and in the esophagus with transesophageal, creating a more detailed image.

traumatic brain injury Damage to the brain caused by trauma to the head.

triage The process of using a set of pre-determined criteria for sorting and determining the priority of patient care.

triggering Describes how the ventilator changes from exhalation to inspiration.

trocar tube thoracostomy A sharp instrument for the insertion of a chest tube.

tromethamine (THAM) A non-bicarbonate buffer for metabolic acidosis that directly reduces the H^+ ion concentration and indirectly reduces the CO_2 level.

U

underwater seal Used to allow air to escape through the drain but not to reenter the thoracic cavity.

V

vallecula With regard to the upper airway, it is a depression in the lining of the throat just behind the root of the tongue.

vasodilators Medicines that work by relaxing smooth muscle of the vasculature, allowing blood to flow more easily through the vessels.

venous admixture A mixture of unoxygenated venous blood and oxygenated arterial blood as a result of ventilation/perfusion mismatch.

ventilation-perfusion mismatch This occurs when the ideal proportion of ventilation in a lung area is either greater or lesser than the amount of blood flow.

ventilator weaning/discontinuance The process of liberating a patient from mechanical ventilation.

ventilator-associated events A broad category of clinical conditions to monitor the progression of infections due to use of artificial airway and mechanical ventilation.

ventilatory failure Occurs when the patient's minute alveolar ventilation cannot keep up with the metabolic rate or CO_2 production. Oxygenation failure usually follows when the cardiopulmonary system cannot provide adequate oxygen needed for metabolism.

ventricular fibrillation Rapid, grossly irregular electrical activity with marked variability in ECG waveform, ventricular rate usually >300/min.

ventricular tachycardia Cardiac arrhythmia of three or more consecutive complexes originating in the ventricles at a rate >100/min.

vestibulo-ocular reflex A reflex where activation of the vestibular system of the inner ear causes eye movement. Head movement is transformed into motor commands that normally generate eye movement in the opposite direction of the head movement.

video-assisted thoracoscopic surgery A type of thoracic surgery performed using a small video camera that is introduced into the patient's chest via a scope.

visual analog scale An interval measurement instrument that allows the patient to report a perception (e.g., sleep depth).

vocal cords Delicate, specialized *folds* of tissue in the larynx (voice box) located just above the trachea that are essential for creating the sounds of vocalization.

volume control modes Ventilator modes in which the control variable is volume, and that variable is used as a feedback signal to control inspiration (pressure, volume, or flow).

volume control—continuous mandatory ventilation A mode of ventilation in which the clinician sets the delivered tidal volume, inspiratory flow, and flow pattern.

volume controller A ventilator that measures pressure and uses it as a feedback signal to control inspiration. Pressure varies during inspiration when the patient's resistance and compliance change.

volume cycling Occurs if volume is measured and used as a feedback signal to end the inspiratory phase.

volume targeted Provides automatic weaning of peak pressure in response to improving lung compliance and patient respiratory effort.

volume triggering Volume used as a trigger variable. An external flow sensor that attaches to the patient's artificial airway senses inspiratory volume. Once the trigger volume is met, inspiration begins.

volutrauma A complication of mechanical ventilation in which damage occurs due to overdistension of the alveoli.

vomiting The forcible partial or full emptying of fluid or food from the stomach.

W

water seal chamber This chamber has a one-way valve that allows air to exit the pleural cavity during exhalation but does not allow it to reenter during inhalation.

waveform analysis Interpretation of the graphical output produced by most mechanical ventilators.

weaning failure Indicates either the failure of an SBT or the need for reintubation within 48 hours following extubation.

weaning protocol A well-defined decision-making process that starts with a standardized assessment of each patient's readiness to *wean* from mechanical ventilation and uses evidence-based steps to guide a patient to liberation from a ventilator as quickly as possible with appropriate monitoring.

weaning success Persistence of spontaneous breathing for at least 48 hours following extubation.

work of breathing (WOB) The effort expended for breathing expressed as the product of pressure and volume.

Index

Note: Locators followed by '*f*' and '*t*' refer figures and tables, respectively.